Cardiovascular/ Thoracic Words and Phrases

by Health Professions Institute

Third Edition

Health Professions Institute · Modesto, California · 2004

Cardiovascular/Thoracic Words and Phrases
Third Edition

Published by

Health Professions Institute
P. O. Box 801
Modesto, CA 95353
Phone (209) 551-2112
Fax (209) 551-0404
Web Site: http://www.hpisum.com
E-mail: hpi@hpisum.com

Sally Crenshaw Pitman
Editor & Publisher

Printed by
Parks Printing & Lithograph
Modesto, California

ISBN 0-934385-48-3

Last digit is the print number: 9 8 7 6 5 4 3 2 1

To the very best sister

Peggy Crenshaw Langley

Preface

Cardiovascular/Thoracic Words and Phrases, third edition, is an update of *Cardiology Words and Phrases*, second edition (1995). This new book, however, with over 55,000 entries in 660 pages, is far more than a mere revision of the second edition.

When we decided to update the cardiology book this year and to provide a more inclusive title, we thought it would be useful to expand the pulmonary, thoracic, and vascular words to topics closely related to the chest, heart, lungs, and vascular system, including pediatric cardiology, diagnostic cardiology, therapeutics and rehabilitation, medications and drug-related terms, and syndromes, diseases, and anomalies. We have added hundreds of surgical instruments and therapeutic devices and systems.

To streamline the book and make it most useful to medical transcriptionists and other healthcare professionals, we have deleted hundreds of obsolete terms and outdated pharmaceuticals while adding over 10,000 new entries from diagnostic, surgical, and therapeutic procedures as well as imaging agents and medications. We've culled abbreviations, coined words, medical slang, and words and phrases from hundreds of transcripts of cardiovascular/thoracic medical and surgical dictation, as well as medical databases, scholarly journals, textbooks, and other electronic and printed references.

In unclear medical dictation, the transcriptionist can sometimes understand only a single word in a phrase; thus, we have extensively cross-referenced phrases by each important word in the phrase. We've listed many common phrases beginning with adjectives as they are dictated (50 entries beginning with *alveolar*, 38 with *diffuse*, 8 with *absence of*, 12 with *absent*). Another useful feature is phonetic renderings of difficult or foreign terms, such as *coup sur coup*, *en face*, *en masse*, *psyllium*, and *phthisis*. Other unusual entries list phrases related to the entry rather than adjectives: *allergy-causing pollens*; *angina, descriptions of*; *cardiac risk factors*; *drug-related terms*; *MRI terms*; *pathogens*; *pulmonary function abbreviations*; *pain relieved by*; *pneumonia, bacterial and viral, caused by*; *pulmonary function tests*; and *SMA chemical panel*. We have dozens of terms not in other reference books, and many new or hard-to-find syndromes and diseases.

This new edition was made possible by the fine scholarly research of Ellen Drake, CMT, and Linda Campbell, CMT. Invaluable assistance in verifying the accuracy of entries and reconciling discrepancies from various authoritative references was provided by John H. Dirckx, M.D.

Sally Crenshaw Pitman, M.A.
Editor & Publisher

How to Use This Book

The words and phrases in this book are alphabetized letter by letter of all words in the entry, ignoring puntuation marks and words in parentheses. The possessive form (*'s*) is omitted from eponyms for ease in alphabetizing. Numbers are alphabetized as if written out, with the exception of subscripts and superscripts which are ignored.

Eponyms may be located alphabetically as well as under the nouns they modify; for example, *Wooler-plasty* may also be found under *operation*. A list of over 220 subentries under *prosthesis* (artificial valves) includes trademarked valves and descriptive terms, whereas the subentries for *valve* are restricted to descriptive adjectives and phrases related to anatomical valves.

The main entry *drug-related terms* includes descriptive terms related to drugs, not the names of pharmaceuticals. The names of hundreds of medications (generic and brand names) used in cardiology and pulmonary medicine appear under the main entry *medications*.

The main entries *artery* and *vein* include many phrases and descriptive terms related to arteries and veins as they are dictated in patient reports, rather than only the names of anatomical terms readily available in medical dictionaries. Physicians dictate many abbreviations, especially for anatomical groups, and those terms frequently abbreviated in medical dictation are listed as main entries with their translations and as subentries.

In medical dictation physicians arbitrarily refer to a diagnostic, therapeutic, or operative procedure (both invasive and noninvasive) as an *approach, method, operation, procedure, repair*, or *technique*, or by the type of procedure, such as *angioplasty*. Thus, surgical procedures are listed alphabetically by the eponym or noun as well as under the type of procedure and under the main entry *operation*.

Instruments used in operative, therapeutic, and diagnostic procedures may also be referred to variously as an *apparatus, device, instrument, system*, or a particular type of device, such as a *catheter*. Thus, instruments are listed under the type when there are many examples given, and those devices or instruments or machines that do not fit neatly under their own categories are listed under the general term *device* or *system*. Important main entries include the following:

angina	forceps	pathogen	sound
aorta	graft	pneumonia	stenosis
bypass	heart	pressure	stent
cardiac	imaging agent	procedure	suture
catheter	lead (electrode)	prosthesis	syndrome
clamp	lung	pulmonary	system
defibrillator	medications	pulse	technique
device	murmur	pump	test
disease	operation	shunt	valve
dressing	pacemaker	sign	ventilator

A, a

"a" (augment)(ed)
AA (ascending aorta)
AA curve
A_1A_2 curve
AA interval
A_1A_2 interval
AAA ("triple A") (abdominal aortic aneurysm)
AACD (abdominal aortic counter-pulsation device)
A-a (alveolar-arterial) gradient
A-a (alveolar-arterial) pO_2 gradient
AAH (atypical adenomatous hyperplasia)
AAI (atrial demand inhibited) pacemaker
AAI pacing mode
AAI rate-adaptive mode
AAI rate-modulated mode
AAI rate-responsive mode
AAIR pacemaker syndrome
AAIR pacing (atrial rate adaptive)
AAMI (Association for the Advancement of Medical Instrumentation)
AAMI validation criteria
A&B (apnea and bradycardia)
a/A ratio

AASV (ANCA-associated systemic vasculitis)
AAT (atrial demand triggered) pacemaker
A bands of sarcomere
Abbott artery
Abbott radioimmunoassay kit
Abbreviated Injury Scale (AIS)
abbreviated interval
A-B-C (airway, breathing, circulation) sequence (cardiopulmonary resuscitation)
abdomen, protuberant
abdominal aneurysm
abdominal aorta, infrarenal
abdominal aorta thrombosis
abdominal aortic aneurysm (AAA)
abdominal aortic aneurysmectomy
abdominal asthma
abdominal bruit
abdominal coarctation
abdominal heterotaxy
abdominal left ventricular assist device (ALVAD)
abdominal mass
  nonpulsatile
  pulsatile

1

abdominal respirations
abdominojugular reflux
ABE (acute bacterial endocarditis)
aberrant conduction
aberrant coronary artery
aberrant depolarization of ventricular
  muscle
aberrant left pulmonary artery
aberrantly conducted beats
aberrant QRS complex
aberrant vascular channels
aberration
  intraventricular
  metabolic
  nonspecific T-wave
  ventricular
ABG, ABGs (arterial blood gas)(es)
  (see *blood gas)*
ABI (ankle-brachial index)
Abigram vascular diagnostic test
ability, cardiac pumping
AbioCor total artificial heart
Abiomed biventricular support (BVS)
  system
Abiomed cardiac device
ablated myocardium
ablation
  accessory conduction (ACA)
  accessory pathway
  atrial flutter
  atrioventricular nodal
  bilateral epicardial radiofrequency
  bundle of His
  catheter
  continuous wave
  cryosurgical
  direct current (DCA)
  electrode catheter
  endocardial
  endocardial catheter
  epicardial
  His bundle

ablation *(cont.)*
  intracoronary ethanol
  intraoperative laser
  Kent bundle
  laser
  microwave atrial
  myocardial
  open-heart endocardial
  radiofrequency
  percutaneous radiofrequency
  catheter
  percutaneous transluminal septal
    myocardial
  pulsed laser
  radiofrequency (RFA)
  radiofrequency thermal
  transaortic radiofrequency
  transapical endocardial
  transcatheter radiofrequency
  transcatheter His bundle
  transcoronary chemical
  transmural atrial
  transseptal radiofrequency
  transvenous
ablation of arrhythmogenic areas in
  myocardium
ablation of myocardium
ablation of pathway
ablation surgery in congenital vascular
  defect
ablation therapy arrhythmia
ablative device
abnormal airways stretch
abnormal bleeding
abnormal chest cage
abnormal gradient
abnormal heart sound
abnormal hemoglobin
abnormal physiologic splitting
abnormal pulmonary venous drainage
abnormalities of platelet function
abnormalities of small blood vessels

abnormality, abnormalities
  akinetic wall motion
  baseline ST-segment
  brisk wall motion
  conduction
  ectopic wall motion
  electrophysiological
  exercise-induced wall motion
  focal wall motion
  global
  intraventricular conduction
  LV (left ventricular) wall motion
  nonspecific T-wave
  occult circulatory
  perfusion
  persistent wall motion
  regional wall motion
  segmental perfusion
  subsegmental perfusion
  transient wall motion
  wall motion
abnormality of arch of aorta
abnormally loud first heart sound
ABO hemolytic disease of the newborn
ABO incompatibility
abolished by breath-holding
abolition of ventricular tachycardia
abortive shock capability
ABPA (allergic bronchopulmonary
  aspergillosis)
ABPM (ambulatory blood pressure
  monitoring)
abrade, abrasion
Abrahams sign
Abrams needle
abrupt onset
abrupt tapering
abrupt vessel closure
abscess (see also *empyema*)
  anular
  aortic root
  blood-streaked drainage from

abscess *(cont.)*
  brain
  foul-smelling
  infected
  lung
  metastatic
  parapharyngeal
  percutaneous
  pulmonary
  putrid
  retropharyngeal
  subphrenic
abscess drainage
abscess formation
absence
  angiographic
  congenital pericardial
  partial pericardial
absence of endoleak
absence of left side of pericardium
absence of left ventricular dysfunction
absence of overt heart failure
absence of recognizable structural
  disease
absence of rheumatic heart disease
absence of sweating
absence of ventricular activity
absent aortic knob on chest x-ray
absent apex pulse
absent apical impulse
absent breath sounds
absent bronchial cartilage
absent pericardium, congenital
absent peripheral veins
absent pulmonary valve syndrome
absent P waves
absent respirations
absent runoff
absent tactile fremitus
absolute artery dimensions
absolute blood eosinophil count
absolute cardiac dullness (ACD)

absolute eosinophilia
absolute neutrophilia
absolute QT interval
absolute refractory period (ARP)
absorbable suture
abundant collateral circulation
AC (aortic closure) interval
ACA (accessory conduction ablation)
ACAD (atherosclerotic carotid artery
  disease)
Acapella chest physical therapy device
ACAS (Asymptomatic Carotid
  Atherosclerosis Study) criteria
ACAT 1 Plus intra-aortic balloon
  pump
accelerated atherosclerosis
accelerated atrioventricular conduction
accelerated atrioventricular junctional
  rhythm
accelerated ejection
accelerated hypertension
accelerated idioventricular rhythm
  (AIVR)
accelerated respirations
acceleration
acceleration map
acceleration of ventricular tachycardia
accelerator globulin (AcG) blood
  coagulation factor
Accent-DG balloon
accentuated pulmonic component
accentuated second pulmonic sound
accentuation
access
  arteriovenous
  ventricular
access artery
access graft failure
accessible lesion
Access MV beating-heart bypass
  system
accessory atrioventricular conduction

accessory atrioventricular pathway
accessory blood supply
accessory hemiazygos vein
accessory lobes
accessory lungs
accessory muscles of respiration
accessory pathway (AP)
  ablation of
  concealed
accessory pathway potentials
accessory pathway reentrant PSVT
  (paroxysmal supraventricular
  tachycardia)
accessory respiratory muscle activity
accessory segments
accessory sinuses
accident
  cardiovascular (CVA)
  cerebrovascular (CVA)
accidental murmur
accordioning of stent coils
Accucap CO_2/O_2 monitor
Accucom cardiac output monitor
Accufix pacemaker lead
Accuguide central venous catheter
Accuguide peripherally inserted central
  catheter
AccuLase excimer laser
Acculink self-expanding stent
Acculith pacemaker
accumulation
  dependent extracellular fluid
  fluid
  lactic acid
accumulation of air in interlobar spaces
accumulation of gas under serous tunic
  of intestine
AccuNeb (albuterol sulfate)
AccuNet embolic protection system
Accupril (quinapriol HCl)
Accutorr monitor
Accu-Vu sizing catheter

ACD (active compression-
decompression) resuscitator
ACE (angiotensin-converting enzyme)
ACE challenge
ACE inhibitor
ACE (asymptomatic complex ectopy)
ACE fixed-wire balloon catheter
ace of spades sign on angiogram
acetaminophen overdose
AcG (accelerator globulin) blood
coagulation factor
ACG (apexcardiogram,
apexcardiography)
achalasia, cricopharyngeal
achalasia of thoracic esophagus
Achieva portable ventilator
Achieve off-pump system
Achiever balloon dilatation catheter
Achromobacter
acid
arachidonic
epsilon-aminocaproic
epoxyeicosatrienoic
gadolinium-diethylenetriamine–
pentaacetic (Gd-DTPA)
glycyrrhetinic
hydrocyanic
lactic
nicotinic
omega-3 fatty
para-aminosalicylic
acid aspiration pneumonitis
acid-base balance
acid-base equilibrium
acid-base imbalance
acid-base status
acidemia
metabolic
moderate respiratory
acid-fast bacilli (AFB) stain
acid-fast bacillus (AFB)

acid-fast culture
acid lipase deficiency
acid maltase deficiency
acidosis
extracellular
hypoxia without
intracellular
lactic
metabolic
moderate
refractory lactic
renal tubular
respiratory
severe
tissue
acidotic
acid phosphatase, histamine
acid pulmonary aspiration syndrome
acid reflux
acid regurgitation
acid release, hydrocyanic vanillylmandelic
Acinetobacter baumannii
ACA (anticardiolipin antibody)
aCL (anticardiolipin) antibody
Acland-Banis arteriotomy set
ACLS (advanced cardiac life support)
protocol
ACM (automated cardiac flow
measurement) technology
Acolysis ultrasound intravascular
thrombolysis system
Acorn nebulizer
acoustic backscatter characteristics of
blood
acoustic impedance
acoustic quantification, left ventricular
ejection fraction
acoustical shadowing
acoustic shadowing
acoustic window
acquired aneurysm

acquired bronchiectasis
acquired disease
acquired heart murmur
acquired hemolytic anemia
acquired lesion
acquired lymphedema
acquired mitral stenosis
acquired multidrug resistance
acquired prolonged Q-T interval
acquired tracheobronchomalacia
acquired tufted angioma
acquired unilateral hyperlucent lung
acquired ventricular septal defect
  (AVSD)
acquisition, data
acquisition technique
Acrobat heart stabilization device
acrocyanosis
acromegalic
acromegaly
acroparesthesia
  Schultze
  simple
acrylates in vaso-occlusive angiotherapy
ACS (Advanced Catheter Systems;
  Cardiovascular Systems)
ACS anchor exchange device
ACS angioplasty Y connector
ACS Concorde over-the-wire catheter
  system
ACS Endura coronary dilatation
  catheter
ACS guidewire
ACS Hi-Torque Balance middle-
  weight guidewire
ACS Indeflator
ACS JL4 (Judkins left 4) French
  catheter
ACS LIMA guide
ACS Mini catheter
ACS Multi-Link catheter

ACS Multi-Link coronary stent
ACS OTW (over-the-wire) HP
  (high pressure) coronary stent
ACS OTW Lifestream coronary
  dilatation catheter
ACS OTW Photon coronary dilatation
  catheter
ACS RX (rapid exchange)
ACS RX Comet catheter
ACS RX Comet coronary dilatation
  catheter
ACS RX coronary dilatation catheter
ACS RX Lifestream coronary
  dilatation catheter
ACS RX Multi-Link stent
ACS RX Rocket catheter
ACS SULP II balloon
ACS Tourguide II guiding catheter
ACT (activated clotting time)
ACT (activated coagulation time)
Actalyke activated clotting time (ACT)
  test
ACTH (adrenocorticotropic hormone)
ACTH hypersecretion
ACTH secretion
Actinobacillus endocarditis infection
Actinobacillus pleuropneumoniae
actinomycete, thermophilic
actinomycosis
actinomycotic pericarditis
action
  defibrillatory
  prolonged
action potential, cardiac
action potential duration (APD)
activated clotting time (ACT)
activated coagulation time (ACT)
activated partial thromboplastin time
  (APTT)
activation
  complement
  Hageman factor
  inappropriate (of ICD)

activation of fibrinolysin
activator
  plasminogen
  recombinant tissue type plasmino-
    gen (rt-PA)
  tissue plasminogen (t-PA)
active bleeding site
Active Cath condom catheter
active compression-decompression
  (ACD) resuscitator
active congestion
active emptying fraction (left atrium)
active fixation lead
active hyperemia
active mode
Activitrax variable rate pacemaker
activity
  breathlessness after
  defibrillatory
  ectopic atrial
  inappropriately elevated plasma
    renin
  inotropic
  pulseless electrical
  respiratory burst
  sympathomimetic
  triggered
activity sensor modulated atrial rate
  adaptive pacing (AAIR)
ACT protocol
actuator component
actuator, double-acting
AcuNav ultrasound catheter
Acuson computed sonography
Acuson echocardiographic equipment
Acuson V5M multiplanar TEE
  (transesophageal echocardiographic)
  monitor
acute alveolar hypoperfusion
acute aortic regurgitation syndrome
acute aortic thrombosis
acute arteritis

acute attack of bronchospasm
acute bacterial endocarditis (ABE)
acute benign pericarditis
acute blood loss
acute bronchitis
acute cerebrovascular insufficiency
acute chest syndrome
acute compression triad
acute coronary insufficiency
acute coronary syndrome
acute eosinophilic pneumonia
acute exacerbation
acute febrile mucocutaneous lymph
  node syndrome (MCLS)
acute heart failure
acute hemodynamic overload
acute hypercapnic respiratory failure
  (AHRF)
acute idiopathic pericarditis
acute infectious bronchitis
acute inhalation injury
acute interstitial myocarditis
acute intramural hematoma
acute intraoperative arterial elongation
acute irritative bronchitis
acute laryngotracheal bronchitis
acute left heart failure
acute lung injury (ALI)
acute massive lung collapse
acute mediastinitis
acute mesenteric artery occlusion
acute mountain sickness
acute myocardial infarction (AMI)
acute nonspecific pericarditis
acute pericarditis
acute pharyngitis
acute pleurisy
acute pneumonitis
acute pulmonary edema
acute radiation syndrome
acute renal failure
acute respiratory arrest

acute respiratory center paralysis
acute respiratory distress syndrome
   (ARDS)
acute respiratory failure (ARF)
acute rheumatic endocarditis (ARE)
acute rheumatic fever (ARF)
acute rheumatic myocarditis (ARM)
acute rheumatic pericarditis (ARP)
acute tracheitis
acute tracheobronchitis
acute traumatic rupture of aortic
   isthmus
acute tuberculosis
acute type B aortic dissection
acute ventilatory failure
acute vessel closure
a, c, v (positive) waves on jugular
   pulse wave tracing
acyanosis
acyanotic congenital heart disease
acyl coenzyme A deficiency
acyl-CoA dehydrogenase, deficiency of
   long chain
AD (aortic diameter)
Adalat CC (nifedipine)
Adamkiewicz artery
Adams-DeWeese vena caval clip
Adams-Stokes disease
Adams-Stokes syncope
Adams-Stokes syndrome
adapter
   butterfly
   side-arm (also, sidearm)
   sleeve
adaptive burst pacing
adaptive hypertrophy
adductor magnus muscle
AddVent atrioventricular pacemaker
adenocarcinoma, papillary
adenoma
   adrenal cortical
   aldosterone-producing
   bronchial

adenomatoid malformation
adenomatous hyperplasia
adenomatous polyp
adenopathy
   axillary
   hilar
   mediastinal
   symmetrical mediastinal
Adenoscan
adenosine diphosphate (ADP) platelet
   adhesiveness
adenosine echocardiography
adenosine stress test
adenosine triphosphate (ATP)
adenosquamous carcinoma
adenovirus
adequate air exchange
adequate cardiac output
adequate collateral circulation
adequate coronary perfusion
adequate heparinization
adequate stroke volume
ADH (antidiuretic hormone) secretion
adherent pericardium, rheumatic
adherent thrombus
adhesion, adhesions
   fibrous pleural
   freeing up of
   inflammatory
   lysed
   lysis of
   pericardial diaphragmatic
   pleural
   pleuropulmonary
   taking down of
adhesion barrier
adhesion-inducing agent
adhesions between lung and
   pericardium
adhesive (glue)
   adjunctive biological
   autologous fibrin
   BioGlue

adhesive *(cont.)*
   CollaTape
   cyanoacrylate (Superglue) tissue
   Dermabond skin
   Elastikon elastic tape
   fibrin
   Glycoprene tissue
   Hemaseel HMN biological
     tissue
   Max-Prene tissue
   Osteoprene tissue
   Surfit ("sure-fit")
   Tissucol biologic
   Vitex tissue
adhesiveness, platelet
adhesive pericarditis
adhesive phlebitis
adhesive pleurisy
ad hoc (improvised)
"a" dip on echocardiogram
Adkins strut
adjunctive anticoagulation
adjunctive biological glue
adjunctive technique
adjunctive therapy
adjunctive treatment
adjuvant chemotherapy
adjuvant therapy
administration
   fluid
   heparin
   volume
admixture, obligatory (of systemic
   venous and pulmonary venous
   blood)
Adolph's Salt Substitute
ADP (adenosine diphosphate)
ADR Ultramark 4 ultrasound
adrenal cortical adenoma
adrenal disease
adrenal gland hyperfunction
adrenal gland hypofunction

adrenal hyperplasia, congenital
adrenal medulla
adrenal steroidogenesis
adrenal steroids
adrenal vein sampling
adrenal venous aldosterone level
adrenalectomy
adrenalin
adrenergic blockade
adrenergic drive
adrenergic receptor
adrenocortical carcinoma
adrenocortical hyperplasia
adrenocorticotropic hormone
adrenomedullary triad
Adriamycin cardiotoxicity
Adson forceps
Adson hook
Adson maneuver
Adson test
adult fibroelastosis
adult-onset reactive airways disease
adult respiratory distress syndrome
   (ARDS)
adult sudden death
adult tuberculosis
Advair Diskus (fluticasone propionate
   and salmeterol inhalation powder)
advanced cardiac life support (ACLS)
advanced cardiac mapping
advanced cardiogenic shock
advanced tuberculous constrictive
   pericarditis
Advantx LC+ cardiovascular imaging
   system
adventitia
   thickened
   tunica
adventitial cystic disease
adventitious breath sounds
adventitious heart sounds
adventitious lung sounds

adverse cardiac event (ACE)
adverse complications
adverse event
AEC (aortic ejection click)
AECG (ambulatory ECG)
AED (automatic external defibrillator)
Ae-H interval (anterograde conduction)
AEI (atrial escape interval)
A_2 equal to P_2
Aegis aortic cannula
Aeon catheter
Aeon vascular access port
Aequitron pacemaker
aeration disturbances
aerobic exercise
aerobic gram-positive bacilli
AerobiCycle (powered treadmill)
aerobullosis
Aerocel pulmonary delivery system
AeroChamber aerosol holding chamber
Aerochamber face mask
AeroDose inhaler
Aerodyne bicycle
aeroembolism
aerogenic tuberculosis
aerophagia
aerosol
    metered-dose
    radioactive
aerosol therapy
aerosolized lidocaine
aerosolized pentamidine
AeroTech II nebulizer
Aerotrol inhalation aerosol device
AERx electronic inhaler
Aestiva/5 MRI anesthesia machine
Aescula left ventricular (LV) cardiac
    lead
AET (automatic ectopic tachycardia)
AF (aortic flow)
AF (atrial fibrillation)
A_2, false

A-FAIR (arrhythmia-insensitive flow-
    sensitive alternating inversion
    recovery) imaging
AFB (acid-fast bacilli) stain
AFBG (aortofemoral bypass graft)
afferent conduit
afferent nerve stimulation syncope
affixed
A fib, A-fib (atrial fibrillation) pattern
a-fiX cannula seals
AFl (atrial flutter)
AFP pacemaker
African trypanosomiasis
AF (axillofemoral) stem
after-depolarizations
afterload
    cardiac
    increased ventricular
    left ventricular
    ventricular
afterload agent
afterload reduction
Afzelius syndrome
AG (anion gap)
Agar-IF (immunofixation in agar) of
    blood serum
Agatston score
AGB+ catheter
agenesis
    lobar
    lung
    pulmonary artery
    segmental
agent
    afterload
    antiarrhythmic
    antiplatelet
    beta-adrenergic receptor blocking
    beta-adrenoceptor blocking
    defibrillatory
agglutination factor
    Duffy
    Kell

agglutination *(cont.)*
  Kidd
  Lewis
  Lutheran
agglutinins, febrile
aggravated by deep inspiration
aggregated eosinophil granules
aggregation, platelet
aggressive interstitial infiltrate
aggressive perivascular infiltrate
aggressive pulmonary toilet
aggressive surgical approach
agitation
agonal (or agony) clot
agonal phase, bradycardic
agonal tracing (on EKG)
agonist
  beta
  selective dopamine
agony clot
agony thrombus
agraphia
A_2 greater than P_2
Agrylin (anagrelide HCl)
ague, brass-founder's
AHA (American Heart Association)
AHA low-fat diet
AHC (apical hypertrophic cardiomyopathy)
A-H curve
A_2 heart sound (aortic valve closure)
AH/HA or AH-HA ratio
AHG (antihemophilic globulin)
AHI (apnea/hypopnea index)
A-H interval
"ahn mahs" (en masse)
Ahn thrombectomy catheter
AHR (airway hyperreactivity)
AHRF (acute hypercapnic respiratory
  failure)
AHT (arterial hypertension)
AI (aortic insufficiency) pacing

AICA (anterior inferior communicating
  artery)
AICD (automatic implantable
  cardioverter-defibrillator)
AICD-B pacemaker
AICD-BR pacemaker
AICD pacemaker
AICD plus Tachylog
AICD shocks
AID (automatic implantable or
  internal defibrillator)
AID-B pacemaker
AIHA (autoimmune hemolytic anemia)
A_2 incisural interval
AIOD (aortoiliac obstructive disease)
air
  ambient
  intracardiac
  room
air boluses
air bronchogram
air cell
air column, corrugated
air-conditioner lung
air crescent sign (on chest x-ray)
air-driven artificial heart
air embolism or embolus
air exchange
air-filled lungs
air-fluid level
air hunger
air in lung connective tissue
air in pleural cavity on x-ray
air interface on x-ray
air leak
airless lung
airlessness, alveolar
airless state
Airozin dietary supplement
air pocket
air-powered nebulizer
air pollutant

air sac
air space
  apical
  lung
  terminal
air-trapping
airway, airways
  artificial
  asthmatic
  clear
  dynamic compression of
  emergency
  esophageal obturator
  hypertonic
  large
  mucoid plugging of
  natural
  oral
  oropharyngeal
  reactive
  small
airway caliber
airway collapse
airway conductance and resistance
airway control
airway constriction
airway epithelial cell
airway epithelial irritant receptors
airway hyperreactivity (AHR)
airway hyperresponsiveness
airway inflammation
airway ischemia
airway narrowing (asthma)
airway obstruction caused by
  asthma
  chronic bronchitis
  cystic fibrosis
  emphysema
  mucoviscidosis
airway opening pressure
airway pressure release ventilation
airway resistance (R_{AW})

airway responsiveness
airway sensitivity
airways stretch, abnormal
AIS (Abbreviated Injury Scale)
AIVR (accelerated idioventricular
  rhythm)
AK (atrial kick)
akinesia, akinesis
  apical
  global
  inferior wall
  lateral wall
  regional
  septal
  wall
akinetic left ventricle
akinetic mutism
akinetic posterior wall
akinetic segmental wall motion
Akutsu III TAH (total artificial heart)
alae nasi, flaring of the
Alagille syndrome
alar chest
alar flaring
alba dolens, phlegmasia
Albini nodule
Albright disease
Albumin Cobalt Binding test
albumin concentration
albumin solution
Albuminar blood volume expander
albuminized woven Dacron tube graft
albuminoid sputum
Albunex (sonicated human albumin)
albuterol bronchodilator
ALCAPA (anomalous origin of left
  coronary artery from the pulmonary
  artery) syndrome
Alcock catheter plug
alcohol ablation therapy for arrhythmias
alcohol ablation to treat cardiomyopathy
alcoholic cardiomegaly-emphysema

alcoholic cardiomyopathy
alcoholic cardiomyopathy with beriberi
alcoholic dilated cardiomyopathy
alcoholic heart
aldosterone
    circadian rhythm of plasma
    postural stimulation of
aldosterone level
    adrenal venous
    circulating
aldosterone production, autonomous
aldosterone secretion, autonomous
aldosterone secretion rate
aldosterone-producing adenoma (APA)
aldosteronism
    primary
    pseudoprimary
    secondary
Aldrete needle
Aldrich-Mees line
Aldrich syndrome
Aldurazyme (laronidase)
ALEC (artificial lung-expanding
    compound)
Alert catheter
Alert Companion II defibrillator
Alexander-Farabeuf rib rasp
Alexander rib raspatory
Alexander rib stripper
Alexander syndrome
Alfieri mitral valve procedure
Alfieri mitral valve repair
Alfieri-plasty (also bow-tie repair;
    double orifice repair)
Alfred M. Large vena cava clamp
algorithm
ALI (acute lung injury)
aliasing phenomenon in Doppler
    studies
A-line (arterial line)
aliquot dose
alkaline phosphatase

alkaline phosphatase-antialkaline phos-
    phatase (APAAP) antibody test
alkalosis
    acapnial
    compensated
    hypokalemic
    metabolic
    respiratory
alkaptonuria
allantoic vessel thrombosis
Allen-Brown criteria
Allen-Brown vascular access shunt
Allen circulatory test
Allen test prior to radial artery
    cannulation
allergen (respiratory)
    airborne
    cockroach
    grass pollen
    house dust mite feces
    mold spores
    Parietaria judaica
    pet dander
allergen extract, lyophilized
allergenic exposure
allergen-induced bronchial hyper-
    responsiveness
allergen-induced bronchial reaction
allergic airway inflammation
allergic alveolitis
allergic alveolitis syndrome
allergic angiitis
allergic angiitis and granulomatosis
allergic asthma
allergic bronchopulmonary
    aspergillosis (ABPA)
allergic bronchopulmonary fungal
    disease
allergic exposure
allergic granulomatosis
allergic granulomatous angiitis
allergic myocardial granulomatous
    disease

allergic reaction
  type I (atopic or anaphylactic)
  type II (cytotoxic)
  type III (immune-complex-
    mediated)
  type IV (cell-mediated or delayed)
allergic respiratory disease
allergic rhinitis
allergy, allergies
  bronchopulmonary
  dust
  mold
  pollen
  respiratory
allergy-causing pollens from
  grasses: timothy, Bermuda,
    orchard, sweet vernal, red top,
    some blue grasses, and others
  trees: oak, western red cedar, elm,
    birch, ash, hickory, poplar,
    sycamore, maple, cypress,
    walnut, and others
  weeds: ragweed, sagebrush, pig-
    weed, tumbleweed, Russian
    thistle, cockleweed, and others
alleviated
ALLHAT (Antihypertensive and
  Lipid-Lowering Treatment
  to Prevent Heart Attack Trial)
alligator pacing cable
Allis grasping forceps
Allis-Adair clamp
Allison lung retractor
allogeneic transplantation
allograft
  cardiac
  cryopreserved human aortic
  lung
allograft coronary artery disease
allograft reaction
allotransplantation

All-Terrain Balloon (ATB) PTA dilatation catheter
ALMD (asymptomatic left main
  disease)
alobar holoprosencephaly
Aloka color Doppler blood flow
  imaging system
Aloka echocardiograph machine
AL-1 catheter
$alpha_1$ or alpha-1
$alpha_1$-adrenergic blocking agent
alpha-adrenoreceptor blockers
alpha-adrenoreceptor stimulant
alpha-agonists, central
$alpha_1$ antitrypsin
$alpha_1$ antitrypsin deficiency
alpha-blockade
alpha-fetoprotein (AFP)
alpha-galactosidase A deficiency
alpha-1,4-glucosidase deficiency,
  lysosomal
$alpha_1$ proteinase inhibitor (a_1PI)
  deficiency
alpha receptor
alpha-stat strategy
alpha thalassemia
alpha-2 antiplasmin functional assay
Alport syndrome
ALT (alanine aminotransferase),
  elevated
Altace (ramipril)
Altaire open MR imaging system
alteration, ST-segment
altered consciousness
alternans
  electrical
  pulsus
  total
alternans noninvasive cardiac
  diagnostic test
alternating blue and white mattress
  sutures

alternating current
alternative modality
alternative respiratory pathway
alternatives, feasible
altitude anoxia
altitude sickness
AL-II guiding catheter
aluminosis of lung
aluminum oxide inhalation
Alupent breathing treatments via
 machine
ALVAD (abdominal left ventricular
 assist device)
alveolar airlessness
alveolar-arterial oxygen pressure
 difference
alveolar-arterial oxygen tension
 gradient
alveolar atrophy
alveolar capillaries
alveolar-capillary block
alveolar capillary block syndrome
alveolar-capillary membrane
alveolar-capillary membrane damage
alveolar carcinoma
alveolar cell (type I or II)
alveolar cell carcinoma
alveolar cell ghosts
alveolar cell tumor
alveolar collapse
alveolar consolidation
alveolar cysts
alveolar destruction
alveolar dilatations of lung tissue
alveolar distention
alveolar duct emphysema
alveolar ducts
alveolar edema
alveolar emphysema
alveolar eosinophilia
alveolar exudate
alveolar gas

alveolar glands
alveolar hydatid disease
alveolar hypocarbia
alveolar hypoplasia
alveolar hypoventilation, primary
alveolar macrophages
alveolar microlithiasis
alveolar necrosis
alveolar overventilation
alveolar pneumonopathy
alveolar proliferation
alveolar proteinosis, pulmonary
alveolar pulmonary edema
alveolar rupture
alveolar sac
alveolar septa
 scarred
 thickened
alveolar septal inflammation
alveolar stability
alveolar underventilation with
 hypercapnia
alveolar ventilation, reduced
alveolar volume
alveolar wall edema
alveolar wall tension
alveoli (pl. of *alveolus*)
alveoli pulmonis (also pulmonum)
alveolitis
 allergic
 cryptogenic fibrosing
 desquamating fibrosing
 desquamative
 extrinsic allergic
 fibrosing
 generalized
 lymphoid
 neutrophil
 T-helper lymphocyte
alveolitis with honeycombing
alveolitis with hyaline membrane
alveolocapillary block

alveolocapillary membrane
alveolus (pl. alveoli), pulmonary
ALVs (arm and lesser saphenous veins)
Alzate catheter
AMA-Fab (antimyosin monoclonal antibody with Fab fragment)
AMA-Fab scintigraphy
Amato body
amaurosis fugax
Amazr catheter
amber-colored pulmonary secretions
Amberlite particles
ambient air
ambient ozone exposure
ambiguus, situs
Ambrose criteria for thrombotic lesions
Ambu bag
ambued, ambuing (slang)
ambulant
ambulatory blood pressure monitoring (ABPM)
ambulatory electrocardiogram, electrocardiography
ambulatory equilibrium angiocardiography
ambulatory monitoring (Holter)
ambulatory status
AMC needle
amebiasis pericarditis
amelioration of tumor
amenable to surgery
amenable to wedge resection
American Heart Association (AHA) classification of stenosis
American Heart Association (AHA) diet for hypercholesterolemia
American Optical oximeter
Amersham radioimmunoassay kit
AMI (acute myocardial infarction)
AMI (anterior myocardial infarction)

Amicus separator blood collection device
aminocaproic acid
aminoglycosides
aminophylline
amiodarone (now cordarone)
AML (anterior mitral leaflet)
ammonium chloride
amniotic fluid embolism (embolus)
A-mode echocardiography
amp (amplitude)
amphoric breath sounds
amphoric breathing
amphoric respirations
Amplatz cardiac catheter
Amplatz dilator
Amplatzer ductal occluder
Amplatzer septal occluder (ASO)
Amplatz femoral catheter
Amplatz right coronary catheter
Amplatz Super Stiff guidewire
Amplatz technique
Amplatz torque wire
Amplatz tube guide
Amplatz ventricular septal defect device
Amplicor *Mycobacterium tuberculosis* test
Amplified *Mycobacterium tuberculosis* direct (MTD) test
amplitude
 aortic
 apical IVS (interventricular septum)
 C-A mitral valve
 cardiac signal
 D-E
 decreased P-wave
 diminished wave
 EKG wave
 low
 mid-IVS (interventricular septum)
 posterior LV (left ventricular) wall

amplitude *(cont.)*
  precordial impulse
  P-wave
  pulse
  QRS complex
  R-wave
  S_1
  septal
  valve opening
  variance
amplitude of motion
amputation sign
AMR (acute rheumatic myocarditis)
AMS (automatic mode switching) in
  cardiac pacemaker
AMT-25-enhanced MR images
AMVL (anterior mitral valve leaflet)
A_2/MVO interval (aortic valve closure
  to mitral valve opening)
amyloid heart disease
amyloidoma
amyloidosis
  cardiac
  familial
  primary
  senile cardiac
  systemic
amyloidotic cardiomyopathy
ANA (antinuclear antibody) test
anacrotic limb of carotid arterial pulse
anacrotic notch of carotid arterial pulse
anaerobic aspiration
anaerobic lung infection
anaerobic threshold
analogous
analysis (see also *assay, test*)
  arterial blood gas
  Doppler spectral
  immunohistochemical
  Northern blot
  PCR (polymerase chain reaction)
  pressure waveform

analysis *(cont.)*
  quantitative
  slot blot
  Southern blot
  Western blot
analyzer
  Beckman O_2
  DMI (Diagnostic Medical
    Instruments)
  FastPack blood
  Medigraphics
  pacemaker system
  pacing
  pacing system (PSA)
  Piccolo blood chemistry
  PSA (pacing system)
  SMA (Sequential Multiple
    Analyzer) chemistry panel
    (SMA-6, SMA-12, SMA-17,
    SMA-20)
  Stat Profile pHOx blood gas critical
    care
anaphylactoid reaction
anaphylatoxins
anaphylaxis
anasarca
Anastaflo intravascular shunt
anastomoser
anastomosis (anatomical or surgical)
  aorta-to-vein
  aortic
  aorticopulmonary or aorto-
    pulmonary
  arterial
  arterioarterial
  arteriolovenular
  arteriovenous
  ascending aorta to pulmonary artery
  atriopulmonary
  beveled
  bidirectional cavopulmonary
  Blalock-Taussig

anastomosis *(cont.)*
    Cabrol I
    caval-pulmonary artery
    cavoatrial
    cavopulmonary
    cobra-head
    Cooley intrapericardial
    Cooley modification of Waterston
    diamond
    diamond-shaped
    distal
    end-to-end
    end-to-side
    end-to-side internal mammary
        artery to coronary
    end-to-side portacaval
    Glenn
    glomiform arteriovenous
    glomiform arteriolovenular
    heterocladic
    homocladic
    intercoronary
    internal mammary artery to
        coronary artery
    Kugel
    laser-assisted microvascular
        (LAMA)
    left pulmonary artery to
        descending aorta
    LIMA (left internal mammary
        artery)
    Martin-Gruber
    mesocaval
    microvascular
    outflow
    portacaval
    portoportal
    portosystemic
    Potts
    Potts-Smith side-to-side
    precapillary
    proximal

anastomosis *(cont.)*
    right atrium to pulmonary artery
    right internal mammary artery
    right pulmonary artery to
        ascending aorta
    right subclavian to pulmonary
        artery
    Riolan
    side-to-end
    side-to-side
    simple arteriovenous
    simple arteriolovenular
    splenorenal
    Sucquet-Hoyer
    superior vena cava to distal right
        pulmonary artery
    superior vena cava to pulmonary
        artery
    systemic to pulmonary artery
    tensionless
    terminoterminal
    tracheal
    vascular
    Waterston-Cooley
    Waterston extrapericardial
anastomosis [is] probe-patent
anastomosis stapler
anastomotic defect
anastomotic device, converge
anastomotic disruption
anastomotic hemorrhage
anastomotic pseudoaneurysm
anastomotic stricture
anastomotica magna, arteria
anatomical dead space
anatomically dominant
anatomic pulmonary resection
anatomic shunt flow
anatomy
    distorted
    left-dominant coronary
    right-dominant coronary

ANCA (antineutrophilic cytoplasmic antibody)
ANCA (antineutrophil cytoplasm antibody) associated systemic vasculitis (AASV)
anchor
  Anchorlok soft-tissue
  Glycoprene suture
  Lactoprene suture
  Max-Prene suture
  Osteoprene suture
  TwinFix suture
anchored
Anchorlok soft-tissue anchor
ancillary
Ancure catheter
Ancure EZ Path catheter sheath
Ancure minimally invasive endovascular system
Ancure stent
Ancure vascular graft
aneuronal respiratory epithelium
Ancylostoma braziliense infection
Ancylostoma duodenale infection
Ancylostoma infection
Anderson-Keys method for total serum cholesterol
Andral decubitus
Andrews Pynchon suction tube
Andrews suction tip
Androflo monitor
Androgram
Androscope i-Stethos
Androscope Stethos
Androsonix biological sound monitor
anecdotal relationship
anecdotal response
anechoic mantle
Anel method
anemia
  achylic
  acquired hemolytic

anemia *(cont.)*
  acute
  acute posthemorrhagic
  anhematopoietic
  aplastic
  apparent
  aregenerative
  autoimmune hemolytic (AIHA)
  Blackfan-Diamond
  congenital (of newborn)
  congenital hypoplastic
  congenital pernicious
  Cooley
  cow's milk
  deficiency
  Diamond-Blackfan
  dilution
  drug-induced immune hemolytic
  folic acid deficiency
  hemolytic
  hemorrhagic
  hereditary hemolytic
  hereditary iron-loading
  hereditary sideroblastic
  hypochromic
  hypochromic microcytic
  hypoplastic
  immune hemolytic
  immunohemolytic
  iron-deficiency
  juvenile pernicious
  macrocytic
  Malin
  Mediterranean
  microangiopathic
  microangiopathic hemolytic
  microcytic
  normochromic
  normocytic
  nutritional
  nutritional macrocytic
  osteosclerotic

anemia *(cont.)*
  pernicious
  physiologic
  physiological
  polar
  posthemorrhagic (of newborn)
  progressive
  scorbutic
  sickle cell
  sideropenic
  splenic
  spur-cell
  tropical macrocytic
  vitamin B_{12} deficiency
  X-linked
anemic phlebitis
anergy panel
anesthesia
  angiospastic
  blow-by
  crash induction of
  Dyclone gargle
  epidural
  hypotensive
  induction of
  mask
aneuploidy
AneuRx stent-graft system
AneuRx tube graft
aneurysm
  abdominal
  abdominal aortic (AAA)
  acquired
  ampullary
  aortic
  aortic arch
  aortic sinus
  aortic sinusal
  aortoiliac
  arterial
  arteriosclerotic
  arteriovenous

aneurysm *(cont.)*
  arteriovenous pulmonary
  ascending
  ascending aortic
  atherosclerotic
  atrial septal
  axillary
  bacterial
  berry
  berry intracranial
  bland aortic
  brain
  cardiac
  carotid artery
  catheter-related false
  cerebral
  Charcot-Bouchard
  circumscript
  cirsoid
  compound
  congenital
  congenital aortic sinus
  congenital cerebral
  coronary artery
  coronary vessel
  Crawford technique
  cylindroid
  DeBakey technique
  debulking of the
  descending thoracic
  dissecting
  dissecting aortic
  distal aortic arch
  ductal
  ectatic
  embolic
  false
  fusiform
  hernial
  iliac artery
  imperforate
  infected

aneurysm *(cont.)*
    innominate
    intracranial
    intramural coronary artery
    isthmus
    juxtarenal aortic
    late false
    lateral
    left ventricular
    luetic aortic
    mesh-wrapping of aortic
    miliary
    mixed
    mural
    mycotic
    mycotic suprarenal
    nodular
    orbital
    pararenal aortic
    Park
    pelvic
    postcatheterization false
    postinfarction ventricular
    Potts
    pulmonary arteriovenous
    pulmonary artery compression
        ascending aorta
    pulmonary artery mycotic
    racemose
    Rasmussen
    renal
    renal artery
    Richet
    Rodriguez
    ruptured
    ruptured atherosclerotic
    sacciform
    saccular
    sacculated
    serpentine
    sinus of Valsalva
    spindle-shaped

aneurysm *(cont.)*
    spontaneous infantile ductal
    spurious
    suprasellar
    syphilitic
    thoracic
    thoracic aorta
    thoracoabdominal
    traumatic
    true
    tubular
    Valsalva sinus
    varicose
    venous
    ventricular
    ventricular septal
    windsock
    worm
    wrapping of abdominal aortic
aneurysmal bruit
aneurysmal bulging
aneurysmal cough
aneurysmal dilatation
aneurysmal hematoma
aneurysmal phthisis
aneurysmal rupture, contained
aneurysmal sac, wrapped
aneurysmal varix
aneurysmal wall, sliver of
aneurysm cavity
aneurysm clipping
aneurysmectomy
    abdominal aortic
    apicoseptal
    descending thoracic
    emergent
    left ventricular
    off-pump
    retroperitoneal
    simultaneous
    thoracoabdominal aortic
aneurysmoplasty, Matas

aneurysmorrhaphy, popliteal artery
aneurysm resection
ANF (atrial natriuretic factor)
AngeFlex leads
AngeLase combined mapping-laser
  probe
Angelchik antireflux prosthesis
Angell-Shiley bioprosthetic valve
Angell-Shiley xenograft prosthetic
  valve
Angelman syndrome
angel wing sign
Anger-type scintillation camera
angiitis
  allergic granulomatous
  Churg-Strauss
  hypersensitivity
  isolated
  necrotic
  necrotizing
  necrotizing granulomatous
  primary (of central nervous system)
  pulmonary
  varicella-associated focal
  vasculitic
angina (angina pectoris)
  accelerated
  atypical
  bandlike
  chronic stable
  classic
  clinical
  cold-induced
  coronary spastic
  coronary vasospastic
  crescendo
  crescendo-decrescendo
  crescendo pattern
  de novo
  eating-induced
  effort
  emotional

angina *(cont.)*
  esophageal
  esophageal spasm mimicking
  excruciatingly painful
  exercise-induced
  exertional
  focal
  gradual onset of
  Heberden
  hypercyanotic
  intractable
  Ludwig
  mixed
  new onset
  nocturnal
  pacing-induced
  post-AMI (acute myocardial
    infarction)
  postinfarction
  postinfarction unstable
  postprandial
  preinfarction
  Prinzmetal variant
  progressive
  recurrent
  refractory
  rest
  rest-related
  retrosternal heaviness with
  Rougnon-Heberden
  stable
  sudden onset of
  treadmill-induced
  typical
  typical effort
  unstable
  variable threshold
  variant
  vasomotor
  vasospastic
  vasotonic
  walk-through

angina after meals
angina at low workload
angina at rest
angina cordis
angina cruris
angina decubitus syndrome
angina, descriptions of
  brought on or precipitated by,
    anxiety
    cold weather
    eating a heavy meal
    emotional stress or upset
    exercise
    exertion
    exposure to cold
    heavy meals
    sexual intercourse
    smoking
    straining at the stool
    stress
    worry/anxiety
  burning feeling
  crushing chest pain
  elephant on chest feeling
  feeling of impending doom
  gradual onset
  heartburn-type feeling
  heaviness in chest
  indigestion-like feeling
  pinching chest pain
  precordial chest pain
  pressure-like sensation
  radiation down/into arm
  radiation down/into epigastrium
  radiation down/into fingers
  radiation down/into left arm
  radiation down/into scapula
  radiation up/into jaw
  radiation up/into left shoulder
  radiation up/into neck
  referred chest pain

angina *(cont.)*
  retrosternal burning; heaviness
  smothering sensation
  squeezing chest discomfort
  substernal burning
  sudden onset
  suffocating chest pain
  tightness of chest
angina equivalent
angina-equivalent dyspnea
angina inversa
anginal episode
anginal equivalent
anginalike
anginal spell
anginal syndrome
angina of first effort
angina pectoris (see *angina*)
angina pectoris sine dolore
angina pectoris variant
angina precipitated by exertion
angina provoked by ergonovine
  maleate
angina relieved by rest
angina syndrome
angina unrelieved by nitroglycerin
angina vasomotoria
angina with recent increase in
  frequency
anginosa, syncope
anginosus, status
angiocardiographically
angiocardiography (see *angiogram*)
  ambulatory equilibrium
  equilibrium radionuclide
  first-pass radionuclide exercise
  gated equilibrium radionuclide
  transseptal
Angiocath Autoguard shielded
  IV catheter
angiocatheter (see *catheter*)

Angiocath PRN flexible catheter
angio contrast
Angiocor prosthetic valve
AngioDynamics angiography catheter
angiodysplasia
angiodysplastic lesion
angioedema
  hereditary
  Milton
angiogram, angiography
   (also angiocardiogram)
  adrenal
  aortic root
  balloon occlusion pulmonary
  biplane left ventricular
  biplane orthogonal
  blood-pool radionuclide
  Brown-Dodge method for
  cardiac
  carotid
  celiac
  cerebral
  cine
  computerized tomographic hepatic
   (CTHA)
  contrast
  coronary
  digital subtraction pulmonary
  dobutamine thallium
  DSA (digital subtraction)
  electrocardiogram-synchronized
   digital subtraction
  equilibrium radionuclide
  first-pass nuclide rest and exercise
  first-pass radionuclide
  fluorescein
  gadolinium-enhanced subtracted
   MR angiography, 3-D
  gated blood pool
  gated nuclear
  gated radionuclide
  IDIS (intraoperative digital
   subtraction)

angiogram *(cont.)*
  intra-arterial DSA
  intravenous DSA
  Judkins coronary
  left ventricular
  mesenteric
  MSCTA (multislice computed
   tomographic)
  postangioplasty
  post-tourniquet occlusion
  power-injector
  PTCA coronary
  pulmonary
  pulmonary artery wedge
  pulmonary vein wedge
  pulmonary wedge
  radionuclide (RNA)
  rest and exercise gated nuclear
  selective coronary cine
  single plane
  sitting-up view
  3-D CE (three-dimensional
   contrast-enhanced) magnetic
   resonance
  3-D FT magnetic resonance
  3-D gadolinium-enhanced MR
  transvenous digital subtraction
  ventricular
angiogram (or angiography) suite
angiographically mild coronary artery
  disease
angiographically occult vascular
  malformations (AOVM)
angiographically occult vessel
angiographically overlapping structures
angiography (see *angiogram*)
AngioGuard embolic protection filter
angiohemophilia
AngioJet Rheolytic thrombectomy
  system
AngioJet XMI Rheolytic thrombectomy system

angioid streaks, retinal
angiokeratoma corporis diffusum
angiokeratoma corporis diffusum
  universale
Angio-Kit catheter
angiolithic degeneration
angioma
  acquired tufted
  capillary
  cavernous
  cherry
  petechial
  spider
  superficial
  telangiectatic
  venous
angioma arteriale racemosum
angioma cavernosum
angioma serpiginosum
angiomata, spider
angioma venosum racemosum
Angiomedics catheter
angioneurotic edema
angio-osteohypertrophy syndrome
angiopathy
  microvascular (MVA)
  peripheral
angioplastiable
angioplasty
  balloon
  boot-strap two-vessel
  carotid artery balloon
  carotid (with stenting)
  coronary artery
  coronary balloon
  Dotter-Judkins technique for
    percutaneous transluminal
  excimer laser coronary (ELCA)
  facilitated
  Gruentzig balloon catheter
  iliac artery

angioplasty *(cont.)*
  LAIS excimer laser for coronary
  laser
  laser balloon
  laser thermal coronary
  laser-assisted balloon (LABA)
  microwave thermal balloon
  multilesion
  multivessel
  one-vessel
  patch
  patch-graft
  percutaneous laser
  percutaneous transluminal (PTA)
  percutaneous transluminal coronary
    (PTCA)
  peripheral
  peripheral excimer laser (PELA)
  peripheral laser (PLA)
  primary
  single-vessel
  smooth excimer laser coronary
    (SELCA)
  supported
  synthetic patch
  transluminal
  transluminal balloon
  transluminal coronary artery
  vein patch
angioplasty catheter, high-speed
  rotation dynamic
angioplasty laser, Lastec System
angioplasty sheath
angioplasty technique, Gruentzig
Angioport angiographic vascular
  introducer
AngiOptic microcatheter
angioreticuloendothelioma of heart
angiosarcoma, cavernous
angiosarcoma of heart
Angioscale diagnostic catheter

angioscope, angioscopy
  fiberoptic
  flexible
  percutaneous intracoronary
  Mitsubishi
  Olympus
angioscope for in-situ bypass
angioscopy (see *angioscope*)
Angio-Seal hemostatic puncture
  closure device
AngioStent balloon-expandable stent
Angiotech adhesion barrier
Angiotech angioplasty balloon
Angiotech cardiovascular port
Angiotech catheter
Angiotech implant
Angiotech stent
Angiotech vascular graft
Angiotech vascular wrap
angiotensin-converting enzyme (ACE)
  inhibitor
angiotensin II antagonist
angiotensin II receptor blocker
angiotripsy
Angiovist 370
angle
  cardiodiaphragmatic
  cardiohepatic
  cardiophrenic
  costal
  costophrenic
  duodenojejunal
  Ebstein
  infrasternal
  Louis
  Ludovici
  Ludwig
  nail-to-nailbed (clubbing)
  phase
  phrenopericardial
  Pirogoff
  QRST

angle *(cont.)*
  sternal
  sternoclavicular
  substernal
  venous
  xiphoid
angled pleural tube
angle of jaw, jugular venous distention
  of the
angor pectoris (variant of angina
  pectoris)
angry appearance
Angstrom MD implantable single-lead
  cardioverter-defibrillator
angulated lesion
angulated segment
anhidrosis
Anichkov (or Anitschkow)
Anichkov cell
Anichkov myocyte
Animal House fever
anion gap (AG)
anisotropic reentry
anisoylated plasminogen streptokinase
  activator complex (APSAC)
anistreplase thrombolysis
ankle-arm index (AAI)
ankle-brachial index (ABI)
ankle-brachial systolic pressure index
ankle swelling
ankylosing spondylitis
anniversary phenomenon
AnnuloFlo anuloplasty ring system
annulus (see *anulus*)
anodal block
anodal patch electrode, anterior
anode, transvenous
anomalous accessory pathway
anomalous atrioventricular conduction
  pathways
anomalous atrioventricular excitation
anomalous conduction

anomalous distribution
anomalous drainage
anomalous origin of left coronary
    artery
anomalous origin of left coronary
    artery from the pulmonary artery
    (ALCAPA) syndrome
anomalous pathway
anomalous pulmonary artery and
    vascular sling
anomalous pulmonary origin of the
    coronary artery
anomalous pulmonary venous
    connection
        partial
        total
anomalous pulmonary venous drainage
anomalous pulmonary venous return
anomalous retroesophageal right
    subclavian artery
anomalous vein of scimitar syndrome
anomalous vessel
anomaly
    aortic arch
    cardiac
    congenital cardiac
    conotruncal congenital
    cutaneous vascular
    DiGeorge
    Ebstein
    extracardiac
    Freund
    May-Hegglin
    Shone
    Taussig-Bing
    tricuspid valve
    Uhl
anorexia
anoxia
    altitude
    cerebral
anoxic arrest

ANP (atrial natriuretic polypeptide)
Anrep effect
ansa subclavia
antacids, relieved by
antagonist
    angiotensin II
    beta
    calcium
    calcium channel
antagonist therapy, vitamin K
antecedent history
antecubital approach for cardiac
    catheterization
antecubital approach for catheter
    insertion
antecubital brachial approach
    for angiography
antecubital crease
antecubital fossa
antecubital fossa cutdown
antecubital space
antecubital vein
antegrade (forward)
antegrade blood flow
antegrade conduction
antegrade fashion, catheter advanced in
antegrade fast pathway
antegrade filling of vessels
antegrade flow
antegrade infusion (of cardioplegia)
antegrade transseptal approach
    in valvuloplasty
antegrade perfusion
antegrade refractory period
antegrade transseptal approach
    in valvuloplasty
antemortem clot
anterior anuloplasty (Konno
    procedure)
anterior anodal patch electrode
anterior aorta with transposition
    of great arteries

anterior aortic sinus
anterior axillary line
anterior basal bronchi
anterior basal segment
anterior border of lung
anterior border of sternocleidomastoid
  muscle
anterior bowing of sternum
anterior bronchi
anterior cardiac vein
anterior chest wall syndrome
anterior chest wall thrombophlebitis
anterior commissure
anterior coronary plexus (of heart)
anterior cusp
anterior descending artery, superdominant left
anterior descending occlusion
anterior fascicular block
anterior inferior communicating artery
  (AICA)
anterior intercostal artery
anterior internodal pathway
anterior internodal tract of Bachman
anterior interventricular groove
anterior leaflet
anterior leaflet prolapse
anterior magna, arteria radicularis
anterior mediastinal compartment
anterior mediastinal space
anterior mediastinum
anterior mitral valve leaflet
anterior motion
  palpable
  visible
anterior motion of posterior mitral
  valve leaflet
anterior papillary muscle
anterior parasternal motion, sustained
anterior/posterior (AP)
anterior pulmonary plexus
anterior rectus sheath divided
  transversely

anterior semilunar valve
anterior septal myocardial infarction
anterior surface of the right ventricle
anterior table
anterior tracheal displacement
anterior wall dyskinesis
anterior wall myocardial infarction
anteroapical wall myocardial infarction
anterograde conduction
anterograde percutaneous aortic
  valvotomy
anterolateral incision
anterolateral muscle-sparing lateral
  thoracotomy
anterolateral wall myocardial infarction
anteroposterior diameter
anteroseptal commissure
anteroseptal wall myocardial infarction
anteverted nares
anthelminthic therapy
anthracosilicosis
anthracosis tuberculosis
anthracyclines
anthraquinones
Anthron heparinized antithrombogenic
  catheter
antiadrenergic agent
antiaggregant, platelet
antianginal agent
antianginal drug
antianginal therapy
antiarrhythmia agent
antiarrhythmic drugs, classes I-V
antiarrhythmics
antibacterial therapy
antibiotic
  broad-spectrum
  perioperative
  postoperative
  preoperative
  prophylactic
  quinolone

antibiotic solution
antibiotic therapy
antibody, antibodies
    anticardiolipin (ACA, aCL, ACL)
    anti-cytokeratin 8 (anti-CK8)
    anti-D (WinRho SD)
    anti-human cardiac myosin
    antimyosin
    antimyosin monoclonal (with Fab
      fragment) (AMA-Fab)
    antineutrophilic cytoplasmic
      (ANCA)
    antinuclear (ANA)
    antiphospholipid
    CD5+ monoclonal
    CD18
    circulating immune complex
    cytokeratin 8:anti-cytokeratin 8
    cytokeratin 8 (CK8)
    heterophile
    IgM anti-human parvovirus
    indium
    indium-labeled antimyosin
    OKT3 monoclonal
    monoclonal
    perinuclear antineutrophil
      cytoplasmic (pANCA)
    polyclonal anticardiac myosin
    precipitating
    7E3 monoclonal antiplatelet
    sheep antidigoxin Fab
    SS-A (Ro)
    SS-B (La)
    teichoic acid
    38-kDa
    whole blood monoclonal
antibody-antigen complex
anticardiolipin (aCL) antibody (ACA)
anticholinergic syndrome
anticoagulant
    coumarin-type
    hirudin (recombinant)
    oral

anticoagulant drugs
anticoagulant prophylaxis
anticoagulant protein S
anticoagulant therapy
anticoagulation
    adjunctive
    appropriate
    bivalrudin
    citrate regional
    extended
    full
    heparin
    intensive
    lifelong
    long-term
    oral
    prolonged
    postdevice
    short-term
    systemic heparin
    therapeutic
    warfarin
anticoronary diet
anti-cytokeratin 8 (anti-CK8) antibody
anti-D antibody (WinRho SD)
antidepressants, tricyclic
antidiuretic hormone (ADH)
antiDNase B (anti-deoxyribonuclease
    B)
antidromic AV (atrioventricular)
    reciprocating tachycardia
antidromic circus movement
    tachycardia
antidromic conduction
antidromic tachycardia
antiembolic stockings
antifibrin antibody imaging
antifibrinolytic drugs
antifilarial drug
antigen
    Aspergillus
    autogenous
    carcinoembryonic (CEA)

antigen *(cont.)*
  histocompatibility
  HLA-B27
  human leukocyte, B27
  kDa
  purified 38-kDa protein
  serum cryptococcal
antigen challenge, nasal
antiglomerular basement membrane
  antibody disease
antihemophilic blood coagulation factor
antihemophilic globulin (AHG)
antihistamines
antihyperlipidemic drug
antihypertensive drug
antihypertensive therapy
anti-inflammatory drug
anti-ischemic
antilymphocyte globulin
antimicrobial drugs
antimicrobial therapy
antimony
Anti-MPO (p-ANCA) ELISA
  autoimmune test
antimyosin antibodies
antineutrophilic cytoplasmic antibody
antineutrophil cytoplasm antibody-
  associated systemic vasculitis
  (AASV)
antineutrophilic cytoplasmic antibody
  (ANCA)
antinuclear antibody (ANA)
antiphospholipid (aPL) antibody
antiphospholipid-antibody syndrome
antiphospholipid syndrome (APS)
antiplatelet agent
antiplatelet drug
antirejection regimen
antisense oligonucleotides, respirable
  or radiolabeled (RASON)
antiseptic drug
antispasmodic drug

antistreptolysin O
antitachycardia pacemaker
antitachycardia pacing therapy
antithrombin III (ATnativ)
antithrombin III antigen
antithrombin III deficiency
antithymocyte globulin
antitubercular
antituberculosis drugs
antitussives
antiviral drugs
antiviral therapy
Antrin (motexafin lutetium)
antritis, acute
Antyllus method
anular abscess
anular calcification
anular cartilage, bronchial
anular constriction
anular dilatation
anular dilatation and reconstruction
anular disruption
anular foreshortening
anular fracture
anular hypoplasia
anular placement of sutures
anular plication
anuli fibrosi cordis
anuloaortic ectasia
anuloplasty
  anterior
  Carpentier
  De Vega
  Frater
  Kay
  Kay-Reed-Wooler
  mitral
  Paneth
  patch graft
  prosthetic ring
  Puig-Massana
  septal

anuloplasty *(cont.)*
  subcommissural suture
  tricuspid valve
  Wooler
  Wooler-Kay
anuloplasty ring
  Carpentier-Edwards Physio
  Puig Massana-Shiley
  Sculptor flexible
anuloplasty with ring
anuloplasty without ring
anulorrhaphy
anulus
  aortic
  aortic valve
  atrioventricular
  calcified
  friable
  mitral
  mitral valve
  noncoronary
  pulmonary
  pulmonary valve
  redundant scallop of posterior
  septal tricuspid
  tricuspid valve
  valve
anulus fibrosus
anulus ovalis
anulus overriding the ventricular
  septum
anulus plication
anuria
anxiety and insomnia
anxiety, profound
anxiety syndrome
anxiolytic
anxious
Ao, AO (aorta)
AO (aortic opening)
AO/AC or AO-AC (aortic valve open-
  ing/aortic valve closing) ratio

AoBP (aortic blood pressure)
AOC (aortic opening click)
Aorfix stent-graft
Aorfix vascular graft
aorta
  abdominal
  arch of
  ascending (AA)
  bifurcation of the
  biventricular origin of
  biventricular transposed
  calcified
  central
  cervical
  coarctation of
  coarcted
  cross-clamping of
  D-malposition of
  descending
  descending thoracic
  dextroposed
  dextropositioned
  double-barreled
  dynamic
  eggshell
  elongation of
  idiopathic necrosis of
  incision of
  infrarenal abdominal
  kinked
  L-malposition
  overriding
  palpable
  pericardial
  porcelain
  preductal coarctation of
  recoarctation of the
  reconstruction of
  root of
  sclerosis of
  small feminine
  supraceliac

aorta *(cont.)*
  supradiaphragmatic
  terminal
  thoracic
  thoracoabdominal
  transection of
  transposed
  unfolded
  unwinding of
  ventral
aorta abdominalis
aorta ascendens
aorta clamped cephalad to aneurysm
aorta-iliac-femoral bypass
aorta-ostium
aorta-renal bypass
aorta sacrococcygea
aorta-subclavian-carotid bypass
aorta-to-aorta conduit
aorta-to-vein anastomosis
aortic allograft
aortic anastomosis
aortic bifurcation graft
aortic anular reconstruction
aortic anular region
aortic anulus
aortic-aortic conduit
aortic arch
  congenital interruption of
  double
  elongated
  penetrating injury to
  uncoiled
aortic arch anomaly
aortic arch arteritis
aortic arch atresia
aortic arch calcification-osteoporosis-
  tooth-buds hypoplasia syndrome
aortic arch hypoplasia syndrome
aortic arch interruption
aortic arch lesion
aortic arch obstruction

aortic arch syndrome
aortic arteritis
aortic atherosclerosis
  juxtarenal
  pararenal
aortic atresia
aortic bifurcation
aortic bifurcation graft, Edwards
  woven Teflon
aortic bifurcation syndrome
aortic blood pressure (AoBP)
aortic bulb
aortic button technique
aortic cannulation
aortic cartilage
aortic clamp
aortic closure (AC)
aortic coarctation, juxtaductal
aortic coarctation-related hypertension
aortic coarctation syndrome
aortic component of murmur
aortic configuration of cardiac shadow
  on x-ray
aortic connector system
aortic cross-clamp
aortic cusp
  perforated
  ruptured
aortic cusps separation
aortic diameter (AD)
aortic diastolic murmur
aortic dilatation
aortic dissection
  DeBakey classification of
  thoracic
  type B
aortic ejection click (AEC)
aortic ejection sound, palpable
aortic elongation
aortic hiatus
aortic homograft
aortic impedance

aortic incisura
aortic incompetence
aortic insufficiency (AI)
aortic insult
aortic isthmus, hypoplasia of
aortic knob, blurring of
aortic knob contour
aortic knuckle
aortic leaflets, redundant
aortic-left ventricular pressure
    difference
aortic-left ventricular tunnel
aortic nipple sign
aortic opening (AO)
aortic opening click (AOC)
aorticopulmonary anastomosis
aorticopulmonary defect
aorticopulmonary septal defect
aorticopulmonary shunt
aorticopulmonary trunk
aorticopulmonary window
aorticopulmonary window operation
aortic orifice
aortic override
aortic oxygen saturation
aortic paravalvular leak
aortic pressure
aortic pseudoaneurysm
aortic pullback
aortic-pulmonary shunt
aortic regurgitation (AR)
    chronic
    congenital
    isolated
    massive
    preoperative
    severe
    syphilitic
aortic resection
aortic root angiogram
aortic root dilatation
aortic root, dilated

aortic root enlargement
aortic root homograft
aortic root perfusion needle
aortic root pressure
aortic root ratio
aortic root replacement
aortic runoff
aortic rupture
aortic second sound
aortic segment
    intradiaphragmatic
    intramuscular
aortic septal defect
aortic shag
aortic sinus
aortic sinus aneurysm
aortic sinus to right ventricle fistula
aortic sound
aortic spindle
aortic stenosis (AS) (also *aortic valve*
    stenosis)
    acquired
    calcific
    congenital
    congenital subvalvular
    congenital valvular
    hypercalcemia-supravalvular
    supravalvar
    supravalvular (SAS, SVAS)
    uncomplicated supraclavicular
aortic stenosis secondary to bicuspid
    aortic valve
aortic stent graft
aortic stiffness
aortic stump blowout
aortic subvalvular ring
aortic-superior mesenteric bypass
aortic systolic murmur
aortic takeoff
aortic thrill
aortic thromboembolism
aortic thrombosis, terminal

aortic tract complex
aortic tract complex hypoplasia
aortic transection, traumatic
aortic tube graft
aortic valve (see *valve*)
  bicommissural
  bicuspid
  composite
  floppy
  native
  tricuspid
  unicommissural
  unicuspid
aortic valve anulus
aortic valve area
aortic valve atresia
aortic valve calcification
aortic valve disease
aortic valve endocarditis
aortic valve incompetence
aortic valve insufficiency
aortic valve leaflet
aortic valve obstruction
aortic valve pressure gradient
aortic valve prosthesis (see *prosthesis*)
aortic valve regurgitation
aortic valve repair
aortic valve replacement (AVR)
aortic valve re-replacement (AVreR)
aortic valve resuspension
aortic valve stenosis (see *aortic stenosis*)
aortic valve thickening
aortic valvotomy, closed transventricular
aortic valvular incompetence
aortic valvular insufficiency
aortic valvulotomy
aortic vasa vasorum
aortic vent suction line
aortic vestibule
aortic vestibule of ventricle
aortic wall

aortic window node
aortic wrap
aortitis
  Döhle-Heller (or Doehle)
  giant cell
  luetic
  nummular
  rheumatic
  syphilitic
  Takayasu
aortoarteritis (types I-IV)
  nonspecific
  nonspecific inflammatory
aortobifemoral bypass graft
aortobifemoral reconstruction
aortobiprofunda bypass graft
aortocarotid bypass
aortocaval fistula
aortoceliac bypass
aortocoronary saphenous vein bypass graft
aortocoronary snake graft
aortocoronary valve
aortoduodenal
aortoenteric fistula
aortoesophageal
aortofemoral arteriography with runoff views
aortofemoral bypass graft (AFBG)
aortogastric
aortogram, aortography
  abdominal
  arch
  biplanar
  contrast
  digital subtraction supravalvular
  flush
  retrograde
  retrograde femoral
  retrograde transaxillary
  supravalvular
  thoracic
  thoracic arch

aortogram *(cont.)*
   translumbar
   ultrasonic
aortogram with distal runoff
aortography
aortoiliac aneurysm
aortoiliac bypass
aortoiliac disease
aortoiliac obstruction
aortoiliac obstructive disease (AIOD)
aortoiliac occlusive disease
aortoiliac-popliteal bypass
aortoiliac thrombosis
aortoiliofemoral arteries
aortoiliofemoral bypass
aortoiliofemoral endarterectomy
aortomegaly, diffuse
aorto-ostial Y saphenous vein graft
aortopathy, idiopathic medial
aortoplasty
   balloon
   patch-graft
   posterior patch
   subclavian flap
aortoplasty with patch graft
aortopopliteal bypass
aortopulmonary anastomosis
aortopulmonary collaterals
aortopulmonary fistula
aortopulmonary shunt
aortopulmonary tunnel
aortopulmonary window
aortopulmonary window operation
aortorrhaphy
aortosclerosis
aortotomy
   circular
   curvilinear
   Goosen
   longitudinal
   punch
   transverse
   trapdoor-type

aortovelography, transcutaneous (TAV)
aortoventriculoplasty
AoV (aortic valve)
AOVM (angiographically occult
   vascular malformations)
Ap (apical)
AP (accessory pathway)
AP (anterior/posterior)
APA (aldosterone-producing adenoma)
APACHE CV risk predictor
APB (atrial premature beat)
APC (atrial premature complex)
APC (atrial premature contraction)
APD (action potential duration)
Apert syndrome
aperture
apex (pl. apices)
   cardiac
   displaced left ventricular
   heart
   left ventricular
   lung
   systolic retraction of
   uptilted cardiac
apex beat
apexcardiogram (ACG)
apexcardiography (ACG)
apex cordis (of heart)
apex of heart
apex of Koch triangle
apex of left ventricle
apex of lung
apex of ventricle
apex pulse, absent
Apgar score
apheresis of autoantibodies
apheresis of cold precipitable serum
   proteins
apheresis of erythrocytes
apheresis of leukocyte fractions
apheresis of plasma
apheresis of platelets

aphonic pectoriloquy
API (ankle-arm pressure index)
apical air space (on x-ray)
apical and subcostal four-chambered
    view
apical aortic valved conduit
apical beat, displaced
apical beat displacement, inferolateral
apical cap sign
apical four-chamber view
apical hypertrophic cardiomyopathy
apical hypoperfusion on thallium scan
apical impulse
    absent
    double systolic
    downward displacement
    hyperdynamic
    sustained
apical impulse displaced to the left
apical infiltrate
apical-lateral wall myocardial
    infarction
apically directed chest tube
apical midsystolic click
apical pleural capping
apical posterior artery
apical posterolateral region of left
    ventricle
apical pulse
apical scar
apical scarring
apical segment
apical short-axis slice
apical surface of heart
apical thrust
apical tissue
apical two-chamber view
apical window
apices (pl. of apex)
apico-abdominal bypass
apicoaortic (abdominal) conduit
apicoaortic shunt
apicoaortic valved conduit

apicoposterior bronchi
apicoseptal aneurysmectomy
aPL (antiphospholipid) antibody
aplasia
    pure red cell
    red cell
    right ventricular myocardial
aplasia of the deep veins
aplastic anemia
APM (anterior papillary muscle)
apnea
    central
    end-tidal-volume
    idiopathic obstructive sleep
    mixed
    obstructive sleep
    sleep
    transient
apnea and bradycardia (A&B)
apnea/hypopnea index (AHI)
apnea neonatorum
apnea of prematurity
apneic episodes, intermittent
apneustic breathing
Apo A1 LDL-cholesterol subfraction
Apo-Atenol (atenolol)
Apo A2 LDL-cholesterol subfraction
Apo B LDL-cholesterol subfraction
Apo-Furosemide (furosemide)
Apogee CX 200 echo system (ablation)
Apo-Hydro (hydrochlorothiazide)
A point
Apollo cannula
Apollo papillotome
Apollo 3AC cannula
Apollo 3AC papillotome
apolipoprotein
Apo-Metoprolol L (metoprolol)
aponeurosis, bicipital
apoplectiform
apoplexy
    pulmonary artery
    pulmonary vein

apoprotein (A-E)
A-port implant infusion port
Apo-Salvent (salbutamol)
apparatus
  breathing
  Endo-Flo endoscopic irrigation
  En Garde closure
  enlarged valve
  mitral
  RESPeRATE
  respiratory
  tensor
  valvular
  Volutrol control (for IV infusion)
apparatus respiratorius
appearance
  angry
  beavertail (of balloon profile)
  bullneck
  coarse
  cobra-head
  cushingoid
  fine-speckled
  fish-flesh
  Florence flask
  frondlike
  ground-glass
  heterogeneous
  homogeneous
  lobulated saccular
  plucked chicken
  reticulogranular
  shocky
  string-of-beads
  toxic
  trilayer
  whorled
appearance and exclusion, normal
appendage
  atrial
  left atrial (LAA)
  right atrial (RAA)

appendage *(cont.)*
  truncated atrial
  wide-based blunt-ended right-sided
    atrial
appendogram
applesauce sign
appliance, removable Herbst
application of vessel loops
applier, VCS clip
appose
apposition
apposition of leaflets
apprehension
apprehensive
approach (see also *operation*)
  aggressive surgical
  antecubital
  antecubital brachial
  axillofemoral
  brachial
  cephalic
  deltopectoral
  external jugular
  femoral venous
  femorofemoral
  groin
  internal jugular
  left subcostal
  median sternotomy
  percutaneous transfemoral
  retrograde femoral arterial
  retroperitoneal
  subclavicular
  subcostal
  subxiphoid
  thoracoabdominal
  transaortic
  transatrial
  transdiaphragmatic
  transpectoral
  transperitoneal
  transthoracic

approach *(cont.)*
  transtricuspid
  transvenous
  transventricular
  transxiphoid pacemaker lead
  umbilical venous
appropriate anticoagulation
appropriately matched donor
appropriately sized donor
approximated
approximate, loosely
approximation
approximator
  Lemmon sternal
  Pilling Wolvek sternal
  rib
  Wolvek sternal
aprikalim
APSAC (anisoylated plasminogen
  streptokinase activator complex)
APTT (activated partial thromboplastin
  time)
Apt test
APUD (amine precursor uptake and
  decarboxylation) cell
apudoma
AquaSens irrigation fluid monitor
AR (atrial rate)
AR (aortic regurgitation)
arachidonic acid cascade
araneus, nevus
Arani double loop guiding catheter
Arantii, ductus
Arantius body
Arantius canal
arborization, Purkinje
arbutamine
arc
ARC (argon beam electrocoagulator)
  laser
arcade
  mitral
  septal

arcade of collaterals
arch
  aortic
  bifid aortic
  distal aortic
  double aortic
  hypoplastic
  mid aortic
  right aortic
  right-sided
  transverse
  transverse aortic
  Zimmerman
arch and carotid arteriography
arch hypoplasia
Archer syndrome
arching of mitral valve leaflet
architecture
  lung
  mural
arch of aorta
arch repair, concomitant
arch study (imaging study of aortic
  arch)
Arco pacemaker
Arco lithium pacemaker
arcuate arteries
arcuate vessels
arcus, corneal
arcus senilis
arc welder's lung
ARDS (adult respiratory distress
  syndrome)
ARE (acute rheumatic endocarditis)
area
  aortic
  aortic valve (AVA)
  arrhythmogenic
  artery
  Bamberger
  body surface (BSA)
  cardiac frontal
  cross-sectional (CSA)

area *(cont.)*
  echo-free
  effective balloon dilated (EBDA)
  Erb
  hilar
  luminal cross-sectional
  midsternal
  mitral valve (MVA)
  perihilar
  peroneal
  pulmonic
  sonolucent
  stenosis
  subcarinal
  subclavicular
  subglottic
  tricuspid
  valve
area-length method for ejection fraction
areas of denudation
areolar tissue
ARF (acute respiratory failure)
ARF (acute rheumatic fever)
arginine vasopressin
argon laser
Argyle chest tube
Argyle Sentinel Seal chest tube
Argyle Turkel safety thoracentesis
  system
Argyll Robertson pupils
Aria coronary artery bypass graft
Arixtra (fondaparinux sodium)
arm and lesser saphenous veins
  (ALSVs)
arm ergometry stress test
ArmorGlide coating for intra-aortic
  balloon (IAB) catheters
armor heart
arm-to-tongue time
Army-Navy retractor
Arneth syndrome
Arnold-Chiari deformity

Arnold-Chiari malformation
Arnold-Chiari syndrome
arousal, episodic
ARP (absolute refractory period)
ARP (acute rheumatic pericarditis)
array electrode
arrest
  anoxic
  asystolic cardiac
  bradyarrhythmic cardiac
  cardiac
  cardioplegic
  cardiopulmonary
  cardiorespiratory
  circulatory
  cold cardioplegia
  cold potassium solution-induced
    cardiac
  deep hypothermic circulatory
  electrical circulatory
  episodic cardiac
  heart
  hypothermic
  hypothermic circulatory
  hypothermic fibrillating
  intermittent sinus
  profound hypothermic circulatory
    (PHCA)
  recurrent cardiac
  respiratory
  sinus
  transient sinus
arrested circulation
arrhythmia
  atrioventricular junctional
  AV (atrioventricular) nodal
    Wenckebach
  baseline
  complex atrial
  continuous
  drug-refractory
  exercise-aggravated

arrhythmia *(cont.)*
  exercise-induced
  extrasystolic
  high-density ventricular
  inducible
  intermittent
  juvenile
  lethal
  life-threatening
  malignant
  malignant ventricular
  nodal
  nonlethal
  nonrespiratory sinus
  pacing-induced termination of
  paroxysmal supraventricular
  perpetual
  phasic
  postmalignant
  postperfusion
  reentrant
  reperfusion
  respiratory sinus (RSA)
  sinus
  spontaneous
  stress-related
  supraventricular (SVA)
arrhythmia circuit
arrhythmia classification
arrhythmia detection
arrhythmia focus
arrhythmia-induced syncope
arrhythmia mapping system
Arrhythmia Net arrhythmia monitor
arrhythmogenic area of ventricle
arrhythmogenic area in myocardium
arrhythmogenic border zone
arrhythmogenic disease
arrhythmogenic pulmonary vein
arrhythmogenic right ventricular
  cardiomyopathy
arrhythmogenic right ventricular
  dysplasia (ARVD) syndrome
arrhythmogenic scar
arrhythmogenic site
arrhythmogenic ventricular activity
  (AVA)
Arrow-Berman balloon angioplasty
  catheter
Arrow Cannon catheter
Arrow catheter
Arrow-Clarke Pleura-Seal thoracentesis kit
Arrow-Flex percutaneous sheath introducer
ArrowGard Blue Line catheter
ArrowGard Blue Line FlexTip catheter
ArrowGard Blue Line Quad-Lumen
  catheter
ArrowGard Blue Line two-lumen
  catheter
ArrowGard Blue Line triple-lumen
  catheter
ArrowGard Blue Line five-lumen
  catheter
ArrowGard Blue Plus catheter
ArrowGard central venous catheter
arrowhead-shaped
Arrow-Howes multilumen catheter
Arrow-Howes triple-lumen catheter
Arrow multi-lumen access (MAC)
  catheter
Arrow needleless injection cannula
Arrow Percutaneous Sheath Introducer
  kit
Arrow pneumothorax kit
Arrow pulmonary artery catheter
Arrow Raulerson syringe
Arrow-Trerotola percutaneous
  thrombolytic device
Arrow Twin Cath multilumen
  peripheral catheter

arteria anastomotica magna
ArteriA embolic protection device
arterial access site
arterial-alveolar CO_2 tension difference
arterial anastomosis
arterial aneurysm
arterial avulsion
arterial bleeding
arterial blood gases (ABGs) (see
   blood gas)
arterial blood gases on 100% oxygen
arterial blood gases on room air
arterial blood pressure (BP)
arterial brachiocephalic trunk
arterial bruit
arterial cannula, peripheral
arterial cannulation
arterial capillaries
arterial circulation
arterial cutoff
arterial degenerative disease
arterial dilatation and rupture
arterial embolectomy catheter
arterial endothelium
arterial fibromuscular dysplasia
arterial fibromuscular hyperplasia
arterial gradient
arterial hyperemia
arterial hypertension
arterial hypocarbia
arterial hypoplasia
arterial hypoxemia
arterial hypoxia
arterial intima, diffuse thickening of
arterial ischemia index
arterialization of venous blood
arterial limb
arterial line (A-line)
arterial lumen
arterial malformation (AM)
arterial obstruction
arterial oxygen content

arterial oxygen saturation (SaO_2)
arterial oxygen unsaturation
arterial partial pressure of CO_2
   (mm Hg) ($PaCO_2$)
arterial partial pressure of O_2 (mm Hg)
   (PaO_2)
arterial patency
arterial peak systolic pressure
Arterial Plug catheter
arterial pressure
arterial pulsation
arterial recoil
arterial return, central
arterial runoff
arterial rupture and dilatation
arterial sclerosis
arterial segment
arterial sheath
arterial spasm
arterial spasm adjacent to plaque
arterial steal
arterial supply of parietal pleura
arterial switch operation
arterial thrill
arterial thrombosis
arterial topography
arterial tree
arteria lusoria
arteria magna
arterial varices
arterial wall dynamics
arterial wall thickness, preacinar
arterial wedge pressure, pulmonary
arteria radicularis anterior magna
arterioarterial anastomosis
arteriocapillary sclerosis
arteriogram, arteriography
   aorta and runoff
   aortofemoral (with runoff views)
   arch
   balloon occlusion
   biplane pelvic

arteriogram *(cont.)*
 biplane quantitative coronary
 bronchial
 carotid
 celiac
 cine
 completion
 coronary
 delayed phase of
 intraoperative
 Judkins selective coronary
 left coronary cine
 thrombotic pulmonary (TPA)
arteriography
arteriolar sclerosis
arteriole
arteriopathy
 idiopathic regressing
 thrombotic pulmonary (TPA)
arterioplasty
arteriorenal
arteriosclerosis
 calcific
 cerebral
 coronary
 generalized
 hyaline
 hypertensive
 infantile
 intimal
 medial
 Mönckeberg (Moenckeberg)
 obliterative
 peripheral
 presenile
 pulmonary
 senile
arteriosclerosis obliterans (ASO)
arteriosclerotic cardiovascular disease
 (ASCVD)
arteriosclerotic dementia

arteriosclerotic deposits
arteriosclerotic heart disease (ASHD)
arteriosclerotic lining of narrowed
 arteries
arteriosclerotic peripheral vascular
 disease
arteriosclerotic plaques
arteriostenosis
arteriosum, ligamentum
arteriosus
 persistent truncus
 pseudotruncus
 true truncus
 truncus
arteriotomy
 Acland-Banis
 brachial
 longitudinal
 transverse
arteriotomy closure device, Cohiba
arteriovenous (AV)
arteriovenous access
arteriovenous anastomosis
arteriovenous aneurysm
arteriovenous fistula (AVF), coronary
arteriovenous fistula formation
arteriovenous fistula of lung
arteriovenous malformation (AVM)
arteriovenous microshunt
arteriovenous nicking
arteriovenous oxygen content
 difference
arteriovenous oxygen difference
 (AVD O_2)
 pulmonary
 systemic
arteriovenous pressure gradient
arteriovenous shunt defects
arteriovenous varix
arteritis
 acute
 aortic

43 **arteritis • artery**

arteritis *(cont.)*
    aortic arch
    brachiocephalic
    cerebral
    coronary
    cranial
    giant cell
    granulomatous
    Horton giant cell
    infantile
    infectious
    innominate artery
    localized visceral
    necrotizing
    obliterative
    para-arterial angiomatosis
    pulmonary
    rheumatic
    supra-aortic Takayasu
    syphilitic
    Takayasu
    temporal
    tuberculous
    young female aortic arch
arteritis obliterans
arteritis umbilicalis
artery, arteries (see also *branch*)
    Abbott
    aberrant coronary
    aberrant left pulmonary
    access
    Adamkiewicz
    anomalous origin of
    anterior descending branch of left
        coronary
    anterior inferior communicating
        (AICA)
    aortoiliofemoral
    apical posterior
    arcuate
    atrioventricular node
    AV (atrioventricular) nodal

artery *(cont.)*
    beading of
    brachial
    brachiocephalic
    calcified
    caliber-persistent
    celiac
    cerebral
    circumflex (circ, CF, CX)
    circumflex groove
    common carotid (CCA)
    common femoral
    common iliac
    communicating
    conus
    corduroy
    coronary
    descending septal
    diagonal branch of
    diagonal branch of left anterior
        descending coronary
    diagonal coronary
    dilated
    distal circumflex marginal
    dominant coronary
    dominant left coronary
    dominant right coronary
    Drummond marginal
    eccentric coronary
    epicardial coronary
    external carotid
    external iliac
    familial fibromuscular dysplasia of
    first diagonal branch
    first obtuse marginal
    gastroepiploic
    high left main diagonal
    hilar
    hypogastric
    inferior mesenteric
    infragenicular popliteal
    infrageniculate

artery *(cont.)*
   innominate
   intercostal
   intermediate coronary
   internal carotid (ICA)
   internal iliac
   internal mammary (IMA)
   internal maxillary (IMax, IMAX)
   internal thoracic
   intra-acinar pulmonary
   Kugel
   LAD (left anterior descending)
     coronary
   LCA (left coronary)
   LCF or LCX (left circumflex)
   left anterior descending
   left circumflex coronary
   left common femoral
   left coronary (LCA)
   left internal mammary (LIMA)
   left main coronary (LMCA)
   left pulmonary (LPA)
   LIMA (left internal mammary)
   LMCA (left main coronary)
   main pulmonary (MPA)
   mainstem coronary
   mammary
   marginal branch of left circumflex
     coronary
   marginal branch of right coronary
   marginal circumflex
   medial plantar
   middle cerebral (MCA)
   musculophrenic
   native coronary
   obtuse marginal (OM) coronary
   OM (obtuse marginal)
   overriding great
   patent
   PDA (posterior descending)
   perforating
   peripancreatic

artery *(cont.)*
   peroneal
   phrenic
   pipestem
   plaque-containing
   popliteal
   posterior descending (PDA)
   posterior descending branch of
     right coronary
   posterior descending coronary
   posterior inferior communicating
     (PICA)
   posterior intercostal
   profunda femoris
   proximal anterior descending
   proximal left anterior descending
   proximal popliteal
   pulmonary (PA)
   radicular
   ramus intermedius
   ramus medialis
   reperfused
   resilient
   retroesophageal right subclavian
   right coronary (RCA)
   right femoral
   right pulmonary (RPA)
   right ventricular branch of right
     coronary
   septal perforator
   sinoatrial node
   sinus nodal
   stenotic coronary
   subclavian
   subcostal
   superficial femoral (SFA)
   superior epigastric
   superior genicular
   superior intercostal
   superior mesenteric
   superior thyroid
   temporal

artery *(cont.)*
   thyroid
   truncal
   vertebral
   weakened
artery (arterial) patency
artery system, iliac
artery takeoff
artery-vein-nerve bundle
arthralgias and myalgias
arthritis
   acute rheumatic
   chronic post-rheumatic fever
   Jaccoud
   rheumatoid
   subacute rheumatic
arthropathy-camptodactyly syndrome
articular capsule
articular rheumatism
articulation of thorax
artifact
   acoustic
   attenuation
   baseline
   catheter
   catheter impact
   catheter tip motion
   catheter tip position
   catheter whip
   end-pressure
   linear
   mirror image
   mitral regurgitation
     (cineangiography)
   mosaic
   motion
   muscle
   pacemaker
   pacing
artifact due to body contour orbit
artifact due to partial volume effect
artifact image

artifacts mimicking intimal flaps
artifactual
artificial blood (see *blood substitute*)
artificial cardiac pacemaker
artificial cardiac valve
artificial heart (see also *heart*)
   AbioCor total
   air-driven
   Akutsu III total (TAH)
   ALVAD (intra-abdominal left
     ventricular assist device)
   Baylor total
   CardioWest total
   electromechanical
   Jarvik VII or Jarvik-7
   Liotta total (TAH)
   Symbion J-7 70-mL ventricle
   Symbion Jarvik-7
   University of Akron
   Utah total (TAH)
artificial left ventricular assist device
   (LVAD)
artificial lung
artificial lung-expanding compound
   (ALEC)
artificial lung, IVOX (intravascular
   oxygenator)
artificial pacemaker
artificial pneumothorax
artificial respiration
artificial vascular access graft,
   Credent
artificial ventilation
AR 2 diagnostic guiding catheter
ARVD (arrhythmogenic right ventricu-
   lar dysplasia)
Arvidsson dimension-length method
   for ventricular volume
Arzco pacemaker
Arzco TAPSUL pill electrode
AS (aortic stenosis)

ASA (American Society of Anesthesia) risk classification (I-IV)
ASA (asthma, nasal polyps, aspirin) triad
asbestos
asbestos bodies
asbestos exposure
asbestos-induced pleural fibrosis
asbestosis
asbestos pleural plaques
asbestos-related pleural disease
Ascaris infection
Ascaris lumbricoides infection
Ascaris pneumonitis
Ascaris suum infection
ASCD (aborted sudden cardiac death)
ascending aneurysm replacement
ascending aorta (AA)
ascending aorta-abdominal aorta bypass graft
ascending aorta hypoplasia
ascending aortic aneurysm
ascending contrast phlebography
ascending hypoplasia of aorta
ascending phlebography
Ascent guiding catheter
ascertain, ascertained
Aschner phenomenon
Aschoff body
Aschoff cell
Aschoff node
Aschoff nodules
Aschoff-Tawara node
ascites
    chylous
    massive
ascorbate dilution curve
ASCVD (arteriosclerotic cardiovascular disease)
ASCVD (atherosclerotic cardiovascular disease)
ASD (atrial septal defect)

ASD (atrioventricular septal defect)
ASD, transcatheter occlusion of (with button device)
aseptic myocarditis of newborn
aseptic technique
ASH (asymmetric septal hypertrophy)
ASHD (arteriosclerotic heart disease)
ashen
Ashman beat
Ashman index
Ashman phenomenon
Ask-Upmark kidney
ASM (atrial systolic murmur)
ASO (Amplatzer septal occluder)
ASO (arteriosclerosis obliterans)
ASO (antistreptolysin-O) titer test
aspartate aminotransferase (AST)
aspartylglycosaminuria
aspergilloma
aspergillosis
    allergic bronchopulmonary (ABPA)
    invasive pulmonary
Aspergillus antigen
Aspergillus fumigatus
Aspergillus niger
Aspergillus pneumonia
Aspergillus precipitins, serum
Aspergillus terreus
asphyxia, neonatal
asphyxial membrane
asphyxiating thoracic dystrophy
aspirate
aspirated acid vomitus
aspirated debris
aspirated foreign body
aspiration
    anaerobic
    CT-guided
    CUSALap
    foreign-body
    percutaneous (of pericardial cyst)
    percutaneous transthoracic

aspiration *(cont.)*
  percutaneous transtracheal
  pericardial fluid
  pulmonary
  tracheal
  transtracheal
  ultrasound-guided transthoracic
    needle
aspiration biopsy
aspiration of air
aspiration of blood from pleural cavity
aspiration of foreign body
aspiration of pus from pleural cavity
aspiration of serous fluid from pleural
  cavity
aspiration pneumonia
aspiration pneumonitis
aspiration-tulip device
aspirator
  Bovie ultrasonic
  Cavitron ultrasonic (CUSA)
  Cavitron ultrasonic surgical
    (CUSA)
  CUSA ultrasonic
aspirin challenge, inhalation
aspirin inhalation provocation
aspirin, prophylactic use of
aspirin therapy
aspirin-intolerant asthmatic
aspirin-precipitated asthma
aspirin-sensitive asthmatic
asplenia
ASPVD (atherosclerotic pulmonary
  vascular disease)
assay (see also *analysis*, *test*)
  Abbott radioimmunoassay
  alpha-2 antiplasmin functional
  Amersham radioimmunoassay
  Bioclot protein S
  cake mix kit for hematopoietic
    progenitor
  Cardiac STATus rapid

assay *(cont.)*
  Cardiac T rapid
  Coulter HIV-1 p24 antigen
  Elecsys proBNP immunoassay
  endotoxin
  enzyme-linked immunosorbent
    (ELISA)
  factor III multimer
  hematopoietic progenitor
  limulus amebocyte lysate
  MAIPA (monoclonal antibody-
    specific immobilization
    of platelet antigens)
  NT-proBNP immunoassay
  Opus cardiac troponin I
  recombinant immunoblot (RIBA)
  reverse
  three-antigen recombinant
    immunoblot
assessment
  invasive
  noninvasive
  regional wall motion
assist
  mechanical cardiac
  mechanical respiratory
assistance
  extracorporeal hepatic
  ventilatory
assist/control mode ventilation
assisted breathing
assisted circulation
assisted-mode ventilator
assisted ventilation
Assmann focus
assumed Fick method for cardiac
  output
AST (aspartate aminotransferase)
asthenia
  neurocirculatory
  neuroregulatory
asthenic habitus

asthma (reversible obstructive airway
   disease)
  abdominal
  allergic
  alveolar
  aspirin-intolerant
  atopic
  bacterial
  blitz
  bronchial
  bronchitic
  cardiac
  cat
  catarrhal
  childhood
  cotton-dust
  cutaneous
  detergent
  diisocyanate
  dust
  Elsner
  emphysematous
  eosinophilic
  essential
  exercise-induced
  extrinsic
  food
  grinder's
  hay
  Heberden
  horse
  humid
  hypercapnic acute
  infective
  intrinsic
  irritant-induced
  isocyanate
  Kopp
  late-onset
  meat wrapper's
  Millar
  miller's

asthma *(cont.)*
  miner's
  nasal
  nervous
  nocturnal
  nocturnal worsening of
  nonallergic
  occupational
  platinum
  pollen
  potter's
  red-cedar
  reflex
  refractory
  Rostan
  Sequoia (sequoiosis)
  sexual
  sodium-induced
  spasmodic
  steam-fitter's
  stone
  stripper's
  summer
  symptomatic
  thymic
  triad
  true
  Wichmann
  wood
asthma attack caused by
  allergenic exposure to airborne
      pollens and molds
  allergenic exposure to animal
      danders
  allergenic exposure to house dust
  emotional upset
  exercise
  exposure to specific allergens
  inhalation of cigarette smoke
  inhalation of cold air
  inhalation of fresh paint
  inhalation of gasoline fumes

asthma *(cont.)*
  inhalation of irritants
  inhalation of noxious odors
  nonspecific factors
  stress
  viral respiratory infection
asthma convulsivum
asthma crystals
asthma-like symptoms
asthma precipitated by aspirin
asthma precipitated by NSAIDs
asthmatic airways
asthmatic bronchitis
asthmatic crisis
asthmaticus, status
asthmatoid respirations
asthmatoid wheeze
Astra lab tests
Astra pacemaker
Astrand treadmill
ASTZ (antistreptozyme) test
Asuka over-the-wire PTCA catheter
ASVIP (atrial synchronous ventricular
  inhibited pacemaker)
asymmetric crying facies
asymmetric hypertrophy of septum
asymmetric pulmonary congestion
asymmetric septal hypertrophy (ASH)
asymmetrical thorax
asymmetry
  characteristic right and left lung
  chiral
  conducting airway (of lung)
  facial
  flow (in airway tree)
  flow volume (in aortic arch)
  functional
  geometrical
  hemodynamic stress
  inherent
  inspiration-to-expiration
  lateral hemispheric (in heart rate
    modulation)

asymmetry *(cont.)*
  left-right
  limb
  lung volume (on x-ray)
  marked
  respiratory airway
  stent
  striking
  thoracic
  thoracoabdominal
asymptomatic
Asymptomatic Carotid Atherosclerosis
  Study (ACAS) criteria
asynchronism
asynchronous pacemaker
asynchrony
asyneresis/dyskinesis
asynergic myocardium
asynergy
  infarct-localized
  left ventricular
  regional
  segmental
asystole
  Beau
  cardiac
  complete atrial and ventricular
  ventricular
asystolic cardiac arrest
asystolic pauses
atactic breathing
ataxia
  Friedreich
  spinocerebellar
ATB (All-Terrain Balloon) PTA dilatation catheter
atelectasis
  absorption
  acquired
  acute
  acute massive
  apical

atelectasis *(cont.)*
  basilar
  bibasilar discoid
  chronic
  compression
  confluent areas of
  congenital
  congestive
  discoid
  disklike
  initial
  linear
  lobar
  lobular
  lower pulmonary lobe
  middle pulmonary lobe
  obstructive
  patchy
  perpetuation of
  platelike
  primary
  reabsorption
  relaxation
  resorption
  round
  secondary
  segmental
  slowly developing
  subsegmental lower lobe
  upper pulmonary lobe
atelectasis treated by lobectomy
atelectasis treated by segmental
  resection
atelectatic lung
atelectatic rales
atenolol
atherectomized vessel
atherectomy
  directional
  directional coronary
  extraction
  high-speed rotational

atherectomy *(cont.)*
  percutaneous coronary rotational
    (PCRA)
  retrograde
  rotational (RA)
  rotational coronary
  transcutaneous extraction catheter
atherectomy catheter
atherectomy cutter
atherectomy device
  directional
  extraction
  PET balloon Simpson
  rotational
atherectomy technique
  double-wire
  kissing
AtheroCath, Simpson
atheroembolism
atherogenesis
atherogenic LDL cholesterol
atherogenic process
atherolytic guidewire
atherolytic reperfusion guidewire
atheroma, coral reef
atheroma formation, exuberant
atheroma molding
atheromata
atheromatous cholesterol crystal
  embolization
atheromatous debris
atheromatous degeneration
atheromatous material
atheromatous embolism
atheromatous plaque
atheromatous plaque breakup by
  balloon catheter
atheromatous stenosis, femoropopliteal
athero-occlusive disease
atherosclerosis
  accelerated
  calcific

atherosclerosis *(cont.)*
  extracranial carotid artery
  fatty streak
  fibrous plaque
  intimal
  intracranial carotid artery
  juxtarenal aortic
  native
  pararenal aortic
  virulent
atherosclerosis obliterans
atherosclerotic aortic ulcer, penetrating
atherosclerotic cardiovascular disease
  (ASCVD)
atherosclerotic carotid artery disease
  (ACAD)
atherosclerotic debris
atherosclerotic fatty streaks
atherosclerotic gangrene
atherosclerotic narrowing
atherosclerotic occlusive syndrome
atherosclerotic plaque, redeposition
atherosclerotic stenosis
atherothrombotic
atherothrombotic brain infarction
Athlete coronary guidewire
athletic heart
athrombia
Atkins diet
ATL (anterior tricuspid leaflet)
Atlantis SR intravascular ultrasound
  imaging catheter
Atlas LP PTCA balloon dilatation
  catheter
Atlas ULP balloon dilatation catheter
ATL duplex scanner
ATL real-time Neurosector scanner
atm. (atmospheres)
atmospheres of pressure
ATnativ (antithrombin III)
atopic asthma
atopy

ATP (adenosine triphosphate)
ATP (antitachycardia pacing)
ATPase
ATRAC multipurpose balloon catheter
ATRAC-II double balloon catheter
Atraloc needle
Atrauclip hemostatic clip
atraumatic Hasson grasper
atraumatic occlusion of vessels
atraumatic vascular clamp
Atraumax surgical clamp
atresia
  aortic
  aortic arch
  aortic valve
  bony choanal
  choanal
  esophageal
  familial
  infundibular
  mitral
  mitral valve
  pulmonary
  pulmonary valve
  pulmonary vein
  pulmonic
  tricuspid
  valvular
  ventricular
atresic
atretic
atria (pl. of atrium), situs ambiguus
atrial activation mapping, retrograde
atrial activation time
atrial appendage
atrial arrhythmia
atrial asynchronous pacemaker
atrial baffle
atrial capture
atrial cardioverter-defibrillator,
  implantable automatic
atrial compliance

atrial conduction
atrial couplets
atrial cuff
atrial demand inhibited pacemaker
atrial demand triggered pacemaker
atrial disk
atrial dysrhythmia
atrial ectopic automatic tachycardia
atrial ectopy
atrial effective refractory period
atrial escape interval
atrial escape rhythm
atrial-femoral bypass
atrial fibrillation (AF)
   ablation of refractory
   chronic
   hyperthyroidism-induced
   paroxysmal (PAF)
   refractory
atrial fibrillation with high-rate
   ventricular response
atrial fibrillation with rapid ventricular
   response
atrial flutter (AFl)
atrial flutter ablation
atrial focus
atrial gallop
atrial gallop rhythm
atrial gallop sound
atrial infarction
atrial irritability
atrial isomerism
atrialization
atrialized ventricle
atrial kick
atrial lead
atrial myocytes
atrial myxoma
atrial natriuretic factor (ANF)
atrial natriuretic peptide
atrial natriuretic polypeptide (ANP)
atrial overdrive pacing

atrial paced beat
atrial paced cycle length
atrial pacing
atrial pacing stress test
atrial pacing wire, temporary
atrial paroxysmal tachycardia (APT)
atrial partition
atrial premature complex (APC)
atrial premature contractions
atrial premature depolarizations
atrial rate (AR)
atrial reentrant PSVT (paroxysmal
   supraventricular tachycardia)
atrial reentry
atrial repolarization wave
atrial right-to-left shunting
atrial screw
atrial sensed event
atrial septal aneurysm
atrial septal defect (ASD)
atrial septal defect occlusion
   (buttoned device)
atrial septal defect with mitral stenosis
atrial septal umbrella
atrial septectomy
atrial septostomy
   balloon
   transcatheter knife blade
atrial septotomy, balloon
atrial septum
atrial single and double extrastimulation
atrial situs
atrial situs solitus
atrial sound
atrial standstill
atrial suture line
atrial synchronous ventricular
   pacemaker
atrial systole
atrial systolic murmur (ASM)
atrial tachycardia

atrial thrombosis
atrial transposition
Atrial View Ventak AV implantable
    cardioverter-defibrillator
Atricor pacemaker
Atricure bipolar radiofrequency clamp
    for intraoperative ablation of atrial
    fibrillation
atriocaval junction
atriofascicular tract
atriography, negative contrast left
atrio-His bypass tract
atrio-Hisian (also atriohisian)
atrio-Hisian bypass tract
atrio-Hisian fiber
atrio-His pathway
atrioplasty, V-Y
atriopulmonary patch
atriopulmonary anastomosis
atrioseptoplasty
atriotomy orifice
atriotomy, transseptal extended
atrioventricular (AV)
atrioventricular anulus
atrioventricular block (A-V block)
    congenital
    first-degree
    Mobitz classification of
    Mobitz I and II
    second-degree
    third-degree
atrioventricular blockage
atrioventricular (AV) bundle in heart
atrioventricular canal
atrioventricular canal defects
atrioventricular concordance
atrioventricular concordant connection
atrioventricular conduction pathways
atrioventricular conduction system
atrioventricular delay
atrioventricular discordance
atrioventricular discordant connection

atrioventricular dissociation,
    isorhythmic
atrioventricular excitation, anomalous
atrioventricular groove
atrioventricular heart block
atrioventricular interval
atrioventricular junction
atrioventricular junctional escape beat
atrioventricular junctional escape
    junction
atrioventricular junctional pacemaker
atrioventricular junctional premature
    contraction
atrioventricular junctional rhythm
atrioventricular junctional tachycardia
atrioventricular nodal artery
atrioventricular nodal bypass tract
atrioventricular nodal conduction
atrioventricular nodal delay
atrioventricular nodal pathway
atrioventricular nodal reentrant PSVT
    (paroxysmal supraventricular
    tachycardia)
atrioventricular nodal reentry
    tachycardia (AVNRT)
atrioventricular nodal rhythm
atrioventricular nodal tachycardia
    (AVNT)
atrioventricular nodal Wenckebach
    arrhythmia
atrioventricular node
atrioventricular node artery
atrioventricular node conduction
    abnormality
atrioventricular node mesothelioma
atrioventricular orifice
atrioventricular ostium
atrioventricular reciprocating
    tachycardia
atrioventricular ring
atrioventricular septal defect (ASD)
atrioventricular septum

atrioventricular sequential pacing
atrioventricular synchrony
atrioventricular tachycardia,
   reciprocating
atrioventricular time
atrioventricular valves (mitral and
   tricuspid)
atrioventriculare commune, ostium
Atrioverter
Atri-pace I bipolar flared pacing
   catheter
atrium (pl. atria)
   common
   dome of left
   giant left
   high right
   left (LA)
   low septal right
   nontrabeculated
   oblique vein of left
   pulmonary
   right (RA)
   single
   thin-walled
   trabeculated
Atrium Blood Recovery System
atrium cordis
atrium dextrum/sinistrum cordis
atrium pulmonale
atrium sinistrum
atrophic emphysema
atrophic rhinitis
atrophic thrombosis
atrophy
   alveolar
   brown
   cutaneous
   lobular lung
   multiple system (MSA)
   patchy (of renal cortex)
   renal
   vascular

atrophy of alveoli
atropine flush
atropine via endotracheal tube
Atrovent (ipratropium bromide)
ATS Open Pivot bileaflet heart valve
attachment
   commissural
   costal
   epicardial
   intimate (of diseased vessel)
   vascular
attack
   Adams-Stokes
   heart
   Morgagni-Adams-Stokes
   proteolytic
   Stokes-Adams
   syncopal
   transient ischemic (TIA)
   vagal
   vasovagal
attenuate
attenuated image
attenuated QT prolongation and
   dispersion
attenuation
   aortic
   breast
   expiratory
attenuation artifact (on x-ray)
attenuation by breast tissue
attenuation by hemidiaphragm
attenuation scan
atypical adenomatous hyperplasia
   (AAH)
atypical angina
atypical aortic valve stenosis
atypical chest pain
atypical coarctation
atypical interstitial pneumonia
atypical mycobacteriosis
atypical subisthmic coarctation

atypical tuberculosis infection
atypical verrucous endocarditis
audibility
audible breath sounds
audible expiratory splitting of S_2
audible splitting
audible S_3
audible wheezing
audible wheezing without a stethoscope
Auenbrugger sign
augment
augmentation
   inspiratory
   mechanical
   pressure
augmented bipolar limb leads
augmented cardiac output
augmented EKG leads
augmented filling of right ventricle
augmented stroke volume
augmented V waves
auricle
   left
   right
auricular rate
Aurora dual-chamber pacemaker
Aurora pulse generator
Ausculscope
auscultation and percussion
auscultation of lungs
auscultation, pulmonary
auscultatory cadence, rhythmic
auscultatory crackles
auscultatory findings
auscultatory gap
auscultatory sounds
Austin Flint murmur
Austin Flint murmur of relative mitral
   stenosis
Austin Flint phenomenon
Austin Flint respirations
Austin Flint rumble (murmur)

Autima II dual-chamber cardiac
   pacemaker
Autima II pacemaker
autoantibodies to phospholipid
AutoCat (AutoCAT) intra-aortic
   balloon pump with AutoPilot
autoclave
autoclaved, steam
autoclot
autoerythrocyte sensitization syndrome
autoerythrophagocytosis
autogenous antigen
autogenous blood transfusion
autogenous graft
autogenous saphenous vein graft
autograft
Autohaler, Maxair
autoimmune
autoimmune disorder
autoimmune hemolytic anemia (AIHA)
autoimmunity
autologous blood transfusion
autologous clot
autologous fat graft
autologous fibrin glue
autologous graft
autologous patch graft
autologous pericardium
autologous reversed vein graft
autologous transfusion of blood
autologous vein graft
automated border detection by echocardiography
automated edge detection
automatic atrial tachycardia
automatic external defibrillator (AED)
automatic implantable cardioverter-
   defibrillator (AICD)
automatic implantable defibrillator
   (AID)
automatic interval limit

automatic mode switching (AMS)
in cardiac pacemaker
automatic pacemaker
automatic tachycardia, atrial ectopic
automaticity
enhanced
pacemaker
sinus node
triggered
autonomic dysfunction
autonomic insufficiency
autonomic nerves
autonomic neuropathy
autonomous production of aldosterone
autonomous secretion of aldosterone
AutoPilot
Autoplex Factor VIII inhibitor bypass
product
autopsy request granted
autopsy request not granted
autoregulation of cerebral blood flow
autosomal dominant ectopia lentis
autosome
autosuture
Auto Suture Premium TA 55 surgical
stapler
Auto-Suture surgical stapler
autotransfusion system
Cobe BRAT
Electromedics AT 750EF
Haemonectics Cell Saver I
Haemonectics Cell Saver III
Haemonectics Cell Saver IV
Haemonectics Cell Saver Plus
Haemonectics Haemolite
Shiley 795 A
autotransfuser, Cell-Saver
auxiliary ventricle
AVA (aortic valve area)
AVA (arrhythmogenic ventricular
activity)

AVA HF catheter
AVA HF dilator
AVA HF introducer
AVA HF obturator
Avanti angiographic catheter
introducer
avascularity
AVA 3XI catheter
AVA 3XI dilator
AVA 3XI introducer
AVA 3XI obturator
AVCO aortic balloon
AV (aortic valve) repair
AV (arteriovenous) graft
AV (arterial/venous) oxygen difference
AV (atrioventricular)
AV block
AV bundle in heart
AV groove
AV nodal conduction
AV nodal reentry tachycardia
AV sequential pacemaker
AVD (aortic valvular disease)
AVD (atrioventricular dissociation)
AVDH (atrioventricular delay
hysteresis)
AVDI (atrioventricular delay interval)
AVD O_2 (arteriovenous oxygen differ-
ence)
Avea esophageal catheter
Avea monitor
Avea nebulizer
Avea tracheal catheter
Avea ventilator
Avenue insertion tool
AVF (arteriovenous fistula)
aVF (augmented lead, left foot) EKG
lead
AVG (aortic valve gradient)
avian tuberculosis (transmissible to
humans)

Avitene collagen
Avitene topical hemostatic material
avium-intracellulare, Mycobacterium
    (MAI)
Avius sequential pacemaker
aVL (augmented lead, left arm) EKG
    lead
AVM (arteriovenous malformation)
AVNR (atrioventricular nodal rhythm)
AVNRT (atrioventricular nodal
    reentrant tachycardia)
AVNT (atrioventricular nodal tachycar-
    dia)
AV100 balloon catheter
AV2000 balloon catheter
AVP (ambulant venous pressure)
AV-Paceport thermodilution catheter
AVR (aortic valve replacement)
aVR (augmented lead, right arm) EKG
    lead
AVreR (aortic valve re-replacement)
AVRT (atrioventricular reciprocating
    tachycardia)
AVSD (acquired ventricular septal
    defect)
avulsion
    arterial
    iatrogenic
    venous
awareness of heartbeat
a wave (jugular venous pulse)
    cannon
    giant
    intermittent cannon
A wave (on EKG)
A wave larger than V wave
A wave of cardiac apex pulse
A-wave pressure on atrial catheter-
    ization
axillary-axillary bypass graft
axillary-brachial bypass graft
axillary electrode

axillary-femoral bypass graft
axillary-femorofemoral bypass graft
axillary vein traumatic thrombosis
axillobifemoral bypass graft
axillofemoral approach
axillofemoral bypass graft
axillofemoral stem
Axiom DG balloon angioplasty
    catheter
axis (pl. axes)
    arterial
    clockwise rotation of electrical
    electrical
    heart
    horizontal
    indeterminate
    J-point electrical
    junctional
    left
    long
    mean electrical
    mean QRS
    normal
    normal QRS
    P-wave
    QRS vertical
    right
    superior QRS
    twisting on the electrical
    variable
    vertical
axis deviation on EKG
    horizontal
    left
    vertical
axis of EKG lead
axis of heart
Axius Vacuum retractor blade
Axius Vacuum shunt
Axius Vacuum surgical blower
Axius Vacuum surgical retractor
Axius Vacuum 2 stabilizer

Ayerza-Arrillaga disease

Ayerza disease or syndrome

Azmacort (triamcinolone acetonide)

azygos lobe of lung

azygos system of veins

azygos vein

B, b

Babcock grasping forceps
Babesia bovis
Babesia divergens
Babesia, intraerythrocytic
Babesia microti
babesiosis
Babinski syndrome
BABYbird respirator (see *ventilator*)
BABYbird II respirator (see *ventilator*)
Babyflex ventilator
Baccelli sign of pleural effusion
Bachmann
    anterior internodal tract of
    pathway of
Bachmann bundle of fibers
Bachmann bundle reentry
bacillary embolism
bacillary epithelioid angiomatosis
    (BEA)
bacille Calmette-Guérin (BCG)
bacilli, enteric gram-negative
bacillus Calmette-Guérin (BCG)
    vaccine
bacitracin-kanamycin solution
back-bleeding
backflow
backflow from arterial line

backflow of blood into atria
backrush of blood into left ventricle
backscatter characteristics of blood
BackStop disposable waste collection
    container (used in angiography)
back stroke volume
backup of blood
backward flow
backward heart failure
BacT/Alert automated blood culture
    system
BacTec (BACTEC) automated blood
    culture system
bacteremia
    catheter-induced
    cryptogenic
    pulmonary artery catheter-related
bacteremic shock
bacteria (see *pathogen*)
bacterial bronchitis
bacterial contamination
bacterial endocarditis, subacute (SBE)
bacterial endotoxins, gram-negative
bacterial infection, chronic indolent
bacterial myocarditis
bacterial pericarditis
bacterial pneumonia or pneumonitis

59

bacterial vegetation
bactericidal drugs
bacteriostatic drugs
Bacteroides fragilis
Bacteroides intermedius
bad cholesterol
baffle
  atrial
  construction of intra-atrial
  endoaortic
  Fontan
  heart-shaped
  hemi-Mustard pericardial
  interatrial
  intra-atrial
  intracardiac
  intrapulmonary artery
  left ventricle to aorta
  Mustard
  pericardial
  pulmonary vein to left atrium
  right ventricle to aorta
  Senning type of intra-atrial
  total cavopulmonary connection
baffled tunnel
baffle fenestration
baffle leak
bag
  Ambu
  Douglas
  Lahey
  manual resuscitation
bag-and-mask ventilation
bagasse (sugar cane) worker's
  syndrome
bagassosis
BagEasy respirator
BAGF (brachioaxillary bridge graft
  fistula)
bagged (ventilated)
bagging
bagpipe sign

Bahnson aortic clamp
Bailey aortic clamp
Bailey aortic valve cutting forceps
Bailey-Gibbon rib contractor
Bailey-Glover-O'Neill commissur-
  otomy knife
Bailey rib approximator
Bailey rib contractor
Bailey rib spreader
bailout catheter
bailout stenting
bailout valvuloplasty
Baim pacing catheter
Baim-Turi cardiac device
Baim-Turi monitoring/pacing catheter
Bainbridge reflex
Bair Hugger warming units and
  blankets
Baladi Inverter device
BAL (bronchoalveolar lavage)
BALF (bronchoalveolar lavage fluid)
Balint syndrome
Balke protocol for cardiac exercise
  stress testing
Balke treadmill exercise protocol
Balke-Ware treadmill exercise (stress
  testing) protocol
ball-and-seat valve
ballistocardiography
ball-occluder valve
balloon
  ACS SULP II
  Angiotech angioplasty
  ArmorGlide coating on
    intra-aortic
  AVCO aortic
  bifoil
  Blue Max
  Extractor three-lumen retrieval
  Fogarty
  Grüntzig (Gruentzig)
  Hartzler angioplasty

balloon *(cont.)*
  Innovante
  Inoue
  intra-aortic (IAB)
  kissing
  Kontron intra-aortic
  LPS
  Mansfield
  Outcomes by Design
  Percor
  Percor Stat
  Percor Stat-DL (dual-lumen)
    intra-aortic
  Percor-Stat intra-aortic
  PET
  pulsation
  Rapid-Trak
  Raptor PTCA
  SciMed Express Monorail
  self-positioning
  slave
  Soto USCI
  Stack autoperfusion
  trefoil
  waist in the
balloon and blade septostomy
balloon and coil embolization
balloon aortoplasty
balloon atrial septostomy
balloon atrial septotomy
balloon catheter fenestration
balloon catheter, Monorail
balloon counterpulsation
balloon embolization (therapeutic)
balloon-expandable flexible coil stent
balloon-expandable intravascular stent
balloon-expandable, fixed tubular
  mesh stainless steel stent
balloon-expandable stainless steel (BE-
  SS) stent
balloon fenestration procedure
balloon-flotation pacing catheter

balloon inflation
  sequential
  simultaneous
balloon-injured carotid intimal thickening
balloon into left atrium during systole
balloon (verb) mitral valve leaflets
balloon mitral valvotomy
balloon mitral valvuloplasty
balloon occlusion
balloon occlusion arteriography
balloon occlusion pulmonary
  angiography
Balloon-on-a-Wire cardiac device
balloon pump (see *intra-aortic*
  balloon pump, IABP)
balloon septostomy
balloon sizing
balloon-tipped aortic occlusion/
  cardioplegia catheter
balloon-tipped catheter
balloon-tipped, dual-channel fiberoptic
  bronchoscope
balloon-tipped end-hole catheter
balloon-tipped flow-directed
  pulmonary artery catheter
balloon tuboplasty
balloon valvotomy
balloon valvuloplasty
balloon wedge pressure catheter
balloon wedge-type catheter
ball poppet of prosthetic valve
ball valve thrombus
ball-valve-type valve prosthesis
ball-wedge catheter
Bamberger disease
Bamberger-Marie disease
Bamberger sign
bamboo bodies
band
  CPK-MB
  moderator

band *(cont.)*
  parietal
  septal
  septum
bandage, Esmarch
bandbox sound
band cell
banding, pulmonary artery
Bandit balloon catheter
band-1
Bannister angioedema disease
BAR (biofragmentable anastomotic
  ring)
barbed epicardial pacing lead
Barbero-Marcial method of truncus
  arteriosus repair
Bard arterial cannula
Bard cardiopulmonary support pump
Bard cardiopulmonary support system
Bard Clamshell Septal Umbrella
Bard CPS system
Bard guiding catheter
Bardic cannula
Bardic cutdown catheter
Bard nonsteerable bipolar electrode
Bard PDA (patent ductus arteriosus)
  Umbrella
Bard percutaneous cardiopulmonary
  support system
Bard-Parker knife
BardPort implanted port
Bard sign on cardiac palpation
Bard SpermaTex preshaped mesh
Bard Stinger S ablation catheter
Bard TransAct intra-aortic balloon
  pump
Bard XT coronary stent
barium-impregnated poppet
barking cough
Barlow syndrome
baroreceptor, carotid
baroreceptor-mediated response

baroreceptor sensitivity
baroreflex
  carotid
  sinoatrial
baroreflex sensitivity
barotrauma, pulmonary
barrel chest
barrel-chested appearance
barrel-shaped chest
barrel-shaped thorax
barrier, blood-brain
Bartter syndrome
basal chordae
basal crepitation
basal-lateral wall myocardial infarction
basal movements (on x-ray)
basal panacinar emphysema
basal short-axis slice
basal systolic murmur
basal temperatures
basal tuberculosis
basal zone
base deficit
base excess
base of heart
base of lung
baseline artifact
baseline EKG
baseline levels (of drugs or lab values)
baseline pulmonary function
baseline, return to
baseline ST-segment abnormality
baseline standing blood pressure
baseline standing pulse rate
basement membrane
base of heart
base of lung
basic blood pressure (BP)
basic cardiac life support (BCLS)
basic cycle length (BCL)
basic drive cycle length (BDCL)
basic rate

basilar artery insufficiency
basilar artery syndrome
basilar carotid murmur
basilar infiltration
basilar intracerebral hemorrhage
basilar rales
basilar zone infiltration
basilic vein
basis, noncardiac
Basix pacemaker
basket cell
basketlike calcification
basket, pericardial
basting stitch or suture
Bate floating embolic protection filter
bathing suit area, telangiectasias in the
Batista left ventriculectomy
Batista myoplasty
bat's wing shadow (on x-ray)
Batten disease
battery
    external pacemaker
    pacemaker
    test
battery voltage
Baumgarten portal hypertension variant
bauxite fibrosis of lung
bauxite lung
bauxite pneumoconiosis
Baxter catheter
Baxter mechanical valve
Bayes theorem in exercise stress testing
Bayliss effect
Baylor bleeding score
Baylor total artificial heart
bayonet bipolar forceps
bayonet-type incision
Bazett formula
Bazin disease
Bazin erythema induratum
BBB (bundle branch block)
BBBB (bilateral bundle branch block)

BBR (bundle branch reentry)
B bump on echocardiogram
BCG (bacillus Calmette-Guérin)
    vaccine
BCL (basic cycle length)
BCLS (basic cardiac life support)
BDCL (basic drive cycle length)
BD First Midcath midline catheter
BD First Midcath single-lumen
silicone midline catheter
BD First PICC catheter
BD First PICC single-lumen silicone
    peripherally inserted central
    catheter
BD Insyte Autoguard shielded intra-
    venous catheter
BD Insyte-N Autoguard shielded IV
    catheter
BD Introsyte-N Autoguard shielded
    introducer
BD L-Cath EX midline catheter
BD L-Cath single-lumen polyurethane
    peripherally inserted central
    catheter
BD Neo PICC neonatal peripherally
    inserted central catheter
BEA (bacillary epithelioid angioma-
    tosis)
beading of artery
beads, suture (on cannula ports)
Beale ganglion cell
Beall circumflex artery scissors
Beall disk valve prosthesis
Beall mitral valve prosthesis
Beall prosthetic mitral valve
Beall-Surgitool ball-cage prosthetic
    valve
Beall-Surgitool disk prosthetic valve
beam, M-mode
bean bag was placed over the incision
Bear Cub infant ventilator
Bear NUM-1 tidal volume monitor

Bear respirator (see also *ventilator*)
beat, beats (see also *heartbeat*)
  aberrantly conducted
  apex
  apical
  Ashman
  asynchronous
  atrial escape
  atrial fusion
  atrial paced
  atrial premature (APB)
  atrioventricular (AV) junctional
    escape
  automatic
  captured
  coupled
  coupled premature
  downward displaced apical
  Dressler fusion
  dropped
  echo
  ectopic
  ectopic ventricular
  entrained
  escape
  forced
  fusion
  interpolated
  junctional escape
  malignant
  missed
  missing
  paced
  paired
  postectopic
  premature atrial (PAB)
  premature ventricular (PVB)
  pseudofusion
  reciprocal
  skipped
  summation
  sustained ventricular apex
  triplet

beat *(cont.)*
  twinned
  ventricular paced
  ventricular ectopic (VEB)
  ventricular escape
  ventricular fusion
  ventricular premature (VPB)
beating at a fixed rate
beating heart, empty
beating-heart bypass system, Access
  MV
beating-heart surgery
beats per minute (BPM or bpm)
beat-to-beat variability
beat-to-beat varying bifidity
Beatty-Bright friction sound
Beau asystole
Beau disease
Beaver blade
Beaver knife
beavertail appearance of balloon profile
Beck clamp
Becker disease
Becker muscular dystrophy
Becker sign
Becker syndrome
Beckman O_2 analyzer
Beckman retractor
Beck miniature aortic clamp
Beck-Potts clamp
Beck triad
Beck vascular clamp
beclomethasone dipropionate (QVAR)
Becton-Dickinson introducer
Becton-Dickinson Teflon-sheathed
  needle
bed
  capillary
  monitor
  pulmonary
  pulmonary vascular
  vascular
bedside commode

beef-lung heparin
beefy red color
beep-o-gram
beer and cobalt syndrome
beer-drinker's syndrome
beer-drinker's cardiomyopathy
behavioral changes
Behçet syndrome
bell of stethoscope
bell sound
Belos VR-T ICD home monitoring
   system
below-knee popliteal to distal peroneal
   reversed vein graft
bend, hand-shaped
bends (noun)
BeneFix hemophilia B blood clotting
   factor drug
Benestent or BENESTENT (named for
   Belgium Netherlands stent study)
Bengolea arterial forceps
benign hypertension
benign idioventricular rhythm runs
benign pericarditis, acute
benign pneumoconiosis
benign vascular hamartoma
Bennett PR ventilator
Bentall inclusion technique
Bentall operation for coronary ostial
   revascularization
Bentall wrap-inclusion composite valve
   graft procedure
Bentley Duraflo II extracorporeal
   perfusion circuit
Bentley oxygenator
Bentley transducer
Bentson guidewire
beractant
beriberi cardiomyopathy
beriberi with alcoholic cardiomyopathy
Berlin Heart ventricular assist device
Berman angiographic balloon catheter

Berman aortic clamp
Bernard-Soulier disease or syndrome
Bernheim syndrome
Bernheim-Schmincke syndrome
Bernoulli equation
Bernoulli formula (equation) of
   velocity
Bernoulli theorem
Bernstein acid infusion test
Bernstein catheter
Bernstein study
berry aneurysm, intracranial
Berry sternal needle holder
berylliosis
beryllium disease
BE-SS (balloon-expandable stainless
   steel)
beta-adrenergic blockade
beta-adrenergic blocker therapy
beta-adrenergic blocking agent
beta-adrenergic reception blockade
beta-adrenergic receptor
$beta_1$-adrenergic receptor
$beta_2$-adrenergic receptor
beta-adrenergic receptor blocking agent
beta-adrenoreceptor blocking agent
beta agonist
beta antagonist
beta-blockade
beta blocker
Beta-Cath intracoronary catheter
   system
Betadine prep (preparation)
beta lipoprotein fraction
$beta_2$-microglobulin level
beta thalassemia
beta-thromboglobulin plasma level
Bethea sign
Bethune rib shears
Bethune rongeur
Better Breathing HEPA-tech half-mask
   respirator

Beuren syndrome
bevel
beveled anastomosis
beveled thin-walled needle
beveled transection
beveling
Bezold-Jarisch reflex
BFE (blood flow enhancement) device
Biad SPECT imaging system
Bianchi nodules
Bianchi valve
biatrial myxoma
biatriatum, cor triloculare
bibasilar crackles
bibasilar discoid atelectasis
bibasilar rales
bibeveled
BICAP unit
bicarbonate (HCO_3)
bicaval cannulation
Biceps bipolar coagulator
Bichat fat pad
Bichat membrane
bicipital aponeurosis
bicommissural aortic valve
bicuspid aortic valve
bicuspid atrioventricular valve
bicuspid valvular aortic stenosis
bicycle
    AerobiCycle I, II, III
    Aerodyne
    Collins
    Siemens-Albis
    Tredex powered
bicycle ergometer exercise test
bicycle ergometry (exercise stress
    testing)
bicycle exercise radionuclide ventricu-
    lography
bicycle exercise test
bidirectional cavopulmonary
    anastomosis

bidirectional Glenn procedure
bidirectional lead configuration
bidirectional ventricular tachycardia
Biermer change of sound
Biermer sign
bifascicular heart block
bifidity
    beat-to-beat varying
    pulmonary artery
bifid precordial impulse
bifid T waves
bifoil balloon
bifoil balloon catheter
bifurcate
bifurcated extension
bifurcated graft
bifurcated J-shaped tined atrial pacing
    and defibrillation lead
bifurcation
    aortic
    carotid
    iliac
    low-lying
    patent
    posterior descending artery (PDA)
    pulmonary artery
bifurcation graft
bifurcation lesion
bifurcation of aorta
bifurcation of posterior descending
    artery (PDA)
bifurcation of pulmonary trunk
bifurcation of trachea
bigeminal rhythm
bigeminus, pulsus
bigeminy
    atrial
    atrioventricular nodal
    escape-capture
    nodal
    reciprocal
    ventricular

bigeminy bisferious pulse
BiLAP bipolar cautery unit with
    cutting and coagulation functions
bilateral anterior chest bulge
bilateral anterior thoracotomy
bilateral epicardial radiofrequency
    ablation of pulmonary veins
bilateral interstitial pulmonary
    infiltrates
bilateral juxtafoveal telangiectasis
    (BJT)
bilateral saphenous varices
bilateral staged thoracotomies
bilateral synchrony
bilateral upper lobe cavitary infiltrates
bilateral venous engorgement
bile acid sequestrants
bilevel positive airway pressure
    (BLPAP)
bilharziasis
    cardiopulmonary
    portopulmonary
billowing mitral valve
bilobectomy
BIMA (bilateral internal mammary
    artery) reconstruction
binomial distribution
Binswanger dementia (or disease)
bioabsorbable closure device
BioBypass PVD (peripheral vascular
    disease) angiogen (gene-based
    therapy)
Bioclot protein S assay
Bioclusive transparent dressing
Biocor porcine stented aortic valve
Biocor porcine stented mitral valve
Biocor stentless porcine aortic valve
Biocor 200 oxygenator device
BiodivYsio phosphorylcholine-coated
    coronary stent
biodegradable stent
Biofilter hemoconcentrator

biofragmentable anastomotic ring
    (BAR)
BioGlide coating
BioGlue surgical adhesive for repair
    of aortic dissections
Biograft stabilized human umbilical
    vein
bioimpedance, thoracic electrical (TEB)
Biojector 2000 jet injection system
    for drug delivery
biological tissue valve
Bio-Medicus pump
Biomer (segmented polyurethane)
Bionit vascular prosthesis
Biopatch foam wound dressing
biophysical profile (BPP)
BioPolyMeric graft for femoropopliteal
    bypass
bioprosthesis (see *prosthesis*)
biopsy
    aspiration
    bronchial
    closed lung
    closed pleural
    CT-scan directed needle
    diagnostic thoracoscopic lung
    drill
    endomyocardial
    excision(al)
    fine needle
    incisional
    lung
    needle
    open
    open lung
    percutaneous endomyocardial
    percutaneous pericardial
    pericardial
    pleural
    plugged
    reexcisional (re-excisional)
    right ventricular endomyocardial

biopsy *(cont.)*
  scalene node
  stereotactic aspiration (SAB)
  transbronchial (TBB)
  transbronchial lung
  transfemoral liver
  transthoracic needle (TNB)
  transthoracic needle aspiration
  transvenous endomyocardial
biopsy and washings
biopsy cup forceps
biopsy forceps
bioptome
  Caves-Schulz
  Fehling
  Kawai
  King
  Konno
  Olympus
  Stanford left ventricular
Bio-Pump centrifugal blood pump
Biorate pacemaker
Biot breathing
Biot respirations
Biot sign
Biostent
Biosyn suture
Biotrack coagulation monitor
Biotronik pacemaker
Bio-Vascular Probe
BioZ system digital noninvasive
  cardiac function monitoring system
BiPal biopsy forceps
BiPAP ventilator
biphasic complex on EKG
biphasic electrical shock
biphasic helical CT scan
biphasic P wave
biphasic shock
biplanar aortography
biplane area-length method (echocar-
  diography)

biplane left ventricular angiogram
biplane fluoroscopy
biplane orthogonal views
biplane pelvic arteriography
biplane pelvic oblique study
biplane transesophageal echocardiography (TEE)
bipolar atrial pacing
bipolar coagulation
bipolar endocardial lead
bipolar generator
bipolar lead
bipolar limb lead
bipolar pacemaker
bipolar pacing electrode catheter
bipolar sensing, integrated
bipolar temporary heartwire
bipolar temporary pacemaker catheter
bird breeder's lung
bird fancier's lung
bird fancier's syndrome
bird handler's lung
Bird Mark ventilator
Bird respirator (see *ventilator*)
Bird sign
Bird's Nest filter (BNF)
Bird's Nest percutaneous IVC filter
Bird's Nest vena caval filter,
  Gianturco-Roehm
birthmark, varicosities, and limb
  enlargement
bisferiens pulse
bisferiens, pulsus
bisferious pulse
bishop's nod
Bisping electrode
bites, suture
BiVAD, BVAD (biventricular assist
  device)
bivalrudin anticoagulation
biventricular assist device (BVAD)
biventricular global systolic
  dysfunction

biventricular heart failure
biventricular hypertrophy
biventricular pacing
biventricular support system, Abiomed
biventricular transposed aorta
biventricularly
Bivona tracheostomy tube
bizarre QRS complexes
Björk-Shiley aortic valve prosthesis
Björk-Shiley floating disc prosthesis
Björk-Shiley monostrut valve
Björk-Shiley valve prosthesis
BJT (bilateral juxtafoveal
    telangiectasis)
black lung disease
Blackfan-Diamond syndrome
blackout
blade
    Bard-Parker
    Beaver
    electrosurgical
    Eschmann
    5-prong (or five-prong) rake
    Hancock trocar
    knife
    3-prong (or three-prong) rake
blade atrial septostomy
Blakemore-Sengstaken tube
Blalock-Hanlon atrial septectomy
Blalock-Hanlon operation
Blalock pulmonary clamp
Blalock running horizontal mattress
    suture
Blalock shunt
Blalock-Taussig anastomosis
Blalock-Taussig procedure for blue
    baby syndrome
Blalock-Taussig shunt
blanch
blanching, skin
bland aortic aneurysm
bland edema

bland embolism
Bland-Garland-White syndrome
blanket
    Bair Hugger
    circulating water
    cooling
    hypothermia
blast chest
blastomycosis endocarditis
BLB mask
bleb
    emphysematous
    ruptured emphysematous
    subpleural
bleed (noun)
bleeding
    abnormal
    arterial
    excessive
    intrapericardial
    massive intracranial
    postoperative
    retroperitoneal
bleeding control
bleeding diathesis
bleeding disorder
bleeding into the infarct
bleeding site, active
bleeding tendency
bleeding time (see also *time*)
    Duke
    Ivy
blender, Sechrist Air/O$_2$
blew off due to arterial pressure
blind dimple in floor of left atrium
blind endarterectomy
blind nasal intubation
blind percutaneous puncture of
    subclavian vein
blind pouch
blind tibial outflow tracts
blindness, transient monocular

BlisterFilm transparent dressing
blitz asthma
bloater, blue
block (see also *heart block*)
   acquired symptomatic AV
   air
   alveolar-capillary (alveolocapillary)
   anodal
   anterior fascicular
   anterograde
   arborization
   atrioventricular (AV) heart
   AV (atrioventricular)
   AV Wenckebach heart
   BBB (bundle branch)
   BBBB (bilateral bundle branch)
   bifascicular
   bifascicular bundle branch
   bifascicular heart
   bilateral bundle branch (BBBB)
   bundle branch (BBB)
   bundle branch heart
   complete AV (CAVB)
   complete congenital heart
   complete heart (CHB)
   conduction
   congenital complete heart
   congenital heart
   congenital symptomatic AV
   cutting
   deceleration-dependent
   divisional
   donor heart-lung
   entrance
   exit
   false bundle-branch
   familial heart
   fascicular
   first-degree AV
   first-degree heart
   fixed third-degree AV
   heart

block *(cont.)*
   high-grade AV
   incomplete atrioventricular (IAVB)
   incomplete heart
   incomplete left bundle branch
     (ILBBB)
   incomplete right bundle branch
     (IRBBB)
   inflammatory heart
   infra-His
   intercostal nerve
   intermittent third-degree AV
   interventricular
   intra-atrial
   intra-His
   intra-Hisian or intrahisian
   intranodal
   intravenous (IV)
   intraventricular conduction
   intraventricular heart
   ipsilateral bundle branch
   left anterior fascicular (LAFB)
   left anterior hemiblock
   left bundle branch (LBBB)
   left posterior fascicular (LPFB)
   Mobitz I or II second-degree AV
   Mobitz type I or II AV
   Mobitz type I on Wenckebach heart
   paroxysmal AV
   partial heart
   peri-infarction (PIB)
   posterior fascicular
   pseudo-AV
   retrograde
   right bundle branch (RBBB)
   second-degree AV
   second-degree heart
   sinoatrial (SAB)
   sinoatrial exit
   sinus
   sinus exit
   sinus node exit

block *(cont.)*
  supra-Hisian or suprahisian
  third-degree AV
  third-degree heart
  transient AV
  3:2 ("three to two") AV
  trifascicular
  2:1 ("two to one") AV
  unidirectional
  unifascicular
  VA (ventriculoatrial)
  ventricular
  vesicular
  Wenckebach AV
  Wilson
blockade
  adrenergic
  alpha-
  alpha-adrenergic
  beta-
  beta-adrenergic
  beta-adrenergic reception
  complete atrioventricular
  neuromuscular
blockage of bronchus
blockage of pulmonary artery
Block cardiac device
blocked APC (atrial premature
  contraction)
blocked artery
blocked bronchus
blocked pleurisy
blocker
  alpha-adrenergic
  alpha-adrenoreceptor
  angiotensin II receptor
  beta-
  calcium channel
  calcium entry
  potassium channel
  sodium channel
  slow channel

blocking agent, beta-adrenoceptor
blocking of histamine receptors
Block right coronary guiding catheter
blood
  arterial
  artificial (100% O_2 + fluorocarbons)
  autologous
  clotted
  coagulability of
  cord
  defibrinated
  deoxygenated
  egress of
  expectoration of
  extravasated
  frank blood cardioplegia
  heparinized
  laky
  nonoxygenated
  normally oxygenated
  occult
  oxygenated
  peripheral
  shunted
  sludged
  type and crossmatch
  unoxygenated
  venous
  whole
blood bank
blood-brain barrier
blood cardioplegia
blood clot
blood-clotting mechanism
blood coagulability, increased
blood coagulation
blood coagulation factors (see *factors*)
blood-conservation techniques
blood count
  complete (CBC)
  differential white
  Schilling

blood dyscrasia
blood flow
  antegrade
  high shear
  superior mesenteric
  superior mesenteric artery
blood flow at capillary level
blood flow enhancement (BFE) device
blood flow on Doppler echocardiogram
blood flow stagnation
blood flow to tissue beyond obstruction
blood flow velocity
blood gas(es) (arterial) panel
  base excess
  bicarbonate
  HCO_2
  O_2 saturation (percent)
  $PaCO_2$
  PaO_2
  pCO_2
  pH
  pO_2
  venous
blood gases on oxygen
blood gases on room air
blood group
  ABO
  Auberger
  Cartwright
  Diego
  Dombrock
  Duffy
  high frequency
  I
  Kell
  Kidd
  Lewis
  low frequency
  Lutheran
  MNS
  P
  Rh

blood leak into interstitial space
blood leak into intra-alveolar space
bloodless fluid
blood lipids
blood loss, nil
blood perfusion
blood perfusion monitor (BPM),
  Laserflo
blood plasma
blood plate thrombus
blood-pool imaging
blood-pool radionuclide angiography
blood-pool radionuclide echocardiography
blood pool, white-appearing
blood pressure (BP)
  arterial
  baseline
  baseline standing
  basic
  diastolic (DBP)
  high
  labile
  low
  maximum
  mean
  minimum
  orthostatic
  standing
  supine
  systolic (SBP)
  systolic/diastolic (SDBP)
  zero diastolic
blood pressure discrepancy in upper
  and lower extremities
blood pressure monitor, Nellcor
  Symphony
blood pressure response
blood sample
blood serum
Blood Shield
blood speckle

blood-streaked drainage from abscess
blood-streaked sputum
blood stream, bloodstream
blood substitute (artificial blood)
   Fluosol plasma expander
   HemAssist
   Hemolink
   100% O_2+ fluorocarbons
   oxygenated perfluorocarbon
   recombinant hemoglobin (rHb1.1)
   SFHB (stroma-free hemoglobin,
     pyridoxylated)
blood supply, accessory
blood supply of thymus
blood test, cold agglutinins
blood-tinged expectoration
blood-tinged sputum
blood transfusion
   autogenous
   autologous
   homologous
   multiple
blood type
blood-type diet
blood urea nitrogen (BUN)
blood vessel thermography
blood viscosity
blood volume
   central
   circulating
Bloodwell forceps
bloody
bloody exudate
bloody fluid
bloody nasal mucus
bloody pericardial effusion
bloody pericardial fluid
bloody sputum
Bloom DTU 201 external stimulator
Bloom programmable stimulator
blooming, signal
blow-by, anesthesia

blowing murmur
blowing pansystolic murmur
blowing pneumothorax
blowout, aortic stump
BLPAP (bilevel positive airway
   pressure)
blue and white Tycron sutures
blue baby
blue bloater
blue finger syndrome
Blue FlexTip catheter
Blue Max balloon
Blue Max triple-lumen catheter
Bluemyst aerosol spray device
blue of Gregoire syndrome (Gregoire's
   blue leg)
blue phlebitis
blue sclerae
Blue Scout guidewire
blue toe syndrome (trash foot)
blue velvet syndrome
bluish coloration of sclerae
bluish nail lacunae
bluish skin color (cyanosis)
blunt border of lung
blunt chest trauma
blunt dissection
blunted chronotropic response
blunt forceps
blunt Hasson grasper
blunt injury
blunt stylet
blunt thoracic trauma
blunt-tip trocar
blurring of aortic knob
blurring of costophrenic angle
   (on x-ray)
BML (billowing mitral leaflet)
B-mode (B-scan)
B-mode echocardiography
B-mode echography
B-mode, pseudocolor

BNF (Bird's Nest filter)
body, bodies
  Amato
  aortic
  Arantius
  asbestos
  Aschoff
  bamboo
  Bracht-Wächter
  central fibrous
  coccoid x
  Deetjen
  ferruginous
  fibrin (of pleura)
  foreign
  gelatin compression
  Heinz
  Howell-Jolly
  inclusion
  Levinthal-Coles-Lillie (LCL)
  Masson
  multilaminar
  Pappenheimer
  Reilly
  Zuckerkandl
body box/plethysmography
body box for lung volume
  measurement
body contour orbit, body artifacts
  due to
BodyFlex catheter
BodyFlex port
Body Glue for faster wound healing
body habitus
body of sternum
body surface area (BSA)
body surface potential mapping
Boeck sarcoid
Boettcher artery forceps
Bohr effect
bolster, Teflon felt

bolus-chase technique in angiography
  and MRI scan
bolus, intravenous
bolus intravenous injection
bolus of medication
boluses of air
Bondek absorbable suture
bone-cutting forceps
bone marrow embolism
bone wax
Bonnie angioplasty catheter
bony choanal atresia
bony landmarks
Bookwalter retractor
booming diastolic rumble
BOOP (bronchiolitis obliterans
  organizing pneumonia)
booster phenomenon
boot, boots
  circulator
  compression
  gelatin
  gelatin compression
  Kerra
  sheepskin
  Unna
  Venodyne compression
boot-shaped heart
boot-strap two-vessel angioplasty
border, borders
  anterior
  cardiac
  ciliated
  clearly demarcated
  inferior (of heart)
  lower sternal (LSB)
  mid-left sternal border
  sternocleidomastoid muscle
  upper sternal
borderline hypertension
borderline severe rejection

border of heart
  anterior
  inferior
  left
  posterior
  right
  superior
Borg scale (1-5) for programming
  pacers
Borg scale of perceived exertion
Borg scale of treadmill exertion
boring pain
Bornholm disease
Borrelia burgdorferi
Bosch ERG 500 ergometer
bottle nose forceps
bottle sound
bottle, suction
Bouillaud disease
Bouillaud sign
Bouillaud syndrome
bounding arterial pulse
bounding peripheral pulses
bounding water-hammer pulse
Bourns Bear 1 ventilator
bouts of tachycardia
Bouchut respirations
Boutin thoracoscope
Bouveret disease
Bouveret-Hoffmann syndrome
Bovie ultrasonic aspirator
bovine allograft
bovine heterograft
bovine lavage extract surfactant
bovine pericardial bioprosthesis
bovine pericardial patch augmentation
  of aortic arch
bovine pericardium (BP)
bovine pericardium strips
bovine respirations
bovine tuberculosis (transmissible to
  humans)

bovine valve
bovine valve prosthesis
bovinum, cor
Bowditch effect
Bowditch staircase phenomenon
Bowditch, treppe (staircase)
Bowen wire cutter
Bowen wire holder
Bowen wire tightener
bowing of mitral valve leaflet
bow-tie repair
Boyd formula
Boyd perforating vein
Boynton needle holder
Bozzolo sign
BP (blood pressure)
BP (bovine pericardium)
BPD (bronchopulmonary dysplasia)
BPM or bpm (beats per minute)
B-port implant infusion port
BPP (biophysical profile)
BPV (balloon pulmonary valvuloplasty)
brachial approach
brachial artery
brachial artery compression
brachial artery cuff pressure
brachial artery pressure
brachial artery pulse pressure
brachial artery to axillary vein dialysis
  graft
brachial-basilar insufficiency
brachial bypass
brachial plexus
brachial plexus compression
brachial plexus injury
brachial pulse
brachioaxillary bridge graft fistula
  (BAGF)
brachioaxillary interposition graft
brachiocephalic arteriovenous fistula
brachiocephalic arteritis

brachiocephalic artery
brachiocephalic ischemia
brachiocephalic lymph nodes
brachiocephalic systolic murmur
brachiocephalic trunk
brachiocephalic vein
brachiocephalic vessels
brachiocrural symptoms
brachiosubclavian bridge graft fistula
  (BSGF)
Bracht-Wächter bodies
brachytherapy, endovascular radiation
Bradbury-Eggleston syndrome
Bradbury-Eggleston triad
bradyarrhythmia
  cardiac
  digitalis-induced
  symptomatic
  vasovagal
bradyarrhythmic cardiac arrest
bradycardia
  Branham
  central
  essential
  fetal
  idioventricular
  intermittent junctional
  junctional
  nodal
  postinfective
  pulseless
  sinoatrial
  sinus (SB)
  symptomatic
  vagal
bradycardia pacing
bradycardia pacing zone
bradycardia-tachycardia syndrome
bradycardic agonal phase
brady down
bradydysrhythmia
bradykinin

bradypnea
bradypneic
bradysphygmia
bradytachycardia syndrome
bradytachydysrhythmia syndrome
braided lead
braided polyester sutures
braided suture
braided tape
brain abscess
brain anoxia
branch, branches (see also *artery*)
  acute marginal
  AV (atrioventricular) groove
  bifurcating
  bronchial
  caudal
  diagonal
  first diagonal
  first major diagonal
  first septal perforator
  inferior wall
  large obtuse marginal
  left bundle
  marginal
  midmarginal
  nonlingular
  obtuse marginal (OMB)
  posterior descending
  posterior intercostal
  posterior ventricular
  ramus
  ramus intermedius artery
  ramus medialis
  right bundle
  second diagonal
  septal
  septal perforating
  side
  subcostal
  superior phrenic
  venous side
  ventricular

branching, mirror-image brachiocephalic
branching mucoid bronchial casts
Branham bradycardia
Branham sign (arteriovenous fistula)
Branhamella catarrhalis
Brasdor method
brass-founder's ague
brass-founder's disease
brass-founder's fever
brassy bruit
brassy cough
BRAT cell saver
Braunwald-Cutter ball prosthetic valve
Braunwald sign
brawny edema
brawny induration
bread-and-butter heart
bread-and-butter pericarditis
BreakAway absorptive wound dressing
break, lead insulation
breakthrough vasodilatation
breast, pigeon
breast thrombophlebitis
breast tissue, attenuation by
breathe (verb)
breath excretion test
breath-hold, five-second
breath-holding
breathing
   amphoric
   apneustic
   assisted
   atactic
   Biot
   bronchial
   bronchovesicular
   cavernous
   Cheyne-Stokes
   cogwheel
   continuous positive pressure
     (CPPB)

breathing *(cont.)*
   diaphragmatic
   frog
   glossopharyngeal
   intermittent positive pressure
     (IPPB)
   Kussmaul
   labored
   mouth
   periodic
   positive-negative pressure (PNPB)
   pursed-lip
   rapid shallow
   resistive (through fixed orifice)
   shallow
   sighing
   skeletal
   sleep-disordered (SDB)
   spontaneous
   stertorous
   stridulous
   tidal
   tubular
   vesicular
breathing apparatus
breathing pattern, tachypneic
breathing reserve (BR) ratio
breathing treatments via machine
breathlessness after activity
breathlessness at rest
breathlessness on waking
breathless when wheezing
breath pentane measurement
breath, shortness of
breath sounds (see also *sounds*)
   absent
   adventitious
   amphoric
   audible
   bronchial
   bronchovesicular
   cavernous

breath sounds *(cont.)*
  coarse
  cogwheel
  decreased
  distant
  faint
  inspiratory-expiratory
  muffled
  normal
  reduced
  sibilant
  tubular
  vesicular
Brechenmacher fiber
Brechenmacher tract
Brecher and Cronkite technique for platelet counting
brephoplastic
Brescia-Cimino AV (arteriovenous) fistula
Bretschneider-HTK cardioplegic solution
Brett syndrome
Bridge Assurant biliary stent delivery system
bridge, Wheatstone
bridging, muscular
brief anterior thrust
bright, highly mobile echoes
bright red flush
Brio pacemaker
Brisbane method of aortic valve and ascending aorta replacement
brisk bifid arterial pulse
brisk drainage
BriteMax catheter
BriteMax sheath introducer
Broadbent inverted sign
broadened P waves
broadened T wave
broad maxillary ridge
broad-spectrum antibiotic

Brock cardiac dilator
Brock clamp
Brock commissurotomy knife
Brockenbrough-Braunwald sign
Brockenbrough cardiac device
Brockenbrough catheter, modified bipolar
Brockenbrough mapping catheter
Brockenbrough needle
Brockenbrough sign
Brockenbrough transseptal catheter
Brockenbrough transseptal method for commissurotomy
Brockenbrough transseptal needle
Brock middle lobe syndrome
Brock transventricular closed valvotomy
Brodie-Trendelenburg test for varicose veins
Brom repair of aortic stenosis
Brom repair of congenital supravalvular aortic stenosis
bronchi (pl. of bronchus) (see *bronchus*)
bronchial adenoma
bronchial anular cartilage
bronchial arteriography
bronchial artery
bronchial artery embolization
bronchial asthma
bronchial biopsy
bronchial branch
bronchial breath sounds
bronchial brushing
bronchial bud
bronchial calculus
bronchial caliber
bronchial candidiasis
bronchial carcinoma myasthenia syndrome
bronchial cartilage absence-bronchiectasis-bronchomalacia syndrome

bronchial cartilage, absent
bronchial cast syndrome
bronchial collapse on forced expiration
bronchial collateral circulation
bronchial cyst
bronchial dehiscence
bronchial distortions
bronchial hyperreactivity to TDI
  (toluene diisocyanate)
bronchial hyperresponsiveness
  allergen-induced
  persistent
bronchial irritation
bronchial kinkings
bronchial lumen
bronchial mucosa
bronchial mucosal edema
bronchial murmur
bronchial nocardiosis
bronchial obstruction
bronchial provocation
  HDM (house dust mites)
  methacholine
bronchial provocation testing
bronchial reactivity
bronchial rejection
bronchial respirations
bronchial secretions
bronchial septum
bronchial sleeve resection
bronchial smooth muscle spasm
bronchial spasm
bronchial stenosis
bronchial stricture
bronchial stump coverage
bronchial suctioning
bronchial tree
bronchial type B disease
bronchial vessels
bronchial washings
bronchial washings cytology
bronchic cell

bronchiectasis
  acquired
  capillary
  chronic
  congenital
  cylindrical
  cystic
  dry
  follicular
  fusiform
  Polynesian
  postinfectious
  Pseudomonas
  recurrent
  saccular
  tuberculous
  varicose
bronchiectasis-ethmoid sinusitis
bronchiectasis-like quantities of
  purulent material
bronchiectasis-megaesophagus-
  osteopathy syndrome
bronchiectatic pattern
bronchi lobares
bronchiloquy
bronchiocele
bronchiogenic
bronchiolar carcinoma
bronchiolar edema
bronchiolar emphysema
bronchiolar epithelium
bronchiolar narrowing, irreversible
bronchiolar obstruction
bronchiolar passages, narrowing of
bronchiole, bronchioles
  alveolar
  lobular
  patchy inflammation of
  respiratory
  terminal
bronchiolectasis
bronchioli (pl. of bronchiolus)

bronchiolitis
  exudative
  proliferative
  RSV (respiratory syncytial virus)
  vesicular
bronchiolitis-associated interstitial lung
  disease, respiratory
bronchiolitis exudativa
bronchiolitis fibrosa obliterans
bronchiolitis obliterans organizing
  pneumonia
bronchiolitis obliterans syndrome
  (BOS)
bronchiolitis obliterans with organizing
  pneumonia (BOOP)
bronchiolus (pl. bronchioli)
bronchiospasm (bronchospasm)
bronchiostenosis
bronchi principales dexter/sinister
  (right and left main bronchi)
bronchi principalis dexter (right main
  bronchus)
bronchi principalis sinister (left main
  bronchus)
bronchi segmentales
bronchismus
bronchi, surgical stumps of
bronchitic
bronchitis
  acute
  acute infectious
  acute irritative
  acute laryngotracheal
  arachidic
  asthmatic
  bacterial
  capillary
  Castellani
  catarrhal
  cheesy
  chemical
  chronic

bronchitis *(cont.)*
  chronic obstructive
  croupous
  dry
  emphysematous
  Enterobacter aerogenes
  ether
  exudative
  fetid
  fibrinous
  Haemophilus influenzae
  hemorrhagic
  infectious asthmatic
  infectious avian
  irritative
  laryngotracheal
  membranous
  mucopurulent
  necrotizing
  obstructive
  phthinoid
  plastic
  pneumococcal
  productive
  pseudomembranous
  purulent
  putrid
  secondary
  septic
  staphylococcal
  streptococcal
  suffocative
  vesicular
  viral
bronchitis obliterans
bronchitis with bronchospasm
Bronchitrac L flexible suction catheter
bronchoadenitis
bronchoalveolar cell carcinoma
bronchoalveolar lavage (BAL)
bronchoalveolar lavage fluid (BALF)
bronchoalveolitis

bronchoaspergillosis
bronchoblastomycosis
bronchoblennorrhea
Broncho-Cath double-lumen endo-
    tracheal tube
bronchocavernous
bronchocele
bronchocentric granulomatosis
bronchocentric inflammatory infiltrate
bronchoconstriction
    exercise-induced
    isocapnic hyperventilation-induced
bronchoconstrictor
bronchocutaneous fistula
bronchocutaneous fistulectomy
bronchodilatation
bronchodilation
bronchodilator
    inhaled
    long-acting
    nebulized
    parenteral
    short-acting
    weaned off
bronchodilator effect
bronchodilator therapy
bronchoegophony
bronchoesophageal fistulectomy
bronchoesophagoscopy
bronchofiberscope
bronchofiberscopy
bronchogenic carcinoma
bronchogram, bronchography
    air
    tantalum
bronchographic
broncholith
broncholithiasis
bronchology
bronchomalacia
bronchomediastinal lymph trunk
bronchomotor effects

bronchomucotropic
bronchomycosis
bronchopathy
bronchophony
    pectoriloquous
    sniffling
    whispered
bronchoplasty, fiberoptic
bronchoplegia
bronchopleural fistula
bronchopleural fistula with empyema
bronchopleuromediastinal fistulectomy
bronchopleuropneumonia
bronchopneumonia (see *pneumonia*)
    bibasilar
    hemorrhagic
    hypostatic
    inhalation
    postoperative
    subacute
    tuberculous
    virus
bronchopneumonitis
bronchopneumopathy
bronchoprovocation testing
bronchopulmonary allergy
bronchopulmonary aspergillosis,
    allergic
bronchopulmonary dysplasia (BPD)
bronchopulmonary lavage
bronchopulmonary lymph node
bronchopulmonary segment
bronchoradiography
bronchorrhagia
bronchorrhaphy
bronchorrhea
bronchoscope (see also *bronchoscopy*)
    balloon-tipped, dual-channel
        fiberoptic
    directable tip of
    Evis Exera video
    fiberoptic

bronchoscope *(cont.)*
  flexible
  Jackson
  Jackson-Olympus
  Karl Storz
  Olympus BF1G10
  Olympus BF3C4
  Olympus BF4B2
  Olympus BF-10
  Olympus BF-20
  Olympus BF-20D
  Olympus BF-40
  Olympus BF-160 video
  Olympus BF-240 video
  Olympus BFP-10
  Olympus BF-1T10
  Olympus BF-1T20
  Olympus BF-1T20D
  Olympus BF-1T160 video
  Olympus BF-1T200
  Olympus BF-1T240 video
  Olympus BF-3C20
  Olympus BF-3C40 fiber
  Olympus BF-3C160 video
  Olympus BF-N20
  Olympus BF-P 200
  Olympus BF-P10
  Olympus BF-P160 video
  Olympus BF-P200
  Olympus BF-P20D
  Olympus BF-P240
  Olympus BF-P240 video
  Olympus BF-P40 fiber
  Olympus BF-XP40 fiber
  Olympus BF-XT40
  Olympus BF1T40 fiber
  Olympus Evis Exera video
  Olympus fiberoptic
  Olympus LF-DP portable intubation
    fiberscope
  Olympus LF-GP portable intubation
    fiberscope

bronchoscope *(cont.)*
  Olympus LF-TP portable intubation
    fiberscope
  Pentax EB-1830
  rigid
  Storz
  Storz infant
  ultrathin
bronchoscopic shuttle technique
bronchoscopy (see also *bronchoscope*)
  diagnostic flexible fiberoptic
  fiberoptic
  flexible
  flexible fiberoptic
  rigid
  therapeutic
bronchoscopy lavage
bronchosinusitis
bronchospasm
  exercise-induced (EIB)
  paradoxical
  uncontrolled
bronchospastic effects
bronchospirometry
bronchostaxis
bronchostenosis
bronchostomy
bronchotome
bronchotomy
bronchotracheal
bronchovesicular breath sounds
bronchovesicular breathing
bronchovisceral fistulectomy
bronchus (pl. bronchi)
  anterior
  anterior basal
  apical
  apicoposterior
  beaded
  cardiac
  contracted
  dilated

bronchus *(cont.)*
  edematous
  eparterial
  extrapulmonary
  flaccid
  granulomatous inflammation of
  hyparterial
  inflamed
  intermediate
  intrapulmonary
  lateral basal
  left main stem
  lingular
  lobar
  medial
  medial basal
  medium-sized
  narrowed
  normal-appearing
  posterior basal
  primary (right and left)
  right main stem
  secondary
  secretion-filled
  segmental
  stem
  subapical
  subsegmental
  superior
  tracheal
bronchus closure
bronchus intermedius
bronchus principalis dexter (right main
  bronchus)
bronchus principalis sinister (left main
  bronchus)
Broviac atrial catheter
Brown Adson forceps
brown atrophy
Brown-Dodge method for angiography
brown induration of the lung
brown lung

brown lung disease
brown pulmonary induration
BR (breathing reserve) ratio
Bruce protocol (exercise stress testing)
  modified
  standard
  treadmill exercise
brucellosis
Brugada syndrome
Brugia malayi infection
bruit, bruits (see also *murmur*, *sound)*
  abdominal
  aneurysmal
  audible
  buzzing venous murmur
  carotid
  carotid artery
  clashing noise
  clear ringing musical (brassy) note
  crackling pericardial
  crackling pleural
  creaking noise
  dull wooden nonmusical note
  epigastric
  false
  flank
  flapping rustle
  grating
  interscapulovertebral arterial
  palpable
  rasping
  rattling
  renal artery
  Roger
  rubbing sound
  rustling murmur from pericardial
  seagull
  skodaic
  slowing sound
  splashing
  subclavian
  supraclavicular

bruit *(cont.)*
  systolic
  to-and-fro
  Traube (gallop)
  Verstraeten
  waterwheel
bruit d'airain (brass)
bruit de bois (wood)
bruit de canon (cannon)
bruit de choc (shock, clash)
bruit de clapotement (rippling)
bruit de craquement (crackling)
bruit de cuir neuf (new leather)
bruit de diable (humming top)
bruit de drapeau (flag)
bruit de felé (cracked)
bruit de froissement (clashing)
bruit de frolement (rustling)
bruit de frottement (friction)
bruit de galop (gallop rhythm)
bruit de grelot (rattle)
bruit de lime (file)
bruit de moulin (mill)
bruit de parchemin (parchment)
bruit de piaulement (whining)
bruit de pot felé (cracked-pot sound)
bruit de rape (grater)
bruit de rappel (drum beating to arms)
bruit de Roger
bruit de scie (saw)
bruit de soufflet (bellows)
bruit de tabourka (drum)
bruit de tambour (drum)
bruit de triolet (a little trio)
bruit placentaire (placental)
bruit skodique
Brunnstróm stage
Brunschwig artery forceps
Brushfield spots
brushing, bronchial
brush, nasal
BSA (body surface area)

BSA ejection fraction
B-scan (also called B-mode) ultrasound
BSGF (brachiosubclavian bridge graft
  fistula)
Buckley syndrome
bucrylate collagen
bud, buds
  bronchial
  capillary
  vascular
bubbling cough
bubbling rales
bubbly lung syndrome
Buchbinder Omniflex catheter
Buckberg cardioplegia
Buckberg solution
buckled innominate artery syndrome
buckling of mitral valve, midsystolic
bucrylate
Budd-Chiari syndrome
budgie (shell parakeet)-fancier's
  disease
Buerger symptoms
Buerger thromboangiitis obliterans
  disease
buffer
buffy coat positive
buffy coat smear
Bugbee electrode
bulb
  aortic
  carotid
  internal jugular
bulbar intracerebral hemorrhage
bulbar septum
bulb of heart
bulb of inferior jugular vein
bulb of superior jugular vein
bulbous-tip electrode
bulboventricular foramen, restrictive
bulbus aortae
bulbus arteriosus

bulbus cordis
bulge
    bilateral anterior chest
    late systolic
    palpable presystolic
    parasternal
bulging precordium
bulging, suprasternal
bulla (pl. bullae), emphysematous
bulldog clamp
bulldog Hasson grasper
bull neck appearance
bullous emphysema
bullous lung disease
bull's eye images
bump, ductus
BUN (blood urea nitrogen)
bundle
    artery-vein-nerve
    AV (atrioventricular)
    Bachmann
    common
    fascicular
    Gierke respiratory
    His
    intercostal
    intercostal neuromuscular
    James
    Keith sinoatrial
    Kent
    Kent-His
    Mahaim
    main
    sinoatrial
    Thorel
    vascular
bundle branch block (BBB)
bundle branch heart block (on EKG)
bundle branch reentrant ventricular
    tachycardia
bundle branch reentry (BBR)
bundle of His

bundle of His ablation
bundle of Kent accessory bypass fibers
bundle of Stanley Kent
bur (also *burr*)
    atherectomy
    diamond-coated
    elliptical
    high-speed
    rotating
Burchard-Liebermann reaction
Burchard-Liebermann test
Burford-Finochietto rib spreader
Burford retractor
Burford rib spreader
Burghart symptoms
Burhenne steerable catheter with basket
    inserted
Bürker chamber for macrophage
    counting
Burke syndrome
burning, substernal
Burns space
burr (see *bur*)
burst cycle length
burst
    multicapture
    respiratory
burst of arrhythmia
burst of ventricular ectopy
burst of ventricular tachycardia
burst pacing, adaptive
burying of P_2 sound
Buselmeier shunt
butterfly pattern of infiltrates
butterfly shadow (on x-ray)
butterfly, silicone
buttock claudication
button device for transcatheter
    occlusion of atrial septal defect
buttonhole opening
buttonhole stenosis
button of aorta

button, skin
buttress, staple-line reinforcement
button technique
buttressed mattress sutures
buttress staple line
buttress suture line
buzzing murmur
BVAD, BiVAD (biventricular assist
    device)
BVM (bag-valve-mask) resuscitating
    device
BVS (biventricular support system)
BV2 needle
BX Agile balloon catheter
BX Agile stent
Bx Sonic balloon expandable stent
BX Velocity Rx with Hepacoat
    balloon-expandable stent
Bx Velocity sirolimus-coated coronary
    stent
bypass (see also *bypass graft*, *graft*)
    aorta-iliac-femoral
    aorta-renal
    aorta-subclavian-carotid
    aorta-subclavian-carotid-axillo-
        axillary
    aorta to first obtuse marginal
        branch
    aorta to LAD
    aorta to marginal branch
    aorta to posterior descending
    aortic-femoral
    aortic-superior mesenteric
    aortobifemoral
    aortocarotid
    aortoceliac
    aortocoronary
    aortocoronary-saphenous vein
    aortofemoral
    aortofemoral-thoracic
    aortoiliac
    aortoiliac-popliteal

bypass *(cont.)*
    aortoiliofemoral
    aortopopliteal
    aortorenal
    apico-abdominal
    atrial-femoral
    atrial-femoral artery
    axillary
    axillary-brachial
    axillary-femoral
    axilloaxillary
    axillobifemoral
    axillofemoral
    axillopopliteal
    brachial
    cardiopulmonary (CPB)
    carotid-axillary
    carotid-carotid
    carotid-subclavian
    common hepatic-common iliac-
        renal
    coronary
    coronary artery (CAB)
    cross femoral-femoral
    crossover
    distal arterial
    DTAF-F (descending thoracic
        aortofemoral-femoral)
    extra-anatomic
    extracranial-intracranial (EC-IC)
    fem-fem (femoral-femoral)
    femoral-above-knee popliteal
    femoral crossover
    femoral to tibial
    femoral vein-femoral artery
    femoral-femoral
    femoral-popliteal
    femoral-tibial-peroneal
    femoral venoarterial
    femoroaxillary
    femorodistal
    femorofemoral

bypass *(cont.)*
 femorofemoral crossover
 femorofemoral partial
 femorofemoral to popliteal
 femoroperoneal
 femoropopliteal
 femoropopliteal saphenous vein
 femorotibial
 fem-pop (femoral-popliteal)
 heart-lung
 hypothermic cardiopulmonary
 iliofemoral
 iliopopliteal
 infracubital
 infrainguinal stenosis
 in-situ
 ipsilateral nonreversed greater
  saphenous vein
 left atrium to distal arterial aortic
 left heart
 lesser saphenous vein in situ
 Litwak left atrial-aortic
 mammary-coronary artery
 marginal circumflex
 microscope-aided pedal
 minimally invasive direct bypass
  coronary artery bypass
  (MIDCAB)
 nodo-Hisian (nodohisian)
 nonreversed translocated vein
 normothermic cardiopulmonary
 obtuse marginal
 partial
 partial cardiopulmonary
 percutaneous femoral-femoral
  cardiopulmonary
 popliteal
 popliteal in situ
 popliteal to distal in situ
 pulsatile cardiopulmonary
 renal artery-reverse saphenous vein
 reversed

bypass *(cont.)*
 right heart
 sequential in situ
 subclavian-carotid
 subclavian-subclavian
 superior mesenteric artery
 temporary aortic shunt
 tibial in situ
 total cardiopulmonary
 totally endoscopic coronary artery
  (TECAB)
 upper extremity in-situ
 venovenous
bypass circuit
bypass conduit
bypass graft
 aortobifemoral
 aortobiprofunda
 aortocoronary saphenous vein
 ascending aorta-abdominal aorta
 axillary-axillary
 axillary-femorofemoral
 axillobifemoral
 axillofemoral
 carotid-carotid venous
 femoral-femoral
 femoral-distal popliteal
 femoroperoneal
 femorotibial
 hepatorenal
 hepatorenal saphenous vein
 iliac-renal
 ilioprofunda
 infrainguinal vein
 saphenous vein
 sequential
 splenorenal arterial
 supraceliac aorta-femoral artery
 supraceliac aortic
 supraceliac aortofemoral
 thoracic aorta-femoral artery

bypass tract
 atrio-His
 atrio-Hisian or atriohisian
 AV (atrioventricular) nodal
 concealed
 cryosurgical interruption of AV
  (atrioventricular)
 fasciculoventricular
 James atrionodal
 nodo-Hisian (nodohisian)

bypass tract *(cont.)*
  nodoventricular
  right ventricular
bypass-tract-mediated AV (atrioventricular) nodal reentrant
 tachycardia
Byrel SX pacemaker
Byrel-SX/Versatrax pacemaker
byssinosis

C, c

C (click)
C-A, CA (cardiac-apnea) monitor for newborns
C-A amplitude of mitral valve
CA (cardiac arrest)
CA (coronary artery)
CAB (coronary artery bypass)
"cabbage" (pronunciation of CABG)
CABG (coronary artery bypass graft)
cabinet respirator
cable
    alligator pacing
    fibrillator
    percutaneous
    stripper
Cabot-Locke murmur
Cabrol I anastomosis
Cabrol I shunt
Cabrol I tube graft
Cabrol II coronary ostial revascularization
Cabrol II interposition coronary prosthetic graft
Cabrol II modification of Bentall procedure
CABS (coronary artery bypass surgery)

cachectic endocarditis
cachectic patient
cachexia, cardiac
CAD (coronary artery disease)
cadaverous
Cadence AICD (automatic implantable cardioverter-defibrillator)
Cadence biphasic ICD (implantable cardioverter-defibrillator)
Cadence ICD (implantable cardioverter-defibrillator)
cadence, rhythmic auscultatory
Cadence TVL nonthoracotomy lead
cadmium iodide detector
CADs (computer-assisted diagnostics)
CADD (computerized ambulatory drug delivery) pump
CADD-Prizm pain control system (PCS)
Cadet cardioverter-defibrillator
CAEP (chronotropic assessment exercise protocol)
caerulea dolens, phlegmasia
Cafcit (caffeine citrate)
caffeine
caffeine heart syndrome
caisson syndrome

cake mix kit for hematopoietic
   progenitor assay
calcareous deposits in pericardium
calcific aortic stenosis
calcific arteriosclerosis
calcific artery
calcific atherosclerosis
calcification
   anular
   aortic
   aortic valve
   basketlike
   coronary
   dystrophic
   eggshell
   idiopathic pleural
   intracardiac
   linear
   mitral anular
   mitral ring
   mitral valve
   Mönckeberg (Moenckeberg)
   subanular
   valve
   valvular
calcification of myocardium
calcification of pericardium
calcific constrictive pericarditis
calcific spur
calcified artery
calcified clot
calcified granulomatous disease
calcified irregular mass, polypoid
calcified pericardium
calcified plaque
calcified thrombus
calcified valvular leaflets
calcium antagonist
calcium channel antagonists
calcium channel blocker (CCB)
calcium deposit
calcium entry blocker

calcium, intracardiac
calcium layering at aortic knob
calculus
   bronchial
   hemic
   lung
Caldwell cannula
Caldwell needle
calf claudication
calf muscle tenderness
calf vein thrombus
caliber
   good
   excellent
   internal
   luminal
   medium
   modest
   normal
   tracheal
   vessel
   wide
caliber of bronchus
caliber of vessel, borderline
caliber of vessel, suitable
caliber-persistent artery
California disease
caliper
callused elbows from repeated
   assumption of tripod position
Calman carotid artery clamp
Calman ring clamp
Calypso Rely catheter
camera
   Anger-type scintillation
   gamma
   GE Starcam single-crystal
     tomographic
   multicrystal gamma
   scintillation
   Starcam
cameral fistula

CAMIS (computer-assisted minimally invasive surgery)
CAM tent
CAMV (congenital anomaly of mitral valve)
Canadian Class system (I-IV) for severity of angina
Canadian Society of Cardiology criteria for effort angina
canal
  Arantius
  arterial
  atrioventricular (AV)
  common atrioventricular
  complex atrioventricular
  Cuvier
  Hunter
  perivascular
  persistent common atrioventricular
  pulmoaortic
  Sucquet-Hoyer
canalization
canalize
cancer embolus
Cancion pump
Candela 405-nm pulsed dye laser
candidal esophagitis
candidate for transplant
  excellent
  marginal
  suitable
candidemia, pulmonary artery catheter-related
candidiasis, bronchial
cannon A wave of jugular venous pulse
Cannon formula
cannon wave
cannula (pl. cannulae, cannulas)
  Aegis aortic
  Apollo
  Apollo 3AC
  Arrow needleless injection

cannula *(cont.)*
  Bard
  aortic arch
  apex
  arterial
  atrial
  Bard arterial
  Bardic
  Caldwell
  CooperSurgical balloon
  Cope needle introducer
  coronary artery
  coronary perfusion
  DirectFlow arterial cannula
  double-stage venous
  Embol-X arterial
  Entree thoracoscopy
  external jugular venous
  flexible suction
  femoral artery
  Flexicath silicone subclavian
  Gregg-type
  Grinfeld
  high-flow
  infusion
  inlet
  internal jugular venous
  intra-arterial
  introducer
  Litwak
  low-profile balloon
  LV (left ventricular) apex
  metallic tip
  nasal (for oxygen)
  needleless injection
  Opti-Clear
  outlet
  Pacifico venous
  perfusion
  peripheral arterial
  peripheral venous
  Polystan perfusion

cannula *(cont.)*
Portnoy ventricular
QuickDraw venous
remote access perfusion (RAP)
Sarns aortic arch
Sarns two-stage
Sarns venous drainage
single-bore
Storz needle
thoracoscopy
Trocan disposable CO_2 trocar and
two-stage Sarns
two-stage venous
USCI
vena cava
Venflon
venous
ventricular
Wallace Flexihub central venous
   pressure
washout
Webster infusion
cannulate, percutaneously
cannulated central vein
cannulation
aortic
arterial
atrial
bicaval
direct caval
left atrial
ostial
single-cannula atrial
two-stage venous
venoarterial
venous
venovenous
cannulization
selective
subselective
CaO_2 (arterial oxygen content)

cap
hilar
pleural
pleural apical hematoma
thin fibrous
capacious veins
capacitance
capacity
carbon monoxide diffusion
cardiac functional
closing (CC)
decreased diffusing
decreased exercise
decreased ventilatory
diffusing
exercise
exertional
forced vital (FVC)
functional residual (FRC)
impaired exercise
inspiratory vital (IVC)
maximal expiratory flow at 25%
   vital capacity (V25)
maximal expiratory flow at 50%
   vital (V50)
maximal expiratory flow at 75%
   vital capacity (V75)
O_2 carrying
reduced diffusing
total lung (TLC)
ventilatory
vital
capacity for work, maximal
CAPD (continuous ambulatory
   peritoneal dialysis)
Capetown aortic prosthetic valve
capillary, capillaries
arterial
lymph
Meigs
permeability of
venous

capillary angioma
capillary bed
capillary blood sugar (CBS)
capillary blood volume
capillary bud
capillary congestion
capillary electrophoresis (CE)
capillary embolism
capillary endothelium
capillary filling, compensatory
capillary filtration coefficient (CFC)
capillary fragility test
capillary hemangioma (strawberry
    mark)
capillary hemangiomas with (or with-
    out) extensive purpura
capillary hydrostatic pressure
capillary hyperpermeability
capillary leak (or leakage), generalized
capillary leak syndrome
capillary malformation (CM)
capillary permeability, increased
capillary pneumonia
capillary pressure
capillary pulsation
capillary refill
capillary resistance test
capillary stick
capillary stick on warmed heel
    of neonate
capillary walls
capillary wedge pressure, pulmonary
capillary-lymphatic malformation
    (CLM)
capillary-venous malformation (CVM)
Capio suture capturing device
Capiox-E bypass system oxygenator
Caplan syndrome
capnograph
capping, apical pleural
Caprosyn suture
capsular thrombosis

CapSure lead
Captiva blood containment device
Captiva needle (for vascular access)
captopril-stimulated renal scan
Captura floating embolic protection
    filter
capture
    atrial
    failure to
    lack of pacemaker
    1:1 retrograde
    pacemaker
    resistance
    retrograde atrial
    ventricular
capture threshold
Carabello sign
CarboFlex wound dressing
carbohydrate-inducible hyperlipemia
CarboMedics prosthetic heart valve
    (CPHV)
CarboMedics valve device
carbonaceous material
carbonated saline solution
carbon dioxide (CO_2), extracorporeal
    removal of
carbon dioxide narcosis
carbon dioxide retention
carbon monoxide diffusion capacity
carbon monoxide diffusion, decreased
carbon-11 (^{11}C)
carbon-11-labeled fatty acids
carbon-11-labeled tracer
carbon-11 palmitic acid radioactive
    tracer
carbonic acid deficit
Carbo-Seal cardiovascular composite
    graft
carboxyhemoglobin
carcinoembryonic antigen (CEA)
carcinoid heart disease
carcinoid syndrome

carcinoid tricuspid valve disease
carcinoid tumor of bronchus
carcinoma
    adenosquamous
    adrenocortical
    alveolar
    alveolar cell
    bronchiolar
    bronchoalveolar cell
    bronchogenic
    cavitating
    clear cell
    endobronchial
    esophageal
    giant cell
    large cell
    large cell neuroendocrine lung
    non-small cell lung
    oat cell
    small cell of the lung
    squamous cell
carcinoma en cuirasse
carcinomatosis, pulmonary
carcinosis, pulmonary
Cardarelli sign
cardiac action commences in sinus
    rhythm
cardiac action potentials
cardiac allograft
cardiac allograft vascular disease
    (CAVD)
cardiac amyloidosis
Cardiac Angioplasty Analysis System
    (CAAS)
cardiac anomaly, Ebstein
cardiac apex
cardiac-apnea (CA) monitor for
    newborns
cardiac-arm syndrome
cardiac arrest (CA)
    asystolic
    bradyarrhythmic

cardiac arrest *(cont.)*
    recurrent
    sudden
cardiac arrhythmia with Stokes-Adams
    attack
Cardiac Arrhythmic Suppression Trial
    (CAST)
Cardiac Assist intra-aortic balloon
    catheter
cardiac asthma
cardiac ballet
cardiac blood pool imaging
cardiac borders
cardiac bradyarrhythmia
cardiac branch
cardiac cachexia
cardiac catheter
cardiac catheterization (see *catheterization*)
cardiac cirrhosis
cardiac compression
cardiac contractility, depressed
cardiac contractions
cardiac cycle
cardiac death
    recurrent, not-so-sudden
    sudden
cardiac decompensation
    end-stage
    fetal
cardiac decompression
cardiac decortication
cardiac denervation
cardiac device (see *device*)
cardiac dilatation
cardiac dullness during respiration
cardiac dynamics
cardiac dysrhythmia
cardiac ectopy
cardiac efficiency
cardiac electromotive force generation
cardiac enlargement

cardiac enzymes (see *isoenzymes*)
cardiac failure (see *heart failure*)
cardiac fibroma
cardiac fibrosarcoma
cardiac filling pressure
cardiac fossa
cardiac function
cardiac function tests (CFTs)
cardiac functional capacity
cardiac glycogenosis
cardiac glycosides
cardiac hamartoma
cardiac hemangioma
cardiac histiocyte
cardiac hybrid revascularization
   procedure
cardiac hypertrophy
cardiac hypokinesis
cardiac imaging, VScore with
   AutoGate high-quality
cardiac impression
cardiac index (CI) (pl. indices)
cardiac infarct
cardiac insufficiency
cardiac irritability
cardiac isoenzymes, serial
cardiac laminography
cardiac leads (see *lead*)
cardiaclike chest pain
cardiac-limb syndrome
cardiac lipoma
cardiac lung
cardiac lymphangioma
cardiac mapping
cardiac margins on x-ray
cardiac massage
cardiac monitor, MemoryTrace AT
cardiac murmur of unknown type
cardiac muscle fibers
cardiac myxoma
cardiac neurosis syndrome
cardiac node

cardiac notch
cardiac output (CO) (see also *output*)
   adequate
   augmented
   inadequate
   reduced
   reduced systemic
   thermodilution
cardiac output measurement
   Fick oxygen method of
   indicator-dilution method of
   indocyanine green dye method of
   thermodilution method
cardiac output monitor, ICG-Pulsion
cardiac overload (or overloading)
cardiac oxygenation
cardiac paraganglioma
cardiac perforation
cardiac plexus
cardiac profile
Cardiac Protect
cardiac psychosis
cardiac pumping ability
cardiac radiation syndrome
cardiac recovery
cardiac referred pain
cardiac reflexes
cardiac rehabilitation program
cardiac reserve, suboptimal
cardiac resynchronization therapy
   (CRT)
cardiac retraction clip
cardiac rhabdomyoma
cardiac rhabdomyosarcoma
cardiac rhythm
cardiac rhythm disturbance
cardiac risk assessment
cardiac risk factors
   age
   alcohol consumption
   alcoholism
   behavior

cardiac *(cont.)*
> blood pressure
> caffeine consumption
> cigarette smoking
> coffee drinking
> diabetes mellitus, type I
> diabetes mellitus, type II
> diet
> elevated cholesterol
> elevated blood lipids
> elevated triglycerides
> environment
> familial disposition
> family history
> gender (male more than female
> > until menopause)
> genetic
> heredity
> high blood pressure (HBP)
> high plasma LDL (low-density
> > lipoproteins)
> hypercalcemia
> hypercholesterolemia
> hypercoagulability
> hyperlipidemia
> hypertension
> hypertriglyceridemia
> hyperuricemia
> lack of exercise
> lipidemia
> low plasma HDL (high-density
> > lipoproteins)
> menopause
> obesity
> oral contraceptive use
> personality type A
> physical inactivity
> race
> saturated fat consumption
> sedentary lifestyle
> smoking of cigarettes
> stress

cardiac *(cont.)*
> tobacco use
> type A personality
> vasectomy
> water hardness

cardiac risk profile
cardiac rupture
cardiac sarcoma
cardiac series (x-rays)
cardiac shadow
cardiac shape
cardiac shock wave therapy (CSWT)
cardiac shunt
cardiac silhouette (on x-ray)
> borderline-enlarged
> enlarged
> large thymus shadow obscuring

cardiac sling
cardiac souffle
cardiac source
cardiac standstill
Cardiac STATus rapid assay
cardiac steady state
Cardiac Stimulator
cardiac stroke volume
cardiac surgery intensive care unit
> (CSICU)

cardiac sympathectomy
cardiac sympathomimetic amines
cardiac syncope
cardiac syphilis
cardiac tamponade, low-pressure
cardiac teratoma
cardiac thrombosis
cardiac thrust
cardiac tone
cardiac transplant donor (CTD)
cardiac transplant recipient (CTR)
cardiac transplant (allograft) rejection
Cardiac T rapid assay
cardiac trauma
cardiac troponin T protein

cardiac troponin T test
cardiac tumor embolization
cardiacus, plexus
cardiac valvar operation
cardiac valve mucoid degeneration
cardiac valve prosthesis, Omniscience
    single leaflet
cardiac valves
cardiac vasculature
cardiac vein, great
cardiac waist
cardialgia
Cardia Salt Alternative
cardiasthma
Cardica anastomotic device
cardiectasis
Cardifix EZ pacing lead
Cardima Pathfinder microcatheter
cardinal event
cardinal physical finding
cardinal signs of inflammation
cardinal symptom
cardioangiography
cardioangioscope
cardioarterial interval carcinoid
cardioauditory syndrome
Cardiobacterium hominis
CardioBeeper CB-12L monitoring
    device
Cardiocap 5 patient monitor
CardioCard digital electrocardiogram
    storage
cardiocele
cardiocentesis
cardiochalasia
cardiocirrhosis
CardioCoil coronary stent
cardiocutaneous syndrome
Cardio Data MK3 Holter scanner
cardiodefibrillator, Endotek
CardioDiary heart monitor
cardiodilator

cardiodiosis
cardiodynamics
cardiodynia
cardioesophageal
cardiofacial defect
cardiofacial syndrome
CardioFix Pericardium patch
Cardiofreezer cryosurgical system
cardiogenesis
cardiogenic embolic stroke
cardiogenic embolism
cardiogenic pulmonary edema
cardiogenic shock, advanced
cardiogenic shock heart
cardiogram
    apex (ACG)
    electro-
    precordial
    ultrasonic (UCG)
    vector
cardiograph, cardiography
Cardio-Green dye
cardiohemic system
cardiohepatic
cardiohepatomegaly
cardioinhibitor
cardioinhibitory
cardioinhibitory carotid sinus syncope
cardioinhibitory carotid sinus
    syndrome
cardioinhibitory responses
cardioinhibitory/vasodepressor
cardiointegram (CIG)
cardiokinetic
cardiokymographic test
cardiokymography (CKG)
Cardiolite (^{99m}Tc sestamibi) scan
cardiologist
cardiology, invasive
cardiolysis
cardiomalacia
Cardiomed Bodysoft epidural catheter

Cardiomed endotracheal ventilation
  catheter
Cardiomed thermodilution catheter
cardiomegaly
  alcoholic
  familial
  globular
  hypertensive
  iatrogenic
  idiopathic
  postoperative
cardiomotility
cardiomyoliposis
cardiopathia nigra syndrome
cardiomyopathic carnitine deficiency
cardiomyopathic lentiginosis,
  progressive
cardiomyopathy
  alcoholic
  alcoholic dilated
  amyloidotic
  apical hypertrophic (AHC)
  arrhythmogenic right ventricular
  beer-drinker's
  beriberi
  concentric hypertrophic
  congenital dilated
  congestive
  constrictive
  diabetic
  diffuse symmetric hypertrophic
  dilated (DCM)
  end-stage
  familial
  familial hypertrophic (FHC)
  Friedreich ataxic
  histiocytoid
  hypertrophic (HCM)
  hypertrophic obstructive (HOC
    or HOCM)
  idiopathic
  idiopathic dilated (IDC)

cardiomyopathy *(cont.)*
  idiopathic restrictive
  infantile
  infantile histiocytoid
  infectious
  infiltrative
  ischemic
  ischemic congestive
  left ventricular
  metabolic
  mucopolysaccharidosis
  myotonia atrophica
  noncoronary
  nonischemic congestive
  nonischemic dilated (NIDCM)
  nonobstructive
  obliterative
  obscure
  obstructive
  obstructive hypertrophic
  peripartum
  peripartum dilated
  postmyocarditis dilated
  postpartum
  primary
  radiation-induced
  restrictive (RCM)
  right ventricular
  right-sided
  secondary
  tachycardia-induced
  thyrotoxicotic
  toxic
  viral
cardiomyopathy with restrictive
  component
cardiomyoplasty
cardiomyotomy
cardionecrosis
cardionephric
cardioneural
cardio-omentopexy

Cardio-Pace Medical Durapulse
  pacemaker
CardioPass vascular graft
cardiopathia nigra (Ayerza syndrome)
cardiopathic
cardiopathy
  hypertensive
  infarctoid
  obscure
cardiopericardiopexy
cardiopericarditis
cardiopexy, ligamentum teres
cardiophobia
cardiophrenia
cardiophrenic angle
cardiophrenic junction
cardioplasty
cardioplege (verb)
cardioplegia (see also *cardioplegic
    solution*)
  blood
  Buckberg
  cold
  cold blood
  cold blood hyperkalemic
  cold crystalloid
  cold potassium
  cold retrograde blood
  cold sanguineous
  continuous warm blood
  crystalloid potassium
  hyperkalemic
  nutrient
  O_2 crystalloid
  potassium chloride
  St. Thomas Hospital
  warm continuous retrograde
cardioplegic arrest, hypothermic
cardioplegic needle
cardioplegic solution (see also
    cardioplegia)
  Bretschneider-HTK
  Buckberg

cardioplegic *(cont.)*
  hyperkalemic crystalloid
  infusion of
  leukocyte-depleted terminal blood
  retrograde
  St. Thomas
cardiopneumatic
Cardiopoint
Cardiopoint cardiac surgery needles
cardioprotective
cardioptosis, Wenckebach
cardiopulmonary arrest
cardiopulmonary bilharziasis
cardiopulmonary bypass (CPB)
cardiopulmonary bypass time
cardiopulmonary deterioration
cardiopulmonary exercise testing
    device, Viasys
cardiopulmonary insufficiency
cardiopulmonary obesity
cardiopulmonary resuscitation (CPR)
cardiopulmonary schistosomiasis
cardiopulmonary support pump
    (see *pump*)
cardiopulmonary support system (CPS)
cardiopulmonary support, temporary
    percutaneous
cardiopuncture
cardiopyloric
cardiorenal disease
cardiorespiratory distress
cardiorespiratory sign
cardiorrhaphy
cardiorrhexis (rupture of heart)
cardiosclerosis
cardioscope U system
CardioSEAL septal occluder
CardioSEAL septal occlusion system
cardioselective agent
cardioselective beta-blocker drug for
    hypertension and angina
cardiospasm

cardiosplenopexy
cardiotachomety
cardiotachometry
Cardio Tactilaze peripheral angioplasty
   laser catheter
CardioTec or Cardiotec (^{99m}Tc teboroxime) scan
cardiotherapy
cardiothoracic index
cardiothoracic ratio (CTR)
cardiothoracic surgeon
cardiothyrotoxicosis
cardiotocograph, cardiotocography
cardiotomy
cardiotomy reservoir
cardiotonic drug
cardiotopometry
cardiotoxic
cardiotoxicity
   Adriamycin
   digitalis
   doxorubicin
cardiouremia
cardiovalvular
cardiovalvulitis
cardiovalvulotome
cardiovalvulotomy
Cardiovasc stent
cardiovascular accident (CVA)
cardiovascular anomalies
cardiovascular collagenosis
cardiovascular hemodynamics
cardiovascular radioisotope scan and
   function study
cardiovascular renal disease
cardiovascular resuscitation
cardiovascular shunt
cardiovascular silk suture
cardioversion
   DC (direct-current)
   electrical
   endocavitary
   pharmaceutical

cardioversion *(cont.)*
   spontaneous
   synchronized DC
cardioversion zone
cardiovert, attempt to
cardioverted patient
cardioverter, cardioverter-defibrillator
   (see also *pacemaker* and *pulse*
     generator)
   Angstrom MD implantable
    single-lead
   Atrial View Ventak AV implant-
    able
   automatic implantable (AICD)
   Belos VR-T internal (ICD)
   Contour MD implantable single-
    lead
   Contour V-145D and LTV-135D
    implantable
   InSync implantable
   internal
   implantable
   implantable automatic atrial
   LifeVest WCD 3000 external
   Medtronic GEM implantable
   nonthoracotomy
   PCD Transvene implantable
   Photon DR dual-chamber
    implantable
   Phylax AV dual chamber
    implantable
   Powerheart automatic external
   Res-Q AICD
   Res-Q ACD (arrhythmia control
    device)
   Res-Q Micron implantable
   Sentinel implantable
   tiered-therapy programmable
    (PCD)
   Ventak AV III DR
   Ventak Mini II (and III) AICD
   Ventritex Angstrom MD
    implantable

cardioverter-defibrillator implantation
cardiovocal syndrome
CardioWest total artificial heart (TAH)
carditis
    Lyme
    rheumatic
    streptococcal
    verrucous
Cardizem (diltiazem HCl)
Cardizem CD (diltiazem HCl)
Cardizem LA (diltiazem HCl)
Cardizem SR (diltiazem HCl)
Cardura (doxazosin mesylate)
care, kangaroo
Carey Coombs murmur
carina of trachea
carinatum, pectus
Carmalt forceps
C-arm digital fluoroscopy
Carmeda bioactive surface (CBAS)
Carmeda Bio-Pump centrifugal blood
    pump
carnitine deficiency
carnitine deficiency syndrome
Carolina rocker
carotid angioplasty with stenting
carotid arterial dissection
carotid arterial pulse, synchronous
carotid artery aneurysm
carotid artery balloon angioplasty
carotid artery bruit
carotid artery-cavernous sinus fistula
carotid artery kinking
carotid artery pulsations, transmitted
carotid artery, redundant
carotid baroreceptor
carotid bifurcation
carotid bruit
carotid bulb
carotid-carotid venous bypass graft
carotid-cavernous fistula
CarotidCoil stent

carotid duplex study
carotid ejection time
carotid endarterectomy (CEA)
carotid glomectomy
carotid intima-media thickness (c-IMT)
carotid intimal thickening, balloon-
    injured
carotid massage, chest pain relieved by
carotid occlusive disease
carotid phonoangiography
carotid pulse
carotid pulse collapse
carotid pulse peak
carotid pulse tracing
carotid pulse upstroke
carotid shudder
carotid sinus
carotid sinus hypersensitivity (CSH)
carotid sinus massage
carotid sinus reflex, hyperactive
carotid sinus syncope
carotid sinus syndrome
carotid steal
carotid string sign
carotid system, extracranial
carotid-subclavian bypass
carotid upstroke, brisk
carotids, equal
carotidynia
Carpenter syndrome
Carpentier anuloplasty ring prosthesis
Carpentier-Edwards (CE)
Carpentier-Edwards aortic valve
Carpentier-Edwards bioprosthetic
    valve
Carpentier-Edwards glutaraldehyde-
    preserved porcine xenograft
    bioprosthesis
Carpentier-Edwards mitral anuloplasty
    valve
Carpentier-Edwards pericardial valve

Carpentier-Edwards Perimount Plus
pericardial bioprosthesis
Carpentier-Edwards Perimount RSR
pericardial bioprosthesis
Carpentier-Edwards Physio anulo-
plasty ring
Carpentier-Edwards Porcine
SupraAnnular valve (SAV)
Carpentier-Edwards ring
Carpentier method
Carpentier ring
Carpentier technique
Carpentier tricuspid valvuloplasty
CAR (carotid arterial) pulse
CarraSmart foam dressing
Carra Sorb H wound dressing
Carra Sorb M wound gel
Carrasyn hydrogel wound dressing
Carrel button
Carrel patch
Carrel technique
Carrel, triangulation of
Carswell's grapes seen in pulmonary
tuberculosis
Carter equation
Carter-Thomason suture passer
Cartia XT (diltiazem HCl)
Cartilade shark cartilage used for
inhibition of angiogenesis
cartilage
absent bronchial
aortic
bronchial anular
costal
costal interarticular
cricoid
hyaline
laryngeal
main stem bronchial
pulmonary
sternal
thyroid

cartilage *(cont.)*
tracheal
xiphoid
Carvallo sign in tricuspid regurgitation
CAS (coronary artery spasm)
by Ultrafast CT
cascade
arachidonic acid
coagulation
cascade of abdomen
caseating tuberculosis with cavity
formation
CASE computerized exercise EKG
system
caseous necrosis
CASS (Coronary Artery Surgery
Study)
CASS scoring of left ventricular
function
CAST (Cardiac Arrhythmic
Suppression Trial)
Castaneda anastomosis clamp
Castaneda vascular clamp
Castellani bronchitis
Castellani disease
Castellino sign
Castillo catheter
Castroviejo-Colibri forceps
Castroviejo needle holder
casts
branching mucoid bronchial
intrabronchial
cast syndrome
CATCH 22 syndrome (cardiac defects,
abnormal facial features, thymic
hypoplasia, cleft palate, and
hypocalcemia)
cat-eye syndrome (or cat's eye)
CAT (computed axial tomography)
catacrotic
catacrotism
catadicrotism

catadicrotic pulse
catatricrotism
catarrhal croup
catarrhal laryngitis
catarrhal tracheitis
catastrophe, vascular
catch
catching feeling
catechol excess
catecholamines, circulating
catgut absorbable suture material
cath (catheterization)
cathed or cath'd (catheterized)
catheter
    Accuguide central venous
    Accuguide peripherally inserted
      central
    Accu-Vu sizing
    ACE
    Achiever balloon dilatation
    ACS (Advanced Catheter or
      Cardiac Systems)
    ACS angioplasty
    ACS balloon
    ACS Concorde over-the-wire
    ACS Endura coronary dilatation
    ACS JL4 (Judkins left 4 French)
    ACS mini
    ACS Multi-Link
    ACS OTW Lifestream coronary
      dilatation
    ACS OTW (over-the-wire) Photon
      coronary dilatation
    ACS RX (rapid exchange) Comet
    ACS RX (rapid exchange) coronary
      dilatation
    ACS RX Rocket
    ACS Tourguide II guiding
    Active Cath condom
    AcuNav ultrasound
    Aeon
    AGB+

catheter *(cont.)*
    Ahn thrombectomy
    Alert
    All-Terrain Balloon (ATB) PTA
      dilatation
    AL-1
    AL II guiding
    Alzate
    Amazr
    Amplatz cardiac
    Amplatz femoral
    Amplatz right coronary
    Ancure
    Angiocath Autoguard shielded IV
    Angiocath PRN flexible
    AngioDynamics angiography
    angiographic balloon occlusion
    Angio-Kit
    Angiomedics
    angiopigtail
    angioplasty balloon
    AngiOptic microcatheter
    Angioscale diagnostic
    Angiotech
    angled balloon
    angulated
    Anthron heparinized antithrombo-
      genic
    aortogram
    AR-2 diagnostic guiding
    Arani double loop guiding
    Arrow
    Arrow-Berman balloon
    Arrow Cannon
    ArrowGard Blue Line
    ArrowGard central venous
    Arrow-Howes multilumen
    Arrow multi-lumen access (MAC)
    Arrow pulmonary artery
    Arrow Twin Cath
    Arrow Twin Cath multilumen
      peripheral

catheter *(cont.)*
   arterial embolectomy
   Arterial Plug
   Ascent guiding
   Asuka over-the-wire PTCA
   ATB (All-Terrain Balloon) PTA
     dilatation
   atherectomy
   atherectomy, peripheral
   AtheroCath
   Atlas LP PTCA balloon dilatation
   Atlantis SR intravascular ultrasound
     imaging
   Atlas ULP balloon dilatation
   ATRAC multipurpose balloon
   ATRAC-II double balloon
   Atri-pace I bipolar-flared pacing
   Auth atherectomy
   AVA HF
   AVA 3XI
   Avea esophageal
   Avea tracheal
   AV100 balloon
   AV-Paceport thermodilution
   AV2000 balloon
   Axiom DG balloon angioplasty
   bail-out
   Baim pacing
   Baim-Turi monitor/pacing
   BAL Cath
   balloon biliary
   balloon dilatation
   balloon dilating
   balloon embolectomy
   balloon flotation
   balloon septostomy
   balloon-flotation pacing
   balloon-tipped angiographic
   balloon-tipped aortic occlusion/
     cardioplegia
   balloon-tipped end-hole
   balloon-tipped flow-directed
     pulmonary artery

catheter *(cont.)*
   ball-wedge
   balloon wedge pressure
   balloon wedge-type
   Bandit balloon
   Bard guiding
   Bardic cutdown
   Bard Stinger S ablation
   Baxter
   BD First MidCath midline
   BD First Midcath single-lumen
     silicone midline
   BD First PICC
   BD First PICC single-lumen
     silicone peripherally inserted
     central
   BD Insyte Autoguard shielded
     intravenous
   BD Insyte-N Autoguard shielded IV
   BD L-Cath EX midline
   BD L-Cath single-lumen
     polyurethane peripherally
     inserted central
   BD Neo PICC neonatal peripherally
     inserted central
   Berman angiographic balloon
   Bernstein
   Beta-Cath intracoronary
   bicoudate
   bifoil balloon
   bipolar pacing electrode
   bipolar temporary pacemaker
   Block right coronary guiding
   Blue FlexTip
   Blue Max triple-lumen
   BodyFlex
   Bonnie angioplasty
   BriteMax
   Brockenbrough
   Brockenbrough mapping
   Brockenbrough modified bipolar
   Brockenbrough transseptal
   bronchial

catheter *(cont.)*
- Bronchitrac L
- bronchospirometric
- Broviac
- Broviac atrial
- Buchbinder Omniflex
- Burhenne steerable catheter with basket inserted
- BX Agile balloon
- Calypso Rely
- Camino microventricular bolt
- cardiac
- Cardiac Assist intra-aortic balloon
- Cardima Pathfinder
- Cardiomarker
- Cardiomed Bodysoft epidural
- Cardiomed endotracheal ventilation
- Cardiomed thermodilution
- Cardio Tactilaze peripheral angioplasty laser
- Castillo
- Cath-Finder
- Cath-Finder tracking system
- Cath-Gard
- Cathmark suction
- CCOmbo
- Celsius control endovascular
- central venous (CVC)
- Cerebrence guiding
- Certofix central venous
- Charger balloon
- Cheetah angioplasty
- Chemo-Cath
- Chemo-Port
- Clean-Cath single use
- CliniCath peripherally inserted
- Cloverleaf
- coaxial
- Cobra
- Cobra over-the-wire balloon
- cobra-shaped
- coil-tipped

catheter *(cont.)*
- Comfort Cath I or II
- Concise balloon
- conductance
- Constant
- Constellation advanced mapping
- Cook arterial
- Cook pigtail
- Cook TPN
- Cool Tip
- Cordis
- Cordis Brite Tip guiding
- Cordis Ducor I (or II, III) coronary
- Cordis Ducor pigtail
- Cordis high-flow pigtail
- Cordis Predator PTCA balloon
- Cordis Son-II
- Cordis Trakstar PTCA balloon
- coronary dilatation
- coronary guiding
- coronary sinus flow
- coronary sinus thermodilution
- Corpac diagnostic
- corset balloon
- coudé
- Cournand cardiac
- CR Bard
- Crista Cath II electrophysiology
- Critikon
- Critikon balloon wedge pressure
- Critikon thermodilution and pressure
- CrossSail coronary dilatation
- cryoablation
- cutdown
- Cutting Balloon
- CVP (central venous pressure)
- Dacron
- Dale Foley
- Datascope DL-II percutaneous translucent balloon
- decapolar

catheter *(cont.)*
    deflectable quadripolar
    diagnostic
    Diasonics
    dilatation balloon
    dilating
    DLP cardioplegic
    Doppler coronary
    Dorros brachial internal mammary
        guiding
    Dorros infusion/probing
    Dorros infusion and probing
    Dotter
    Dotter caged balloon
    Dotter coaxial
    Double J indwelling
    Double J ureteral
    double-lumen
    Driver
    Ducor balloon
    Duette
    DVI Simpson Atherocath
    EAC (expandable access catheter)
    EchoMark
    EchoMark angiographic
    Edwards diagnostic
    Elecath thermodilution
    electrode
    11 French JCL 3.5 guiding
    El Gamal coronary bypass
    Elite
    Elmhurst Curve
    embolectomy
    Endeavor
    end-hole
    EndoCPB (endovascular cardio-
        pulmonary bypass)
    endosound (endoscopic ultrasound)
    Endotak C lead
    enhanced torque 8F (8 French)
        guiding
    Eppendorf angiocatheter

catheter *(cont.)*
    EPT-Dx steerable diagnostic
    Erythroflex
    Erythroflex hydromer-coated
        central venous
    e-TRAIN 110 AngioJet
    Evert-O-Cath drug delivery
    expandable access (EAC)
    Explorer 360° rotational diagnostic
    Explorer ST fixed curve diagnostic
    Express
    Express PTCA
    extended dwell
    extraction
    extrusion balloon
    FACT (Focal Angioplasty Catheter
        Technology) coronary balloon
        angioplasty
    Falcon coronary
    FAST (flow-assisted, short-term)
        balloon
    Fast-Cath introducer
    Feldman ventriculography
    femoral guiding
    Finesse large-lumen guiding
    Fino vascular
    Flexguard Tip
    Flexi-Cath balloon
    Flexi-Torque thermodilution
        balloon
    FloCath
    FloControl
    flotation
    flow-directed
    flow-oximetry
    Fluency
    Fluency XX stent graft delivery
    fluid-filled
    Fogarty adherent clot
    Fogarty arterial embolectomy
    Fogarty balloon
    Fogarty balloon biliary

catheter *(cont.)*
  Fogarty embolectomy
  Fogarty graft thrombectomy
  Fogarty occlusion
  Fogarty venous thrombectomy
  Fogarty-Chin extrusion balloon
  Force balloon dilatation
  Fountain
  Freeway PTCA
  Freezor cryocatheter
  French
  French 5 (5 French) angiographic
  French MBIH
  FR4 guiding
  Friend
  Fulcrum
  Ganz-Edwards coronary infusion
  Gensini coronary
  Gentle-Flo suction
  Glidecath
  Gold Probe bipolar hemostasis
  Goodale-Lubin cardiac
  Gorlin pacing
  Gould PentaCath 5-lumen thermo-
    dilution
  graft-seeking
  Grollman
  Grollman pigtail
  Groshong
  Groshong double-lumen
  Gruentzig (Grüntzig)
  Grüntzig arterial balloon
  guiding
  Halo
  Hanafee
  Hands-Off balloon pacing
  Hands-Off thermal dilution (or
    thermodilution) (TD)
  Hartzler ACX-II or RX-014 balloon
  Hartzler LPS dilatation
  Hartzler Micro II
  Hartzler Micro XT dilatation

catheter *(cont.)*
  Hattler respiratory support (artificial
    lung device)
  headhunter visceral angiography
  HealthShield antimicrobial
    mediastinal wound drainage
  Heartport Endoclamp aortic
  helical-tip Halo
  helium-filled balloon
  Hemo-Cath
  Hemo-Stream dialysis
  Hemo-Stream vascular
  Hemosplit
  hexapolar
  Hickman indwelling right atrial
  Hidalgo
  Hieshima Taper Select
  high-fidelity
  high-flow
  high-speed rotation dynamic
    angioplasty
  Hohn central venous catheter,
    single- and double-lumen
  hot-tip
  HydraCross TLC PTCA
  Hydrolyser microcatheter
  IAB (intra-aortic balloon)
  Illumen-8 guiding
  ILUS (intraluminal ultrasound)
  indwelling
  Infiniti
  Infuse-A-Cath
  Innovante
  Inoue balloon
  internal jugular acute hemodialysis
  In-Time
  intra-aortic balloon
  intra-aortic balloon double-lumen
  Intracath
  intracoronary guiding
  intracoronary perfusion
  intravascular ultrasound

catheter *(cont.)*
    intravenous pacing
    Intrepid PTCA angioplasty
    introduction of
    ITC balloon
    Jackman orthogonal
    Jelco intravenous
    JL4 (Judkins left 4 cm curve)
    JL5 (Judkins left 5 cm curve)
    Jocath coronary balloon
    Jocath diagnostic
    Jography angiographic
    Jography balloon
    Jography diagnostic
    Joguide balloon
    Joguide coronary guiding
    Joguide diagnostic
    JR4 (Judkins right 4 cm)
    Judkins left 4 cm (JL4)
    Judkins left coronary
    Judkins right 4 cm (JR4)
    Judkins right coronary
    Judkins USCI
    Kaye tamponade balloon
    KDF-2.3
    Kensey
    Kensey atherectomy
    Kifa
    King multipurpose coronary graft
    Kinsey atherectomy
    kissing balloon
    Kontron balloon
    large-bore
    large-lumen
    laser
    left coronary
    left heart
    left Judkins
    left ventricular sump
    Lehman
    Lehman ventriculography
    Lifestream coronary dilatation

catheter *(cont.)*
    Litespeed
    Logocath electrophysiology
    Lo-Profile balloon
    Lo-Profile II balloon
    Lo-Profile steerable dilatation
    Longdwel Teflon
    low-speed rotation angioplasty
    LPS
    Lubri-Sil
    LubriCath
    Luer-Slip IAB
    Lumaguide
    MAC (multi-lumen access)
    Mallinckrodt angiographic
    manometer-tipped cardiac
    Mansfield
    Mansfield Atri-Pace 1
    Mansfield orthogonal electrode
    Mansfield Scientific dilatation
        balloon
    MapCath
    Marathon guiding
    Max Force balloon
    Maverick Monorail balloon
    Maverick over-the-wire balloon
    Maverick PTCA
    Maverick XL PTCA
    Maverick2 Monorail
    McGoon coronary perfusion
    McIntosh double-lumen
    Medtronic balloon
    Metricath catheter and transducer
    Micro-Driver balloon
    Micro-Guide
    micromanometer-tip
    MicroMewi multiple sidehole
        infusion
    MicroMewi occlusion/infusion
    microtipped Millar
    midstream aortogram
    Mikro-tip micromanometer-tipped

catheter *(cont.)*
  Millar
  Millar micromanometer
  Millar MPC-500
  Millar pigtail angiographic
  Millenia balloon
  Miller septostomy
  Mini-Profile dilatation
  minocycline-rifampin-impregnated
  Mirage over-the-wire balloon
  Mistique
  Mitsubishi angioscopic
  Molina needle
  Mongoose PTCA
  Monorail angioplasty
  Monorail balloon
  More-Flow double-lumen
    hemodialysis
  MPF
  MS Classique
  Mullins transseptal
  Multicath
  multi-electrode impedance
  Multi-Med triple-lumen infusion
  multifiber
  multilumen
  multipolar electrode
  multipolar impedance
  multipurpose
  multi-sideport infusion
  MVP
  Mylar
  Myo-Star injection
  Mystic Mongoose PTCA
  NarrowFlex intra-aortic balloon
  NarrowFlex prewrapped double-
    lumen IAB
  Navi-Star diagnostic/ablation
    deflectable tip
  Navi-Star mapping
  Navius
  NBIH

catheter *(cont.)*
  NC Raptor PTCA dilatation
  Neostar vascular access
  Nexus 2 linear ablation
  Niagara dialysis
  NIH (National Institutes of Health)
  NIH cardiomarker
  NIH left ventriculography
  9 F JL 4 guiding (9 French Judkins
    left 4 guiding)
  Ninja FX PTCA dilatation
  nontraumatizing
  NoProfile balloon
  No Torque Right coronary
    angiography
  NovaCath multi-lumen infusion
  Nycore
  Nycore angiography
  Nydex
  octapolar
  Olbert
  OmniCath atherectomy
  Omniflex balloon
  Omni Flush shape Accu-Vu
  OmniMesh ablation
  OmniMesh bidirectional
  OmniMesh braided-tip
  one-hole angiographic
  OpenSail balloon
  Opta
  Opti-Flow angiography
  Opti-Flow dialysis
  Opti-Plast XT balloon
  Optiscope
  Optiva intravenous
  Oracle Focus PTCA
  Oracle Megasonics PTCA
  Oracle Micro
  Oracle Micro Plus PTCA
  Orbiter PV
  Orion balloon dilatation
  Outcomes by Design

catheter *(cont.)*
over-the-wire balloon
oximetric
Pace bipolar pacing
Paceport
Pacewedge dual-pressure bipolar
pacing
pacing
Parahisian pacing electrode
Parodi anti-embolization (PAEC)
Pathfinder
PA Watch position-monitoring
PentaCath 5-lumen thermodilution
PE Plus II balloon dilatation
Percor DL balloon
Percor DL-II balloon
Percor-Stat-DL
Percuflex APD all-purpose catheter
with Fader Tip
percutaneous
Performa angiographic
perfusion
Periflow peripheral balloon
peripherally inserted central (PICC)
PermCath double-lumen ventricular
access
pervenous
Phantom V Plus
PIBC (percutaneous intra-aortic
balloon counterpulsation)
Pico-ST II low-profile balloon
pigtail
PolarCath
Polaris-Dx steerable diagnostic
Polaris X steerable diagnostic
polyethylene
PolyFlo
Polystan venous return
Positrol II
Possis
PowerPICC
Predator angioplasty balloon

catheter *(cont.)*
preformed
preshaped
Primopac diagnostic
probing
ProCross Rely over-the-wire
balloon
Profile Plus dilatation
Proflex 5 dilatation
Pro-Flo
Propac diagnostic
Pruitt-Inahara balloon-tipped
perfusion
PTCA (percutaneous transluminal
coronary angioplasty)
pulmonary artery
pulmonary flotation
pulmonary triple-lumen
Pulse Spray infusion
quadpolar electrode
QuadraPulse radiofrequency
quadripolar electrode
quadripolar steerable electrode
Quantum Maverick coronary
balloon dilatation
Quantum PTCA
Quanticor
QuickFlash radial artery
Quinton
Qwikstart
Raaf Cath vascular
radial artery
Radius coronary stent delivery
RadPICC
Ranger PTCA
rapid-exchange PTCA balloon
angioplasty
Rapid-Trak
RaptorRail PTCA dilatation
Rashkind balloon
Rashkind septostomy balloon
Rebar microcatheters

catheter *(cont.)*

  recessed balloon septostomy
  RediFurl TaperSeal IAB
  RediGuard flexible IAB
  Rentrop infusion
  Resolve drainage
  Response electrophysiology
  retroperfusion
  Revelation microcatheter
  reverse Berman angiographic
    balloon
  RF (radiofrequency-generated
    thermal) balloon
  RF-Performr electrophysiology
    (*not* Performer)
  Rhythm, The
  RIC fluid exchange resuscitation
  right coronary
  right heart
  right Judkins
  Rivas vascular
  Robinson
  Rodriguez
  Rodriguez-Alvarez
  R1 Rapid Exchange balloon
  Royal Flush angiographic flush
  Rumel
  Sable balloon
  Samuels Micro-Scler
  Sarns wire-reinforced
  Schneider
  Schneider-Shiley
  Schoonmaker femoral
  Schoonmaker multipurpose
  Schwarten balloon
  Schwarten balloon dilatation
  SciMed NC Ranger PTCA
  SciMed SSC Skinny
  Scoring Balloon
  Select Performance balloon
    dilatation
  sensing

catheter *(cont.)*

  SET three-lumen thrombectomy
  serrated
  Shaldon
  shaver
  sheathless, flexible, pre-wrapped
    double-lumen IAB
  Shaldon
  Sherpa guiding
  Shiley guiding
  Shiley-Ionescu
  Skinny
  SHJR4s (side-hole Judkins right,
    curve 4, short)
  side-hole
  sidewinder
  Silastic
  Silicore
  silver-iontophoretic
  Simmons-type (sidewinder)
  Simplus PE/t dilatation
  Simpson peripheral AtheroCath
  Simpson Ultra Lo-Profile II balloon
  Simpson-Robert
  single-stage
  Sirius
  Slalom balloon dilatation
  SLIC
  sliding rail
  Slim-Cath
  Slinky PTCA (percutaneous
    transluminal coronary
    angioplasty)
  Smec balloon
  snare
  soaker
  Soft-Cell
  Softip arteriography
  Softip diagnostic
  Softouch guiding
  Soft-Vu Omni flush
  Sones cardiac

catheter *(cont.)*
Sones Cardio-Marker
Sones Hi-Flow
Sones Positrol
split sheath
Sprinter balloon
Spyglass angiography
Stack perfusion coronary dilatation
standard Lehman
StatLock hemodialysis
steerable electrode
Steri-Cath suction
Steerocath
Steerocath-A ablation
Steerocath-Dx octapolar and valve
mapping
Steerocath-T ablation
Stertzer brachial guiding
Stertzer guiding
Stimucath continuous nerve block
stimulating
Stinger
Stinger S ablation
Stinger SL
St. Jude 4F Supreme
Stormer balloon
Stormer over-the-wire balloon
dilatation
straight flush percutaneous
Sub-Microinfusion
SULP II
sump
Super Arrow-Flex central venous
SuperTorque diagnostic
SuperTorque Plus diagnostic
Supreme electrophysiology
surgically implanted hemodialysis
(SIHC)
Swan-Ganz balloon-flotation
pulmonary artery
Swan-Ganz flow-directed
Swan-Ganz Guidewire TD

catheter *(cont.)*
Swan-Ganz Pacing TD
Swan-Ganz thermodilution
swan-neck
Symbiant
Syntel latex-free embolectomy
TAC atherectomy
Tactilaze angioplasty laser
Tango
Tecothane
Teflon
temporary pacing
Tennis Racquet angiographic
tetrapolar esophageal
Texas
thermistor
thermodilution balloon
thermodilution pacing
thermodilution Swan-Ganz
thoracic
Thor angioplasty dilatation
three-way
thrombectomy
Thruflex PTCA balloon
Tiason
Titan Mega PTCA dilatation
Titan PTCA dilatation
toposcopic
Torcon NB selective angiographic
torque-directed nonballoon
torque tube
Tracker
Tracker-18 Soft Stream
transcutaneous extraction
transducer-tipped
transluminal extraction (TEC)
transseptal
transvenous pacemaker
trefoil balloon
Trellis infusion catheter and system
Trifusion
Triguide

catheter *(cont.)*
triple-lumen central venous
triple thermistor coronary sinus
tripolar
tripolar electrode
Twin Cath multiple peripheral
Tygon
ULP (ultra-low profile)
Ultra 8 balloon
Ultraflex intra-aortic balloon
UltraLite flow-directed micro
ultra-low profile fixed-wire balloon
    dilatation
UMI
universal IAB
U-Pass balloon
USCI Bard
USCI guiding
USCI Mini-Profile balloon
    dilatation
valvuloplasty balloon
Van Andel
Van Tassel pigtail
Vaxcel peripherally inserted central
V-Cath
V-Cath ML
Vector large-lumen guiding
VectorX large-lumen guiding
Venaport guiding
VenaSonix ultrasound
venous
venous thrombectomy
venting
Ventra
ventricular
ventriculography
Veripath peripheral guiding
vessel-sizing
VIPER PTA
Visa II PTCA
VisCath fiberoptic imaging
Visease angiographic

catheter *(cont.)*
Vision PTCA
Vista Brite Tip guiding
Vitesse E-II eccentric, rapid-
    exchange coronary
VNUS Closure
VNUS Restore
Voda
Vueport balloon-occlusion guiding
Was-Cath catheter for percutaneous
    thromboendarterectomy
Webster Compli diagnostic
Webster coronary sinus
Webster orthogonal electrode
Wexler
Williams L-R guiding
Wilton-Webster coronary sinus
Wishard
Workhorse percutaneous
    transluminal angioplasty balloon
XMI
Xpeedior 60
Xpeedior 100
X-Sept
Xtent
X-Trode electrode catheter
    for intravenous insertion
    into a heart cavity
Zipper angioplasty
Zipper balloon
Z-Med catheter
Zucker
Zuma guiding
catheter ablation with use of pulsed
    fluoroscopy
catheter advanced under fluoroscopic
    guidance
catheter artifact
catheter balloon valvuloplasty
catheter-based intervention
catheter coated with cefazolin
catheter damping

catheter deployment
catheter-directed thrombolysis
catheter electrode
catheter embraced by plaque
catheter exchanged over a guidewire
catheter impact artifact
catheter inched up the artery
catheter-induced bacteremia
catheter-induced coronary artery spasm
catheterization
  antegrade transseptal left heart
  cardiac
  central venous (CVC)
  femoral artery (or arterial)
  Fogarty balloon
  heart
  left heart
  Mullins modification of transseptal
  PTCA (percutaneous transluminal
    coronary angioplasty)
  retrograde
  retrograde arterial
  retrograde left heart
  right heart
  selective cardiac
  simultaneous right and left heart
  subclavian vein
  transseptal cardiac
  transseptal heart
  transseptal left heart
  transvenous
catheterizing
catheter kinking
catheter locator system, CathTrack
catheter mapping
catheter migration
catheter passage, tortuosity precluding
catheter-related false aneurysm
catheter sheath
catheter-skin interface
catheter tip hockey-stick appearance
catheter tip motion artifact

catheter-tipped manometer
catheter-tissue contact
catheter vitrector
catheter whip artifact
catheter with preformed curves
CathLink implantable vascular access
  device
Cathmark suction catheter
cathodal lead
cathodal patch electrode, posterior
cathode
  defibrillation
  epicardial patch
CathScanner ultrasound imaging
  system
CathTrack catheter locator system
caudad
caudal branch
caudal collaterals
caudal view
causative organism
causative virus
cautery
cautious dissection
cava (pl. cavae)
  inferior vena
  juxtarenal
  superior vena
caval-atrial (or cavoatrial) junction
caval-pulmonary artery anastomosis
caval snare
caval thrombolysis
caval tourniquet
CAVB (complete atrioventricular
  block)
CAVD (cardiac allograft vascular
  disease)
cavernous angioma
cavernous angiosarcoma
cavernous breath sounds
cavernous breathing
cavernous hemangioma

Caves-Schulz bioptome
CAVH (continuous arteriovenous hemofiltration)
cavitary lung mass
cavitary mass
cavitary tuberculosis
cavitating carcinoma
cavitation
Cavitron ultrasonic aspirator (CUSA)
Cavitron ultrasonic surgical aspirator (CUSA)
cavity
  coexistent
  pericardial
  pseudoaneurysm
  pulmonary
  thoracic
cavity in the lung
cavoatrial (cavo-atrial) anastomosis
cavoatrial (caval-atrial) junction
cavogram
cavopulmonary anastomosis, bidirectional
cavopulmonary connection
cavopulmonary connection baffle, total
Cayler syndrome
CBAS (Carmeda bioactive surface)
CBAS external or implantable ventricular assist device (VAD)
CBAS stent-graft
CBAS vascular graft
CBAS vascular stent
CBC (complete blood cell count)
  hematocrit
  hemoglobin
  MCH (mean corpuscular hemoglobin)
  MCHC (mean corpuscular hemoglobin concentration)
  MCV (mean corpuscular volume)
  RBC (red blood cell) count
  WBC (white blood cell) count

CBC with diff (differential)
CBC with WBC and differential
CBFV (cerebral blood flow velocity)
CBG (cord blood gases)
CBS (capillary blood sugar)
CBV (catheter balloon valvuloplasty)
CC (closing capacity)
CCA (common carotid artery)
CCB (calcium channel blocker)
C-C (convexo-concave) heart valve
CCO (continuous cardiac output)
CCOmbo catheter
cc/min. (cubic centimeters per minute)
C, C, or E (clubbing, cyanosis, or edema)
CCU (coronary care unit) protocol
CCU (critical care unit) protocol
CD (conduction defect)
CD (color Doppler)
CD5+ monoclonal antibody
CD18 antibodies
CDI blood gas-monitoring system
CDP (computerized dynamic posturography)
CDP (continuous descending pressure)
CDP (continuous distending pressure)
C_{dyn} (dynamic lung compliance)
CE (capillary electrophoresis)
CE (conjugated estrogens)
CEA (carcinoembryonic antigen)
CEA (carotid endarterectomy)
C-E amplitude of mitral valve
CEAP (clinical, etiologic, anatomic, pathophysiologic) classification
CECG (continuous electrocardiographic monitoring)
Cedars-Sinai classification of pump failure
Ceelen-Gellerstedt syndrome
cefazolin and dextrose treatment of respiratory tract infections
cefazolin, catheter coated with

Cegka sign
celer, pulsus (quick pulse)
C-11 (^{11}C) (carbon-11)
C-11 acetate imaging
C-11 hydroxylase deficiency
C-11 palmitate uptake on PET scan
celiac angiography
celiac artery
celiac artery compression syndrome
celiac axis syndrome
cell, cells
    adventitial
    air
    airway epithelial
    alveolar (type I or II)
    Anichkov (or Anitschkow)
    APUD (amine precursor uptake and
        decarboxylation)
    Aschoff
    automatic
    basket
    Beale ganglion
    bend
    blood
    bronchic
    caterpillar
    chicken-wire myocardial
    Clara
    dust
    endothelioid
    epithelioid
    FACS (fluorescence-activated cell
        sorter)-sorted
    foamy myocardial
    goblet
    heart-disease
    heart-failure
    heart-lesion
    large undifferentiated (LUCs)
    Marchand
    mast
    mononuclear

cell *(cont.)*
    multidrug resistance-associated
        protein (MRP)-positive tumor
    multinucleate giant
    myocardial
    oat
    oat-shaped
    P
    pacemaker
    packed red blood
    perithelial
    perivascular
    plasma
    pleomorphic mononuclear
    pulmonary capillary endothelial
    pulmonary epithelial
    Purkinje
    spider
    strap
    T
    tennis racquet
    transitional
    vascular smooth muscle (VSMCs)
    virus-infected
Cellano phenotype
cell count
CellGen electrotherapy device
cell necrosis, myocardial
cellophane rales
Cell-Saver autotransfuser
cell saver, BRAT
Cell-Saver Haemolite
Cell-Saver Haemonetics Auto-
    transfusion System
cell seeding (of vascular grafts)
Celltrifuge
cellular debris
cellular hypo-osmolality
cellular infiltrates
cellular infiltration
cellulitis
cellulitis-phlebitis

cell washings for cytologic study
Celsior organ preservation solution
Celsius control endovascular catheter
Cenflex central monitoring system
centistoke
central alpha-agonists
central aortic pressure
central aortic pulse pressure
central aortopulmonary shunting
central apnea
central arterial return
central blood volume
central cyanosis
central fibrous body
central hilar structures
central hypoventilation
central intra-aortic pressure curve
central jet
central lesion
central splanchnic venous thrombosis
   (CSVT)
central vein, cannulated
central venous catheter (CVC)
central venous line
central venous line placement
central venous pressure (CVP)
central venous pressure elevation
centriacinar emphysema
centrifugal mechanical assist (CMA)
centrifugal pump system
   Medtronic/Bio-Medicus 520
   Medtronic/Bio-Medicus 540
   Sarns Delphin 9000
   Sarns 7800
centrilobular emphysema
cephalad
cephalic vein, cutdown over
cephalization of pulmonary flow
   pattern
CeQUAL protocol
ceramidase deficiency
ceramide trihexosidase deficiency

cerebellar intracerebral hemorrhage
cerebral aneurysm
cerebral anoxia
cerebral arteries
cerebral arteriovenous fistula
cerebral blood flow velocity (CBFV)
cerebral edema
cerebral palsy (CP)
cerebral perfusion pressure (CPP)
Cerebrence guidewire
Cerebrence guiding catheter
Cerebrence stent
cerebrocardiac syndrome
Ceredur vascular access port
Ceresine
Ceretec technetium 99m (Tc-99m)
   imaging agent
Certofix central venous catheter
cervical aortic arch
cervicomediastinal venous trauma,
   penetrating
chagoma
chain, respiratory
chamber, superficial pseudoaneurysm
Chameleon guidewire
Champ cardiac device
chaotic ventricular depolarization,
   diffuse
characteristic right and left lung
   asymmetry
Charger balloon catheter
Chaux retractor
Checkmate intravascular brachytherapy
   system
Checkmate system, Cordis
Cheetah angioplasty catheter
Chemo-Cath catheter
chemoradiation protocol
chemostat culture
chemotherapy, induction
cherry angioma
cherry-red endobronchial lesions
   of Kaposi sarcoma

chest
  alar
  barrel
  blast
  cobbler's
  congestion in the
  cylindrical
  flail
  flat
  foveated
  funnel
  globular
  heaviness in the
  hollow
  keeled
  pain in the
  paralytic
  phthinoid (flat)
  pigeon
  pounding
  pressure in the
  pterygoid (flat)
  rawness in the
  symmetrical
  tetrahedron
  tightness in the
chest drainage unit
chest physiotherapy (PT)
chest PT (physical therapy)
chest shell
chest thoracostomy site infection
chest tightness, waking with
chest tomograms
chest tube (see *tube*)
chest tube breakage upon removal
chest wall
  anterior
  lower
  upper
chest wall compliance
chest wall fixation
chest wall flattening

chest wall invasion
chest wall pain
chest wall paradoxical motion
chest wall phlebitis
chest wall tenderness
chest wall retractions
chest x-ray (CXR) (see *position*; *view*)
  AP (anteroposterior)
  baseline
  contralateral decubitus
  lateral
  PA (posteroanterior)
  portable
chevron incision
Cheyne-Stokes breathing
Cheyne-Stokes respiration
CHF (congestive heart failure)
CH50 or CH_{50} (total hemolytic
  complement)
Chiari-Budd syndrome
Chiari I malformation
Chiari syndrome
chicken fat clot
chicken-wire myocardial cell
Child class (A, B, and C) classification
  system for esophageal varices
Child classification of hepatic risk
  criteria
Child-Pugh class A, B, or C hepatic
  disease
Child-Turcotte hepatic surgery classification
Child-Turcotte-Pugh classification
  of cirrhosis
childhood asthma
childhood tuberculosis
chills
  brass
  brazier
  creeping
  fever and
  periodic

chills *(cont.)*
  shaking
  spelter
  teeth-chattering
  zinc
chiral asymmetry
Chlamydia pneumoniae
Chlamydia trachomatis
Chlamydia psittaci
Chloraprep One-Step (chlorhexidine
  gluconate; isopropyl alcohol)
chloral hydrate
chloride, chlorides
chlorotic phlebitis
chlorpromazine
choking
Cholestagel (colesevelam hydrochloride)
Cholestech LDX system with the TC
  (total cholesterol) and glucose panel
cholesterol
  bad
  good
  serum
  total plasma
cholesterol-carrying lipoproteins
cholesterol cleft
cholesterol crystal embolization,
  atheromatous
cholesterol debris
cholesterol effusion
cholesterol embolism
cholesterol embolization
  diffuse
  disseminated
cholesterol embolization syndrome
  peripheral
  renal
  visceral
cholesterol ester storage disease
Cholesterol Manager home cholesterol
  management kit

cholesterol microembolization in toes
Cholesterol 1,2,3 noninvasive testing
  device
cholesterol pericarditis syndrome
cholesterol pleurisy
CholesTrak test kit
chondromatous hamartoma
chondrosternal junction
chordae (pl. of chorda)
  basal
  cleft
  commissural
  elongation of
  first order
  redundant
  ruptured
  second order
  shortening of
  strut
  third order
chordae tendineae cordis
  redundant
  ruptured
chordae tendineae rupture
chordal insertion
chordal length
chordal rupture
chorditis, fibrinous
chorditis nodosa
chorditis tuberosa
chorea
  cordis
  rheumatic
  Sydenham
choreiform movements, postoperative
choreoathetosis, postoperative
chorioangiosis
Chorus dual-chamber pacemaker
Chorus II dual-chamber pacemaker
Chorus RM rate-responsive dual-
  chamber pacemaker
CHRF (chronic hypercapnic respiratory failure)

Christmas blood coagulation factor
Christmas coagulation factor IX
Christmas disease (hemophilia B)
chromatography, gas
chromic catgut sutures
chromic suture
chromosome 22q11-13 deletion
chromosome 22q11.2 deletion
chronic airways obstruction
chronic allergic rhinitis
chronic allograft dysfunction
chronic arterial occlusive disease of
    extremities
chronic asthmatic diathesis
chronic atrial fibrillation with slow
    ventricular response
chronic bronchiectasis
chronic bronchitis
chronic constrictive pericarditis
chronic discoloration of skin
chronic effusive pericarditis
chronic emphysema
chronic emphysematous mountain
    sickness
chronic eosinophilic pneumonia
chronic erythremic mountain sickness
chronic granulomatous disease
    of childhood
chronic heart failure
chronic hemodynamic overload
chronic humoral rejection
chronic hypercapnic respiratory failure
    (CHRF)
chronic hypertensive disease
chronic hypertrophic emphysema
chronic hypertrophic myocarditis
chronic hyperventilation syndrome
chronic hypoxia
Chronicle implantable hemodynamic
    monitor
chronic indolent bacterial infection
chronic interstitial myocarditis

chronic intractable cough
chronic lead placement
chronic lung embolization by blood-
    borne eggs
chronic lunger
chronic mountain sickness
    emphysematous-type
    erythremic-type
chronic myeloid leukemia (CML)
chronic myelomonocytic leukemia
    (CMML)
chronic nasopharyngitis
chronic necrotizing infection of
    bronchi
chronic obstructive bronchitis
chronic obstructive emphysema
chronic obstructive lung disease
    (COLD)
chronic obstructive pulmonary disease
    (COPD)
chronic parenchymal hemorrhage
chronic passive congestion of the lung
chronic pericarditis
chronic pernicious myocarditis
chronic pleural empyema
chronic pleurisy
chronic pneumonitis
chronic post-rheumatic fever arthritis
chronic pulmonary disease
chronic pulmonary emphysema (CPE)
chronic rejection of transplanted lung
chronic renal failure
chronic respiratory decompensation
chronic rheumatic heart disease
    (CRHD)
chronic rheumatic mediastinoperi-
    carditis
chronic rheumatic myopericarditis
chronic salicylate ingestion
chronic thromboembolic hypertension
chronic thromboembolic pulmonary
    hypertension

chronic venous insufficiency (CVI)
chronic vessel closure
Chronocor IV external pacemaker
Chronofusor infusion pump
chronotropic assessment exercise
    protocol (CAEP)
chronotropic effect
chronotropic incompetence
chronotropic response, blunted
chronotropic therapy
CHUK (conserved helix-loop-helix
    ubiquitous kinase) protein
chunky sputum
Churchill-Cope reflex
Church scissors
Churg-Strauss angiitis
Churg-Strauss syndrome
Churg-Strauss vasculitis
chyle
    effused
    pericardial
chyliform pleurisy
chylocele, nonfilarial
chyloid pleurisy
chylomicron
chylomicronemia, familial
chylopericardium
chylothorax (pl. chylothoraces)
chylous ascites
chylous pleurisy
CI (cardiac index)
Ciaglia percutaneous tracheostomy
    introducer
Cibatome
CIC (circulating immune complex)
ciclesonide
CIE (counterimmunoelectrophoresis)
    of sputum
CIG (cardiointegram)
cigarette abuse
cigarette smoking, pack-years of

cilia
    dyskinetic
    immotile
ciliated border
Cinch QR steerable guidewire
cinchonism
cineangiocardiography
cineangiogram, cineangiography
    biplane
    coronary
    left anterior oblique (LAO)
    left posterior oblique (LPO)
    left ventricular (LV)
    radionuclide
    right anterior oblique (RAO)
    right posterior oblique (RPO)
    selective coronary
    Sones technique for
    ventricular
cinecardioangiography
cine CT (computed tomography)
    scanner
cinefluorography
cine loop (noun), cine-loop (adj.)
cine magnetic resonance, tagging
cineradiographic views
cineradiography
cine view in MUGA (cinematograph in
    multiple gated acquisition) scan
circ, CF, CX (circumflex artery)
Circadia dual-chamber rate-adaptive
    pacemaker
circadian event recorder
circadian periodicity
circadian rhythm of plasma aldosterone
circle of Vieussens
circle of Willis
CircPlus compression dressing
circuit
    arrhythmia
    Bentley Duraflo II extracorporeal
        perfusion

circuit *(cont.)*
  bypass
  Fontan
  macroreentrant
  microreentrant
  reentry
  shunting
circular aortotomy
circular cherry-red lesion
circular muscles
circular plane
circular shape factor
circular syncytium
circulating aldosterone level
circulating blood
circulating blood cells
circulating blood volume
circulating catecholamines
circulating fibrinogen pool
circulating immune complex (CIC)
circulating immune complex antibodies
circulating lymphocytes
circulating renin
circulating water blanket
circulation
  abundant collateral
  adequate collateral
  allantoic
  arrested
  assisted
  balanced coronary
  bronchial collateral
  codominant
  codominant coronary
  collateral
  compensatory
  derivative
  extracorporeal
  fetal
  greater
  intervillous
  left circumflex-dominant

circulation *(cont.)*
  left-dominant coronary
  lesser
  parasitic
  peripheral
  persistent fetal
  placental
  poor collateral
  portal
  precarious
  pulmonary
  pulmonary arterial
  reduced
  right-dominant coronary
  systemic
  thebesian
circulation time
Circulon dressing or wrap
circulatory abnormalities, occult
circulator boot therapy
circulatory arrest
  profound hypothermic (PHCA)
  profoundly hypothermic total
circulatory assist devices
circulatory collapse
circulatory compromise
circulatory disturbances
circulatory embarrassment
circulatory failure
circulatory hyperkinetic syndrome
circulatory impairment
circulatory shock
circulatory stasis
circulatory support device, Elecath
circulatory support, mechanical
circumferential dissection
circumferential echodense layer
circumferential suture
circumflex (circ, CF, CX)
circumflex artery
circumflex branches
circumflex coronary artery

circumflex coronary system
circumflex groove artery
circumflex system
circumflex vessels
circumoral cyanosis
circumoral flush
circumoral pallor
circumscribed edema
circumscribed pleurisy
circumscript aneurysm
circumscript lesion
circus movement
circus-movement tachycardia (CMT)
CIRF (cocaine-induced respiratory
   failure)
CirKuit-Guard device
cirrhosis
   cardiac
   congestive
   liver
   lung
   pulmonary
   vascular
cirsenchysis
cirsocele
cirsodesis ("sur-sod-ee-sis")
cirsoid aneurysm
cirsotome
cirsotomy
citrate regional anticoagulation
Citrobacter
CK (creatine kinase)
CK/AST or CK-AST ratio
CK isoenzymes (see *isoenzymes*)
CKG (cardiokymography)
CK-MB (creatine kinase-muscle band)
CL (cycle length)
clamminess
clammy skin
clamp or clip
   Adams-DeWeese vena caval clip
   Alfred M. Large vena cava

clamp *(cont.)*
   Allis
   Allis-Adair
   anastomosis
   angled peripheral vascular
   aortic
   aortic aneurysm
   aortic occlusion
   appendage
   atraumatic vascular
   Atrauclip hemostatic
   Atraumax
   Atricure bipolar radiofrequency
   Bahnson aortic
   Bailey aortic
   Beck
   Beck aortic
   Beck miniature aortic
   Beck-Potts
   Beck vascular
   Berman aortic
   Blalock pulmonary
   Brock
   bulldog
   Calman carotid artery
   Calman ring
   Castaneda
   Castaneda anastomosis
   Castaneda vascular
   celiac
   coarctation
   Cooley
   Cooley anastomosis
   Cooley aortic
   Cooley-Beck
   Cooley coarctation
   Cooley-Derra anastomosis
   Cooley iliac
   Cooley partial occlusion
   Cooley patent ductus
   Cooley pediatric
   Cooley renal

124

clamp *(cont.)*
  Cooley-Satinsky
  Cooley vascular
  Cooley vena cava catheter
  Crafoord aortic
  Crafoord coarctation
  Crile
  curved
  curved Cooley
  Davidson vessel
  Davis aneurysm
  DeBakey aortic aneurysm
  DeBakey arterial
  DeBakey-Bahnson vascular
  DeBakey-Bainbridge
  DeBakey-Beck
  DeBakey bulldog
  DeBakey coarctation
  DeBakey cross-action bulldog
  DeBakey-Derra anastomosis
  DeBakey-Harken
  DeBakey-Howard
  DeBakey-Kay
  DeBakey patent ductus
  DeBakey pediatric
  DeBakey peripheral vascular
    bulldog
  DeBakey-Reynolds anastomosis
  DeBakey ring-handled bulldog
  DeBakey-Semb
  DeBakey tangential occlusion
  DeBakey vascular
  DeMartel vascular
  Demos tibial artery
  DeWeese vena cava
  double-occluding
  exclusion
  Fogarty
  Fogarty Hydragrip
  Fogarty-Chin
  Garcia aortic
  Gerbode patent ductus

clamp *(cont.)*
  Glassman
  Glover coarctation
  Glover patent ductus
  Glover vascular
  Glycoprene surgical
  Goldblatt
  Grant aneurysm
  Gregory baby profunda
  Gregory carotid bulldog
  Gregory external
  Greyhound surgical spring
  Gross coarctation occlusion
  Grover
  Gutgeman
  Harken auricle
  Heifitz
  hemostatic
  Henley vascular
  Hopkins aortic
  Hufnagel aortic
  Intelli-Clamp vascular occlusion
  Intelli-Clip vascular occlusion
  Jacobson-Potts
  Jahnke anastomosis
  Javid carotid artery
  Johns Hopkins coarctation
  Jones thoracic
  Kapp-Beck
  Kapp-Beck-Thomson
  Kay aortic
  Kindt carotid artery occlusion
  Lactoprene surgical
  Lambert aortic
  Lambert-Kay aortic
  Lambert-Kay vascular
  Lee microvascular
  Leland-Jones vascular
  Liddle aorta
  Ligaclip
  long Péan
  Mason vascular

clamp *(cont.)*
 Mattox aorta
 Max-Prene surgical
 metal
 metallic
 Michel aortic
 microvascular
 Mixter
 Mixter right-angle
 Morris aorta
 mosquito
 Muller pediatric
 noncrushing vascular
 Noon AV fistula
 occluding
 Omed bulldog vascular
 Osteoprene surgical
 partially occluding vascular
 partial-occlusion
 patent ductus
 Péan
 pediatric bulldog
 pediatric vascular
 portal venous
 Potts aortic
 Potts coarctation
 Potts patent ductus
 Potts-Satinsky
 Potts-Smith aortic occlusion
 Raney
 Reinhoff
 Reynolds vascular
 Right Clip
 right-angle
 Rumel myocardial
 Rumel thoracic
 Sarot bronchus
 Satinsky aortic
 Satinsky vascular
 Satinsky vena cava
 Schnidt *(not* Schmidt)
 Schwartz

clamp *(cont.)*
 Sehrt
 Selverstone carotid
 side-biting
 silver
 sponge
 spoon
 stainless steel
 Stille-Crawford
 straight
 Subramanian
 Sugita right-angle aneurysm
 Swan aortic
 Thompson carotid artery
 tissue occlusion
 tube-occluding
 tubing
 vascular
 VCS clip applier
 Wangensteen anastomosis
 Wangensteen patent ductus
 Weber aortic
 Weck
 Wister vascular
 Wylie carotid artery
 Yasargil carotid
clamp-and-sew technique
clamping
 endoaortic balloon
 prolonged aortic
clamshell incision
Clamshell Occluder
clapping
Clara cells
Clarinex (desloratadine)
Clarke-Hadefield syndrome
Clarke-Reich micro knot pusher
Clark oxygen electrode
classical angina
classical hemophilia
classical triad of symptoms
classic Glenn procedure

classic interstitial pneumonia
classification (see also *criteria, index, score*)
  AHA (American Heart Association)
  AHA stenosis
  ASA (American Society of Anesthesia) risk
  Canadian system (I-IV) for severity of angina
  CEAP (clinical, etiologic, anatomic, pathophysiologic)
  Cedars-Sinai pump failure
  Child's class (A, B, and C)
  Child's classification of hepatic risk criteria
  Child-Turcotte hepatic surgery
  Child-Turcotte-Pugh cirrhosis
  Croften (for pulmonary eosino-philia)
  DeBakey (type I, II, III) (of aortic dissection)
  Dexter-Grossman mitral regurgitation
  Dubin and Amelar varicocele
  Fredrickson and Lees hyperlipo-proteinemia (types I-V)
  Fredrickson hyperlipoproteinemia
  Goldman
  Heath-Edwards
  Keith-Wagener-Barker (arteriolo-sclerosis, group 1-4)
  Killip heart disease
  Killip-Kimball heart failure
  Killip pump failure
  Lev complete AV (atrioventricular) block
  Levine-Harvey heart murmur
  Liebow and Carrington (for pulmonary eosinophilia)
  Lown ventricular arrhythmia
  Lown ventricular premature beat
  Minnesota EKG

classification *(cont.)*
  Mobitz atrioventricular block
  NYHA (New York Heart Association)
  NYHA angina (I-IV or A-D)
  NYHA congestive heart failure
  NYHA heart block, I-IV
  Pulec and Freedman (of congenital aural atresia)
  Stanford (type A, B, etc.) (of aortic dissection
  TIMI (thrombolysis in myocardial infarction) (II, IIA, etc.)
  Vaughan-Williams antiarrhythmic drugs
classification of aortic dissection
classification of cardiomyopathy
Classix pacemaker
claudicant
claudication
  buttock
  calf
  hip
  intermittent
  intermittent venous
  leg
  lifestyle-limiting
  lower extremity
  non-lifestyle-limiting
  one-block
  one-flight
  progressive
  thigh
  three-block
  two-block
  two-flights-of-stairs
  venous
Clauss modified method of plasma fibrinogen measurement
claustrophobic anxiety
claviclotomy technique
claviculectomy technique

claviculotomy technique
claw grasper
Claybrook sign
CLE (congenital lobar emphysema)
Clean-Cath single use catheter
cleanser (see *wound cleanser*)
clear airway
clearance, creatinine
clear cell carcinoma of kidney
ClearCut 2 device
clearly demarcated borders
ClearSite borderless dressing
ClearSite Hydro Gauze dressing
clear to auscultation and percussion
  (CTAP)
ClearView CO_2 laser
clear viscous sputum
clear zone
cleavage plane, subintimal
cleaving, plaque
cleft
  cholesterol
  horizontal chin
  Sondergaard
cleft chordae
cleft mitral valve
Clerc-Levy-Cristeco (CLC) syndrome
click
  aortic
  aortic ejection (AEC)
  aortic opening (AOC)
  apical midsystolic
  ejection (EC)
  fixed aortic ejection
  late systolic
  loud
  low-intensity systolic
  midsystolic
  mitral
  nonejection (NEC)
  nonejection systolic (NESC)
  palpable ejection

click *(cont.)*
  pulmonary ejection (PEC)
  systolic (SC)
  systolic ejection
  systolic nonejection
  valvular
Clickhaler
click louder when patient sits up
click murmur
click of maximal intensity when patient
  stands
clinical diagnosis
clinical disease, manifestation of overt
clinical picture
clinical remission
clinical sequelae
clinically significant
CliniCath peripherally inserted catheter
clinometry
clip (see *clamp*)
clip applier, VCS
Clip On torquer
clipping, aneurysm
CLO (congenital lobar overinflation)
clockwise rotation of electrical axis on
  EKG
clockwise torque, constant (of
  electrode tip)
clonidine
cloning
Clonorchis sinensis infection
closed lung biopsy
closed pleural biopsy
closed transventricular aortic
  valvotomy
closed tube thoracotomy
Closer, The, closure device
CloseSure suture procedure kit
closing capacity (CC)
closing volume (CV)
clostridial infection

closure
  abrupt
  abrupt vessel
  acute vessel
  bronchus
  chronic vessel
  delayed sternal
  double umbrella
  ductus arteriosus
  impending
  patch
  patent ductus arteriosus
  patent ductus arteriosus (by double
    umbrella device)
  primary
  pulmonary valve
  Robicsek
  secondary
  staged
  subcuticular
  subcuticular skin
  threatened vessel, post-PTCA
  tricuspid valve
  valve
  vein patch
closure of defect, spontaneous
closure of native aortic valve
closure system by VNUS
Clo-Sur P.A.D. hemostatic dressing
clot
  agonal (or agony)
  antemortem
  autologous
  blood
  calcified
  chicken fat
  currant jelly
  distal
  fibrin
  heart
  internal
  laminated

clot *(cont.)*
  marantic
  passive
  plastic
  postmortem
  proximal
  preformed
  red
  stratified
  washed
  white
clot-dissolving mechanism
clot-dissolving treatment of coronary
  thrombosis
clot formation
clot lysis
clots and debris
clotted blood
clotting process
clotting time of whole blood
clouded consciousness
clouding of consciousness
cloudy swelling of the heart
Cloverleaf catheter
cloverleaf-shaped lumen
CLC (Clerc-Levy-Cristeco) syndrome
clubbing and cyanosis
clubbing, cyanosis, or edema
  (C, C, or E)
clubbing
  digital
  finger
clubbing of fingernails
clubbing of fingers and toes
clubbing of fingertips
clubbing of nail beds
clumps of sickled red cells
CM (continuous murmur)
CMA (centrifugal mechanical assist)
CM5 lead
CML (chronic myeloid leukemia)
CMML (chronic myelomonocytic
  leukemia)

CMR (congenital mitral regurgitation)
CMT (circus-movement tachycardia)
CMV (cytomegalovirus)
CNT (continuous nebulization therapy)
CO_2 (carbon dioxide)
CO (cardiac output) (L/min)
coags (slang for coagulation studies)
CoaguChek self-testing device
coagulability of the blood
coagulable
coagulase-negative staphylococci
coagulase-positive *Staphylococcus aureus*
Coagulin-B therapy drug for hemophilia B
coagulation
  bipolar
  disseminated (or diffuse) intra-vascular (DIC)
  electric
  endovascular
coagulation cascade
coagulation factors of blood
  I: fibrinogen
  II: prothrombin
  III: thromboplastin
  IV: calcium ions
  V: proaccelerin (or AcG, accelerator globulin)
  VI: no factor VI
  VII: proconvertin (or SPCA, serum prothrombin conversion accelerator)
  VIII: antihemophilic (AHF) (von Willebrand)
  IX: plasma thromboplastin component (PTC) (Christmas)
  X: Stuart (or Stuart-Prower)
  XI: plasma thromboplastin antecedent (PTA)
  XII: Hageman
  XIII: fibrin stabilizing (FSF)

coagulation inhibitors
coagulation monitor, Biotrack
coagulator
  Biceps bipolar
  Concept bipolar
coagulopathic
coagulopathy
  consumption
  disseminated intravascular
coal miner's lung
coal worker's lung
coal worker's pneumoconiosis
Coanda effect
coaptation of valve leaflets
coaptation point
coapted leaflets
coarctation
  aortic
  atypical
  atypical subisthmic
  congenital isthmic
  isthmic
  juxtaductal
  preductal
  reversed
coarctation of aorta
  adult-type
  infantile-type
  juxtaductal
  postductal
  preductal
  reversed
coarctation repair
coarctectomy
coarcted aorta
coarcted segment
CoA reductase
coarse appearance
coarse bronchovascular markings
coarse crackles
coarse friction rub
coarse nodularity

coarse rales
coarse rhonchi
coarse sibilant expiratory rhonchi
coarse streaking
coarse thickening of interstitial
    structures
coated with cefazolin, catheter
coating
    ArmorGlide
    bioactive
    BioGlide
    Hepacoat
    Hydro-Glide
    HydroPlus
    Pro/Pel
coaxial catheter
coaxial catheter tip position
coaxial steering
Coban elastic dressing
cobbler chest syndrome
Cobe BRAT autotransfusion system
Cobe CPS heart-lung machine
Cobe Sentry arterial filter
    with PrimeGard
COBE Spectra Apheresis System
Cobe-Stockert dual head pump module
Cobe-Stockert heart-lung machine
COBE 2991 Cell Processor device
Coblation (trademark coined from
    cool ablation)
Cobra catheter
cobra-head appearance
cobra-head effect
Cobra over-the-wire balloon catheter
cobra venom factor (for myocardial
    ischemia)
cocaine-induced arrhythmias
cocaine-induced myocardial infarcts
cocaine-induced respiratory failure
    (CIRF)
cocaine-related cardiac death
cocaine-related fatal arrhythmias

cocaine-related fatal myocardial
    infarcts
cocci, gram-negative
Coccidioides immitis
coccidioidin test
coccidioidoma
coccidioidomycosis
    asymptomatic
    desert
    disseminated
    latent
    Posadas-Wernicke
    primary
    progressive
    San Joaquin Valley
    secondary
    valley
coccidioidal granuloma
coccidioidosis
coccidiosis
coccoid x bodies
Cockayne syndrome
cocktail, renal
Code Blue
codominant circulation
codominant coronary circulation
codominant system
codominant vessel
CO_2 (carbon dioxide) electrode
CO_2 (carbon dioxide) production
coenzyme Q10
coeur en sabot (on x-ray)
coexistent cavity
coexisting disease
coffee worker's lung
Coffin-Siris syndrome
CoFoam hydrophilic polyurethane
    composite
cognitive dysfunction
cognitive symptoms
cogwheel breathing
Coherent VersaPulse device

Cohiba arteriotomy closure device
Cohn cardiac stabilizer
coil
    defibrillation
    endoesophageal MRI
    Gianturco
    Gianturco occlusion
    Gianturco wool-tufted wire
    High Performance Detach
       embolization
    proximal
    right ventricular
    surface
    SynerG detachable coil system
coil closure of coronary artery fistula
coil embolization (therapeutic),
    percutaneous
coil embolization of fistula to
    pulmonary artery
coil embolization of unwanted vessel
coil occlusion
coil puller, In-Time
coil soaked in thrombin
coil-tipped catheter
coil-to-vessel diameter
coin lesion (on x-ray)
coin sound
coin test for pneumothorax
CO_2 laser
COLD (chronic obstructive lung
    disease)
cold agglutinin titer
cold agglutinins
cold blood cardioplegia
cold blood hyperkalemic cardioplegic
    solution
cold cardioplegia
cold cardioplegia arrest
cold cardioplegic solution
cold crystalloid cardioplegia
cold exposure
cold extremities

cold-induced angina
cold lactated Ringer solution
coldness of lower extremities
cold potassium cardioplegia
cold potassium solution-induced
    cardiac arrest
cold pressor stimulation
cold pressor test (Hines and Brown
    test)
cold retrograde blood cardioplegia
cold spot myocardial imaging (thallium
    imaging, thallium scintigraphy)
cold stimulation test for Raynaud
    syndrome
Cole-Cecil murmur
colesevelam hydrochloride
Colinet-Caplan syndrome
CollaCote collagen wound dressing
collagen (see also *hemostatic material*
    or sponge)
    Avitene
    bucrylate
    Collastat
    Contigen glutaraldehyde cross-
       linked
    cryoprecipitate
    Endo-Avitene
    Helitene fibrils
    Hemaflex sheath
    Hemopad
    Hemotene
    Instat MCH (microfibrillar
       hemostat)
    Surgical Nu-Knit hemostatic
       material
    Surgicel
    Unilab Surgibone
    Zyderm I or II
collagen absorbable suture
collagen degeneration
collagen hemostat
collagen hemostatic material
    for wounds

collagen-impregnated knitted Dacron
  velour graft
collagenosis, cardiac
collagenous deposits in alveolar septa
collagenous fibers
collagenous pneumoconiosis
collagen tissue proliferation
collagen vascular disease
collagen vascular screen (test)
collapse
  airway
  alveolar
  carotid pulse
  circulatory
  complete lung
  hemodynamic
  left lower lobe
  lung field
  massive lung
  partial lung
collapsed lung field
collapsed portion of lung
collapse of alveoli
collapse of jugular venous pressure
collapse of venous pulse, diastolic
collapsing pulse
collar incision
collar prosthesis
collar, tracheostomy
Collastat collagen hemostatic sponge
CollaTape used with wound dressing
collateral, collaterals
  antegrade
  aortopulmonary
  arcade of
  bridging
  caudal
  filled by
  filling via
  gives
  left to right
  persistent congenital stenosed

collateral *(cont.)*
  receives
  retrograde
  right to left
  septal
  venous
collateral blood flow
collateral blood supply
collateral branch
collateral circulation
  abundant
  adequate
  bronchial
collateral hyperemia
collateralization, distal
collateralization of the airways
collateral supply
collateral system
collateral vessel filling
collateral vessels
CollectFirst autotransfusion system
collecting system, engorged
collection, loculated
collection of fluid in pleural cavity
collector, Lukens
Collins bicycle ergometer
Collins cycle ergometer
Collins retractor
collodion surgical wound protectant
colloid osmotic pressure
colloid solution
colloids
color
  blue bloater
  bluish skin
  beefy red
  dusky skin
  pink puffer
color Doppler (CD)
color Doppler imaging
color Doppler recording
color-duplex interrogation

color-duplex ultrasound
Color Flow Doppler real-time imaging
    of blood flow
color-flow Doppler sonographic
    guidance
color-flow duplex scan
color flow mapping
columnae carneae (trabeculae carneae)
columnar epithelium, pseudostratified
CombiDerm absorbent cover dressing
combination flow and pressure loads
combined hyperlipidemia
Combivent (ipratropium bromide)
Comfeel Ulcus dressing
Commander guidewire
comma sign in truncus arteriosus
Command PS pacemaker
commence
commissural attachments
commissural chordae
commissural fusion
commissural incision
commissural leaflets
commissural neuron
commissural plication
commissural point
commissure
    anterior
    anteroseptal
    fused
    scalloped
    valve
    vestigial
commissurotomy
    Brockenbrough transseptal
    closed
    closed mitral
    mitral valve
    open mitral
    percutaneous catheter
    percutaneous transatrial mitral

commissurotomy *(cont.)*
    percutaneous transvenous mitral
        (PTMC)
    pulmonary valve
commissurotomy with ring
commissurotomy without ring
committed defibrillation shocks
committed shock
commode, bedside
common carotid artery
common faint
common femoral artery
common hepatic-common iliac-renal
    bypass
common iliac arteries
common pulmonary vein stenosis
Commucor A+V Patient Monitor
commune, ostium atrioventriculare
communicating artery
communicating vein incompetence
communicating veins
communication, interatrial
communicative disease
communicators, stripping of multiple
community-acquired pneumonia (CAP)
comorbid condition
comp (comparison)
compartment
    anterior mediastinal
    superficial posterior
compartment syndrome
compensated congestive heart failure
compensating emphysema
compensatory enlargement
compensatory hypertrophy
compensatory mechanism
compensatory pause
compensatory polycythemia
competent valve
complaints, constitutional
complement activation

complementary increase in respiratory
   frequency
complement levels
complete atrioventricular block
complete atrioventricular blockade
complete atrioventricular dissociation
complete atrioventricular heart block
complete congenital heart block
complete graft preservation
complete heart block
complete lung collapse
complete occlusion of graft
complete stent expansion
complete transposition of the great
   arteries
completion arteriogram
complex
   aberrant QRS
   anisoylated plasminogen
     streptokinase activator
   anomalous
   aortic tract
   atrial
   atrial arrhythmias
   atrial premature (APC)
   AV (atrioventricular) junctional
     escape
   AV (atrioventricular) junctional
     premature
   biphasic EKG
   circulating immune (CIC)
   cytokeratin 8:anti-cytokeratin 8
     antibody immune
   diphasic EKG
   Eisenmenger
   frequent spontaneous premature
   fusion QRS
   Ghon
   immune
   interpolated ventricular junctional
     premature
   Lutembacher

complex *(cont.)*
   monophasic contour of QRS
   multiform premature ventricular
   Mycobacterium avium (MAC)
   narrow QRS
   normal-voltage QRS
   parasystolic ventricular
   plasminogen streptokinase activator
   preexcited QRS
   premature atrial (PAC)
   premature AV (atrioventricular)
     junctional
   premature ventricular
   QRS
   QRST
   QS
   respiratory chain enzymatic
   RS
   rS
   slurring of QRS
   Steidele
   symptom
   triphasic contour of QRS
   ventricular
   ventricular escape
   ventricular premature (VPC)
   wide QRS
   widening of QRS
complex cardiovascular defects
complex lesion
complexus stimulans cordis
complex ventricular ectopic activity
compliance
   atrial
   chest wall
   decreased dynamic
   decreased lung
   decreased pulmonary vascular
   dynamic
   dynamic lung (C_{dyn})
   excellent
   good

compliance *(cont.)*
  lung
  patient
  poor
  reduced pulmonary
  regional
  static lung (C_{STAT})
  ventricular
complicated hypertension
complicated silicosis
complicating meningitis
complication rate
complications
  adverse
  concomitant
  groin
  iatrogenic
  perioperative
  procedure-related
component
  actuator
  aortic
  first
  loud pulmonic
  markedly accentuated pulmonic
  pulmonic
  second
composite aortic valve
composite aortic valve replacement
composite graft
composite valve graft (CVG)
composite valve graft replacement
composite vein graft
Composix E/X mess
compound
  artificial lung-expanding (ALEC)
  heparinoid
  lipophilic anticancer
compressed Ivalon patch graft
compressible grape-like clusters of
  large venous spaces

compression
  brachial artery
  brachial plexus
  cardiac
  extrinsic
  iliocaval
  instrumental
  manual
  mediastinal
  plaque
  pneumatic
  posterior fossa
  thermal
  ultrasound-guided (to obliterate
    false aneurysm)
  vessel
compression/atelectasis
compression boot
compression cough
Compression Device, Kendall
  Sequential
compression garment, pneumatic foot
compression of tissues with pressure
  effects
compression stockings, Sigvaris
compression ultrasonography
compressor Deschamps
compromise
  circulatory
  respiratory
  systemic circulatory
  vascular
compromised flow
compromised respiratory status
compromised ventricular function
compromising flow
Compuscan Hittman computerized
  electrocardioscanner
computed ejection fraction
computed tomography angiographic
  portography (CTAP)

computed tomography angiography
(CTA)
computed tomography (CT),
electron-beam
computed tomography (CT) scan
computed tomography with linear
accelerator (CT-Linac)
computer-assisted minimally invasive
surgery (CAMIS)
computer-enhanced telemetric mitral
valve repair
computerized dynamic posturography
(CDP)
computerized texture analysis of lung
nodules and lung parenchyma
computerized tomographic hepatic
angiography (CTHA)
conal papillary muscle
conal portion of right ventricle
conal septum
Concato disease
concealed accessory pathway
concealed atrioventricular pathways
concealed bypass tracts
concealed conduction
concealed entrainment
concealed retrograde conduction
concentration
    albumin
    fibronectin
    histamine
    magnesium plasma
    neutrophil
    plasma
    potassium
    serum myoglobin (Mb)
    serum potassium
    24-hour urine creatinine
    24-hour urine potassium
    24-hour urine sodium
concentric atherosclerotic plaque
concentric hypertrophy

concentric left ventricular hypertrophy
concentric lesion
concentric plaque in arterial walls
concentric plaque in carotid arteries
concentric tear
Concept bipolar coagulator
Concise balloon catheter
concomitant
concomitant antiarrhythmic therapy
concomitant arch repair
concomitant chest pain
concomitant complication
concomitant condition
concomitant coronary artery bypass
concomitant defect
concomitant disease
concomitant findings
concomitant infarction
concomitant symptoms
concomitant therapy
concomitant tracheal injury
concordance, atrioventricular
concordant arterial connection
concordant atrioventricular connection
concretio cordis (dense pericardial
    calcification)
concretio pericardii
concurrent infection
condition
    comorbid
    concomitant
    improving
    inherently unstable
    precarious
conductance and resistance
conducting airway asymmetry of lung
conducting system of heart
conduction
    aberrant
    accelerated AV (atrioventricular)
        node
    accelerated atrioventricular

conduction *(cont.)*
  accessory atrioventricular
  anomalous
  antegrade
  anterograde
  atrioventricular node
  AV (atrioventricular) nodal
  concealed
  concealed retrograde
  decremental
  delayed
  fast-pathway
  infranodal
  intra-atrial
  intraventricular
  preexcitation
  preexcitation atrioventricular
  reciprocating
  retrograde
  retrograde VA (ventriculoatrial)
  slow-pathway
  supernormal
  ventriculoatrial (VA)
conduction abnormality
conduction block
conduction defect, intraventricular
conduction delay
conduction disturbance
conduction interval
conduction interval, intra-atrial
conduction ratio (number of P waves to
  number of QRS)
conduction system of heart
conduction time, sinoatrial (SACT)
conductive system of heart
conduit (see also *graft*)
  afferent
  aortic-aortic
  aorta-to-aorta
  apical aortic valved
  apico-aortic (abdominal)
  apico-aortic valved

conduit *(cont.)*
  efferent
  extracardiac
  inferior vena cava to left atrium
  intracaval
  jawed
  left ventricle to pulmonary artery
  left ventricular apical to aorta
    (LV-Ao)
  left ventricular to descending aorta
    (LV-DAo)
  Medtronic Hall rotatable aortic
    valved collagen-impregnated
  right ventricle to pulmonary artery
    (RV-PA)
  valved
conduit graft
conduit valve
cone nose forceps
cone of apical tissue
confabulation
confidence interval
configuration
  bidirectional lead
  fishmouth (of mitral valve)
  inverted Y
  scalloped luminal
  spike-and-dome
  spike-dome
  thoracic cage
  unidirectional lead
confluent consolidation
confluent fibrosis
Conformant contact-layer wound
  dressing
Conform-X aortic prosthetic heart
  valve
confusion following open heart surgery
congenita
  myotonia
  paramyotonia

congenital absence of venous valves as
cause of leg ulcers
congenital absent pericardium
congenital adrenal hyperplasia
congenital anemia of newborn
congenital aneurysm
congenital angiodysplasias of
extremities
congenital anomaly of tricuspid valve
congenital aortic regurgitation
congenital aortic sinus aneurysm
congenital aortic stenosis
congenital arteriovenous fistula
congenital bicuspid aortic valve
congenital bleeding diathesis
congenital bronchiectasis
congenital cardiac anomaly
congenital cardiac defects
congenital cardiac malformation
congenital central hypoventilation
syndrome
congenital cerebral aneurysm
congenital dilated cardiomyopathy
congenital fetal arrhythmia
congenital heart block
congenital heart disease, cyanotic
congenital heart failure
congenital heart murmur
congenital hypoplastic anemia
congenital interruption of aortic arch
congenital isolated hypoplasia
congenital isthmic coarctation
congenital lobar emphysema (CLE)
congenital lobar overinflation (CLO)
congenitally absent pericardium
congenital mitral regurgitation
congenital mitral stenosis
congenital mitral valve disease
congenital pericardial absence
congenital pneumothorax
congenital polyvalvular dysplasia

congenital pulmonary fistula
congenital regurgitation
congenital rings of aortic arch
congenital rubella pneumonitis
congenital rubella syndrome
congenital segmental renal hyperplasia
congenital stenosis of pulmonary vein
congenital subaortic stenosis
congenital subpulmonic obstruction
congenital subvalvular aortic stenosis
congenital supravalvular aortic
stenosis, Brom repair of
congenital transposition, corrected
congenital valvular aortic stenosis
congenital vascular malformation
(CVM)
congenital vascular-bone syndrome
(CVBS)
congenital ventricular tachycardia
congestion
active
asymmetric pulmonary
capillary
chronic passive
hepatic
hypostatic
passive vascular
pulmonary
pulmonary venous
symmetric pulmonary
vascular
venous
congestion stage
congestive atelectasis
congestive cardiomyopathy
congestive cirrhosis
congestive heart failure
conical heart
conjoined leaflet
conjugated estrogens (CE)
conjunctive treatment

connection
  anomalous pulmonary venous
  cavopulmonary
  concordant arterial
  concordant atrioventricular
  discordant arterial
  discordant atrioventricular
  discordant ventriculoarterial
  partial anomalous pulmonary
    venous
  slip-in
  total anomalous pulmonary venous
    (TAPVC)
connective tissue proliferation
connective tissue septa
connector
  Jocath graft
  Jography graft
  Joguide graft
  lock-tip
  Luer-Lok
  Luer-Slip
  slip-tip
  three-way stopcock
Connolly eversion endarterectomy
Conn syndrome
conotruncal anomaly, congenital
conotruncal defect
conotruncal malformation
conotruncal repair
conoventricular defect
Conradi-Hünermann syndrome
consciousness
  altered
  clouded
  diminished
  impaired
  near-loss of
  transient decrease
  transient loss of
consent, written informed
consequences, lethal

consolidated infiltrate
consolidated lung
consolidation
  alveolar
  confluent
  dense
  exudative
  lobar
  lung
  lung parenchyma
  patchy
  pulmonary
consolidation of alveoli
consolidation of lung
consolidative change
consolidative changes on chest x-ray
consolidative pneumonia
consolidative pneumonia due to
  pneumococcus
conspicuous feature
Constant catheter
constant clockwise torque of electrode
  tip
Constant distal protection device
Constant guidewire
Constant stent
Constant stent delivery system
constant rate atrial pacing
constant tilt wave
Constellation advanced mapping
  catheter
constellation of findings
constellation of symptoms
constituent, plaque
constitutional complaints
constitutional disturbance
constitutional symptoms
constriction
  airway
  occult pericardial
  tangential
constriction of coronary arteries by
  cocaine

constriction of ductus arteriosus
constriction of peripheral arterioles
constrictive cardiomyopathy
constrictive lesion
constrictive pericardial disease
constrictive pericarditis
    advanced tuberculous
    effusive
construction of intra-atrial baffle
construction, venous valve
consumption
    myocardial oxygen (MVO_2)
    oxygen
    ventilatory oxygen (VO_2)
consumption coagulopathy
contact-layer wound dressing
contact, stent-vessel wall
contagious disease
contained aneurysmal rupture
container, evacuator
Contak CD CRT-D implantable
    cardioverter-defibrillator
Contak CD 2 defibrillator
contamination
    bacterial
    continued
    exogenous
    low-level
    mediastinal
    membrane oxygenator
    perioperative (not pre-)
    wound
Contigen Bard collagen implant
Contigen glutaraldehyde cross-linked
    collagen
contiguous segment
continuity equation
continuous ambulatory peritoneal
    dialysis (CAPD)
continuous arteriovenous hemo-
    filtration (CAVH)
continuous cardiac output (CCO)

continuous descending pressure (CDP)
continuous electrocardiogram
continuous-flow irrigation
continuous infusion (of cardioplegia)
continuous irrigation
continuous lateral rotation therapy
continuous mammary souffle
continuous mechanical ventilation
continuous monitoring of myocardial
    ischemia
continuous murmur (CM)
continuous positive airway pressure
    (CPAP)
continuous positive pressure ventilation
    (CPPV)
continuous rapid atrial pacing
continuous saline irrigation
continuous sampling of cardiac
    electrical activity
continuous sutures
continuous venovenous hemodialysis
    (CVVHD)
continuous warm blood cardioplegia
continuous wave ablation
continuous wave Doppler examination
continuous wave Doppler recording
continuous wave Doppler ultra-
    sonography
continuous wave laser system
Continuum MR-compatible infusion
    system
contour
    aortic knob
    irregular hazy luminal
    precordial impulse contour
    S
Contour closed end stent
contoured lead
Contour MD implantable single-lead
    cardioverter-defibrillator
Contour stent with HydroPlus coating

Contour V-145D and LTV-135D
   implantable cardioverter-
   defibrillator devices
contractile dysfunction
contractile force
contractile function, depressed right
   ventricular
contractile pattern
contractile performance, depressed
   myocardial
contractile reserve
contractile work index
contractility
   cardiac
   depressed
   depressed cardiac
   deranged left ventricular
   diaphragmatic
   myocardial
contractility effect
contractility index
contracting factor, endothelium-derived
contraction
   atrial premature (APC)
   atrioventricular junctional
     premature
   automatic ventricular
   cardiac
   escaped ventricular
   force of
   isometric heart
   isotonic heart
   isovolumic (IVC)
   left atrial
   left ventricular
   myocardial
   nodal
   nodal premature
   period of isovolumic
   premature atrial (PAC)
   premature junctional (PJC)
   premature nodal (PNC)

contraction *(cont.)*
   premature ventricular (PVC)
   right atrial
   right ventricular
   R-on-T ventricular premature
   spastic
   supraventricular premature (SVPC)
   ventricular premature (VPC)
   ventricular segmental
contraction stress test (CST)
contraction time, isovolumic
contractor
   Bailey-Gibbon rib
   Bailey rib
   rib
contracture
   myocardial
   Volkmann
contraindicated drugs
contraindication to surgery
contralateral decubitus chest x-ray
contralateral hemiparesis
contralateral lung volume reduction
   surgery
contralateral pneumonectomy
contralateral pulmonary function
contralateral vessel
contralateral washout time
contrast
   spontaneous echo
   tissue
contrast agent (see *imaging agent*)
contrast echo agents
contrast echocardiography
contrast laryngogram
contrast material (see *imaging agent*)
contrast medium (pl. media) (see
   imaging agent)
contrast venography
control
   C-arm
   diluent

control *(cont.)*
  distal
  fluoroscopic
  fluoroscopy
  histamine
  radiographic
  roentgenographic
controlled aortic root reperfusion
controlled ventilation
controlled ventricular response
control of hypertension
Control-Release pop-off needle
Control Wire guidewire
contusion
  myocardial
  pulmonary
conus arteriosus
conus artery
conus branch ostia
conus ligament
conus septum
convalesce
convalescence, uncomplicated
convalescent
conventional pulse sequence
Converge anastomotic device
convergence zone
Convergent color Doppler imaging
conversion
  spontaneous
  successful
converting-enzyme inhibitors
convexo-concave disk prosthetic valve
convulsivum, asthma
Cook arterial catheter
Cook deflector
Cook introducer
Cook Micropuncture catheter system
Cook pacemaker
Cook yellow pigtail catheter
Cooley anastomosis clamp
Cooley anemia

Cooley aortic clamp
Cooley atrial retractor
Cooley-Baumgarten aortic forceps
Cooley-Beck clamp
Cooley clamp
Cooley coarctation clamp
Cooley-Cutter disk prosthetic valve
Cooley-Cutter valve prosthesis
Cooley-Derra anastomosis clamp
Cooley Dacron prosthesis
Cooley iliac clamp
Cooley intrapericardial anastomosis
Cooley modification of Waterston
  anastomosis
Cooley partial occlusion clamp
Cooley patent ductus clamp
Cooley pediatric clamp
Cooley renal clamp
Cooley retractor
Cooley-Satinsky clamp
Cooley trait
Cooley valve dilator
Cooley vascular clamp
Cooley vascular forceps
Cooley vena cava catheter clamp
Cooley woven Dacron graft
CoolFlow infusion pump (used in
  electrophysiology procedures)
cooling
  core
  external cardiac
cooling blanket
Cool Tip catheter
Coombs murmur
Coombs test
  direct
  indirect
Cooper ligament
Cooperman event probability
CooperSurgical balloon cannula
  with atraumatic surface disk
coordinates, rectilinear

"coo sur coo" (coup sur coup)
COPD (chronic obstructive pulmonary
    disease), emphysematous
COPD Lung Profiler
Cope biopsy needle
Cope needle introducer cannula
copious amounts of blood
copious irrigation
copiously irrigated
copiously irrigated incision
copious sputum production
copious watery rhinorrhea
copper deficiency
copper wire effect
CoQ10; Co-Q10 (coenzyme Q10)
cord blood gases (CBG)
Cordis catheter
Cordis Bioptome sheath
Cordis Checkmate system
Cordis coronary stent
Cordis-Hakim shunt
Cordis Predator PTCA balloon
    catheter
Cordis Stabilizer steerable guidewire
Cordis Trakstar PTCA balloon
Cordis Wizdom steerable guidewire
Cor-Flex wire guides
Corflo catheter
CorLink device
coronaropathy
    dilated
    three-vessel
coronary anastomotic shunt
coronary artery bypass, minimally
    invasive direct (MIDCAB)
coronary artery scan (CAS)
    by Ultrafast CT
coronary artery scoring
coronary atherectomy
coronary branch ostial lesion
coronary ostium
coronary radiation therapy (CRT)

coronary remodeling
coronary sinus flow catheter
coronary-subclavian steal syndrome
coronavirus
Corpac diagnostic catheter
cor pulmonale
corrected TIMI frame count (CTFC)
Correra line
corridor operation in atrial fibrillation
Corrigan aortic regurgitation disease
Corrigan collapsing pulse
Corrigan disease
Corrigan pulse
Corrigan sign
Corrigan syndrome
corrugated air column
corset balloon catheter
cor sinistrum
cor taurinum
corticale, Cryptostroma
cortical intracerebral hemorrhage
cortical sign
corticobulbar disease
corticospinal disease
corticosteroid
    prenatal
    inhaled
corticosteroid-administration-related
    tuberculosis reactivation
corticosteroid in hemangioma therapy
corticosterone
cortisol production, deficient
cortisone in congenital vascular defect
    therapy
cor triatriatum
cor triatriatum dextrum
cor triloculare
cor triloculare biatriatum
cor triloculare biventriculare
corundum smelter's lung
cor venosum
cor villosum

Corvisart disease
Corvisart syndrome
Corynebacterium infection
Corynebacterium pseudotuberculosis
   infection
coryza
CoSeal resorbable synthetic sealant
Cosgrove-Edwards anuloplasty
   system
Cosmos pulse generator
Cosmos pulse generator pacemaker
Cosmos 283 DDD pacemaker
Cosmos II DDD pacemaker
costal angle
costal cartilage
costal groove
costal interarticular cartilage
costalis, pleura
costal margin
costal margin syndrome
costal pleura
costal pleural reflection
costal pleurisy
costal retractions
costal surface of lung
costectomy
costocervical trunk of subclavian artery
costochondral joint
costochondral junction
costochondral junction syndrome
costochondritis, angina mimicked by
costoclavicular maneuver
costoclavicular test
costodiaphragmatic recess of pleura
costodiaphragmatic recesses
costolateral areas
costomediastinal recess
costophrenic angle, obliteration of
costosternal malformation
costosternal syndrome
costotome
costotransverse joint

costovertebral angle (CVA)
costovertebral joint
costoxiphoid ligament
cotinine level
cottage loaf appearance (on x-ray)
cottage loaf deformity
cotton dust
cotton-mill fever syndrome
cough
   aneurysmal
   barking
   brassy
   bubbling
   chronic intractable
   compression
   croupy
   decubitus
   dog (compression)
   dry
   dry nonproductive
   encouraged to
   hacking
   harsh
   hollow
   loose
   mechanical
   membranous
   metallic
   Morton
   motion
   nocturnal
   nonproductive
   nonproductive dry
   productive
   rasping
   rattling
   reflex
   smoker's
   spasmodic
   Sydenham
   tea taster's
   typical regularity of

cough *(cont.)*
    voluntary (productive of mucus)
    wet
    whooping
    winter
    wracking
cough CPR technique
coughing
    paroxysmal
    repeated bouts of
    voluntary cough productive of
        mucus
coughing and wheezing
coughing sign
coughing up blood
cough productive of phlegm
cough productive of purulent sputum
cough productive of sputum
cough reflex
    depression of
    impaired
    inhibited
    suppressed
cough syncope
cough-thrill
Coulter counter for platelet count
Coulter HIV-1 p24 antigen assay
Coumadin (warfarin sodium)
coumadinization
coumarin-type anticoagulants
count
    absolute blood eosinophil
    cell
    complete blood cell (CBC)
    differential
    needle, sponge, and instrument
    platelet
    RBC (red blood cell)
    reticulocyte
    WBC (white blood cell)
counterclockwise rotation

counterclockwise superiorly oriented
    frontal QRS loop
counterimmunoelectrophoresis (CIE)
    of sputum
counterincision
counter-occluder delivered into right
    atrium
counter-occluder equals buttonhole
counter-occluder threaded over loading
    wire through rubber buttonhole
counterpulsation
    balloon
    diastolic
    intra-aortic balloon (IAB)
    mechanical
    percutaneous intra-aortic balloon
        (PIBC)
countershock
    direct current electrical
    unsynchronized
coupled beats
coupled premature beats
coupler, venous
couplet
    atrial
    ventricular
    ventricular premature contraction
coupling, excitation-contraction
coupling interval
coupling interval decrement
coup sur coup ("coo sur coo")
Cournand cardiac catheter
Cournand catheter
Cournand needle
course
    fulminant
    fulminant disease
    improving
course of the vessel
Covaderm composite wound dressing
coved ST segments
coverage, bronchial stump

covering, musculotendinous
Coverlet adhesive dressing
Cover-Roll adhesive gauze
Cover-Strip wound closure strips
CoverTip safety syringe
coxsackievirus
CO_2 wave forms
Coxiella burnetii (Rickettsia burnetii)
  infection
Cox maze procedure
Coxsackie A virus
Coxsackie B virus
coxsackievirus
coxsackievirus endocarditis
coxsackievirus myocarditis
coxsackievirus pericarditis
Cozaar (losartan potassium)
CP (cerebral palsy)
CPAD (chronic peripheral arterial
  disease)
CPAP (continuous positive airway
    pressure)
  face mask
  nasal
CPB (cardiopulmonary bypass)
CPE (chronic pulmonary emphysema)
CPHV (Carbomedics prosthetic heart
  valve)
CPHV OptiForm mitral valve
CPI (Cardiac Pacemakers, Inc.)
CPI Astra pacemaker
CPI automatic implantable defibrillator
CPI DDD pacemaker
CPI electrode lead
CPI endocardial defibrillation lead
CPI endocardial defibrillation/rate-
  sensing/pacing lead
CPI endocardial rate-sensing/pacing
  lead
CPI Endotak SQ electrode lead
CPI Endotak transvenous electrode
CPI L67 electrode

CPI external cardioverter-defibrillator
  (ECD) for crinkling, patch
CPI pacemaker
CPI porous tined-tip bipolar pacing
  lead
CPI Sweet Tip lead
CPI ULTRA II pacemaker
CPI ventricular lead
CPK (creatine phosphokinase)
CPK isoenzymes (see *isoenzymes*)
CPK-MB (creatine phosphokinase
  of muscle band)
C point of cardiac apex pulse
CPP (cerebral perfusion pressure)
CPP (coronary artery perfusion
  pressure)
CPPV (continuous positive pressure
  ventilation)
CPR (cardiopulmonary resuscitation)
  closed chest
  open-heart
cps (cycles per second)
CPS (cardiopulmonary support) system
c. pulmonale (cor pulmonale)
CPVG (cryopreserved vein graft)
crackles (see also *rales*)
  auscultatory
  coarse
  diffuse
  early inspiratory
  fine
  late inspiratory
  medium
  paninspiratory
  pleural
crackling rales
Crafoord aortic clamp
Crafoord clamp
Crafoord coarctation clamp
Crafoord-Senning heart-lung machine
Crafoord thoracic scissors
Cragg endoluminal graft

Cragg Endopro System 1 stent
Cragg thrombolytic brush
cramped position
cramping, intense disabling
cramps
 calf
 muscle
Crampton test
cranial and caudal angulations
cranial angled view
cranial angulation, anteroposterior
 x-ray projection with
cranial arteritis
cranial nerve palsy
cranial vessels
cranial view
craniofacial overgrowth
cranky
crash induction of anesthesia
craterlike ulcer with jagged edges
Crawford aortic retractor
Crawford-Cooley tunneler
Crawford graft inclusion technique
Crawford suture ring
Crawford technique for thoracoabdominal aneurysm
CR Bard catheter
C-reactive protein
creaking friction rub
crease
 earlobe
 inframammary
creatine kinase (CK) isoenzymes
creatine phosphate
creatine phosphokinase (CPK)
creatinine clearance
creatinine concentration, 24-hour urine
creatinine estimated using modified
 Jaffé rate reaction
creatinine, urinary
Credent artificial vascular access graft
creep of ventricular diastolic pressure

creeping eruption
crepitant rales
crepitation
 basal
 inspiratory
 pleural
 superficial
crepitus indux
crepitus redux
crescendo angina
crescendo-decrescendo murmur
crescendo murmur
crescendo pattern of angina
crescendo rumble
crescendo-systolic thrill
crescendo transient ischemic attacks
crescent sign
crescentic lumen
crest
 infundibuloventricular
 supraventricular
 terminal (of right atrium)
CREST (calcinosis cutis, Raynaud
 phenomenon, esophageal dys-
 motility, sclerodactyly, and
 telangiectasia) syndrome
CRF (chronic renal failure)
CRF (chronic reserve flow)
CRHD (chronic rheumatic heart
 disease)
cricoid cartilage
cri du chat (short arm deletion-5)
 syndrome
cricopharyngeal achalasia
cricothyroid
cricothyroid cartilage, obstetrical
 injury
cricothyroid membrane
cricothyrotomy, emergency
Crile clamp
Crile curved dissecting forceps
Crile curved forceps

Crile curved grasping forceps
Crile hemostat
Crile straight dissecting forceps
Crile straight grasping forceps
Crile-Wood needle holder
crimp
crimper
crimping
cripple, pulmonary
crisis (pl. crises)
  hypertensive
  hypertensive paroxysmal
  rejection
crisscross fashion
crisscross heart
Crista Cath
Crista Cath II electrophysiology
  catheter
crista supraventricularis
crista supraventricularis septal defect
crista terminalis atrii dextri
criteria (see also *classification*, *index*,
    score)
  ACAS (Asymptomatic Carotid
    Atherosclerosis Study)
  Ambrose (for thrombotic lesions)
  Framingham
  Heath-Edwards
  Framingham criteria for heart
    failure
criteria of Martini and Melamed
critical care unit (CCU)
critical lesion
Critikon balloon wedge pressure
  catheter
Critikon catheter
Critikon guidewire
Critikon thermodilution and pressure
  catheter
Crit-Line III blood monitoring system
crochetage on electrocardiogram
Croften classification for pulmonary
  eosinophilia

cromoglycate
crossability
cross-aortic
cross clamp (noun)
cross-clamp, cross-clamped (adj.,
  verb)
cross-clamping of aorta
cross-clamp time
cross-collateralization
crossed embolism
CrossFlex LC coronary stent
crossmatch
  major
  minor
crossmatching
CrossSail coronary dilatation catheter
Cross-Jones disk prosthetic valve
crossover femoral-femoral bypass
crossover graft
cross-pelvic collateral vessel
cross-sectional area, luminal
cross-sectional area stenosis
cross-sectional image
cross-sectional view
crosstalk, pacemaker
croup
  catarrhal
  diphtheritic
  false
  membranous
  pseudomembranous
  spasmodic
croup syndrome
croup tent
croupous bronchitis
croupy cough
CRS (catheter-related sepsis)
CRT (cardiac resynchronization
  therapy)
CRT (cathode ray tube)
CRT (coronary radiation therapy)
cruciate incision
Crump vessel dilator

crunch, Hamman
crura diaphragmatis
crura of the diaphragm (left and right)
cruris, angina
crus, diaphragmatic
crushing chest pain
crushing injury to chest
crushing pain
crushing substernal chest pain
crust
crusting
Cruveilhier-Baumgarten murmur
Cruveilhier-Baumgarten syndrome
Cruveilhier nodule
Cruveilhier sign
crux (pl. cruces)
crux cordis (crux of heart)
cryoablation (see also *ablation*)
  CryoCor cardiac
  encircling endocardial
  Frostline
  Soprano
  transmural
  transvenous
cryoablation catheter
CryoCor cardiac cryoablation system
cryocrit
cryolesions
Cryolife-O'Brien porcine heart valve
Cryolife-Ross porcine heart valve
cryoprecipitate
cryoprecipitate collagen
cryopreservation
cryopreserved allograft
cryopreserved homograft tissue
cryopreserved human allograft conduit
cryopreserved human aortic allograft
cryopreserved vein graft (CVG,
  CPVG)
cryoprobe
cryostat
cryosurgery, map-guided

cryosurgical ablation
cryosurgical lesions
cryosurgical probe
cryotherapy
cryothermia
CryoValve-SG
cryptococcosis
Cryptococcus neoformans pneumonia
cryptogenic bacteremia
cryptogenic fibrosing alveolitis
cryptogenic organizing pneumonia
cryptogenic pulmonary eosinophilia
cryptophthalmos syndrome
Cryptostroma corticale
crystalloid cardioplegic solution
crystalloid fluid
crystalloid prime for heart-lung
  machine
crystals
  asthma
  Charcot-Leyden
  cholesterol
CS (coronary sinus)
CSA (cross-sectional area)
CSH (carotid sinus hypersensitivity)
C-shaped bars of cartilage
C-17 hydroxylase deficiency
CSI (coronary stenosis index)
CSICU (cardiac surgery intensive care
  unit)
CSNRT (corrected sinus node recovery
  time)
CSR (coronary sinus rhythm)
CSS (carotid sinus syndrome)
CST (contraction stress test)
C_{STAT} (static lung compliance)
CSVT (central splanchnic venous
  thrombosis)
CSWT (cardiac shock wave therapy)
CT (computed tomography)
CTA (computed tomography angiog-
  raphy)

CTAP (clear to auscultation and percussion)
CTAP (computed tomography angiographic portography)
CT angiographic portography (CTAP)
CT-directed hook wire localization
CTFC (corrected TIMI frame count)
CT-guided aspiration
CT-Linac (computed tomography with linear accelerator)
CT-scan directed needle biopsy
CT scan, ultrafast
C3a serum level
CTGA (corrected transposition of great arteries)
CTHA (computerized tomographic hepatic angiography)
CTR (cardiac transplant recipient)
CTR (cardiothoracic ratio)
cuboidal epithelium
cuff
   aortic
   atrial
   blood pressure
   finger
   inflow
   pneumatic
   right atrial
cuffed endotracheal tube
cuff pressure
cuff rupture of tube
cuirasse, coeur en
cuirass respirator
culprit lesion
culprit stenosis
culprit vessel
culture
   acid-fast
   chemostat
   sputum
culture and sensitivity, sputum
cultured for aerobes and anaerobes

cumulative effect
cuplike pockets
cupula (pl. cupulae), pleural
cup-shaped semilunar valves
Curaderm hydrocolloid dressing material
Curafil hydrogel dressing
Curafoam foam wound dressing
Curagel hydrogel dressing
Curasorb calcium alginate dressing
Curlin 2000 Plus portable infusion pump
Curosurf (poractant alfa)
currant jelly clot
Currarino-Silverman syndrome
current, alternating
current leak
current of injury
Curschmann spirals
curse, Ondine's
curve
   AA
   AH
   A_1-A_2
   arterial dilution
   ascorbate dilution
   A2-H2
   central intra-aortic pressure
   dye
   indicator dilution
   indicator dye-dilution
   indocyanine dilution
   intracardiac dye-dilution
   left ventricular inflow velocity
   oxyhemoglobin dissociation
   Starling
   time activity (for contrast agent)
   tortuous arterial
   V1-V2
   V2-A2
   venous dilution
   ventricular function

curved Cooley clamp
curved Hasson grasper
curved Kelly forceps
curved mosquito forceps
curves, catheter with preformed
curvilinear aortotomy
curvilinear defect
curvilinear incision
curvilinear lines, subpleural
Curvularia lunata
CUSA (Cavitron ultrasonic aspirator)
CUSA (Cavitron ultrasonic surgical
  aspirator)
CUSALap
Cushing forceps
cushingoid appearance
Cushing phenomenon
Cushing, pressor response of
Cushing reflex
Cushing response
Cushing triad
Cushing rongeur
Cushing syndrome
Cushing vein retractor
cushion defect
cushion, endocardial
cusp
  accessory
  anterior
  aortic
  asymmetric closure of
  conjoined
  coronary
  dysplastic
  fibrocalcific
  fishmouth
  fusion of
  intact valve
  left coronary
  left pulmonary
  mitral valve
  noncoronary

cusp *(cont.)*
  perforated aortic
  posterior
  pulmonary valve
  right coronary
  ruptured aortic
  semilunar valve
  septal
  septic perforation of
  tricuspid valve
  valve
cusp degeneration
cusp fenestration
cuspis anterior valvae atrioventricularis
  dextrae
cuspis anterior valvae atrioventricularis
  sinistrae
cuspis posterior valvae atrioventricularis dextrae
cuspis posterior valvae atrioventricularis sinistrae
cuspis septalis valvae atrioventricularis
  dextrae
cusp motion
cusp shots (films)
cut and cine film
cutaneous atrophy
cutaneous emphysema
cutaneous telangiectasia
cutaneous vascular anomaly
cutaneous vasoconstriction, peripheral
cut, clamp, and tie
cutdown
  antecubital fossa
  brachial
  femoral
cutdown catheter
cutdown intra-aortic balloon pump
  (IABP)
cutdown over cephalic vein
Cutinova Cavity wound filling material
Cutinova Hydro dressing

cutis laxa syndrome
cutis marmorata
cutoff
  arterial
  atherectomy
  Leather valve
  vessel (of contrast material)
  wire
Cutter aortic valve prosthesis
Cutter-Smeloff cardiac valve prosthesis
Cutter-Smeloff heart valve
Cutting Balloon catheter
cutting device
cutting diathermy
cutting loop
cutting mechanism was engaged
Cuvier, canal of
CV (cardioversion)
CV (closing volume)
CVA (cardiovascular accident)
CVA (cerebrovascular accident),
  posterior circulation
CVA (costovertebral angle)
CVBS (congenital vascular-bone
  syndrome)
CVC (central venous catheter)
CVC (central venous catheterization)
CVG (cryopreserved vein graft)
CVI (cerebrovascular insufficiency)
CVI (chronic venous insufficiency)
CVIS imaging device
CVM (congenital vascular malforma-
  tion)
CvO_2 (mixed venous oxygen content)
CVP (central venous pressure) catheter
CV Peri-Guard patch
CVProfilor DO-2020 cardiovascular
  profiling device
CVRI (coronary vascular resistance
  index)
CVVHD (continuous venovenous
  hemodialysis)

cv wave of jugular venous pulse
cv waves, regurgitant
C wave pressure on right atrial
  catheterization
CX (circumflex)
CXR (chest x-ray), baseline
cyanide poisoning
cyanide toxicity
cyanoacrylate (Superglue) tissue
  adhesive
cyanosis
  central
  circumoral
  differential
  false
  frank
  mucous membrane
  nail bed
  perioral
  peripheral
  pulmonary
  reversed differential
  ruddy
  shunt
  slate-gray
  systemic
  tardive
  tardive pulmonary
cyanosis and clubbing
cyanosis, clubbing, or edema
  (C, C, or E)
cyanotic congenital heart disease
cyanotic heart disease
cyanotic hypoxic spells
cyanotic nail beds
CyberKnife Express
Cyberlith multiprogrammable pulse
  generator
Cyberlith pacemaker
Cybertach automatic-burst atrial
  pacemaker
Cybertach 60 pacemaker

cycle
  cardiac
  length of atrial
  length of ventricular
  RR
  sinus length (SLC)
  vicious
cycle-ergometer
cycles per second (cps)
cyclical edema
cyclic idiopathic edema
cyclo-oxygenase inhibitors
cyclosporine toxicity
cyclosporin G
cylindrical bronchiectasis
cylindrical chest
cylindrical thorax
Cypher sirolimus-eluting stent
Cyriax syndrome
cyst
  alveolar
  bronchial
  bronchogenic
  bronchopulmonary
  echinococcal (of lung)
  hydatid
  pericardial
  springwater

cystic disease of lung
cystic emphysema
cystic fibrosis
cystic medial necrosis
cystic medionecrosis, Erdheim
cystic pulmonary emphysema
cystlike foci of hyperaeration
cytocrit
cytoimmunologic monitoring (also
  immunocytologic monitoring)
cytokeratin 8:anti-cytokeratin 8
  (CK8:anti-CK8) antibody immune
  complexes
cytokeratin 8 (CK8) antibody
cytology, bronchial washings
cytomegalic inclusion disease
cytomegalovirus (CMV)
cytomegalovirus infection
cytomegalovirus pneumonitis
cytometer, FACScan (fluorescence-
  activated cell sorter) flow
cytosome
Czaja-McCaffrey rigid stent
  introducer/endoscope

D, d

D (diaphragmatic)
D'Acosta disease (acute mountain
    sickness)
Da Costa syndrome (neurocirculatory
    asthenia)
Dacron catheter
Dacron conduit
Dacron-covered prosthesis
Dacron graft
Dacron mesh
Dacron onlay patch-graft
Dacron outflow graft
Dacron pouch
Dacron patch graft
Dacron preclotted tightly woven graft
Dacron roof
Dacron Sauvage patch
Dacron stent
Dacron suture
Dacron synthetic ligament material
Dacron tape
Dacron tube graft, albuminized woven
Dacron velour tube graft
Dagrofil suture
Daig ESI-II or DSI-III screw-in lead
    pacemaker

Dakin Biograft
Dale Foley catheter holder
Dale forceps
Dallas Classification System for
    diagnosing myocarditis
damage
    alveolar-capillary membrane
    focal myocyte
    myocardial wall
D'Amato sign in pleural effusion
dam, left ventricular
dampened obstructive pulse
dampened pulsatile flow
dampened wave form
damping of catheter tip pressure
Damus-Kaye-Stansel (DKS) operation
Damus-Norwood procedure
Danielson method of tricuspid valve
    repair
Dardik Biograft
dark region
dark sputum
Dash rate-adaptive pacemaker
Dash single-chamber rate-adaptic
    cardiac pacemaker
data acquisition

data log, ICD
Datascope DL-II percutaneous trans-
lucent balloon catheter
Datascope intra-aortic balloon pump
Datascope System 83 intra-aortic
balloon pump
Datascope System 90 intra-aortic
balloon pump
Datascope System 90T intra-aortic
balloon pump
DataVue calibrated reference circle
David operation
Davidson scapular retractor
Davidson shunt
Davidson thoracic trocar
Davidson vessel clamp
Davies-Colley syndrome
Davies endomyocardial fibrosis
Davies myocardial fibrosis
Davies syndrome
da Vinci robot
Davis aneurysm clip
Davis forceps
Davis rib spreader
Davol drain
Davol pacemaker introducer
DBP (diastolic blood pressure)
DC (direct current)
DC cardioversion
DC defibrillator
DC electrical shock
DCA (direct current ablation)
DCA (directional coronary
angioplasty)
DCA (directional coronary
atherectomy)
DCM (dilated cardiomyopathy)
DCS (distal coronary sinus)
DDD mode
DDD pacemaker
DDD pacing mode
dD/dt (derived value on apex
cardiogram)

DDM (delayed diastolic murmur)
de-aired
de-airing maneuvers
de-airing of arch
de-airing of graft
de-airing procedure
de-airing site
de-airing the heart
dead arm syndrome (DAS)
dead space, anatomical
D-E amplitude of mitral valve
Dean Ornish diet
death
    aborted sudden cardiac (ASCD)
    adult sudden
    apparent
    imminent
    infant sudden
    recurrent, not-so-sudden cardiac
    sudden
    sudden cardiac
Deaver retractor
DeBakey aortic aneurysm clamp
DeBakey arterial clamp
DeBakey arterial forceps
DeBakey Autraugrip forceps
DeBakey-Bahnson vascular clamp
DeBakey-Bainbridge clamp
DeBakey ball valve prosthesis
DeBakey-Beck clamp
DeBakey bulldog clamp
DeBakey clamps
DeBakey classification (type I, II, III)
    of aortic dissection
DeBakey coarctation clamp
DeBakey-Cooley retractor
DeBakey cross-action bulldog clamp
DeBakey curved dissecting forceps
DeBakey curved grasping forceps
DeBakey-Derra anastomosis clamp
DeBakey-Diethrich vascular forceps
DeBakey dissecting forceps
DeBakey endarterectomy scissors

DeBakey-Harken clamp
DeBakey-Howard clamp
DeBakey-Kay clamp
DeBakey patent ductus clamp
DeBakey pediatric clamp
DeBakey peripheral vascular bulldog
    clamp
DeBakey peripheral vascular clamp
DeBakey prosthetic valve
DeBakey-Reynolds anastomosis clamp
DeBakey rib spreader
DeBakey ring-handled bulldog clamp
DeBakey-Semb clamp; forceps
DeBakey straight dissecting forceps
DeBakey straight grasping forceps
DeBakey-Surgitool prosthetic valve
DeBakey tangential occlusion clamp
DeBakey technique for thoracoabdomi-
    nal aneurysm
DeBakey tissue forceps
DeBakey type I aortic dissection
DeBakey valve scissors
DeBakey vascular clamp
DeBakey vascular forceps
DeBakey Vasculour prosthesis
DeBakey ventricular assist device
DeBakey woven Dacron
debanding procedure
debanding, pulmonary artery
debilitation
debrancher disease
debris
    aspiration of
    atheromatous
    atherosclerotic
    calcium
    cholesterol
    gelatinous
    grumous
    intimal
    particle
    thallium

debt
    mild oxygen
    moderate oxygen
    oxygen
    severe oxygen
debubbling procedure
debulking, excimer laser
debulking of aneurysm
debulking of atheroma
decannulated
decannulation
decapolar catheter
decay, free induction
deceleration-dependent heart block
deceleration, differential
deceleration time
decelerative injury
decidua
declamping
decompensated congestive heart failure
decompensation
    cardiac
    chronic respiratory
    end-stage adult cardiac
    end-stage fetal cardiac
    hemodynamic
    respiratory
    ventricular
decompress
decompression, cardiac
decompression of heart
decompression of ventricle
decompression sickness
deconditioning
decortication
    cardiac
    chemical
    heart
    lung
decreased arterial hemoglobin
    saturation
decreased beta adrenergic receptor

decreased breath sounds
decreased carbon monoxide diffusion
decreased cerebral blood flow
decreased cerebral perfusion pressure
decreased closing velocity
decreased compliance
decreased diaphragmatic motion
decreased diffusing capacity
decreased dynamic compliance
decreased E-F slope
decreased exchangeable sodium
decreased exercise capacity
decreased I-E (I to E) ratio
decreased inspirated oxygen tension
decreased inspiratory limb (on PFTs)
decreased intensity
decreased left ventricular filling on
    inspiration
decreased lung compliance
decreased P-wave amplitude
decreased peripheral vascular
    resistance
decreased pulmonary vascular
    compliance
decreased stroke volume
decreased systemic resistance
decreased tidal volume
decreased venous return
decreased ventilatory capacity
decreased ventricular preload
decrease in vascular markings
decrease of blood viscosity
decrease of capillary dilatation
decremental conduction
decremental element
decremental pacing
decrescendo holosystolic murmur
decrescendo murmur
decubital ulcer
decubitus
    Andral
    angina

decubitus *(cont.)*
    contralateral
    dorsal
    lateral
decubitus cough
decubitus on the sound side
decubitus position
    left lateral
    right lateral
decubitus ulcer
deep-breathing exercises
deep calf veins
deep cardiac plexus
deep Doppler velocity interrogation
deep hypothermic circulatory arrest
deep limb lead
deep plexus
deep respirations
deep tendon reflex (DTR)
deep thrombophlebitis
deep veins
deep venous aplasia
deep venous hypoplasia
deep venous insufficiency (DVI)
deep venous thromboembolism
deep venous thrombosis (DVT)
deep visceral pain
defecation syncope
defect (see also *deformity*)
    acquired ventricular septal (AVSD)
    anastomotic
    anteroapical
    aortic septal
    aorticopulmonary
    aorticopulmonary septal
    atrial ostium primum
    atrial septal (ASD)
    atrioventricular canal
    atrioventricular septal
    AV (atrioventricular) conduction
    cardiofacial
    concomitant

defect *(cont.)*
  conduction
  conoventricular
  contiguous ventricular septal
  conotruncal
  crista supraventricularis septal
  curvilinear
  cushion
  discrete
  endocardial cushion
  filling (on imaging study)
  fixed
  fixed intracavitary filling
  fixed perfusion
  inferoapical
  infracristal septal
  infracristal ventricular septal
  infundibular ventricular septal
  interatrial septal (septum)
  interventricular conduction
  interventricular septal (IVSD)
  intra-atrial conduction
  intra-atrial filling
  intraluminal
  intraluminal filling
  intraventricular conduction
  junctional
  juxta-arterial ventricular septal
  juxtatricuspid ventricular septal
  linear
  lobulated filling
  luminal
  matched V/Q (ventilation-perfusion)
  membranous ventricular septal
  muscular ventricular septal
  nonuniform rotational (NURD)
  ostium primum
  ostium secundum
  partial AV (atrioventricular) canal
  perfusion
  peri-infarctional
  peri-infarction conduction (PICD)

defect *(cont.)*
  perimembranous ventricular septal
  posteroapical
  postinfarction ventricular septal
  Rastelli type A, B, or C
    atrioventricular canal
  restrictive ventilatory
  reversible
  reversible ischemic
  reversible perfusion
  scintigraphic perfusion
  secundum and sinus venosus
  secundum atrial septal
  secundum-type atrial septal
  septal
  sinus venosus
  spontaneous closure of
  supracristal septal
  supracristal ventricular
  supracristal ventricular septal
  Swiss cheese ventricular septal
  transcatheter closure of atrial
    transient perfusion
  transient perfusion
  truncular congenital vascular
  type I (supracristal) ventricular
    septal
  type II (infracristal) ventricular
    septal
  type III (canal type) ventricular
    septal
  type IV (muscular) ventricular
    septal
  valvular
  ventilation-perfusion
  ventricular septal or (VSD)
defective communication between
  cardiac chambers
defective hemoglobin synthesis
defective platelet function
defective volume regulation
defervesce, defervesced

defibrillation
  endovenous
  external
  rectilinear biphasic waveform
    for external
  rescue
  single pulse
  transvenous
defibrillation cathode
defibrillation coil
defibrillation electrode
defibrillation performed with lungs
  fully inflated
defibrillation shock
defibrillation threshold (DFT)
defibrillation zone
defibrillator (also *cardioverter-
    defibrillator*)
  AICD (automatic implantable [in-
    ternal])
  AICD-B cardioverter-
  AICD-BR cardioverter-
  AID (automatic implantable [or
    internal])
  AID-B
  Alert Companion II
  Angstrom MD implantable single-
    lead
  Atrial View Ventak AV implantable
  Atrioverter
  automatic external (AED)
  automated external (AED)
  automated implantable cardioverter-
    (AICD)
  Belos VR-T internal cardioverter-
    (ICD)
  Cadet
  Contak CD CRT-D implantable
    cardioverter-
  Contak CD 2
  Contour MD implantable single-
    lead

defibrillator *(cont.)*
  Contour V-145D and LTV-135D
    implantable
  CPI automatic implantable
  DC (direct current)
  external cardioverter
  FirstSave automated external
  ForeRunner automatic external
  Gem DR implantable
  GEM II DR/VR implantable
    cardioverter-
  GEM III AT implantable
    cardioverter-
  Heart Aid 80
  Heartstream ForeRunner
    automatic external
  Hewlett-Packard
  implantable
  implantable cardioverter- (ICD)
  InSync implantable cardioverter-
  Intec implantable
  Jewel AF implantable
  LifeVest WCD 3000 external
    cardioverter-
  LifeVest wearable cardiac
  Medtronic Gem automatic
    implantable
  Medtronic GEM implantable
    cardioverter-
  Medtronic Micro Jewel II
    implantable
  Medtronic Physio-Control
    automatic and semiautomatic
  Medtronic Sprint lead for
    cardioverter-
  Metrix atrial
  Micron Res-Q implantable
    cardioverter-
  ODAM
  patient (PDF)
  PCD Transvene implantable
    cardioverter-

defibrillator *(cont.)*
  Photon DR dual-chamber
    implantable cardioverter-
  Phylax AV dual chamber
    implantable cardioverter-
  Physio-Control automatic and semi-
    automatic (Medtronic)
  Porta Pulse 3 portable
  Powerheart automatic external
    cardioverter-
  Res-Q ACD (arrhythmia control
    device)
  Res-Q Micron implantable
  Sentinel implantable cardioverter-
  Ventak AV III DR cardioverter-
  Ventak Mini II (and III) AICD
  Ventak Mini II (and III) AICD
  Ventak Prizm implantable
  Ventritex Angstrom MD
    implantable cardioverter-
  WCD 2000 system wearable
  transvenous lead
  Zoll
defibrillator paddle
defibrillator pads
defibrillator power source
defibrillator unit
defibrillatory action
defibrillatory activity
defibrillatory agent
defibrillatory device
defibrillatory efficacy score
defibrillatory paddle
defibrillatory shock
defibrinating syndrome
defibrination
deficiency
  accessory factor
  acyl coenzyme A (acyl-CoA)
  acid lipase
  acid maltase
  alpha$_1$-antitrypsin

deficiency *(cont.)*
  alpha-galactosidase
  alpha-galactosidase A
  alpha$_1$-proteinase inhibitor (a$_1$PI)
  antithrombin III
  ^{11}C (C-11) hydroxylase
  ^{17}C (C-17) hydroxylase
  cardiomyopathic carnitine
  carnitine
  ceramidase
  ceramide trihexosidase
  coagulation factor XI
  copper
  11 beta-hydroxylase
  glucocerebrosidase
  lipase acid
  lipoprotein lipase
  long chain acyl-CoA dehydrogenase
  lysosomal alpha-1,4-glucosidase
  maltase acid
  methemoglobin reductase
  multiple sulfatase
  phosphorylase kinase
  plasma coagulation factor
  plasminogen
  potassium
  protein C
  prothrombin
  respiratory chain complex I
  17-hydroxylase
  surfactant
  systemic carnitine
  thiamine
  thyroid hormone
  vitamin B complex
  vitamin K
deficient cortisol production
deficient fibrinolysis
deficit
  base
  carbonic acid
  oxygen

deficit *(cont.)*
  peripheral pulse
  pulse
  reversible ischemic neurologic
    (RIND)
  significant residual
  transient neurological
deflectable catheter
deflectable quadripolar catheter
deflectable-tip catheter
deflection
  delta
  His bundle
  intrinsic
  intrinsicoid
  QS
  RS
deflection of normal depolarizing wave
deflector, Cook
deflector wire
deformity (see also *defect*)
  cottage loaf
  gooseneck outflow tract
  hockey-stick tricuspid valve
  hourglass
  parachute mitral valve
  parachute-type
  pulmonary valve
  rolled edge
  scimitar
  snow man
  tricuspid valve
degenerated intima, friable thickened
degeneration
  angiolithic
  atheromatous
  cardiac valve mucoid
  cardiomyopathic
  collagen
  cusp
  fatty

degeneration *(cont.)*
  fibrinoid
  glassy
  hyaline
  hydropic
  hypertensive vascular
  Mönckeberg
  mucoid medial
  mural
  myocardial
  myocardial cellular
  myocardial fibers
  myxoid
  myxomatous
  sclerotic
degeneration of mitral valve,
  myxomatous
degenerative atrioventricular node
  disease
DeGimard syndrome
deglutition syncope
degradation
  fibrinogen
  image quality
degree, noncircularity
degrees of heart block
Dehio test
dehisced
dehiscence
  perivalvular
  prosthesis
  wound
dehiscence of graft anastomosis
dehydroepiandrosterone sulfate
  (DHEA-S)
dehydrogenase, lactic
Deklene suture
Deknatel (Shur-Strip) wound closure
  tape
de la Camp sign
de Lange syndrome

delay
    atrioventricular
    conduction
    intraventricular conduction
delayed diastolic murmur (DDM)
delayed image
delayed phase of arteriogram
delayed sternal closure
delayed xenograft rejection (DXR)
delayed xenon washout
delay time, echo
Delbet sign
deleterious effect
delicate crepitation
delirium, postcardiotomy
delivered energy
Delmege sign of tuberculosis
Delrin frame of valve prosthesis,
    Dacron-covered
delta deflection
delta wave
Delta pacemaker
deltopectoral approach
deltopectoral groove
deltopectoral incision
demand (standby)
demand mode of pacemaker
demand pacemaker battery
demand pulse generator unit
demarcation line
DeMartel scissors
DeMartel vascular clamp
De Martini-Balestra syndrome
dementia
    arteriosclerotic
    Binswanger
    multi-infarct
    vascular
demifacets
demise, imminent
demographic data
Demons-Meigs syndrome

Demos tibial artery clamp
de Musset sign (aortic aneurysm)
denatured homograft
denervation, cardiac
denervation of heart
de novo angina
de novo fenestration
de novo lesion
de novo thrombosis
dense adhesions
dense consolidation
dense scar
densitometry, dynamic spiral CT lung
density, densities
    diffuse reticular
    discrete perihilar
    echo
    hydrogen
    increased
    mottled
    perihilar
    proton
    spin
    wedge-shaped
denudation, areas of
denude
denuded epithelium
denuding
Denver PAK (percutaneous access kit)
Denver pleuroperitoneal shunt
deoxygenated blood
dep (slang for depressed)
dependent
    pacer-
    steroid
dependent edema
dependent edema fluid, resorption of
dependent extracellular fluid accumula-
    tion
dependent rubor
dephasing, signal

depletion
    intravascular volume
    mild volume
    moderate volume
    premature battery
    profound volume
    volume
deployed the graft
deployment
    catheter
    graft-into-graft
    stent
depolarization
    atrial
    atrial premature (APD)
    cardiac
    diffuse chaotic ventricular
    early ventricular (preexcitation)
    graft-into-graft
    His bundle–distal coronary sinus
        atrial (H-DCSA)
    His bundle–middle coronary sinus
        atrial (H-MCSA)
    premature atrial
    premature ventricular
    rapid
    ventricular
depolarization phase, diastolic
depolarization wave
deposit
    glycolipid
    hemosiderin
deposition
    particle
    ultrafine particle
depressed cardiac contractility
depressed contractility
depressed diaphragm
depressed ejection fraction
depressed J point
depressed myocardial contractile
    performance

depressed right ventricular contractile
    function
depressed serum potassium
depressed T waves
depression
    cough reflex
    downhill ST segment
    hemidiaphragm
    hemodynamic
    horizontal ST segment
    marked ST segment
    myocardial
    reciprocal
    respiratory
    sinus node
    ST segment
depression of cough reflex
depressor anguli oris muscle
deranged left ventricular contractility
derangement
    chemical
    immunologic
Dermabond skin adhesive
Dermacea wound care
Derma-Gel hydrogel sheet
Dermalene suture
Dermalon suture
DermaMend foam wound dressing
DermaMend hydrogel dressing
Dermanet contact-layer wound
    dressing
DermAssist hydrocolloid dressing
    material
DermAssist wound filling material
Dermatell hydrocolloid dressing
    material
dermatitis, stasis
Derra commissurotomy knife
Derra valve dilator
DES (drug-eluting stent)
desaturated phospholipids
desaturation, systemic arterial oxygen

descending aorta
descending aorta–pulmonary artery
   shunt
descending thoracic aneurysmectomy
descending thoracic aorta, penetrating
   wound to
descent
   x
   X′ (X prime)
   y
Deschamps compressor
Deschamps ligature carrier
desensitizing regimen
Deseret angiocatheter
desert fever
desert rheumatism
desiccated
desiccation
desiccation of thrombus, laser
Desilets-Hoffman catheter introducer
desoxycorticosterone (DOC)
d'Espine sign
desquamating fibrosing alveolitis
desquamation, epithelial
desquamative interstitial pneumonia
   (DIP)
destruction, alveolar
destruction of pulmonary parenchyma
destruction of vascular bed
destructive inflammatory bronchial
   changes
detail
   exquisite
   suboptimal
detection, automated edge
detection zone
detector, cadmium iodide
detergent asthma
deterioration
   mild cardiopulmonary
   moderate cardiopulmonary
   profound cardiopulmonary

Determann syndrome
determination of all lung volumes
Detsky modified cardiac risk index
   score
De Vega prosthesis
De Vega tricuspid valve anuloplasty
development, interval (on x-ray)
deviant pathways
deviated septum
deviation
   aortic
   left axis (LAD)
   mediastinal
   right axis (RAD)
   significant axis
   tracheal
device—a quick-reference list of medical devices and systems found in
   cardiovascular/thoracic dictation.
   Common devices such as *catheter,*
   defibrillator, drug delivery devices,
   pacemaker, stent, tube, and *ventric-*
   ular assist devices appear as main
   entries.
   abdominal aortic counterpulsation
      (AACD)
   ablative
   Acapella chest physical therapy
   ACD (active compression-
      decompression) resuscitator
   Acrobat heart stabilization
   ACS anchor exchange
   Acuson V5M multiplanar TEE
      (transesophageal echocardio-
      graphic) monitor
   Adkins strut
   Aerochamber face mask
   Aestiva/5 MRI anesthesia machine
   a-fiX cannula seals
   Amicus separator
   Amplatzer septal occluder (ASO)
   Amplatz ventricular septal defect

device *(cont.)*

Androgram
Androscope i-Stethos
Androscope Stethos
Angio-Seal hemostatic puncture
    closure
Angiotech adhesion barrier
AnnuloFlex anuloplasty ring
Arrow-Clarke Pleura-Seal
    thoracentesis kit
Arrow-Trerotola percutaneous
    thrombolytic
ArteriA embolic protection
aspiration-tulip
Axius Vacuum 2 stabilizer
BackStop disposable waste
    collection container
Baim-Turi
Baladi Inverter (clampless aortic
    partial occlusion)
Balloon-on-a-Wire
Bentley Duraflo II extracorporeal
    perfusion circuit
bioabsorbable closure
Biocor 200 oxygenator
Biofilter hemoconcentrator
Bio-Vascular Probe
Block
blood flow enhancement (BFE)
Blood Shield
Bovie ultrasonic aspirator
Bowel wire cutter
Bowen wire
Bowen wire tightener
Boynton needle holder
Brockenbrough
Bürker chamber for macrophage
    counting
Capio suture capturing
Captiva blood containment
cardiac
Cardica anastomotic

device *(cont.)*

CardioBeeper CB-12L monitoring
Cardiocap 5 patient monitor
Cath-Finder catheter tracking kit
CathLink implantable vascular
    access
Cath-Shield
Cavitron ultrasonic surgical
    aspirator (CUSA)
Champ
Chemo-Port per venam catheter
    system
circulator boot therapy
CirKuit-Guard
Clarke-Reich micro knot pusher
ClearCut 2
CoaguChek self-testing
Cobe CPS heart-lung machine
COBE 2991 Cell Processor
Coherent VersaPulse
Cohiba arteriotomy closure
Cohn cardiac stabilizer
Constant distal protection
Converge anastomotic
COPD Lung Profiler
CorLink
Cournand
Cragg thrombolytic brush
CT-Linac (computed tomography
    with linear accelerator)
cutting
CV Peri-Guard
CVProfilor DO-2020 cardio-
    vascular profiling
CyberKnife Express
da Vinci robot
defibrillatory
Deschamps ligature carrier
DHD CliniFLO exercise
    equipment
Dinamap automated blood pressure
directional atherectomy

device *(cont.)*
    disposable aortic rotating punch
    Doppler
    double umbrella
    D-Prevent
    DSP Micro Diamond-Point
        microsurgery
    D-Stat vascular sealing
    Duet positive airway pressure
        breathing
    Duet vascular sealing
    Duraflo II extracorporeal perfusion
        circuit
    Durathane cardiac
    Elecath circulatory support
    Electro-Mate cutting and
        coagulating
    El Gamal
    Elite vascular hemostasis
    emergency infusion (EID)
    Enclose anastomosis assist
    Endo Babcock surgical grasping
    endocut cautery
    Endodissect
    Endo-Flo endoscopic irrigation
        apparatus
    Endo Grasp
    endoscopic suction cap
    En Garde closure apparatus
    Endo Shears
    Endo Stitch
    EndoWrist
    ENTec Plasma Wands
    Epi-Grip
    Equivas
    Eschmann blade
    Evershears II bipolar curved
        scissors
    Evolve Cardiac Continuum
    eXcel-DR (disposable/reusable)
    eXcel-DR heliX knot pusher
    eXcel-DR pneumo needle

device *(cont.)*
    eXpose retractor
    eXtract specimen bag
    ExtreSafe phlebotomy
    extraction atherectomy
    Fehling bioptome
    Finesse cardiac
    Flo-Thru Intraluminal Shunt
    FloWire Doppler ultrasound
        medical
    Flutter
    Fulcrum distal filter
    Fulcrum distal occlusion
    Gelport
    Gensini
    Glidecath torque
    Glycoprene vascular occlusion
    Goetz
    Goodale-Lubin
    GraftAssist vein and graft holder
    Hall valvulotome
    Harmonic Scalpel
    HeartCard
    HeartQuest
    heliX knot pusher
    Hemochron Response whole blood
        coagulation
    Herbst mandibular advancement
    Hi-Per
    HomeTrak Plus compact cardiac
        event recorder
    HumidAire heated humidifier
    Hydrocoil XT vascular emboliza-
        tion
    ICD-ATP (implantable cardio-
        verter-defibrillator/atrial
        tachycardia pacing)
    Ideal cardiac
    In-Exsufflator cough machine
    Innovante retrieval
    Inspirator
    InspirEase

device *(cont.)*
    intense pulsed light source (IPLS)
    intra-aortic balloon assist
    intracoronary Doppler flow wire
    Itrel 3 spinal cord stimulation
      system
    IVM vascular occluder
    Kendall Sequential Compression
    King
    Lactoprene vascular occlusion
    LaparoSonic coagulating shears
      for autograft harvesting
    Lehman
    LeukoNet Filter
    Ligaclip
    Linx guidewire extension
    Liposorber LA-15 machine
    Lloyd-Davies scissors
    low profile balloon feeding
    L-shaped trocar
    Marlow Primus instrument
      collection
    Master Flow Pumpette
    Maxima Forté blood oxygenator
    Max-Prene vascular occlusion
    MediPort implantable vascular
      access
    Medtronic-Hall
    Medtronic-Hancock
    Medtronic Jewel AF implantable
      arrhythmia management
    Medtronic Octopus stabilizing
    Medtronic Pulsor Intrasound pain
      reliever
    Medtronic tremor control therapy
    Merit Medical stent inflation kit
    Meritrans disposable blood pressure
      transducer
    MicroMed DeBakey ventricular
      assist
    Miltex surgical instruments
    mist stick

device *(cont.)*
    Monarch digital inflation
    multiadjustable fitting
    multi-electrode surgical (MES)
    Myolift heart positioning
    NBIH cardiac
    NB200 vascular access
    Neuroshield cerebral protection
    Nevyas drape retractor arched
      frame
    New Leaf cardiopulmonary
      performance testing
    Nu-Tip disposable scissor tip
    Nycore cardiac
    Octopus stabilizing
    OmniFilter
    Omniscience
    one-shot anastomotic instrument
    Onyx finger pulse
    OptiHaler
    Osciflator balloon inflation syringe
    Osteoprene vascular occlusion
    oxygenator
    Pacesetter APS pacemaker
      programmer
    Pacesetter Trilogy DR+ pulse
      generator
    Padogram
    Papercuff disposable blood pressure
      cuff
    Passager introducing sheath
    Perclose
    Perclose A-T (auto-tie) suture-
      mediated vessel closure
    Perclose closure
    percutaneous closure
    percutaneous thrombolytic (PTD)
    PerDUCER pericardial access
    Performance irrigation
    Peri-Guard
    Peri-Strips
    Peri-Strips Dry

device *(cont.)*
    PET balloon atherectomy
    photonic stimulator
    Physio Partner support mechanism
    Pitié-Salpetrière saphenous vein hook
    Pixsys FlashPoint
    PLAATO (percutaneous left atrial appendage transcatheter occlusion)
    PlegiaGuard
    PlexiPulse
    Pleur-evac
    Port-A-Cath
    Positrol
    Probe
    Proximate flexible linear stapler
    Proximate linear cutter surgical stapler
    PulmoSphere
    pulsatile assist (PAD)
    PulseDose technology
    QuantiFERON-TB
    quickWIT (wire insertion tool)
    RAMP Reader
    Raptor PTCA balloon
    Rashkind
    Raulerson syringe
    Regency SR+ single-chamber, rate-responsive pulse generator
    Reitan catheter pump
    Relia-Flow
    Request (used in heart catheterization)
    RESPeRATE apparatus
    Respironics CPAP (continuous positive airway pressure) machine
    Respironics nasal mask
    Respitrace machine
    Retrox fractal active fixation lead
    Rheolog

device *(cont.)*
    R-Med Plug
    Rotablator
    RotaLink Plus rotational atherectomy
    RotaLink rotational atherectomy
    rotary cutter
    rotational atherectomy
    roticulating endograsper
    Rotoresect
    Ruiz-Cohen round expander
    Rumel tourniquet
    SAPHFinder surgical balloon dissector
    SAPHtrak balloon dissector
    Sarns ABLD system
    Sarns H.E.L.P unit
    Sechrist Air/O_2 blender
    Segura Lock hub
    sewing capsule
    Signa I.S.T. MRI scanner
    Simpson PET balloon atherectomy
    SiPAP
    SmartFlow
    Soft N Dry Merocel sponge
    Sof-Wick drain sponge
    Sorin heart-lung machine
    specimen collecting
    Spectranetics laser sheath (SLS)
    Sphygmocorde
    Spira-Valve
    Stentloc
    St. Jude
    Super-9 guiding
    Supple Peri-Guard
    Surgifoam absorbable gelatin sponge
    suture-ligated embolization microcoils
    Suture Trimmer accessory to The Closer
    Suture/VesiBand organizer

device *(cont.)*
   Symbiant distal protection
   Symbion pneumatic assist
   Syringe Avitene delivery system
      for a collagen hemostat
   Szabo-Berci needle driver
   Tagarno 3SD cine projector
      for angiography
   Tandem
   TandemHeart
   TEC atherectomy
   Techstar percutaneous closure
   The Closer closure
   Thermedics
   third-generation (first-, second-,
      fourth-, etc.)
   Thoracoport
   Titanium VasPort implantable
      vascular access
   Trocan disposable CO_2 trocar
      and cannula
   Tru-Area Determination wound-
      measuring
   TruWave pressure transducer
   TruZone PFM (peak flow meter)
   tunneling instrument
   Ultravas
   Unigrip safety adaptor for stent
      delivery system
   Univas
   Vasconnect
   Vascu-Guard
   VasoSeal VHD (vascular
      hemostatic device)
   VCS clip adapter
   VenaSonix ultrasound therapeutic
   Venodyne compression boots
   Venometer vascular diagnostic
      and monitoring
   ventilation-exchange bougie
   Viasys cardiopulmonary exercise
      testing

device *(cont.)*
   Viasys pulmonary function testing
   videoendoscopic surgical equipment
   Visuflo
   VMax diagnostic
   VM diagnostic
   VNUS radiofrequency generator
   Volutrol control apparatus for
      intravenous infusion
   Voyager aortic
   Wallstent endoprosthesis with
      Unistep catheter delivery system
   Williams
   Wizard disposable inflation
   XT
   Zucker and Myler cardiac
device embolization
Devices, Ltd., pacemaker
DeVilbiss ultrasound nebulizer
devitalized tissue
devoid of circulation
DeWeese vena cava clip
dexamethasone
dexamethasone suppression of adrenal
   tissue
Dexon mesh
Dexon Plus suture
Dexon suture
Dexon II suture
dextrum, cor triatriatum
Dexter-Grossman classification of
   mitral regurgitation
dextran
   high-molecular-weight
   low-molecular-weight
dextran and saline solution
dextran plasma volume extender
dextrocardia, mirror image
dextroposed aorta
dextroposition of the aorta
dextrorotatory

dextrotransposition (D-transposition) of
   great arteries
dextroversion
dextroversion of heart
DF (defibrillation)
DF lead, Telectronics endocardial
D5W, D$_5$W (5% dextrose in water)
DFP (diastolic filling pressure)
DFT (defibrillation threshold)
DG (Davis & Geck) Softgut suture
DHD CliniFLO exercise equipment
DHEA-S (dehydroepiandrosterone
   sulfate)
diabetic peripheral vascular insufficiency
diagnosis
   clinical
   differential
   empirical
   pathologic
   postoperative
   preoperative
   presumptive
   tentative
diagnostic flexible fiberoptic
   bronchoscopy
diagnostic modality
diagnostic ST segment changes
diagnostic thoracentesis
diagnostic thoracoscopic lung biopsy
diagonal branch of artery
diagram, Ladder
dialysis, continuous ambulatory
   peritoneal (CAPD)
diameter (or dimension)
   anteroposterior
   aortic (AD)
   aortic root
   artery
   coil-to-vessel
   increased AP (anterior-posterior)
      (of the chest)

diameter *(cont.)*
   left anterior internal (LAID)
   left atrial
   left ventricular internal (LVID)
   luminal
   minimal luminal
   narrow anteroposterior
   right ventricular internal (RVID)
   satisfactory luminal
   skin wheal
   stenosis
   transverse
   transverse cardiac
   valve
   wide luminal
diamond anastomosis principle
Diamond-Blackfan syndrome
diamond-coated bur
Diamond-Lite titanium surgical
   instrument
diamond-shaped anastomosis
diamond-shaped heart murmur
diamond-shaped sequential vein graft
diaphoresis
diaphoretic
diaphragm, diaphragms
   crura of the
   crus of the
   depressed
   elevated
   free air under the
   muscular crus of
   polyolefin rubber
diaphragmatica, pleura
diaphragmatic breathing
diaphragmatic contractility
diaphragmatic crus
diaphragmatic elevation
diaphragmatic hernia
diaphragmatic lymph nodes
diaphragmatic pacemaker
diaphragmatic pericardium

diaphragmatic pleura
diaphragmatic pleurisy
diaphragmatic surface of heart
diaphragmatic surface of lung
diaphragmatic surface of right ventricle
diaphragmatic wall myocardial
   infarction
diaphragm compressed downward and
   costal margin upward, exposing the
   heart
diaphragm divided at costal attachments
diaphragm flap diaphragmitis
diaphragm of stethoscope
Diasonics catheter
Diasonics transducer
Diastat vascular access graft
diastole
   early
   late
   mid
diastolic blood pressure (DBP)
diastolic cardiac arrest
diastolic collapse of venous pulse
diastolic coronary perfusion pressure
diastolic counterpulsation
diastolic depolarization phase
diastolic diameter of left ventricle
diastolic dysfunction
diastolic filling period
diastolic gallop, prominent ventricular
diastolic gallop sound
diastolic heart failure
diastolic murmur (DM), graded from
   1 to 4
diastolic overload
diastolic perfusion pressure
diastolic perfusion time
diastolic pressure-time index (DPTI)
diastolic regurgitant velocity
diastolic reserve
diastolic rumbling murmur
diastolic thrill

diastolic velocity-time integral
DiaSys Novacor cardiac device
diathermy, cutting
diathesis
   hemorrhagic
   hypertensive
diatrizoate meglumine contrast medium
diatrizoate sodium contrast medium
DIC (disseminated intravascular
   coagulation)
Dick valve dilator
dicrotic notch
dicrotic notch or wave of carotid
   arterial pulse
dicrotic pulse
Dideco arterial filter
diet
   AHA (American Heart Association)
   AHA low-fat
   AHA (for hypercholesterolemia)
   anticoronary
   Atkins
   Dean Ornish
   Kempner
   Kempner rice
   low-cholesterol
   low-fat
   low in saturated fat
   low-salt
   low-sodium
   no-added-salt
   salt-restricted
   Schemm
   sodium-restricted
   Zone
dietary fiber
dietary sodium restriction
dietary supplements
dietary therapy
Diethrich coronary artery instruments
diethylcarbamazine
Dietlen syndrome

Dieulafoy gastric lesion
DIF (digital image fusion) procedure
difference
    aortic-left ventricular pressure
    arteriovenous oxygen (AVD O_2)
    AV (arteriovenous)
    discernible
    pulmonary AV
    resting AV
    systemic AV
differential in white blood cell count:
    eosinophils, basophils, lymphocytes,
    monocytes, polymorphonuclear
    neutrophils
differential cyanosis
differential deceleration
differential diagnosis
differential renal vein renin
differentiation
difficult to wean from cardiopulmonary
    bypass
difficulty in breathing
difficulty swallowing
diffuse aggressive polymorphous
    infiltrate
diffuse alveolar interstitial infiltrates
diffuse angiokeratoma disease
diffuse aortic dilatation
diffuse aortomegaly
diffuse arteriolar spasm
diffuse bilateral alveolar infiltration
diffuse capacity of lungs for carbon
    monoxide (DL_{CO})
diffuse chaotic ventricular depolariza-
    tion
diffuse cholesterol embolization
diffuse crackles
diffuse emphysema
diffuse heart block
diffuse hyperemia
diffuse hypoplasia
diffuse infiltrate

diffuse inspiratory crepitant rales
diffuse interstitial infiltrate
diffuse interstitial lung disease
diffuse interstitial pulmonary fibrosis
diffuse lentiginosis
diffuse lesion
diffuse nodular densities
diffuse perivascular infiltrate
diffuse pleural thickening
diffuse pleurisy
diffuse pulmonary fibrosis
diffuse pulmonary infiltration
diffuse rales
diffuse reticular densities
diffuse reticulonodular infiltrates
diffuse stenosis
diffuse ST-T depression
diffuse subarachnoid hemorrhage
diffuse symmetric hypertrophic
    cardiomyopathy
diffuse thickening of arterial intima
diffuse T-wave inversions
diffuse wheezes
diffusing capacity of alveolar capillary
    membrane
diffusing capacity of lung for CO
    (carbon monoxide) (DL_{CO})
diffusion
    decreased carbon monoxide (CO)
    impaired oxygen
diffusion tensor magnetic resonance
    imaging (DT-MRI)
dig (slang for digitalis)
dig effect
dig level
DiGeorge anomaly
DiGeorge syndrome
digestive-respiratory fistula (DRF)
digital clubbing
digital image fusion (DIF) procedure
digital subtraction
digital vascular imaging (DVI)

digital vessel thrombosis
digitalis effect
digitalis excess
digitalis intoxication
digitalis level
digitalis toxicity
digitalization
digitalize, digitalized
digitalizing dose
digital runoff
digital storage (in cineangiography)
digital subtraction angiography (DSA)
digital subtraction pulmonary
  angiogram
digital videoangiography
digitoxicity
Digitron digital subtraction imaging
  system
digoxin
digoxin-specific Fab antibody
  fragments
dihydropyridine
diisocyanate asthma
Dilantin syndrome
Dilaparel inhaler
dilatation (also *dilation*)
  aneurysmal
  anular
  aortic root
  arterial
  balloon
  cardiac
  chamber
  diffuse aortic
  fusiform
  idiopathic pulmonary artery
  idiopathic right atrial
  intraluminal
  left ventricular
  multiple mural
  percutaneous balloon
  percutaneous transluminal balloon
    (PTBD)

dilatation *(cont.)*
  poststenotic
  poststenotic aortic
  pulmonary artery
  pulmonary trunk idiopathic
  pulmonary valve stenosis
  right ventricular
  sequential
  transient left ventricular
  ventricular
  ventricular wall
dilatation and hypertrophy of left
  ventricle
dilatation of alveoli
dilatation of aorta
dilatation of ascending aorta
dilatation of respiratory bronchioles
dilatation of terminal bronchioles
dilatation of veins
dilated aortic root
dilated bronchi
dilated cardiomyopathy secondary to:
  chronic overload
  toxicity to doxorubicin
  toxicity to ethanol
  toxicity to uremia
dilated coronaropathy
dilated myocardium
dilated pulmonary artery
dilated tortuous veins
dilated vein
dilation (see *dilatation*)
dilation of artery by balloon catheter
dilation of bronchus
dilation of pulmonary artery
dilation of tract
dilator
  aortic
  AVA HF
  AVA 3XI
  Brock cardiac
  Cooley valve

dilator *(cont.)*
    Crump vessel
    Derra valve
    Dick valve
    Garrett vascular
    Gerbode valve
    Glidecath
    Hegar
    Hemo-Cath
    Henley
    Hiebert vascular
    Hohn vessel
    Innovante
    Lucchese mitral valve
    mitral valve
    myocardial
    stepped tissue
    through-the-scope balloon
    transventricular
    Trousseau
    Tubbs mitral valve
    UMI (not HUMI)
    valve
    vein
dilator-sheath
diluent control
dilutional hematocrit
dilutional hyponatremia
dimension
    absolute artery
    aortic root
    end-systolic
    intraluminal
    intrathoracic
    left atrial
    left ventricular end-diastolic (LVEDD)
    left ventricular end-systolic (LVESD)
    left ventricular internal (LVID)
    left ventricular internal diastolic (LVIDD)

dimension *(cont.)*
    left ventricular internal end-diastole (LVIEd)
    left ventricular internal end-systole (LVIDs)
    left ventricular systolic (LVs)
    luminal
    right ventricular (RVD)
diminished consciousness
diminished lung volume
diminished pedal pulses
diminished systemic perfusion
diminution of pulses
diminutive vessel
dimple, blind
Dinamap automated blood pressure device
Dinamap blood pressure monitor and Oxytrak pulse oximeter
Dinamap monitor
Dinamap ultrasound blood pressure manometer
diode, Zener
Diovan (valsartan)
Diovan HCT (valsartan, hydrochlorothiazide)
DIP (desquamative interstitial pneumonia)
dip and plateau phenomenon
dip phenomenon
dip, septal
diphasic complex on EKG
diphasic postcardiotomy syndrome
diphasic P wave
diphasic T wave
diphtheria
diphtheritic croup
diphtheritic membrane
diphtheritic myocarditis
diplopia
Diplos M pacemaker
dipyridamole echocardiography test

dipyridamole handgrip test
dipyridamole infusion test
dipyridamole thallium imaging
dipyridamole thallium scan
dipyridamole thallium stress test
dipyridamole thallium ventriculography
dipyridamole thallium-201 scintigraphy
directable tip (of bronchoscope)
direct caval cannulation
direct current ablation (DCA)
direct current electrical countershock
direct current energy
DirectFlow arterial cannula
directional atherectomy device
directional coronary angioplasty
    (DCA)
directional coronary atherectomy
    (DCA)
direct mechanical ventricular actuation
    (DMVA)
direct myocardial revascularization
    (DMR)
direct puncture phlebography
DirectView CR 900 imaging system
direct vision nasal intubation
direct vision through a mediastinoscope
Dirofilaria immitis infection
DISA S-Flex coronary stent
discernible difference
discernible findings
discernible venous motion
discharge, inappropriate
disklike atelectasis
disk of endocardium
discoid shadow
discolored
discomfort
    burning
    chest
    dull substernal
    ominous chest

discomfort *(cont.)*
    precordial
    substernal burning
discordance, atrioventricular
discordant arterial connection
discordant atrioventricular connection
discordant cellular xenograft
discordant organ xenograft
discordant ventriculoarterial connections
Discovery LS imaging system
Discovery portable monitor
discrepancy in blood pressure in upper
    and lower extremities
discrete defect
discrete lesion
discrete perihilar densities
discrete pulsations
discrete sound
discrete stenosis
discrete subaortic stenosis
discriminate
discrimination
disease
    acquired
    acquired heart
    acute rheumatic endocarditis
    acute rheumatic fever (ARF)
    acute rheumatic pericarditis (ARP)
    acute tuberculosis
    acyanotic congenital heart
    Adams-Stokes
    adrenal
    Albright
    alcoholic heart muscle
    allergic bronchopulmonary
        aspergillosis
    allergic bronchopulmonary fungal
    allergic myocardial granulomatous
    allergic respiratory
    allograft coronary artery
    amyloid heart

disease *(cont.)*
  angiographically mild coronary
    artery
  angiokeratoma corporis diffusum
  antiglomerular basement membrane
    antibody
  aortic valve
  aortic valvular (AVD)
  aorto-occlusive
  aortoiliac
  aortoiliac obstructive valvular
  aortoiliac occlusive
  aortoiliac vascular
  arrhythmogenic
  arterial degenerative
  arteriosclerotic cardiovascular
    (ASCVD)
  arteriosclerotic heart (ASHD)
  arteriosclerotic peripheral vascular
  asbestos-related pleural
  asymptomatic left main (ALMD)
  atheromatous
  athero-occlusive
  atherosclerotic
  atherosclerotic carotid artery
    (ACAD)
  atherosclerotic pulmonary vascular
    (ASPVD)
  atypical aortic valve stenosis
  Ayerza-Arrillaga
  Bamberger
  Bamberger-Marie
  Bannister angioedema
  Batten
  Battey-avium complex
  Bazin
  Beau
  Becker
  Bernard-Soulier
  beryllium
  Binswanger
  bird-fancier's

disease *(cont.)*
  black lung
  Bornholm
  Bouillaud
  Bouveret
  branch
  brass-founder's
  bronchial type B
  bronchiolitis obliterans syndrome
    (BOS)
  brown lung
  budgerigar-fancier's
  Buerger
  Buerger thromboangiitis obliterans
  bullous lung
  calcified granulomatous
  California coccidioidomycosis
  carcinoid heart
  carcinoid tricuspid valve
  cardiac allograft vascular (CAVD)
  cardiorenal
  cardiovascular
  cardiovascular renal
  carotid occlusive
  carotid vascular
  cavitary tuberculosis
  cerebellar
  Chagas
  cheese handler's
  cheese washer's
  Christmas (hemophilia B)
  chronic granulomatous (of
    childhood)
  chronic hypertensive
  chronic obstructive pulmonary
    (COPD)
  chronic peripheral arterial (CPAD)
  chronic rheumatic heart (CRHD)
  chronic thromboembolic
    hypertension
  CLE (congenital lobar emphysema)
  cobalt

disease *(cont.)*
  coexisting
  collagen vascular
  communicative
  Concato
  concomitant
  congenital heart (CHD)
  congenital lobar emphysema (CLE)
  congenital mitral valve
  constrictive pericardial
  contagious
  COPD
  cork-handler's
  coronary artery (CAD)
  coronary heart
  Corrigan aortic regurgitation
  corticobulbar
  corticospinal
  Corvisart
  cyanotic congenital heart
  cyanotic heart
  cystic lung
  cytomegalic inclusion
  debrancher
  degenerative atrioventricular node
  desquamating fibrosing alveolitis
  diffuse
  diffuse angiokeratoma
  diffuse interstitial
  disseminated *Mycobacterium*
    avium-intracellulare (MAI)
  Döhle (Doehle)
  Döhle syphilitic aortitis
  Duroziez congenital mitral stenosis
  eccentric plaque
  effusive pericardial
  ehrlichiosis
  emphysematous type A
  end-stage
  end-stage cardiac
  end-stage cardiopulmonary
  end-stage chronic obstructive
    pulmonary

disease *(cont.)*
  end-stage lung
  end-stage pulmonary
  end-stage renal
  end-stage suppurative lung
  end-stage vascular
  endocardial fibroelastosis
  eosinophilic disseminated collagen
  eosinophilic endomyocardial
  exanthematous
  extracardiac
  extracranial vascular
  extrapulmonary
  extrapyramidal
  Fabry
  factor IX deficiency
  Fallot
  Farber's
  fibrocalcific rheumatic
  flax-dresser's
  Forbes
  Friedländer endarteritis obliterans
  functional cardiovascular
  functional valve
  Gairdner
  gannister
  Gaucher
  Glanzmann
  global cardiac
  glycogen storage
  graft occlusive
  graft versus host (GVHD)
  grain-handler's
  great artery
  Hagner
  Hamman
  hard metal
  Harley
  heart
  Heberden
  Heberden angina pectoris
  Heckathorn

disease *(cont.)*
    Heller-Döhle syphilitic aortitis
    hemoglobin C–thalassemia
    hemoglobin E–thalassemia
    hepatic veno-occlusive
    Heubner
    Hodgkin
    Hodgson
    Hodgson aortic
    Horton
    Huchard
    Hutinel
    hydatid
    hyaline membrane
    hypereosinophilic heart
    hyperkinetic heart
    hypertensive cardiovascular
      (HCVD)
    hypertensive heart (HHD)
    hypertensive renal
    hypertensive vascular
    I-cell
    idiopathic eosinophilic lung
    idiopathic mural endomyocardial
    idiopathic pulmonary fibrosis
    IHD (ischemic heart)
    iliac atherosclerotic occlusive
    infectious
    infiltrative
    infiltrative interstitial
    inflammatory aneurysmal
    infrapopliteal
    infrarenal aortic
    inoperable
    interstitial
    interstitial lung (ILD)
    intimal atherosclerotic
    intrapulmonary
    intrinsic
    intrinsic pulmonary
    invasive pulmonary mycosis
    iron storage

disease *(cont.)*
    ischemic
    ischemic heart (IHD)
    ischemic myocardial
    Johnson-Stevens
    Kawasaki
    Keshan
    Krishaber
    Kussmaul-Maier
    kyphoscoliotic heart
    latent coronary artery
    latent ischemic heart
    left anterior descending coronary
      artery
    left main coronary artery
    left main equivalent
    legionnaires
    Leigh syndrome
    Lenègre
    Letterer-Siwe
    Lev
    Lev acquired complete heart block
    Lewis upper limb cardiovascular
    Libman-Sacks
    Libman-Sacks endocarditis
    Löffler (Loeffler)
    lower respiratory tract
    Lucas-Champonnière
    lunger
    lung fluke
    Lutz-Splendore-Almeida
    Lyme
    lymphoreticular malignant
    Majocchi
    maple bark stripper's
    microvascular
    Milton
    Milton angioedema
    mitral valve
    mitral valve stenosis (MVS)
    mixed connective tissue
    mixed restrictive-obstructive lung

disease *(cont.)*
  Mönckeberg (Moenckeberg)
  Mönckeberg medial sclerosis
  Mondor
  Mondor phlebitis
  Monge
  Moschcowitz
  moyamoya cerebrovascular
  multiple system
  multivalvular
  multivessel
  multivessel coronary artery
  mushroom picker's
  mushroom worker's
  necrotizing arterial
  nephrosclerosis
  Niemann-Pick
  no evidence of (NED)
  nonatherosclerotic coronary artery
  noncritical coronary artery
  nonhypertension-related
  nonoperable
  obstructive small airways
  occlusive
  occlusive peripheral arterial
  occlusive vascular
  occult
  occupational
  one-vessel coronary artery
  Opitz
  organic heart (OHD)
  organic valve
  Osler
  Owren (Factor V deficiency)
  parenchymal
  parenchymal lung
  Patella pyloric stenosis
  pericardial
  peripartal heart
  peripartum
  peripheral air-space
  peripheral arterial

disease *(cont.)*
  peripheral atherosclerotic
  peripheral vascular (PVD)
  Pick (of heart)
  pigeon-fancier's
  pituitary snuff-taker's
  polycystic kidney
  Pompe
  Pompe glycogen storage, type II
  popliteal artery
  Posadas
  Posadas-Wernicke
  post-transplant coronary artery
  primary electrical
  primary myocardial
  pulmonary alveolar proteinosis
    (PAP)
  pulmonary collagen vascular
    (PCVD)
  pulmonary heart
  pulmonary parenchymal
  pulmonary vascular
  pulmonary vascular obstructive
  pulmonary veno-occlusive (PVOD)
  pulseless
  Quincke angioedema
  radiation pericardial
  ragpicker's
  Raynaud
  reactive
  reactive airways (RAD)
  Refsum
  Reiter
  renal parenchymal
  Rendu-Osler-Weber
  renovascular
  reperfusion edema after lung
    transplantation
  respiratory bronchiolitis-associated
    interstitial lung
  respiratory chain complex I
    deficiency

disease *(cont.)*
    restrictive lung
    restrictive myocardial
    rheumatic arthritis
    rheumatic chorea
    rheumatic heart (RHD)
    rheumatic mitral valve
    rheumatic valvular
    rheumatoid lung
    rhizomelic chondrodysplasia
        punctata (RCP)
    right coronary artery
    Roger
    Rokitansky
    Rougnon-Heberden
    San Joaquin Valley fever
    saphenous vein bypass graft
    Schönlein (Schoenlein)
    scleroderma heart
    silo-filler's
    single-vessel
    single-vessel heart
    sinoatrial
    sinus node
    snuff taker's pituitary
    specific heart muscle
    Steinert
    Stokes-Adams
    suppurative lung
    Sydenham chorea
    symptomatic left main (SLMD)
    Takayasu
    thalassemia–sickle cell
    Thomsen
    three-vessel (four-, five-, etc.)
    three-vessel coronary artery
    thromboembolic
    thyrocardiac
    thyrotoxic heart
    tibial artery
    tibioperoneal occlusive
    triple coronary artery

disease *(cont.)*
    triple-vessel
    tsutsugamushi
    tuberculosis
    tungsten carbide
    two-vessel coronary artery
    upper respiratory infection (URI)
    URI (upper respiratory infection)
    valley fever (San Joaquin Valley,
        California)
    valvular (VD)
    valvular heart
    valvulitis
    vasculo-Behçet
    veno-occlusive (VOD)
    von Willebrand (or Willebrand)
    Weil
    Wenckebach
    Werlhof
    wheat weevil
    William syndrome
    Winiwarter-Buerger
    Wolman
    wood pulp worker's lung
    woolsorter's inhalation
disease-free vessel wall
disintegration of plaque by laser pulses
disk (see also *disc*)
    atrial
    Eigon
    intercalated
disk poppet
disklike atelectasis
disk-type valve
dislodgement
    complete
    lead
    partial
disobliteration, carotid
disorder
    autoimmune
    coronary vasomotion

disorder *(cont.)*
  lysosomal storage
  nodal rhythm
  posttransplantation lympho-
    proliferative (PTLD)
  restrictive lung
disorders of conduction
disorders of impulse conduction
disorders of impulse formation
disorientation, right-left
disparate (unequal; dissimilar)
disparity
disparity of maturation
dispersion, QT
displaced apical beat
displaced to left
  apical impulse
  PMI (point of maximal impulse)
displacement
  anterior tracheal
  late systolic
  mediastinum
  ST-segment
displacement of apical beat,
  inferolateral
display
  pseudocolor B-mode
  real-time
disposable aortic rotating punch
disposable electrode
disproportion
disrupted plaque
disruption
  medial
  perivalvular
dissected circumferentially
dissected free
dissecting aneurysm of aorta
dissecting aortic aneurysm
dissecting aortic hematoma
dissecting sponge

dissection
  aortic (type B)
  arterial
  blunt
  carotid arterial
  cautious
  cervicocephalic arterial
  circumferential
  extensive
  extrapericardial
  finger
  infundibular
  intimal
  intimal-medial
  intrapericardial
  meticulous
  SAPHFinder surgical balloon
  sharp
  sharp and blunt
  spiral
  subintimal
  tedious
  thoracic aortic
  type A
  type B
  vertebral arterial
dissection flap
dissection of descending aorta
dissection of mediastinal lymph nodes
dissector
  Holinger
  Jannetta
  Lemmon intimal
  Penfield
  ring
  SAPHtrak balloon
  Spacemaker balloon
  sponge
disseminated atheromatous
  embolization
disseminated cholesterol embolization
disseminated glial hamartoma

disseminated intravascular coagulation
    (DIC) syndrome
disseminated *Mycobacterium avium-*
    intracellulare (MAI) complex
disseminated necrotizing periarteritis
disseminated tuberculosis
dissemination of organisms by blood-
    stream
dissemination, pleural
dissociation
    atrial
    atrioventricular (AVD)
    auriculoventricular
    AV (atrioventricular)
    complete AV
    electromechanical
    Gallavardin
    incomplete atrioventricular (IAVD)
    interference
    intracavitary pressure-electrogram
    isorhythmic AV
    Mobitz-type AV
Distaflo bypass graft
distal anastomosis, parachute technique
    for
distal aortic arch aneurysm
distal arterial bypass
distal circumflex marginal artery
distal clot
distal control
distal coronary sinus (CS)
distal embolization
distal graft anastomosis
distal occlusion device, fulcrum
distant breath sounds
distant heart tones
distant metastases
distended veins at 45°
distended with heparinized blood
distensibility, ventricular
distensible

distention
    atrial presystolic
    jugular vein (or venous) (JVD)
    neck vein
    passive venous
    trigeminus (of neck veins)
    venous
distention of neck veins
distichiasis-heart and vasculature
    abnormalities
distomiasis, pulmonary
distortion of ST segment
distortion, radiographic pincushion
distractibility
distress
    cardiorespiratory
    idiopathic respiratory (of newborn)
    infantile respiratory
    marked respiratory
    mild respiratory
    moderate respiratory
    respiratory (of newborn)
    severe respiratory
distress at rest, respiratory
distribution
    anomalous
    binomial
    peribronchial
    perivascular
    reverse
    rimlike calcium
distributive shock
disturbance
    cardiac rhythm
    conduction
    constitutional
    electrolyte
    rhythm
    visual
disturbance of blood coagulation
disturbance of heart rhythm
diurese, diuresed

diuresis of heart failure
diuretic, diuretics
  high-ceiling
  loop
  mercurial
  osmotic
  potassium-sparing
  potassium-wasting
  thiazide
diuretic drugs
diuretic therapy
diver's syncope
divided doses
Dividose
diving reflex
divisional block
dizziness, periodic
DKS (Damus-Kaye-Stansel)
DKS anastomosis
DKS procedure for congenital heart
  defects
DL_{CO} (diffusing capacity of lungs for
  carbon monoxide)
D-loop, ventricular
D-loop ventricular situs
DLP cardioplegic catheter
DLP cardioplegic needle
DLT (double lung transplant) recipient
DM (diastolic murmur)
D-malposition of aorta
DMI (Diagnostic Medical Instruments)
  analyzer
DMI (diaphragmatic myocardial
  infarction)
DMPE (^{99m}Tc-bis-dimethylphos-
  phonoethane)
DMR (direct myocardial revasculariza-
  tion)
DMVA (direct mechanical ventricular
  actuation)
DNA ploidy pattern

DNA polymerase-alpha tumor marker
DNAR (do not attempt resuscitation)
  orders
DNR (do not resuscitate) status
dobutamine echocardiography
dobutamine exercise stress test
dobutamine stress echocardiography
  (DSE)
dobutamine thallium angiography
DOBV (double outlet both ventricles)
DOC (desoxycorticosterone)
DOC exchange technique
DOC guidewire extension
Docke diastolic murmur
docking wire
dock wire
Dodd perforating vein group
Dodge area-length method for
  ventricular activity
Dodge method for calculating left
  ventricular volume
Dodge method for ejection fraction
DOE (dyspnea on exertion)
Doehle (Döhle)
dog-boning
dog cough
Döhle (Doehle)
Döhle disease
Döhle-Heller aortitis
Döhle-Heller syndrome
Döhle syphilitic aortitis disease
dolens
  phlegmasia alba
  phlegmasia cerulea
  thrombophlebitis cerulea
DOLV (double outlet left ventricle)
dome and dart configuration on cardiac
  catheterization
dome of atrium
dome of diaphragm
dome of left atrium
dome-shaped heart

dome-shaped roof of pleural cavity
dominance
  coronary artery
  mixed
  right ventricular
  shared coronary artery
dominant, anatomically
dominant left coronary artery
dominant left coronary system
dominant left ventricular morphology
dominant right coronary artery
dominant right coronary system
doming, diastolic
doming of leaflets
doming of valve
domino procedure
Donath-Landsteiner test for
  paroxysmal cold hemoglobinuria
D1 (diagonal branch #1)
donor
  appropriately matched
  appropriately sized
donor heart
donor heart failure
donor heart-lung block
donor organ, appropriately sized and
  matched
donor organ ischemic time
donor team
Do Not Attempt Resuscitation (DNAR)
  orders
Do Not Resuscitate (DNR) status
doom, feeling of impending
Doplette
Doppler
  color flow
  continuous wave
  intraoperative
  pulsed
  spectral
Doppler blood flow detector
Doppler blood flow monitor

Doppler blood pressure
Doppler color flow imaging,
  transesophageal
Doppler color flow mapping
Doppler color spectral analysis
Doppler coronary catheter
Doppler derived stroke distance
Doppler echocardiography, epicardial
Doppler fetal heart murmur
Doppler flow probe study
Doppler flow-imaging system,
  real-time, two-dimensional
Doppler flow-meter
Doppler imaging
Doppler Intra-Dop intraoperative
Doppler perfusion index (DPI)
Doppler phenomenon
Doppler pulse
Doppler shift
Doppler signal
Doppler signal enhancers
Doppler spectral analysis
Doppler tissue imaging (DTI)
Doppler ultrasonic blood flow detector
Doppler ultrasonic fetal heart monitor
Doppler ultrasonic velocity detector
  segmental plethysmography
Doppler ultrasonography
Doppler ultrasound flowmeter
Doppler velocimetry
Doppler velocity waveforms (VWFs)
Doppler venous examination
Doppler waveform analysis of blood
  vessels
Dopplette monitor
Doptone monitor of fetal heart tones
Dorendorf sign of aortic arch
  aneurysm
Dor modification
Dor reconstruction
Dor remodeling ventriculoplasty

Dorros brachial internal mammary
  guiding catheter
Dorros infusion and probing catheter
Dor technique
dorsal branch
dorsal pedal pulse
dorsal ramus of spinal nerve
dorsalis pedis pulse
DORV (double outlet right ventricle)
dose, doses
  digitalizing
  divided
  incremental
  loading
  maintenance
  tapering
  titrated
  tracer
dose-escalation schedule
dose-limiting toxicity
dosimetry, nasal
dosing, titrated
Dos Santos needle for aortography
Dos Santos technique
Dotter angioplasty technique
Dotter caged balloon catheter
Dotter catheter
Dotter coaxial catheter
Dotter effect
dottering effect
Dotter Intravascular Retrieval Set
Dotter-Judkins PTA (percutaneous
  transluminal angioplasty)
Dotter method
Dotter system
Dotter technique
double-acting actuator
double aortic arch
double-armed suture
double-barrel aorta
double-barrel lumen
double extrastimuli

double inlet left ventricle/double outlet
  both ventricles
double inlet ventricles
double-lumen 5-cm catheter
double-lung transplant (DLT) recipient
double-occluding clamp
double orifice repair (Alfieri-plasty)
double-orifice repair of mitral regurgitation in Barlow disease
double outlet both ventricles (DOBV)
double outlet left ventricle (DOLV)
double outlet left ventricle syndrome
double outlet right ventricle (DORV)
double outlet right ventricle (I–IV)
  syndrome
double pleurisy
double-stage venous cannula
double systolic apical impulse
double umbrella closure
double umbrella device used in closure
  of a patent ductus arteriosus
double umbrella technique
double-walled fibroserous sac
double-wire atherectomy technique
doubly-armed suture
doubly clamped
doubly-committed ventricular septal
  defect
doughnut configuration on thallium
  imaging
doughnut magnet
doughy mass
Douglas bag method for determining
  cardiac output
Dow method for cardiac output
Down syndrome
downhill ST segment depression
downsloping ST segment depression
downstream sampling method
downward displaced apical beat
downward displacement of apical
  impulse

downward sloping
doxorubicin cardiotoxicity
Doyen clamp grasping forceps
Doyen rib elevator
Doyen rib rasp; raspatory
dP/dt (upstroke pattern on apex
    cardiogram), peak
DPI (Doppler perfusion index)
D point
DPTI (diastolic pressure-time index)
DPT positive skin prick test
Drager Babylog 8000 ventilator
drain
    Davol drain
    Penrose
    Quad-Lumen
    Shirley wound
drainage
    abscess
    anomalous pulmonary venous
    brisk
    bronchial secretions
    closed chest
    extrapleural
    percutaneous abscess and fluid
        (PAFD)
    pulmonary venous
    purulent
    thoracic duct (TDD)
    total anomalous pulmonary venous
    tube
    underwater-seal
draining vein pressure (DVP)
drain sponge, Sof-Wick
drape, iodophor-impregnated adhesive
draw-back stent deployment technique
Drechslera hawaiiensis
drenching sweats
dressing
    Bioclusive transparent
    Biopatch foam wound
    BlisterFilm transparent

dressing *(cont.)*
    BreakAway absorptive wound
    CarboFlex wound
    Carra Sorb H wound
    Carra Sorb M wound gel
    CarraSmart foam
    Carrasyn hydrogel wound
    CircPlus compression
    ClearSite borderless
    ClearSite Hydro Gauze
    Clo-Sur P.A.D. hemostatic
    Coban elastic
    CollaCote collagen wound
    CombiDerm absorbent cover
    Comfeel Ulcus
    Conformant contact-layer wound
    contact-layer wound
    Covaderm composite wound
    Coverlet adhesive
    Curaderm hydrocolloid
    Curafil hydrogel
    Curafoam foam wound
    Curagel hydrogel
    Curasorb calcium alginate
    Cutinova Cavity wound filling
    Cutinova Hydro
    DeBakey woven Dacron
    DermaMend foam wound
    DermaMend hydrogel
    Dermanet contact-layer wound
    DermAssist hydrocolloid
    DermAssist wound filling
    Dermatell hydrocolloid
    DiaB Gel hydrogel
    Dyna-Flex compression
    drip
    Elasto-Gel hydrogel sheet
    Elastomull gauze bandage
    elta dermal hydrogel
    Endo-Avitene
    Epi-Lock polyurethane foam wound
    Flexzan foam wound

dressing *(cont.)*
Intelligent
Iodoflex absorptive
iodoform gauze
Iodosorb absorptive
Kaltostat hydrofiber wound packing
Kerra Boot
Maxorb alginate wound
Medifil collagen hemostatic wound
Medipore Dress-it
Mepitel contact-layer wound
Mepore absorptive
Mesalt
MPM hydrogel
Multidex wound-filling
Multipad absorptive
Normigel hydrogel
N-Terface contact-layer wound
Nu-Derm hydrocolloid
occlusive
OpSite Flexigrid transparent
    adhesive film
Optipore wound-cleaning
OsmoCyte pillow
PanoGauze hydrogel-impregnated
    gauze
PanoPlex hydrogel
PermaMesh
Plast-O-Fit thermoplastic bandage
Polyderm foam wound
PolyMemfoam wound
Polyskin II
PolyWic wound filling
Primaderm semipermeable foam
Primapore absorptive wound
Primer compression
Pro-Clude transparent film wound
ProCyte transparent adhesive film
PuraPly wound
Repel bioresorbable barrier film
RepliCare hydrocolloid
Repliderm collagen-based

dressing *(cont.)*
Reston foam wound
Restore alginate wound
Robert Jones bulky soft dressing
    with Hemovac drainage
SAF-Gel hydrogel
SeaSorb alginate wound
Seprafilm tissue barrier
SignaDress hydrocolloid
Silastic tape
Silverlon wound packing strips
SiteGuard MVP transparent
    adhesive film
SkinTegrity hydrogel
smart foam
Sofsorb absorptive
SoftCloth absorptive
Sof-Wick
SoloSite nonsterile hydrogel
SoloSite wound gel
SorbaView composite wound
SpyroDerm
stent
Steri-Strips
Stratasorb composite wound
SurePress compression
Suresite transparent adhesive film
Synthaderm synthetic (poly-
    urethane) occlusive wound
Tegaderm
Tegagel hydrogel dressing and sheet
Tegagen HG alginate wound
Tegagen HI alginate wound
Tegapore contact-layer wound
Tegasorb hydrocolloid wafer
Teletrast absorbable surgical gauze
Telfa
Thera-Boot compression
THINSite
THINSite with Biofilm
Tielle absorptive
Transeal transparent adhesive film

dressing *(cont.)*
    TransiGel hydrogel-impregnated
        gauze
    Transorbent multilayer
    Ultec hydrocolloid
    Uniflex polyurethane adhesive
        surgical
    Unna-Flex compression
    Vari/Moist wound
    Veingard transparent
    Ventex
    Viasorb
    Vigilon
    Vitacuff
    WDE (wound dressing emulsion)
    wet-to-dry
    wick (usually gauze)
    Woun'Dres hydrogel
    Wound-Span Bridge II
    wet-to-dry
    Xeroform ("zero-form") gauze
    Zipzoc stocking compression
Dressler fusion beat
Dressler post-myocardial infarction
    syndrome
Dressler syndrome
DRF (digestive-respiratory fistula)
drifting wedge pressure
drill biopsy
drip
    I.V., IV (intravenous)
    postnasal
drip dressing
Dripps-American Surgical Association
    score to predict cardiac morbidity
drip test
drive cycle length
Driver catheter
Driver guidewire
Driver stent
Driver stent delivery system
Dromos pacemaker

drooping eyelid
drop attacks
drop heart
droplets, respiratory
drop test for pneumoperitoneum
drowned lung
drowsiness
drug classes (see *drug-related terms*)
drug delivery devices (see also
        medications)
    Aerocel pulmonary delivery system
    AeroChamber aerosol holding
        chamber
    AeroDose inhaler
    Aerotrol inhalation aerosol device
    AERx electronic inhaler
    Autohaler
    Bluemyst aerosol spray
    Clickhaler
    Dilaparel inhaler
    Infamyst aerosol spray
    inhaler
    metered-dose inhaler
    OptiHaler
    Pockethaler
    Pulmios inhaler
    Qdose inhaler
    Rainbow ABC aerosol dispenser
    Respihaler
    Spinhaler turbo-inhaler
    Staccato
    Tempo inhaler
    Transvac transdermal patch
    Turbinaire
    Turbuhaler
    Ventavis inhaler
drug dosage forms
    Dividose
    Perles
    Pulvules
    Rotacaps
drug-eluting stent (DES)

drug-induced leukopenia
drug-induced orthostatic hypotension
drug-induced pericarditis
drug-induced pulmonary eosinophilia
drug-induced syncope
drug of choice
drug-refractory arrhythmia
drug-refractory tachycardia
drug-related terms (see *medication*
    entry for list of drugs)
  ACE (angiotensin-converting
    enzyme) inhibitors
  adrenergic blocker
  adrenergic stimulant
  adjuvant
  agonist
  alpha/beta adrenergic blocker
  aminoglycoside
  angiotensin converting enzyme
    (ACE) inhibitors
  antagonist
  anthracyclines
  anthraquinones
  antiadrenergic agent
  antianginal agent
  antiarrhythmic agent
  antibiotic
  anticoagulant
  antidiuretics
  antifibrinolytic
  antifilarial
  antihistamines
  antihyperlipidemic agent
  antihypertensive
  anti-infective
  anti-inflammatory
  antimicrobial
  antiparasitics
  antiplatelet
  antipruritic
  antiseptic
  antispasmodic

drug-related terms *(cont.)*
  antituberculosis
  antitussives
  antiviral
  bactericidal
  bacteriostatic
  beta-adrenergic receptor blocking
    agent
  beta agonist
  beta blocker
  beta blocking
  bile acid sequestrant
  bronchodilators
  calcium channel antagonist
  calcium channel blocker
  cardioselective agent
  cardioselective beta-blocker
  cardiotonic
  chronotropic agent
  corticosteroid
  cough syrup
  coumarin-type anticoagulant
  cyclo-oxygenase inhibitor
  decongestant
  digitalis
  diuretic
  drug delivery devices
  expectorant
  ganglion blocker
  hemostatics
  histamines
  HMG-CoA reductase inhibitors
  hyperlipidemics
  hypolipidemics
  immunosuppressive
  inhaler
  inotropic agent
  intramuscular
  intravenous
  long-acting
  loop diuretic
  lung surfactant

drug-related terms *(cont.)*
  macrolide
  MAO (monoamine oxidase)
    inhibitor
  medium chain triglyceride (MCT)
  mucolytics
  neuromuscular blocking agent
  nicotinic acid
  nicotine withdrawal aid
  long-acting nitrate
  nitroglycerin
  nitrous oxide
  nonselective beta blocker
  nonsteroidal anti-inflammatory
    drugs (NSAID)
  novel plasminogen activator (NPA)
  oral
  osmotic diuretic
  PDE III (phosphodiesterase, type 3)
    isoenzyme inhibitor
  phosphodiesterase inhibitor
  plasma expanders
  plasma extenders
  platelet concentrate
  platelet inhibitors
  potassium channel openers
  potassium-sparing diuretic
  potassium-wasting diuretic
  pulmonary surfactant replacement
  quinolone antibiotic
  recombinant tissue plasminogen
    activator (rt-PA)
  reductase inhibitors
  respiratory stimulants
  respiratory therapy agents
  selective dopamine agonists
  slow-channel blocking drugs
  smoking deterrent
  statin drugs
  sulfonamide
  sulfonylurea
  surfactant agents

drug-related terms *(cont.)*
  sympathomimetic
  sympathomimetic amine
  thiazide diuretic
  thionamides
  thrombin
  thrombolytics
  topical
  torsemide
  transdermal
  tricyclic antidepressant
  tuberculosis preparations
  vasoconstrictor
  vasoactive
  vasodilator
  vasopressor
  venous insufficiency treatment
drug-refractory atrial tachyarrhythmia
drug-resistant tachyarrhythmia
drugs (see *medication*)
drug refractory atrial tachyarrhythmia
drug therapy
drug tolerance
drumlike percussion note
Drummond marginal artery
Drummond sign of aortic aneurysm
dry-air-induced nasal symptoms
dry cough
dry mucous membranes
dry nonproductive cough
dry pleurisy
DSA (digital subtraction angiography)
DSAS (discrete subvalvular aortic
  stenosis)
DSE (dobutamine stress echocardiography)
D-shaped vessel lumen
DSP Micro Diamond-Point micro-
  surgery instruments
D-Stat vascular sealing device
DTAF-F (descending thoracic
  aortofemoral-femoral) bypass

DTI (Doppler tissue imaging)
DT-MRI (diffusion tensor magnetic
 resonance imaging)
D to E slope on echocardiography
DTPA, technetium bound to
DTR (deep tendon reflex)
D-transposition (dextrotransposition)
 of great arteries
DU (duplex ultrasound)
dual atrioventricular node pathway
dual balloon method
dual chamber Medtronic.Kappa 400
 pacemaker
dual chamber pacemaker
dual chamber pacing
dual-coronary system
dual heart rhythm
dual ventricles
Dubin and Amelar varicocele
Duchenne muscular dystrophy
duckbill forceps
Ducor balloon catheter
Ducor-Cordis pigtail catheter
Ducor HF (high-flow) catheter
Ducor tip
duct
 alveolar
 lymphatic
 thoracic
ductal arch
ductal constriction
ductal remnant
ductile, ductility
ductless
duct of Arantius
duct of Botallo
ductulus
ductus
 friable
 recanalized
 recurrent
 window

ductus Arantii
ductus arteriosus
 patent (PDA)
 persistent
 persistent patency of
 reversed
ductus arteriosus closure, pulmonary
 hypoperfusion unmasked by
ductus arteriosus patency
ductus bump
ductus thoracicus
ductus thoracicus dexter
ductus venosus, persistent patency of
Duet positive airway pressure breathing
 device
Duette catheter
Duet vascular sealing device
Duffield scissors
Duffy blood antibody type
Duke bleeding test
Duke bleeding time
Duke treadmill exercise score
dullness
 cardiac
 Gerhardt
 Grocco triangular
 left border of cardiac (LBCD)
 percussion
 shifting
 tympanitic
dullness to percussion
dull pain
dull percussion note
dull substernal discomfort
dull tympanitic resonance in pleural
 effusion
dumbbell-shaped tip
Dumon tracheobronchial stent
Dunlop thrombus stripper
duodenitis, hemorrhagic
duodenojejunal angle

DuoDerm hydroactive gel for wound
  hydration
Duostat
duplex Doppler ultrasound
duplex imaging
duplex pulsed-Doppler sonography
duplex scan (or scanning)
    color-flow
    renal
duplex study, follow-up
duplex ultrasound (DU)
Duraflo II extracorporeal perfusion
  circuit
Dura-Guard patch
Duran anuloplasty ring
Durapulse pacemaker
Durathane cardiac device
duration
    action potential (APD)
    pulse
duration of EKG wave
duration of exercise
duration of P wave
duration of QRS
Duromedics aortic valve
Duromedics prosthetic heart valve
Duroziez mitral stenosis disease
Duroziez murmur
Duroziez sign
Dusard syndrome
duskiness of skin
dusky skin color
dust
    cotton
    inhalation of environmental
dust cells
Duval-Crile lung forceps
Duval lung forceps
dV/dt (contractility)
DVI (deep venous insufficiency)
DVI (digital vascular imaging)
DVI pacing mode

DVI Simpson Atherocath
DVP (draining vein pressure)
DVT (deep venous thrombosis)
DXR (delayed xenograft rejection)
D wave on EKG
Dyclone gargle anesthesia
dye (see also *imaging agent*)
    Cardio-Green
    Fox green
    indocyanine green
dye curve
Dyna-Flex compression dressing
    or wrap
dynamic apnea
dynamic air therapy, Restcue CC
dynamic compliance
dynamic compression of airways
dynamic helical scan
dynamic lung compliance (C_{dyn})
dynamic lung
dynamic pulmonary hyperinflation
dynamic single photon emission
    tomography
dynamic spiral CT lung densitometry
dynamics, arterial wall
DynaPulse 5000A ambulatory blood
    pressure monitor
dysarthria
dysautonomia
dysbarism syndrome
dysbetalipoproteinemia, familial
dyscontrol, episodic
dyscrasia
    blood
    plasma cell
dysesthesia
dysfibrinogenemia
dysfunction
    autonomic
    biventricular global systolic
    chronic allograft
    cognitive

dysfunction *(cont.)*
   contractile
   exercise-induced left ventricular
   focal ventricular
   global ventricular
   hemodynamic
   left ventricular (LVD)
   mitral valve (MVD)
   papillary muscle (PMD)
   regional myocardial
   sinoatrial node
   sinus node
   sleep
   ventilatory
   ventricular
dyskeratosis
dyskinesia, regional
dyskinesis
   anterior wall
   anteroapical
   left ventricular
dyskinetic cilia
dyskinetic segmental wall motion
dyslipidemia, familial genetic
dysmaturity, pulmonary
dysmodulation
dysphagia lusoria
dysphonia
dysplasia
   arrhythmogenic right ventricular
     (ARVD)
   arteriohepatic
   bronchopulmonary
   congenital polyvalvular
   endocardial
   familial arterial fibromuscular
   fibromuscular
   fibrous
   geleophysic
   multilineage
   perimedial
   primary chordal

dysplasia *(cont.)*
   pulmonary valve (PVD)
   right ventricular
   secondary chordal
   ventricular
   ventriculoradial
dysplastic pulmonary valve
dysplastic tricuspid valve
dyspnea
   angina-equivalent
   cardiac
   episodic
   exertional
   expiratory
   functional
   inspiratory
   mild
   nocturnal
   noncardiac
   nonexpansional
   orthostatic
   paroxysmal nocturnal (PND)
   paroxysmal wheezing
   postural
   profound
   renal
   sighing
dyspnea at rest
dyspnea on exertion (DOE)
dyspnea with cyanosis
dyspnea with tachypnea and hyperventilation
dyspneic
dysproteinemia
dysrhythmia
   atrial
   cardiac
   malignant ventricular
Dysshwannian syndrome
dyssynergia
   regional
   segmental

dyssynergy
dystrophy
    asphyxiating thoracic
    Becker muscular
    Duchenne muscular
    Emery-Dreifuss muscular
    Erb limb-girdle

dystrophy *(cont.)*
    infantile thoracic
    Landouzy-Dejerine
    limb-girdle
    myotonic
    progressive pulmonary
    suffocating thoracic

E, e

E (ejection sound)
EAC (expandable access catheter)
Eagle equation to predict cardiac
  morbidity
E/A or E-A (E to A) ratio on echocardiogram
earlobe crease (probable risk sign for
  coronary artery disease)
early asthmatic response
early inspiratory crackles
early-onset varicose veins
early rapid repolarization
early systolic murmur
early venous filling
early ventricular depolarization
  (pre-excitation)
ear (*not* air) oximetry
EAS (endoscopic articulating stapler)
easily palpable carotid arterial pulse
easy fatigability
Easy Twist steerable guidewire
Eaton agent pneumonia
Eaton-Lambert syndrome
EBDA (effective balloon dilated area)
Eberth line
EBL (estimated blood loss)
Ebstein cardiac anomaly

Ebstein disease of tricuspid valve
Ebstein malformation
Ebstein sign
EC (ejection click)
ECA (external carotid artery)
E-CABG (endarterectomy and
  coronary artery bypass graft)
E-CABG (endoscopic coronary artery
  bypass graft)
ECC (emergency cardiac care)
eccentric atherosclerotic plaque
eccentric atrial activation
eccentric coronary artery
eccentric hypertrophy
eccentric ledge
eccentric lesion
eccentric plaque disease
eccentric restenosis lesion
eccentric stenosis
eccentric tear
eccentric vessel
eccentrically placed lumen
eccentricity index
ecchymosis (pl. ecchymoses)
ECD (endocardial cushion defect)
ECF-A (eosinophil chemotactic factor
  of anaphylaxis)

ECG or EKG (*electrocardiogram*)
ECG asynchronous mode
ECG asynchronous ventricular assist
    device
ECG synchronous mode
ECG synchronous ventricular assist
    device
ECG triggered mode
echinococcal cysts of lung
echinococcosis
echinococcus cysts in pleura
Echinococcus granulosus infection
Echinococcus multilocularis
echo, echoes
    amphoric
    atrial
    bright, highly mobile
    dense
    homogeneous
    inhomogeneous
    linear
    metallic
    shower of
    specular
    spin
    swirling smokelike
    thick
    ventricular (on EKG)
echo (brief form for echocardiogram)
echocardiogram, echocardiography
    A-mode
    akinesis on
    ambulatory Holter
    anterior left ventricular wall motion
    apical
    apical five-chamber view
    apical left ventricular wall motion
        on
    apical two-chamber view
    B bump on anterior mitral valve
        leaflet
    B-mode

echocardiogram *(cont.)*
    biplane transesophageal
    blood pool radionuclide
    cardiac output
    color flow imaging Doppler
    continuous loop exercise
    continuous wave Doppler
    contrast
    contrast-enhanced
    cross-sectional two-dimensional
    CW (continuous wave) Doppler
    D to E slope on
    dipyridamole
    dobutamine stress
    Doppler
    dyskinesis on
    E point on
    echo intensity disappearance rate on
    echo-free space on
    epicardial Doppler
    exercise
    Feigenbaum
    fetal (in utero)
    four-chamber
    hypokinesis on
    inferior left ventricular wall motion
        on
    intracardiac (ICE)
    intracoronary contrast
    intraoperative cardioplegic contrast
    late systolic posterior displacement
        on
    lateral left ventricular wall motion
        on
    left ventricular long-axis
    long-axis parasternal view
    loss of an "a" dip on
    M-mode Doppler
    myocardial contrast (MCE)
    myocardial perfusion
    parasternal long-axis view
    parasternal short-axis view

echocardiogram *(cont.)*
  pharmacologic stress
  postcontrast
  posterior left ventricular wall
    motion on
  postexercise
  postinjection
  postmyocardial infarction
  precontrast
  preinjection
  premyocardial infarction
  pulsed Doppler
  pulsed-wave (PW) Doppler
  real-time
  resting
  right ventricular short-axis
  sector scan
  septal wall motion on
  short-axis view
  signal averaged
  stress
  subcostal short-axis view
  subxiphoid view of
  3D (three-dimensional)
    transesophageal
  transesophageal (TEE)
  transthoracic
  2D (two-dimensional)
  two-chamber
  ventricular wall motion
echocardiogram adenosine
echocardiogram microbubble study
echocardiographic automated border
  detection
echo characteristics on ultrasound
Echo-Coat ultrasound biopsy needles
echo contrast
echo-contrast variability imaging
echo delay time (TE)
echo density
EchoEye 3-D ultrasound imaging
  system

echo-free area
echo-free space
EchoGen (perflenapent; perflisopent)
echogenic mass
echogenic plaque
echogenicity
echogram, mitral valve
echography, B-mode
echoicity
echolucent plaque
EchoMark angiographic catheter
echophonocardiography, combined
  M-mode
echo-planar imaging
echo-planar sequence
echoreflectivity
echo reverberation
echo signature
Echovar Doppler system
echovirus
Echovist-200 (d-galactose)
Eclipse TMR holmium laser system
Eclipse TMR laser
ECLS (extracorporeal life support)
ECMO (extracorporeal membrane
  oxygenation)
ECOM (endotracheal cardiac output
  monitoring)
ECS (cardioplegic solution)
ectasia, anuloaortic
ectasia of coronary artery
ectatic emphysema
Ectocor pacemaker
ectodermosis erosiva pluriorificialis
ectopia cordis abdominalis
ectopia cordis, pectoral
ectopic atrial activity
ectopic atrial focus
ectopic atrial tachycardia
ectopic beat
ectopic focus (pl. foci)
ectopic impulse

ectopic lift
ectopic rest of thyroid tissue
ectopic ventricular beat
ectopic wall motion abnormality
ectopy
    asymptomatic complex (ACE)
    atrial
    bursts of ventricular
    cardiac
    frequent ventricular
    high-density ventricular
    supraventricular
    ventricular
ED (emergency department)
eddy formation
eddy sound of patent ductus arteriosus
edema
    acute pulmonary
    alveolar pulmonary
    angioneurotic
    ankle
    bland
    brawny
    bronchiolar
    brown
    cardiac
    cardiogenic pulmonary
    cardiopulmonary
    cerebral
    chemical pulmonary
    chronic
    circumscribed
    cyclic idiopathic
    cyclical
    dependent
    fingerprint
    flash pulmonary edema with anuria
    florid
    frank pulmonary
    fulminant pulmonary
    generalized pulmonary
    giant

edema *(cont.)*
    gravitational
    hard
    hereditary angioneurotic (HANE)
    high-altitude pulmonary (HAPE)
    idiopathic
    intercellular
    interstitial pulmonary
    laryngeal
    leg
    localized
    lymphatic
    massive
    mild
    Milton
    mushy
    nephrotic
    neurogenic pulmonary
    noncardiac pulmonary
    noncardiogenic pulmonary
    noninflammatory
    nonpitting
    osmotic
    painless
    paroxysmal pulmonary
    passive
    pedal
    perihilar
    periodic
    peripheral
    perivascular
    pitting
    postoperative pulmonary
    pretibial
    pulmonary
    purulent
    Quincke
    reexpansion pulmonary
    reperfusion edema after lung
        transplantation
    sacral
    salt

edema *(cont.)*
   scalp
   solid (of lungs)
   stasis
   subglottic
   supraglottic
   terminal
   trace
   2+ pitting
   venous
   vernal (of lung)
edema fluid
edema neonatorum
edema to groins
edematous tissues
edge
   leading
   shelving
   sternal
   trailing
edge-detection angiography
Edmark mitral valve
EDRF (endothelium-relaxing factor)
EDV (end-diastolic velocity)
EDVI (end-diastolic volume index)
Edwards diagnostic catheter
Edwards-Duromedics bileaflet valve
Edwards-Kerr procedure
Edwards Prima Plus stentless
   bioprosthesis
Edwards syndrome
Edwards woven Teflon aortic
   bifurcation graft
EECP (enhanced external counterpulsation)
EES (expandable esophageal stent)
EF (ejection fraction)
EFE (endocardial fibroelastosis)
effect
   adverse
   Anrep
   artifact due to partial volume

effect *(cont.)*
   Bayliss
   Bohr
   Bowditch
   bronchodilator
   bronchomotor
   cobra head
   contractility
   copper wire
   cumulative
   deleterious
   Dotter
   dottering
   electrophysiologic
   hemodynamic
   inhibitory
   inotropic
   jet
   osmotic
   placebo
   potassium-sparing
   proarrhythmic
   purse-stringing
   silver wire
   snowplow
   tetrodotoxin
   vasodilatory
   Venturi
effective refractory period (ERP)
efferent conduit
efficacious
efficacy of drug therapy
efficacy of treatment
efficiency, valvular
effort
   maximal inspiratory
   respiratory
   ventilatory
effort-dependent
effort syncope
effort thrombosis
effuse

effused chyle
effusion
  bloody
  bloody pericardial
  cholesterol
  cholesterol pericardial
  chyliform
  eosinophilic pleural
  exudative
  hemorrhagic
  loculated
  malignant
  malignant pleural
  milky or chylous pleural
  parapneumonic
  pericardial (PE)
  pleural
  pleurisy with
  pseudochylous
  serofibrinous pericardial
  subpleural
  taut pericardial
  tiny
  turbid
effusion of blood in the pleural cavity
effusive constricting pericarditis
effusive pericardial disease
eggshell aorta
eggshell calcification
egophony at upper border of pleural
  fluid
egress of blood
Ehlers-Danlos syndrome
ehrlichiosis
EIB (exercise-induced bronchospasm)
eicosapentaenoic acid (EPA)
EID (emergency infusion device)
800 Series Blood Gas and Critical
  Analyte System
Eigon disk
Eikenella infection
Einthoven law for EKG

Einthoven reference lines (on EKG
  lead placement)
Einthoven triangle
Eisenmenger complex (congenital heart
  anomaly)
Eisenmenger reaction with septal
  defects
Eisenmenger syndrome
ejection, accelerated
ejection click (EC)
  palpable
  systolic
ejection fraction (EF)
  area-length method for
  basilar half
  blunted
  BSA (body surface area)
  computed
  depressed
  digital
  Dodge method for
  global
  globally depressed
  interval
  Kennedy method for calculating
  left ventricular (LVEF)
  one-third
  regional
  resting left ventricular
  right ventricular (RVEF)
  systolic
  Teichholz
  thermodilution
  well preserved
ejection fraction acoustic quantification, left ventricular
ejectionlike systolic murmur
ejection murmur
ejection phase indices
ejection sound (E)
  palpable aortic
  palpable pulmonic

ejection systolic murmur (ESM)
ejection time
    increased left ventricular
    prolonged
EJV (external jugular vein)
EKG or ECG (electrocardiogram)
EKG-gated multislice MRI technique
EKG-gated spin-echo MRI
EKG lead system
    Frank
    Mason-Likar
EKG rhythm strip
EKG-silent
EKG-synchronized digital subtraction
    angiography
Ekos device
El Gamal cardiac device
El Gamal coronary bypass catheter
Ela pacemaker
elaborate
elaboration, further
ELAS (endoluminal laser ablation
    of the greater saphenous vein)
    procedure
Elastalloy Ultraflex Strecker nitinol
    stent
elastance
    end-systolic
    maximum ventricular (EMAX)
elastase, neutrophil
elastic fibers stain
elastic lamina
elastic recoil
elastic recoil of artery
elastic stockings
elasticity
elasticum, pseudoxanthoma
Elastikon elastic tape
Elasto-Gel hydrogel sheet
Elastomull gauze bandage
elastomyofibrosis
ELCA (excimer laser coronary
    angioplasty)

Elecath circulatory support device
Elecath electrode
Elecath thermodilution catheter
Elecsys proBNP immunoassay
elective cardiac arrest and subsequent
    reperfusion
elective replacement indicators
electrical activity, pulseless
electrical alternans
electrical axis
electrical axis of heart
electrical axis on EKG, J-point
electrical cardioversion
electrical circulatory arrest
electrical defibrillation
electrical events of the EKG
electrical impedance
electrical inactivity
electrically conditioned and driven
    skeletal muscle
electrical potential
electrocardiogram (ECG or EKG)
    ambulatory (AECG)
    baseline
    Burdick
    computerized
    Corometrics-Aloka
    counterclockwise superiorly
        oriented frontal QRS loop
    depressed T waves on
    esophageal
    evolutionary changes on
    exercise
    fetal
    flat
    flatline
    flattened T waves on
    Fourier analysis of
    His bundle
    intracardiac
    intracavitary recording of
    intracoronary
    intramyocardial (during sleep)

electrocardiogram *(cont.)*
  inverted T waves in V_1, V_2, and V_3 on
  Micro-Tracer portable
  normal QRS axis
  normal resting
  persistently upright T waves on
  postconversion
  pre-exercise resting supine
  precordial
  Q-S complex on
  Q waves in right precordial leads on
  resting
  scalar
  serial changes in
  signal-averaged (SaECG)
  signal-averaging technique
  16-lead
  stress
  surface
  telephone transmission of
  three-channel
  three-lead
  12-lead
  upright tilt-testing
  vector
electrocardiogram leads (see *lead*)
electrocardiogram tracing
electrocardiographic gating
electrocardiographic gating with
  electron-beam CT technology
electrocardiographic variant
electrocardiograph machine
electrocardiography (see *electrocardiogram*)
electrocardiophonogram
electrocardioscanner, Compuscan
  Hittman computerized
electrode (see also *lead*)
  active can
  anodal
  anterior anodal patch

electrode *(cont.)*
  array
  Arzco TAPSUL pill
  axillary
  barbed-hook pacemaker
  Biotronik IE 65-I pacemaker
  bipolar pacemaker
  bipolar pacing
  Bisping design
  Bugbee
  bulbous-tip
  catheter
  Clark oxygen
  Cordis
  corkscrew-tip pacemaker
  CPI Endotak transvenous
  CPI porous tine-tipped bipolar
    pacing
  defibrillation
  disposable
  endocardial
  endocardial pacemaker
  endocardial placement of
  Endotak
  epicardial
  epicardial pacemaker
  epicardial patch
  esophageal pill
  external adhesive patch
  flanged
  flanged Silastic tip pacemaker
  floating
  free end of
  free-floating
  handheld
  high right atrium
  His bundle
  impedance
  IVM
  J orthogonal
  J-shaped pacemaker
  Laserdish

electrode *(cont.)*
   Medtronic bipolar
   Medtronic pacemaker
   Medtronic Transvene transvenous
   multilead
   multiple point
   myocardial
   negative pacemaker
   negative pacing
   orthogonal
   pacing
   paddle
   Parahisian pacing
   patch
   pectoral
   permanent pacing
   pill
   platinum
   point
   porous
   porous tip
   positive pacemaker
   positive pacing
   posterior cathodal patch
   precordial surface
   quadripolar catheter
   Quinton
   recording
   ring tip
   roving handheld bipolar
   scalp
   screw-in tip pacemaker
   sensing
   shocking
   Siemens
   Silastic
   skin
   stainless steel
   stimulating
   subcutaneous array
   subcutaneous patch
   subxiphoid

electrode *(cont.)*
   suction-type
   sutureless myocardial
   swallowed
   target tip
   Telectronics pacemaker
   temporary pacemaker
   temporary pacing
   temporary transvenous catheter
   thermistor
   thoracic
   three-turn
   tine-tipped pacemaker
   tined
   transesophageal (TEE)
   transthoracic
   Transvene
   transvenous
   transvenous placement of
   tripolar transvenous screw-in
   two-turn
   unipolar coil
   unipolar pacemaker
   urethane
   USCI Goetz bipolar
   USCI NBIH bipolar
   Vitatron catheter
   VPL (ventroposterolateral) thalamic
   Waterston pacing
   wire
electrode catheter tip
electrode gel
electrode lead
electrode pads
electrode paste
electrode stimulation, transvenous
   (of atrium)
Electrodyne pacemaker
electrogram, electrography
   coronary sinus
   CSos (coronary sinus ostium)
   esophageal

electrogram *(cont.)*
    fractionated ventricular
    His bundle (HBE)
    HRA (high right atrium)
    intra-atrial
    intracardiac
    intracavitary
    intracoronary
    right atrial
    RVA (right ventricular apical)
    sinus node
electrolyte disturbance
electrolyte imbalance
electrolytes, consisting of
    bicarbonate (bicarb; HCO_3)
    calcium (Ca)
    chloride (Cl)
    magnesium
    potassium (K)
    sodium (Na)
electromagnetic blood flow study
electromagnetic flowmeter
electromagnetic interference (EMI)
Electro-Mate cutting and coagulating
    device
electromechanical dissociation (EMD)
    of the heart
electromechanical systole
electromechanical total artificial heart
electromechanically quiescent heart
Electromedics AT 750EF auto-
    transfusion system
electromotive force generation, cardiac
electron-beam angiography of coronary
    arteries
electron-beam computed tomography
    (CT)
electronic portal images (EPI)
electrophoresis, lipoprotein
electrophysiological abnormalities
electrophysiologic effect
electrophysiologic mapping

electrophysiologic study (EPS) to
    assess ventricular arrhythmia
electrotherapy device, CellGen
electrovaporization
electrovectorcardiogram
electrovectorcardiography
Elema-Schonander pacemaker
elements, parenchymal
elephant on chest, feeling of
elephant trunk technique
elev (elevated)
elevated ALT (alanine aminotrans-
    ferase)
elevated AST (aspartate aminotrans-
    ferase)
elevated blood lipids
elevated diaphragms
elevated diastolic plateau
elevated gradient
elevated jugular venous pressure
elevated neck veins
elevated plasma lactate
elevated plasma renin activity,
    inappropriately
elevated pulmonary wedge pressure
elevated RT segment
elevated serum lactate level
elevated ST segment
elevated to the angle of the jaw at 90°
elevated venous pressure
elevation
    central venous pressure
    diaphragmatic
    ST segment
    transient ST segment
elevation of enzymes
elevation of limb
elevation pallor of extremity
elevator
    Doyen rib
    Freer
    Matson rib

elevator *(cont.)*
   Matson-Alexander rib
   Penfield
   rib
11-hydroxylase deficiency
elfin facies syndrome
Elgiloy frame of prosthetic valve
EliSpot method
Elite double-loop catheter
Elite dual-chamber rate-responsive
   pacemaker
Elite guide catheter
Elite vascular hemostasis device
Ellestad protocol for treadmill stress
   test
Ellestad treadmill exercise protocol
Elliotson syndrome
elliptical bur
elliptical lead
elliptical lumen
ellipticity index
Ellis-Garland line
Ellis line
Ellis sign
Ellis-van Creveld syndrome
Elmhurst Curve catheter
Eloesser flap
Eloesser procedure for chest cavity
   drainage
elongated aortic arch
elongated doubly pyramidal structures
elongated heart
elongation
elongation and tortuosity
elongation, aortic
elongation of globe of eye
Elsner syndrome
elta (trademarked lowercase) dermal
   hydrogel dressing
ELVT (endolaser venous therapy)
emaciated
EMAX (ventricular elastance,
   maximum)

embarrassment
   circulatory
   hemodynamic
   respiratory
Embden-Meyerhof-Parnas pathway
embedding of stent coils
embolectomy
   arterial
   pulmonary
   transfemoral Fogarty
emboli (pl. of *embolus*), shower of
embolic event
embolic gangrene
embolic obstruction of pulmonary
   artery
embolic phenomenon
embolic shower
embolic stroke
embolism (also *embolus*)
   air
   amniotic fluid
   arterial
   atheromatous
   bacillary
   bland
   bone marrow
   cancer
   capillary
   cardiogenic
   catheter-induced
   cellular
   cerebral
   coronary artery
   crossed
   direct
   fat
   fibrin platelet
   foam
   gas nitrogen
   infective
   intraluminal
   massive

embolism *(cont.)*
  miliary
  multiple
  obturating
  occluding spring
  oil
  pantaloon
  paradoxical
  peripheral
  plasmodium
  polyurethane foam
  prosthetic valve
  pulmonary (PE)
  pulmonary venous-systemic air
  recurrent
  renal cholesterol
  riding
  septic
  septic pulmonary
  shower of
  straddling
  submassive pulmonary
  trichinous
  tumor
  venous
  visceral
embolism without infarction
embolization
  atheromatous cholesterol crystal
  balloon (therapeutic)
  balloon and coil
  bronchial artery
  cardiac tumor
  cholesterol
  chronic lung (by blood-borne eggs)
  coil (of unwanted vessel)
  coil (therapeutic)
  diffuse cholesterol
  disseminated atheromatous
  disseminated cholesterol
  distal
  endovascular

embolization *(cont.)*
  massive
  percutaneous coil
  septic
  Silastic bead
  stent
  transcatheter arterial (TAE)
embolization coil
  high performance detach
  Hydrocoil XT vascular
embolization of vascular malformation
embolization syndrome
  peripheral cholesterol
  renal cholesterol
  visceral cholesterol
  therapeutic
embolotherapy, catheter
embolus (pl. emboli) (see *embolism*)
embolus trap, Mobin-Uddin
Embol-X arterial cannula and filter
  system
embryonal vein
embryonic aortic arch
embryonic branchial arch
embryonic cell rests in the septum
embryonic infection
EMD (electromechanical dissociation)
  of the heart
Emerald diagnostic guidewires
emergency airway
emergency cardiac care (ECC)
emergency cricothyrotomy
emergency infusion device (EID)
emergent
emergent aneurysmectomy
emergently
Emerson pump
Emerson vein stripper
Emerson ventilator
Emery-Dreifuss muscular dystrophy
EMF (endomyocardial fibrosis)
EMI (electromagnetic interference)

EMI-induced pacemaker failure
Eminase thrombolysis
emotional angina
emphysema
  alcoholic
  alveolar
  alveolar duct
  atrophic
  basal panacinar
  bronchiolar
  bullous
  centriacinar
  centrilobular
  chronic
  chronic hypertrophic
  chronic obstructive
  chronic pulmonary (CPE)
  compensating
  compensatory
  congenital lobar
  cutaneous
  cystic
  cystic pulmonary
  diffuse
  ectatic
  false
  focal-dust
  gangrenous
  generalized
  giant bullous
  glass blower's
  hypoplastic
  idiopathic unilobar
  infantile lobar
  interlobular
  interstitial
  intestinal
  liquefactive
  lobar
  localized obstructive
  mediastinal
  neck

emphysema *(cont.)*
  necrotizing
  neonatal cystic pulmonary
  obstructive
  oxygen-dependent
  panacinar
  panlobular
  paracicatricial
  paraseptal
  postoperative
  postsurgical
  pulmonary
  pulmonary interstitial (PIE)
  senile
  skeletal
  small-lunged
  subcutaneous
  surgical
  traumatic
  unilateral
  unilateral pulmonary
  vesicular
emphysema due to alpha$_1$-antitrypsin
  deficiency
emphysema of lungs
emphysematous bleb
emphysematous bronchitis
emphysematous bulla
emphysematous COPD (chronic
  obstructive pulmonary disease)
emphysematous expansion of left
  upper lobe
emphysematous expansion of lobe
  of lung
emphysematous lungs
emphysematous lung tissue
emphysematous type A disease
empiric bronchodilator therapy
empiric therapy
empirical therapy
emplaced (verb)
empty beating heart

empty beating heart method
empty collapsed lung
emptying, tortuous
empyema (see also *abscess*)
   chest
   chronic pleural
   interlobar
   latent
   left-sided
   loculated
   metapneumonic
   pericardial
   pleural
   pneumococcal
   pulsating
   putrid
   right-sided
   streptococcal
   synpneumonic
   thoracic
   tuberculous
empyema articuli
empyema benignum
empyema necessitatis
empyema of chest
empyema of pericardium
empyema with pachypleuritis
EMS (endoscopic multifeed stapler)
emulsified fat globules
Enabler circulatory support system
en bloc
en bloc vein resection
encapsulated bacteria
encephalocele
encephalopathy, hypertensive
encephalopathy, post-arrest hypoxic
encircled
encirclement
encircling endocardial cryoablation
encircling endocardial ventriculotomy
Encompass cardiac network
Encor pacemaker

Encore inflation device
encroachment, luminal
en cuirasse, coeur
encysted pleurisy
endarterectomized segment
endarterectomy
   aortoiliac
   aortoiliofemoral
   blind
   carotid
   carotid bifurcation
   carotid eversion
   Connolly eversion
   coronary
   eversion
   extraluminal
   gas
   innominate
   laser
   manual core
   open
   profunda
   proximal aortic
   right carotid
   semiclosed
   subclavian
   transaortic
   transaortic extraction
endarterectomy and coronary artery
   bypass graft (E-CABG)
endarteritis obliterans
endartery
end diastole
end-diastolic flow
end-diastolic pressure
end-diastolic pressure-volume relation
end-diastolic velocity (EDV)
end-diastolic volume
Endeavor catheter
Endeavor guidewire
Endeavor stent
Endeavor stent delivery system

end-effectors
end-expiratory lung volume (FRC)
end-expiratory pressure
end-expiratory wheezing
end-inspiratory pressure
end-inspiratory wheezes
endless loop, dual-chamber pacemaker
endoaneurysmorrhaphy
endoaortic baffle
endoaortic balloon clamping
Endo-Avitene collagen
Endo-Avitene hemostatic material
Endo Babcock surgical grasping device
endobronchial carcinoma
endobronchial exudates
endobronchial Kaposi sarcoma
endobronchial lesion
endobronchial mucosa
endobronchial neoplasm
endobronchial obstruction
endobronchial tuberculosis
endobronchial tumor
endocardial ablation
endocardial activation mapping
endocardial catheter ablation
endocardial catheter mapping
endocardial cryoablation, encircling
endocardial cushion defect (ECD)
endocardial cushion malformation
endocardial dysplasia
endocardial electrode
endocardial fibroelastosis (EFE)
endocardial fibrosis, Davies
endocardial hemorrhage, focal
endocardial lead
endocardial lesion, noninfective
endocardial mapping
endocardial pace/sense and
    defibrillation lead
endocardial plaque
endocardial pocket
endocardial resection

endocardial scarring
endocardial sclerosis
endocardial trabeculation
endocardial-to-epicardial resection
endocardiectomy
endocarditis
    atypical verrucous
    acute
    acute bacterial (ABE)
    acute infective
    acute rheumatic
    aortic valve
    atypical verrucous
    bacterial
    blastomycotic
    cachectic
    chronic
    constrictive
    coxsackievirus
    enterococcal
    fungal
    gonococcal
    histoplasmotic
    indeterminate
    infectious
    infective
    infective aneurysmal
    Libman-Sacks
    Loeffler fibroblastic
    Loeffler parietal fibroplastic
    Löffler (Loeffler)
    malignant
    marantic
    marantic infective
    meningococcal
    monilial
    mural
    mycotic
    nonbacterial
    nonbacterial thrombotic (NBTE)
    nonbacterial verrucous
    noninfective verrucous

endocarditis *(cont.)*
  nonrheumatic
  nosocomial infective
  parietal
  parietal fibroplastic
  postoperative
  prosthetic valve
  pulmonary artery catheter-
    associated
  pulmonic
  purulent
  Q fever
  rheumatic
  rickettsial
  right-side
  septic
  staphylococcal
  streptococcal
  subacute
  subacute bacterial (SBE)
  subacute infective
  syphilitic
  thrombotic
  tricuspid valve
  tuberculous
  typhoid
  ulcerative
  valvular
  vegetative
  verrucous
  viridans
endocarditis chordalis
endocarditis infection
endocarditis lenta
endocarditis prophylaxis
endocardium
  disk of
  wafer of
EndoCPB (endovascular cardiopulmonary bypass) catheter
endocrine neoplasia, multiple
endocut cautery device

Endodissect
endoesophageal MRI coil
end of atrial systole
Endo-Flo endoscopic irrigation
  apparatus
Endo-GIA suture stapler
end of systole
endogenous hypertriglyceridemia
endogenous lipoid pneumonia
endograft repair
Endo Grasp device
endolaser venous therapy (ELVT)
endoleak
endoluminal laser ablation
  of the greater saphenous vein
  (ELAS) procedure
endoluminal stent
endoluminal vascular repair
endolymphatic hypertension
endomyocardial biopsy
endomyocardial fibrosis
  mural
  tropical
endophlebitis
endoplasmic reticulum
endoprosthesis, Spotorno
EndoRetract retractor
end-organ
EndoSaph vein harvest system
endoscope (see also *bronchoscope*)
  Boutin thoracoscope
  Fujinon NAP-F nasopharyngoscope
  Pentax FNL-10P2 nasopharyngo-
    scope
  Pentax FNL-13S nasopharyngo-
    scope
  Pentax FNL-15RP2 nasopharyngo-
    scope
endoscopic aspiration mucosectomy
endoscopic coronary artery bypass
  graft (E-CABG)
endoscopic division of incompetent
  perforating veins

endoscopic mitral valve repair
endoscopic suction cap
endoscopic ultrasonography (EUS)
endoscopic ultrasound-guided fine
    needle aspiration (EUS-FNA)
Endo Shears
EndoSonics IVUS/balloon dilatation
    catheter
endosound (endoscopic ultrasound)
    catheter
Endo Stitch
Endotak automatic internal cardio-
    verter-defibrillator (AICD)
Endotak C lead
Endotak electrode
Endotak Picotip cardiac defibrillation
    lead
Endotak nonthoracotomy implantable
    cardioverter-defibrillator (ICD)
Endotak Reliance lead
Endotak SQ lead array
Endotak transvenous ICD
endothelial cells, pulmonary capillary
endothelial proliferation
endothelial surface
endothelialization of stent
endothelialization of vascular graft
endothelialized vascular grafts
endothelin-1
endothelioid cell
endothelioma
endothelium
    arterial
    pulmonary capillary
    squamous
endothelium-derived contracting factor
endothelium-derived relaxing factor
endothoracic fascia
endotoxin assay
endotoxins, gram-negative bacterial
endotracheal cardiac output monitoring
    (ECOM)

endotracheal intubation
endotracheal tube (ETT)
Endotrol tracheal tube
Endo-Tube
endovascular
endovascular coagulation of blood
    vessels
endovascular coil embolization
    procedure
endovascular infection
endovascular grafting system,
    Litespeed
endovascular radiation brachytherapy
endovascular repair of abdominal
    aortic aneurysm
endovascular stent-grafting
endovascular stented graft
endovascular stent placement
endovascular ultrasonography
endovenous defibrillation
endoventricular circular patchplasty
EndoWrist used with the da Vinci
    robot surgical system
endpoint, exercise
end-pressure artifact
end-stage cardiomyopathy
end-stage cardiopulmonary disease
end-stage chronic obstructive
    pulmonary disease
end-stage congestive heart failure
end-stage disease
end-stage fetal cardiac decompensation
end-stage lung disease
end-stage renal disease
end-stage suppurative lung disease
end systole
end-systolic dimension
end-systolic elastance
end-systolic pressure-volume relation
end-systolic reversal
end-systolic volume
end-systolic volume indices

end-tidal-volume apnea
end-tidal carbon dioxide (ETCO$_2$)
end-tidal carbon dioxide monitor
end-to-end anastomosis
end-to-side anastomosis
end-to-side internal mammary artery to
    coronary anastomosis
end-to-side microvascular anastomosis
end-to-side portocaval anastomosis
end-to-side vein anastomosis
endurance exercise
energy, stored
Enertrax pacemaker
en face ("ahn fahss") (Fr., in front,
    head on)
engaged, cutting mechanism was
En Garde closure apparatus
En Garde grasper
En Garde staple
En Garde suture
engorged collecting system
engorged tissues
engorged veins under the tongue
engorgement
    bilateral venous
    neck vessel
    pulmonary artery
    vascular
    venous
engorgement of pulmonary vessels
Engström respirator
enhanced
enhanced external counterpulsation
    (EECP)
Enhanced Torque 8F guiding catheter
enhancement of Doppler flow signals
enlarged cardiac silhouette
enlarged heart
enlarged valve apparatus
enlargement (see also *hypertrophy*)
    cardiac
    chamber

enlargement *(cont.)*
    compensatory
    hilar lymph node
    mediastinal lymph node
en masse lobectomy
EnSite 3000 imaging system
ensuing
ENTec Coblator plasma surgery
    system
ENTec Plasma Wands
enteric gram-negative bacilli
Enterobacter aerogenes bronchitis
Enterobacter agglomerans
Enterobacter cloacae
Enterobacteriaceae infection
enterococcal infection
enteropathy, protein-losing
enteroviral infection
enteroviral pericarditis
entirely chaotic pulse
Entity pacemaker
entrainment
    concealed
    transient
entrance block
entrance heart block
entrapment, popliteal artery
Entree thoracoscopy trocar and
    cannula
EnTré guidewire
entry of air into pleural cavity
enucleated
enveloping fascia
environmental exposure
environmental tobacco smoking
    exposure
enzyme (see also *isoenzyme*)
    angiotensin-converting (ACE)
    cardiac
    elevated
    lysosomal
    myocardial

enzyme levels
enzyme-linked immunosorbent assay
  (ELISA)
enzyme study
EOL (end of life)
EOS (end of service)
eosinophil chemotactic factor of
  anaphylaxis (ECF-A)
eosinophil count, absolute
eosinophilia
  alveolar
  cryptogenic pulmonary
  drug-induced pulmonary
  idiopathic familial
  Löffler (Loeffler)
  profound peripheral
  prolonged pulmonary
  pulmonary
  pulmonary infiltration
  simple pulmonary
  sputum
  tropical
eosinophilia-myalgia syndrome
eosinophilia-pulmonary tuberculosis
  syndrome
eosinophilia with asthma, pulmonary
eosinophilic asthma
eosinophilic disseminated collagen
  disease
eosinophilic endomyocardial disease
eosinophilic endomyocardial
  fibroelastosis
eosinophilic gastroenteritis, primary
eosinophilic granuloma
eosinophilic infiltrate
eosinophilic infiltration
eosinophilic leukemia
eosinophilic lung disease, idiopathic
eosinophilic pleural effusion
eosinophilic pneumonia
  acute
  chronic

eosinophilic *(cont.)*
  improving
  pertussoid
eosinophilic pustular folliculitis
eosinophil lung syndrome
eosinophils
EPA (eicosapentaenoic acid)
EP (electrophysiology) study
eparterial bronchus
EPBF (effective pulmonary blood
  flow)
ephelides
EPI (electronic portal images)
epicanthic fold
epicardial ablation on beating heart
epicardial attachment
epicardial Doppler echocardiography
epicardial Doppler flow transducer
epicardial electrode
epicardial fat, overlying
epicardial fat pad
epicardial imaging
epicardial implantation
epicardial lead
epicardial pacemaker electrode
epicardial pacemaker lead
epicardial patch cathode
epicardial reflection
epicardial space
epicardial surface
epicardial tension
epicardial vessels, vasorelaxation of
epicarditis
epicardium
epidural anesthesia
epiglottidectomy
Epi-Grip
epilepsy, laryngeal
Epi-Lock polyurethane foam wound
  dressing
epimyocardial rate-sensing lead
epinephrine

epipleural fibrinous exudate
episode
  anginal
  apneic
  hypercyanotic
  intermittent apneic
episode log
episode of crushing chest pain
episodic arousal
episodic bleeding
episodic cardiac arrest
episodic dyspnea
episodic hypoxemia
epistaxis
epistenocardiac pericarditis
epithelial desquamation
epithelioid cells
epithelioid hemangioendothelioma
  benign
  malignant
epithelium
  aneuronal respiratory
  bronchiolar
  columnar
  cuboidal
  denuded
  pseudostratified columnar
  respiratory
  stratified squamous
  ventral olfactory
eplerenone
E point of cardiac apex pulse
E point on apex cardiogram
E point on echocardiogram
E point to septal separation (EPSS)
epoxyeicosatrienoic acids
Eppendorf catheter
EPS (electrophysiologic study) to
  assess ventricular arrhythmia
Epsilon-aminocaproic acid
EPSS (E point to septal separation)
Epstein-Barr (EB) virus infection

EPTFE (expanded polytetrafluoroethylene) vascular suture
EPT-Dx steerable diagnostic catheter
eptifibatide
EPT-1000 cardiac ablation system
equal in intensity
equalization of pressure
equalized diastolic pressures
equal respiratory excursions
equation
  Bernoulli
  Carter
  continuity
  Fick
  Hagenbach extension of Poiseuille
  Krovetz and Gessner
  Nernst (cardiac action potential,
    resting phase)
  Teichholz
equilibrium, acid-base
equilibrium angiocardiography,
  ambulatory
equilibrium radionuclide angiocardiography
Equinox occlusion balloon system
equivalent
  angina
  anginal
  metabolic
  migraine
  ventilation
Equivas device
equivocal exercise test
equivocal finding
equivocal results
equivocal symptoms
equivocal test
ER (emergency room)
eradication of varicose veins
Erb area
Erb limb-girdle dystrophy
Erb point (of heart)

Erdheim cystic medionecrosis
Erdheim cystic necrosis of aorta
Erdheim I syndrome
ergometer
    arm
    bicycle
    Bosch ERG 500
    Collins bicycle
    Siemens-Albis bicycle
ergometry
    arm (stress test)
    bicycle (exercise stress testing)
ergonovine infusion
ergonovine test
Ergos O_2 dual-chamber rate-responsive
    pacemaker
Ergos O_2 pacemaker
ERI (elective replacement indicator)
erosion
    bronchial
    graft-enteric
    plaque
erosion of bronchi by tuberculous
    lymph nodes
erosion of pulse generator pocket
erosiva pluriorificialis, ectodermosis
ERP (effective refractory period)
    atrial
    ventricular
error
    margin of
    sampling
    sensing
    standard
ERT (elective replacement time)
ERV (expiratory reserve volume)
erythema induratum, Bazin
erythema marginatum
erythema migrans
erythema multiforme
erythema multiforme exudativum
erythema multiforme majus

erythema nodosum
erythema without induration
erythematosus
    lupus
    systemic lupus (SLE)
erythroblastosis fetalis
erythrocyanosis
erythrocyte autosensitization syndrome
erythrocyte sedimentation rate (ESR)
erythrocyte sodium
erythrocytosis, stress
Erythroflex hydromer-coated central
    venous catheter
erythromelalgia
erythromycin
erythropheresis
erythropoietin
ESAT-6 protein used in diagnosing
    Mycobacterium tuberculosis
escape beat
escape interval after an Rx delivery
escape mechanism, ventricular
escape of air into lung connective
    tissue
escape pacemaker
escape rhythm
Escherichia coli (*E. coli*) pneumonia
Eschmann blade
E sign (on x-ray)
ESM (ejection systolic murmur)
Esmarch bandage
Esmarch tourniquet
esophageal adenocarcinoma
esophageal angina
esophageal atresia
esophageal balloon technique
esophageal electrocardiogram
esophageal lead
esophageal obturator airway
esophageal pain
esophageal pill electrode (disposable
    EKG lead encased in a gelatin
    capsule)

esophageal plexus
esophageal spasm mimicking angina
esophageal spasm mimicking
    myocardial infarction
esophageal temperature
esophageal varices
esophageal window
esophagectomy, transhiatal
esophagitis, candidal
ESP (end-systolic pressure)
ESP/ESV ratio
ESR (erythrocyte sedimentation rate)
essential brown induration of lung
essential hypertension
essential hyponatremia
essential thrombocytosis
EST (extrastimulus testing)
Estes EKG criteria or score
estimated blood loss (EBL)
ESV (end-systolic volume)
ESVI (end-systolic volume index)
ESWI/ESVI (end-systolic wall stress
    index/end-systolic volume index)
ET (ejection time)
ETCO$_2$ (end-tidal carbon dioxide)
ethacrynic acid
Ethalloy TruTaper cardiovascular
    needle
ethanolaminosis
Ethibond suture
Ethicon suture
Ethiflex suture
Ethilon suture
ethmoidal sinusitis
ethmoiditis, Woakes
ethylenediaminetetraacetic acid
    disodium salt
etiology, noncardiac
E to A changes
E to F slope of valve
E to F slope on echocardiogram

ETT (endotracheal tube)
ETT (exercise tolerance test)
E2F Decoy solution
eucapnic voluntary hyperventilation
eukinesis
eupnea, eupneic
EUS (endoscopic ultrasonography)
EUS-FNA (endoscopic ultrasound-
    guided fine needle aspiration).
euthyroid sick syndrome
euvolemic
evacuate air from the aorta
evacuated, air was
evacuation of offending pericardial
    fluid
evacuator container
evaluation of deep veins for patency
    and valvular reflux
evanescent chest pain
evanescent nature
Evans syndrome
even murmur
event
    adverse
    atrial sensed (As)
    cardinal
    embolic
    inciting
    ischemic
    morbid
    precipitating
    untoward
    ventricular sensed
event counter
event marker
event monitor
eventration (peaking)
event recorder
Evershears II bipolar curved scissors
eversion endarterectomy, Connolly
eversion technique

everting mattress sutures
everting sutures
Evert-O-Cath drug delivery catheter
Evis Exera video bronchoscope
evolution of EKG
evolutionary changes on EKG
Evolution XP ultrafast CT scanner
Evolve Cardiac Continuum
Ewart sign
exacerbation, acute
exacerbation of chronic congestive
   heart failure
exaggerated S4
examination
   cardiac
   Doppler venous
   follow-up
   histologic
   lower extremity
   peripheral vascular
   physical
   pulmonary
exanthematous changes of extremities
exanthematous disease
Excalibur Introducer
excavatum, pectus
eXcel-DR (disposable/reusable)
eXcel-DR a-fiX cannula seals
eXcel-DR heliX knot pusher
eXcel-DR pneumo needle
excellent prognosis
excellent thrill
excess
   base
   catechol
   mineralocorticoid
   thyroid hormone
excessive bleeding
excessive salt intake
exchange
   air
   catheter
   guidewire

exchange transfusion
excimer (from "excited dimer") laser
excimer laser coronary angioplasty
   (ELCA)
excimer laser debulking
excision(al) biopsy
excision, keel
excitation
   anomalous atrioventricular
   atrioventricular
   supernormal
excitation-contraction coupling
exciting factor
excrescences, Lambl
excretory intravenous pyelography
excruciating pain
excursion, excursions
   chest
   decreased valve
   equal respiratory
   full respiratory
   jugular venous
   limited respiratory
   respiratory
   venous
exercise, exercises
   active
   active assisted
   active resistive
   aerobic
   breathing
   corrective
   deep-breathing
   endurance
   graduated
   injection at peak
   isometric
   isometric handgrip
   isotonic
   low-level
   peak
   relaxation
   rehabilitation

exercise *(cont.)*
  static
  submaximal
  symptom-limited
  therapeutic
exercise capacity
  decreased
  impaired
  increased
exercise challenge
exercise duration (in minutes)
exercise echocardiography
exercise electrocardiography
exercise endpoint
exercise factor
exercise images
exercise index
exercise-induced angina pectoris
exercise-induced asthma
exercise-induced bronchoconstriction
exercise-induced bronchospasm (EIB)
exercise-induced left ventricular
  dysfunction
exercise-induced myocardial ischemia
Exercise Self-efficacy Scale
exercise testing device, Viasys
  cardiopulmonary
exercise tolerance test (ETT)
exercise-inducible transient myocardial
  ischemia
exercise intolerance
exercise load (kpm/min)
exercise oximetry
exercise regimen
exercise restriction
exercise strain gauge venous
  plethysmography
exercise stress test, positive
exercise stress testing protocol (see
  protocol)
exercise stress-redistribution
  scintigraphy

exercise testing protocol (see *protocol*)
exercise thallium-201 stress test
exercise thallium-201 tomography
exercise therapy
exercise tolerance
  decreased
  increased
  improving
exercise tolerance test (ETT), graded
exertional angina
exertional capacity
exertional chest pain
exertional dyspnea
exertional pain
exertional syncope
exertion, pain precipitated by
exhalation, forced
exhaling into the atmosphere
exit heart block, sinoatrial
exogenous contamination
exogenous glucocorticoid
exogenous invasion
exogenous mineralocorticoid
exogenous pneumonia
Exosurf lung surfactant (colfosceril
  palmitate)
expandable access catheter (EAC)
expandable coronary stent
expandable esophageal stent (EES)
expanded polytetrafluoroethylene
  (ePTFE) vascular graft
expanded reinforced polytetrafluoroethylene (ER-PTFE) vascular graft
expanders, plasma
expanding valvulotome
expansile aortic segment
expansion
  complete stent
  emphysematous
  lung
  rapid fluid
  stent

expansion of upper lobe, emphysematous
expectorant drugs
expectorate (verb)
expectorated from the lungs
expectorated from the trachea
expectorated material
expectoration of blood
expectoration of bloody sputum
expectoration of bronchial casts
expeditious
expiration
 forced
 grunting
 prolonged
 sighing
 tidal
 whining
expiratory attenuation
expiratory dyspnea
expiratory flow limitation
expiratory grunting
expiratory phase
expiratory rales
expiratory reserve volume (ERV)
expiratory resistance
expiratory rhonchi, coarse sibilant
expiratory slowing
expiratory time
expiratory wheezes
expiratory whining
expired gas
explanted
exploration of pseudoaneurysm
Explorer ST fixed curve diagnostic
 catheter
Explorer 360° rotational diagnostic
 catheter
exponential simultaneous waveforms,
 truncated
eXpose retractor

exposure
 ambient ozone
 asbestos
 environmental
 environmental tobacco
 smoking
 extraperitoneal
 extrathoracic
 in utero
 intraperitoneal
 passive smoking
 second-hand smoke
exposure to cold, pain precipitated by
exposure to irritants
exposure to isocyanate
Express over-the-wire balloon catheter
Express PTCA catheter
Express coronary stent
Express2 coronary stent system
exquisite detail
exquisite pain
exsanguinate
exsanguinated
exsanguinating hemorrhage into
 pleural space
exsanguination
 fatal
 massive
 partial
extended anticoagulation
extended collection device
extended dwell catheter
extended vertical transseptal approach
 in mitral valve surgery
extended vertical transseptal approach
 in mitral valve surgery
extension
 basal
 bifurcated
 intracavitary (of tumor)
 hilar

extension *(cont.)*
  medial
  parenchymal
  parietal
extension tubing
extensive dissection
external adhesive patch electrode
external cardiac cooling
external cardiac massage
external carotid artery
external carotid steal syndrome
external defibrillation
external iliac stenosis
external jugular veins
external jugular venous cannula
external penetrating wound of lung
extirpation of saphenous vein
extirpation of valve
extra-adrenal pheochromocytoma
extracardiac anomalies
extracardiac collateral circulation
extracardiac conduit
extracardiac conduit Fontan operation
extracardiac disease
extracardiac malformations
extracardiac right-to-left shunt
extracardiac systolic arterial murmur
extracardiac valved conduit
extracavitary-infected graft
extracavitary prosthetic arterial graft
extracellular acidosis
extracellular fluid
extracellular fluid volume
extracorporeal carbon dioxide (CO_2)
  removal technique
extracorporeal circulation
extracorporeal circulation using heart-
  lung machine
extracorporeal circulatory support
extracorporeal hepatic assistance
extracorporeal life support (ECLS)
extracorporeal membrane oxygenation
  (ECMO)

extracorporeal ultrafiltration
extracranial carotid artery atherosclerosis
extracranial carotid system
extracranial cerebral circulation
extracranial cerebral system
extracranial-intracranial bypass
extraction atherectomy device
extraction catheter atherectomy,
  transcutaneous
extraction catheter, transluminal
extraction endarterectomy, transaortic
extractor, In-Time vascular foreign
  body
Extractor three-lumen retrieval balloon
eXtract specimen bag
extradural vertebral plexus of veins
extraluminal endarterectomy
extrapericardial dissection
extrapericardial patch placement
extraperitoneal exposure
extrapleural drainage
extrapleural hemorrhage
extrapleural organs
extrapolate
extrapolation
extrapulmonary disease
extrapulmonary tuberculosis
extrapyramidal disease
extraskeletal osteosarcoma of the heart
Extra Sport coronary guidewire
extrastimulation
extrastimulus (pl. extrastimuli)
  critically timed
  double
  multiple
  paired
  premature
  single
  triple
extrastimulus pacing
extrastimulus technique

extrastimulus testing (EST)
extrasystole
  atrial
  atrioventricular (AV)
  infranodal
  interpolated
  junctional
  nodal
  nonpropagated junctional
  premature ventricular
  retrograde
  ventricular
extrasystolic arrhythmia
extrathoracic exposure
extrathoracic obstruction
extravasated blood
extravasated red blood cells
extravasation of blood
extravasation of erythrocytes into
  alveoli
extravasation of fluid in alveoli
extravasation of intravascular contents,
  secondary
extravascular granulomas
extravascular mass
extravascular pressure
extremities
  blue
  cold
  cyanotic
  mottled
  numb
  tingling

ExtreSafe phlebotomy device
extrinsic allergic alveolitis
extrinsic asthma
extrinsic compression
extrinsic compression of trachea
extrinsic lesion
extrinsic sick sinus syndrome
extruded Gore-Tex graft
extubate
extubated
extubation
exuberant atheroma formation
exudate
  bloody
  endobronchial
  epipleural fibrinous
  fibrinous
  mucopurulent
  retinal
  sanguineous
  serous
  sticky
  tenacious bronchial
exudation of fibrin-rich fluid
exudative consolidation
exudative effusion
exudative pericardial fluid
exudative pleurisy
exudative tuberculosis
exude
exuding wounds
Exxcel ePTFE soft vascular graft

F, f

Fab fragment, antimyosin
Fabry disease
face, hypercalcemic
face mask CPAP (continuous positive
  airway pressure)
facial asymmetry
facial freckling, myxoma syndrome
  with
facies
  asymmetric crying
  elfin
  mitral
  mitrotricuspid
  moon
facies anterior cordis
facies costalis pulmonis
facies diaphragmatica cordis
facies diaphragmatica pulmonis
facies dolorosa
facies inferior cordis
facies interlobaris pulmonis
facies mediastinalis pulmonis
facies sternocostalis cordis
facilitate
facilitated angioplasty
faciobrachial symptoms

FACScan (fluorescence-activated cell
  sorter) flow cytometer
FACS (fluorescence-activated cell
  sorter)-sorted cells
FACSVantage cell sorter
FACT (Focal Angioplasty Catheter
  Technology) coronary balloon
  angioplasty catheter
factitial
factitious symptoms
Factive (gemifloxacin)
factor, factors (see also *coagulation*
    factors of blood)
  antihemophilic blood coagulation
  atrial natriuretic (ANF)
  blood coagulation
  cardiac risk (see *cardiac risk*)
  Christmas blood coagulation
  circular shape
  coagulation
  cobra venom (for myocardial
    ischemia)
  endothelium-derived contracting
  endothelium-derived relaxing
    (EDRF)
  endothelium-relaxing

factor *(cont.)*
  exciting
  exercise
  Hageman
  histamine-releasing
  inciting
  myocardial depressant
  platelet-activating
  platelet-derived growth
  precipitating
  predisposing
  rheumatoid arthritis
  risk
  tumor necrosis, alpha (TNFa)
  vascular endothelial growth
  von Willebrand (also Willebrand)
  von Willebrand blood coagulation
factor III multimer assay
factor III platelet deficiency syndrome
factor IV platelet
factor V Leiden
factor IX deficiency
Fahr-Volhard syndrome
FAI (functional aerobic impairment)
failure
  access graft
  acute congestive
  acute heart
  acute hypercapnic respiratory
    (AHRF)
  acute renal
  acute ventilatory
  backward heart
  battery
  biventricular heart
  cardiac
  chronic hypercapnic respiratory
    (CHRF)
  chronic renal
  chronic respiratory
  circulatory
  compensated congestive heart

failure *(cont.)*
  congestive heart (CHF)
  decompensated congestive heart
  diastolic heart
  donor heart
  end-stage congestive heart
  end-stage liver
  fetal heart
  forward heart
  heart
  heart forward
  heart power
  high-output cardiac
  high-output circulatory
  high-output heart
  hypercapnic respiratory (HRF)
  hypoxemic respiratory
  intrauterine cardiac
  intrauterine heart
  left heart
  left ventricular
  left-sided congestive heart
  low-output heart
  multiorgan
  pacemaker battery
  peripheral circulatory
  postoperative renal
  primary bioprosthetic valve
  pulmonary
  pump
  refractory congestive heart
  refractory heart
  respiratory
  right heart
  right-sided congestive heart
  right ventricular
  systolic heart
  ventilatory
failure of match test at 3 inches
failure to capture
failure to sense
faint breath sounds

faint, common
faint friction rub
fainting spell
Falcon coronary catheter
Fallot disease
Fallot pentalogy (tetralogy of Fallot
    plus atrial septal defect)
Fallot syndrome
Fallot tetralogy
Fallot trilogy in congenital cyanotic
    heart disease
false A_2
false aneurysm, late
false bruit
false bundle-branch block
false channel
false croup
false cyanosis
false emphysema
false lumen
false-positive test result
false sac
familial amyloidosis
familial anuloaortic ectasia
familial aortic dissection
familial arterial fibromuscular
    dysplasia
familial arteriopathy
familial atresia
familial cardiomegaly
familial cardiomyopathy
familial chylomicronemia
familial dysautonomia
familial dysbetalipoproteinemia
familial elevated triglycerides
familial endocardial fibroelastosis
familial fibromuscular dysplasia of
    arteries
familial genetic dyslipidemia
familial hyperbetalipoproteinemia
familial hypercholesterolemia
familial hyperchylomicronemia

familial hyperlipidemia
familial intracranial hemangioma
familial intracranial hemorrhage
familial myxoma of the heart
familial pulmonary hypertension
familial varicose veins
family history of heart disease
family history of hypertension
family history of myocardial infarction
Family Index of Life Events (FILE)
Fanconi-Hegglin syndrome
fan-shaped view
FAP (femoral artery pressure)
Farber disease
Farber lipogranulomatosis
far field
farmer's lung
fascia (pl. fasciae)
    anterior
    enveloping
    extrapleural
    Gerota
    obturator
    pectoralis
    posterior
    prepectoral
    presternal
    superficial
    thoracic
fascicles
fascicular bundles
fascicular heart block
fascicular heartbeat
fasciculations
fasciculoventricular bypass fiber
fasciculoventricular bypass tracts
fasciotomy, anterior compartment
fashion
    antegrade
    retrograde
F.A.S.T. (First Access for Shock and
    Trauma) 1 System

FAST (flow-assisted, short-term)
FAST balloon catheter
Fast-Cath introducer catheter
fast-flow lesions
fast-flow malformation
fast-flow vascular anomaly
FastPack blood analyzer system
Fast-Pass lead pacemaker
fast-pathway conduction
FasTrac guidewire
fat
    animal (in diet)
    epicardial
    mediastinal
    monounsaturated
    overlying epicardial
    polyunsaturated
    preperitoneal
    properitoneal
    saturated
    unsaturated
fatal exsanguination
fat embolism syndrome (FES)
fatigability, easy
fatigue, progressively severe
fat removed from anterior surface
    of pericardium
fat-suppressed breath-hold technique
fatty acids
fatty degeneration
fatty streak atherosclerosis
Favaloro-Morse rib spreader
Favaloro sternal retractor
favorable prognosis
FBN1 gene
FBN2 gene
[18]FDG (fludeoxyglucose F 18)
FDP (fibrin degradation products)
fear of impending death (or doom)
    from angina
feasible alternatives
feature, conspicuous

febrile agglutinins
Fechtner syndrome
$FeCO_2$ (fraction of expired CO_2)
Federici sign
feeders
feeder veins
feeding mean arterial pressure
    (FMAP)
feeling of impending doom prior to
    myocardial infarction
$FEF_{25-75\%}$ (forced midexpiratory flow)
Feigenbaum echocardiogram
F-18 2-deoxyglucose uptake on PET
    scan
Fehling bioptome
Feldaker syndrome
Feldman ventriculography catheter
felt bolster, Teflon
felt strip
feminine aorta, small
femoral above-knee popliteal bypass
femoral approach for cardiac catheteri-
    zation
femoral artery catheterization
femoral artery cutdown
femoral artery pressure
femoral artery, superficial
femoral-femoral bypass graft
femoral-femoral crossover
femoral-peroneal in situ vein bypass
    graft
femoral-popliteal bypass surgery
femoral-popliteal Gore-Tex graft
femoral (artery) pseudoaneurysm,
    postcatheterization
femoral pulse
femoral thrombophlebitis
femoral vein percutaneous insertion
femoral vein, superficial
femoral venoarterial bypass
femoral venous approach
femoris, profunda

femoroaxillary bypass
femorodistal bypass
femorodistal popliteal bypass graft
femorofemoral approach
femorofemoral bypass
femorofemoral partial bypass
femorofemoral subcutaneous supra-
    pubic graft
femorofemoropopliteal
femoroperoneal bypass graft
femoropopliteal atheromatous stenosis
femoropopliteal bypass surgery
femoropopliteal thrombosis
femoropopliteal vein graft
femorotibial bypass graft
fem-pop (slang for femoral-popliteal)
    bypass
fencing-in of thoracoscopic ports
fenestra (pl. fenestrae)
fenestrated Fontan procedure
fenestrated tracheostomy tube
fenestration
    aortopulmonary
    apical
    baffle
    cusp
    de novo
    interchordal space
    single-punch
    transcatheter
fenestration of dissecting aneurysm
FEP (fluorinated ethylene-propylene)
    polymer
Ferguson forceps
ferruginous bodies
ferrule (on pacemaker wires)
FES (fat embolism syndrome)
fetal bradycardia
fetal cardiac anomalies
fetal cardiac arrhythmia
fetal echocardiography in utero
fetal heart failure

fetal hydrops (hydrops fetalis)
    nonimmune
    nonimmunologic
fetal ultrasonography
fetal umbilical vein injection under
    sonographic guidance
fetalis, hydrops
fetid bronchitis
FEV (forced expiratory volume)
FEV_1 (forced expiratory volume in
    1 second)
FEV_1-FVC, FEV_1 to FVC (forced
    vital capacity) ratio
FEV_3 (forced expiratory volume in
    3 seconds)
FEV_t (forced expiratory volume,
    timed)
fever
    acute rheumatic (ARF)
    Animal House (organic dust
        syndrome)
    atropine
    brass-founder's
    cotton-mill
    desert
    drug
    foundryman's
    hay
    hectic
    histamine
    low-grade
    mahogany
    metal fume
    Monday
    parrot
    perennial
    pneumonic lung
    polymer fume
    Pontiac
    Q
    rheumatic
    Rocky Mountain spotted

fever *(cont.)*
    rose
    San Joaquin Valley
    spiking
    threshing
    valley
fever and chills
fevers, chills, and sweats
FFA (free fatty acid) scintigraphy,
    labeled
FFP (fresh frozen plasma)
FG syndrome
FGF-I (human fibroblast growth
    factor-I)
FHC (familial hypertrophic cardio-
    myopathy)
fiber, fibers
    accelerating
    atrio-Hisian; atriohisian
    Brechenmacher
    bulbospiral
    bystander
    cardiac accelerator
    cardiac depressor
    cardiac muscle
    cardiac pressor
    collagenous
    depressor
    dietary
    fasciculoventricular bypass
    fasciculoventricular Mahaim
    impulse conducting
    intercostal bundle
    James
    Kent
    Mahaim
    Mahaim and James
    muscle
    nodoventricular bypass
    Purkinje
fiberbronchoscope

fiberbronchoscopy
fiberoptic angioscopy
fiberoptic bronchoplasty
fiberoptic bronchoscope
fiberoptic bronchoscopy
FiberScan laser system
fiber-shortening velocity (VCF)
Fiblast (trafermin)
fibrillate
fibrillating heart, hypothermic
fibrillation
    atrial (AF)
    auricular
    idiopathic ventricular
    intermittent cross-clamp (ICCF)
    paroxysmal atrial (PAF)
    refractory atrial
    reversible ventricular
    ventricular (VF)
fibrillation-flutter
fibrillation rhythm
fibrillator, electric
fibrillator source
fibrillatory impulse
fibrillin gene mutation
Fibrimage technetium imaging agent
fibrin bodies of pleura
fibrin clot
fibrin degradation products (FDP)
fibrin glue, autologous
fibrin glue sealant
fibrinogen
    plasma
    radiolabeled
    serum
    technetium 99m-labeled
fibrinogen degradation
fibrinogen determination test
fibrinogen-fibrin conversion syndrome
fibrinoid degeneration
fibrinoid necrosis

fibrinolysis
  deficient
  physiologic
fibrinolysis of thrombi
fibrinolytic system
fibrinolytic therapy
fibrinopeptide A (FPA)
fibrinopurulent pleurisy
fibrinous pleurisy
fibrinous bronchitis
fibrinous chorditis
fibrinous exudate
fibrinous pericarditis
fibrinous pleurisy
fibrinous pleuritis
fibrinous split products
fibrin platelet emboli
fibrin products
fibrin-rich exudate
fibrin-rich thrombus
fibrin split products
fibrin-stabilizing blood coagulation
  factor
fibroblasts, pulmonary airway
fibrocalcific cusps
fibroelastoma of heart valve
fibroelastoma, papillary
fibroelastosis
  adult
  endocardial
  familial endocardial
  primary endocardial
  secondary endocardial
  subendocardial
fibrofatty yellow plaque
fibrogenic dust disease
fibroid lung
fibroid myocarditis
fibroma of heart
fibromuscular dysplasia, familial
  arterial
fibromuscular ridge

fibronectin concentration
fibroplasia
  intimal
  medial
fibrosa, intervalvular
fibrosarcoma of heart
fibrosclerotic
fibroserous pericardial sac
fibrosi cordis, anuli
fibrosiderosis
fibrosing alveolitis associated with
  systemic sclerosis
fibrosing lung diseases
fibrosis
  African endomyocardial
  asbestos-induced pleural
  bauxite (of lung)
  bundle branch
  confluent
  cystic
  Davies endocardial
  Davies endomyocardial
  diatomite
  diffuse interstitial pulmonary
    (DIPF)
  diffuse pulmonary
  endocardial
  endomyocardial (EMF)
  graphite
  His-Purkinje system
  idiopathic pulmonary (IPF)
  interstitial
  interstitial diffuse pulmonary
  interstitial prematurity
  interstitial pulmonary
  intra-alveolar
  mediastinal idiopathic
  myocardial
  nodal
  nonnodular
  perialveolar
  perianeurysmal retroperitoneal

fibrosis *(cont.)*
  periaortic
  peribronchial
  perielectrode
  perivascular
  plexiform
  postinflammatory pulmonary
  postradiation
  progressive interstitial pulmonary
  pulmonary interstitial idiopathic
  pulmonary vein
  radiation
  retroperitoneal
  rheumatic
  tropical endomyocardial
fibrosis and inflammation, periaortic
fibrosis of pericardium
fibrosum, pericardium
fibrotic distortion of valve
fibrotic honeycombing
fibrotic mitral valve
fibrotic nodules
fibrotic plaques
fibrotic scarred media
fibrous cord
fibrous dysplasia
fibrous hyperplasia
fibrous mediastinitis
fibrous pericarditis
fibrous pericardium
fibrous plaque atherosclerosis
fibrous pleural adhesions
fibrous ring
fibrous skeleton of heart
fibrous tab
fibrous trigone, left
Fick cardiac output index
Fick cardiac output method
  assumed
  direct
Fick equation or formula

Fick method for calculating cardiac
  output
Fick oxygen method of cardiac output
Fick principle of cardiac output
Fiedler myocarditis
Fiedler syndrome
field
  bloodless
  collapsed lung
  far
  high-power
  low-power
  lung
  midlung
  near
  rf (radio frequency)
  surgical
field-dependent
fifth intercostal space
fifth left interspace
fifth rib
figure-3 sign
figure-of-8 suture
filamentous fungus
Filcard temporary removable vena
  cava filter
filiform pulse
filipuncture
fillet the wound tract open
filling
  augmented
  capillary
  decreased left ventricular
  left atrial
  left ventricular
  passive
  period of rapid ventricular
  period of reduced ventricular
  period of ventricular
  rapid (RF)
  retrograde

filling *(cont.)*
   right atrial
   right ventricular
   ventricular
filling defect (on x-ray)
filling of right ventricle, augmented
filling phase, rapid
filling pressure
filling rate, peak
films
   manual subtraction
   synthetic absorbable
filter
   AngioGuard embolic protection
   Bate floating embolic protection
   Bird's Nest percutaneous IVC
   Bird's Nest vena caval
   Captura floating embolic protection
   caval
   Cobe Sentry arterial
   E-Trap embolic protection
   Filcard temporary removable vena
      cava
   FilterWire
   FilterWire EX
   fishmouth opening on a
   Fulcrum distal
   Gianturco-Roehm Bird's Nest vena
      caval
   Greenfield vena caval
   Heprotec vascular
   Innovante
   Kimray-Greenfield caval
   leukocyte reduction
   LeukoNet
   Mobin-Uddin umbrella
   Mobin-Uddin vena caval
   Optease permanent vena cava
   percutaneous inferior vena cava
      (IVC)
   prophylactic IVC
   Simon nitinol percutaneous IVC

filter *(cont.)*
   Timeless Performance vena cava
   Trachi-Naze laryngectomy
   Trachi-Naze tracheostomy
   umbrella
   Venatech percutaneous IVC
   Wiener
FilterWire
FilterWire EX
filtration rate, reduced glomerular
final rapid repolarization
Finapres blood pressure monitor
Finesse cardiac device
finding, findings
   auscultatory
   cardinal
   characteristic
   concomitant
   equivocal
   no discernible
   ominous
   pathognomonic
   salient physical
   scanty
   spurious
fine crackles
fine crepitant rales
fine needle biopsy
fine rales
fine-speckled appearance
fine wheezes
Finesse cardiac device
Finesse large-lumen guiding catheter
finger clubbing
finger cuff
finger dissection divides costal
   attachments of diaphragm
finger fracture dissection
fingertip sign
fingerlike projection
finned pacemaker lead
Finochietto forceps

Finochietto retractor
Finochietto rib spreader
Finochietto thoracic scissors
Fino vascular catheter
FiO_2 (forced inspiratory oxygen)
firing of ectopic atrial focus
firm mass
first branch of artery
first component
first-degree atrioventricular (AV) heart
  block
first diagonal branch
first intercostal space
First Midcath single-lumen silicone
  midline catheter
first obtuse marginal artery
first order chordae
first-pass imaging
first-pass radionuclide exercise angiocardiography
first-pass study
first-pass view (in multiple gated
  acquisition scan, or MUGA)
First PICC single-lumen silicone
  peripherally inserted central
  catheter
FirstSave automated external defibrillator (AED)
first septal perforator
first-stage Norwood operation
Fischer sign
Fisher exact test
fish-flesh appearance
fishhook lead
fishmeal worker's lung
fishmouth configuration of mitral
  valve
fishmouth filter opening
fishmouth stenosis
Fisoneb nebulizer
Fissinger-Rendu syndrome

fissure
  horizontal
  lung
  oblique
fist palpation
fistula
  aortic sinus
  aortic sinus to right ventricle
  aortocaval
  aortoenteric
  aorta-left ventricular
  aortopulmonary
  aorta-right ventricular
  arteriovenous (AVF)
  AV (arteriovenous)
  brachioaxillary bridge graft
    (BAGF)
  brachiocephalic arteriovenous
  brachiosubclavian bridge graft
    (BSGF)
  Brescia-Cimino AV
  bronchocutaneous
  bronchopleural
  cameral
  carotid artery-cavernous sinus
  carotid cavernous
  cerebral arteriovenous
  chylous
  coil closure of coronary artery
  congenital pulmonary
  coronary
  coronary arteriosystemic
  coronary arteriovenous
  coronary artery cameral
  coronary artery to right ventricular
  coronary artery-pulmonary artery
  coronary-cameral
  coronary-pulmonary
  graft-enteric
  hepatic arteriovenous
  hepatopleural

fistula *(cont.)*
    intrapulmonary arteriovenous
    lumen of the
    mature
    mediastinal
    microvenoarteriolar
    paraprosthetic-enteric
    persistent bronchopleural
    pleural
    pseudoaneurysm of
    pulmonary arteriovenous
    radial artery to cephalic vein
    thoracic
    tracheobronchial
    tracheoesophageal
    ventriculocoronary arterial
fistulectomy
    bronchocutaneous
    bronchopleuromediastinal
    bronchovisceral
    laryngeal
    laryngotracheal
    thoracicoabdominal
    thoracicogastric
    thoracicointestinal
    tracheoesophageal
Fitzgerald aortic aneurysm forceps
FIVC (forced inspiratory vital
    capacity)
5 French angiographic catheter
5-prong (or five-prong) rake blade
five-second breath-hold
fixation, chest wall
fixed airway obstruction
fixed aortic ejection click
fixed area of narrowing in large airway
fixed defect
fixed intracavitary filling defect
fixed mass
fixed pulmonary valvular resistance
fixed-rate pacing
fixed rate permanent pacemaker

fixed splitting of heart sound
FL4 guide
flabby heart
flaccid bronchi
Flack node
Flack sinoatrial node
flail chest
flail mitral leaflet
flail mitral valve
flange of tracheostomy tube
flank incision
flap
    diaphragm
    dissection
    Eloesser
    intercostal muscle
    intimal
    intraluminal
    muscle
    necrotic
    pectoralis major muscle
    pedicle
    pedicled intercostal muscle
    pericardial
    pleural
    scimitar-shaped
    Waldenhausen subclavian
flaplike valves
flap tracheostomy
flap valve ventricular septal defect
flaring of the alae nasi
FLASH (fast low-angle shot) cardiac
    MRI study
flashlamp-pulsed dye laser
flash pulmonary edema with anuria
flat chest
flat-hand test
flat lined (verb)
flat neck veins
flat P wave
flat percussion note
flat ST segment depression

flattened T waves
flattening of chest wall
flattening of plaque
flattening of ST segment
flat tube pressure sensor
flax-dresser's disease
Fleischner sign
Fletcher coagulation factor
FlexDerm hydrogel sheet
Flexguard tip catheter
Flexguide intubation guide
Flex guidewire
flexibility
flexible angioscope
flexible bronchoscope
flexible cardiac valve
flexible fiberoptic bronchoscopy
flexible J guidewire
flexible steerable guidewire
flexible suction cannula
Flexi-Cath balloon catheter
Flexicath silicone subclavian cannula
Flexi-Torque thermodilution balloon
   catheter
Flexon steel suture
Flextend pacing lead
Flexzan foam wound dressing
FL4 guide
flip-flop of heart
flip-flop sensation in chest
flip, LDH$_1$
flipped LDH
flipped LD$_1$-LD$_2$ (LD$_1$ to LD$_2$) ratio
flipped T wave
floating leaflets
floating trocar tip
FloCath catheter
FloControl catheter with occluding
   mechanism
flopping in chest
floppy aortic valve
floppy mitral valve syndrome

floppy tongue
floppy valves
floppy valve syndrome
flora
   multiple unidentified respiratory
      (MURF)
   normal
Florence flask appearance
Flo-Rester vessel occluder
florid cardiac tamponade
florid complexion
florid edema
florid Hantavirus pulmonary syndrome
florid Marfan syndrome
florid symptoms
FloSeal matrix hemostatic sealant
flotation catheter
Flo-Thru Intraluminal Shunt
flow
   antegrade
   antegrade blood
   antegrade diastolic
   aortic (AF)
   backward
   blood
   cerebral blood (CBF)
   chronic reserve
   collateral
   collateral blood
   compromised
   coronary blood
   coronary reserve (CRF)
   dampened pulsatile
   decreased cerebral blood
   effective pulmonary blood (EPBF)
   effective pulmonic
   forward
   Ganz method for coronary sinus
   great cardiac vein (GCVF)
   high velocity
   intercoronary collateral
   laminar

flow *(cont.)*
  left-to-right
  maximal midexpiratory (MMEF)
  maximum midexpiratory
  midexpiratory tidal
  mitral valve
  myocardial blood (MBF)
  peak
  peak expiratory (PEF)
  peak tidal expiratory
  pulmonary blood (PBF)
  pulmonic output
  pulmonic versus systemic
  redistribution of pulmonary
    vascular
  regional myocardial blood
  regurgitant
  regurgitant systolic
  restoration of
  retrograde
  retrograde systolic
  reversed vertebral blood (RVBF)
  sluggish
  systemic blood (SBF)
  systemic output
  tissue
  total cerebral blood (TCBF)
  transmitral
  tricuspid valve
  turbulent blood
  turbulent intraluminal
flow asymmetry (in airway tree)
flow-compromising lesion
flow-directed catheter
flow-guided Inoue balloon
FlowGun suction/irrigation
flow volume asymmetry (in aortic
  arch)
FloWire Doppler guidewire
FloWire Doppler ultrasound medical
  device
flow-limited expiration

flow mapping technique
flowmeter
  blood
  Doppler
  electromagnetic
  Narcomatic
  Parks 800 bidirectional Doppler
  pulsed Doppler
  Statham electromagnetic
flow rates, rapid inspiratory
flow redistribution
flow stagnation, blood
Flowtron DVT (deep venous
  thrombosis) pump system
Flowtron intermittent compression
  garment
flow velocity profile
flow velocity signals
flow void
flow-volume curve
flow-volume loop (in spirometry
  reports)
flow-volume, tidal inspiratory
Fluckiger syndrome
fluctuant
Fluency and Fluency XX stent
Fluency and Fluency XX stent-graft
  delivery catheter
flu exposure
fluffy infiltrate
fluid
  amniotic
  bloodless
  bloody
  bronchoalveolar lavage (BALF)
  crystalloid
  dependent edema
  edema
  evacuation of offending pericardial
  extracellular
  exudation of fibrin-rich
  exudative pericardial

fluid *(cont.)*
    Fluosol-DA 20% oxygen-transport
    hemorrhagic
    increased interstitial
    interstitial
    mediastinal drainage
    parenteral
    pericardial
    pleural
    purulent
    regurgitation of sour
    serosanguineous
    serous
    straw-colored
    subpulmonic
    thoracentesis
    tissue
    transudation of
    transudative pericardial
    turbid
fluid accumulation, dependent extra-
    cellular
fluid accumulation in tissues
fluid administration
fluid balance
fluid challenge
fluid collection, loculated
fluid expansion, rapid
fluid extravasation
fluid-filled mass
fluid flow between capillaries and
    interstitial tissue
fluidification
fluid intake, restricted
fluid level
fluid overload
fluid resorption
fluid restriction
fluid resuscitation
fluid retention
fluid volume, extracellular
fluid volume, increased extracellular

flu-like illness
flu-like symptoms
FluMist influenza virus vaccine
fluorescein angiography
fluorescence spectroscopy
fluorinated ethylene-propylene (FEP)
    polymer
fluorodeoxyglucose (FDG) radioactive
    tracer
fluorography, spot-film
Fluoropassiv thin-wall carotid patch
FluoroPlus Cardiac imaging
fluoroscope, fluoroscopy
    biplane
    C-arm digital
    chest
fluoroscopic control, advanced under
fluoroscopic guidance
fluoroscopic road-mapping technique
    in angioplastic vascular procedures
Fluosol (artificial blood)
Fluosol oxygen transport medium and
    plasma expander
Fluosol-DA 20% oxygen-transport
    fluid
flush
    bright red
    circumoral
    heparinized saline
    malar
flush aortogram
flushed
flushing of catheter
flushing maneuver
flushing, vascular graft
flush method of taking blood pressure
    in infants
flutter
    atrial (AFl)
    auricular
    coarse atrial
    impure

flutter *(cont.)*
   mediastinal
   pure
   ventricular
Flutter device
flutter-fibrillation
fluttering of valvular leaflet
fluttering sensation
flu vaccine
fluximetry
fluxionary hyperemia
FMAP (feeding mean arterial
   pressure)
foam embolus
foamy appearance of exudate
foamy exudate in the air spaces
foamy lipoid material
focal changes
focal dilatations of air spaces
focal-dust emphysema
focal eccentric stenosis
focal endocardial hemorrhage
focal interstitial infiltrate
focal intimal thickening
focal moderate rejection
focal myocyte damage
focal neurologic signs
focal perivascular infiltrate
FocalSeal
FocalSeal-L
FocalSeal-S
focal stenosis
focal wall motion abnormality
focus (pl. foci)
   Assmann
   atrial
   cystlike
   ectopic
   junctional
   radiolucent
   Simon
Foerster forceps

Foerster sponge forceps
Fogarty adherent clot catheter
Fogarty arterial embolectomy catheter
Fogarty balloon catheter
Fogarty balloon catheterization
Fogarty-Chin clamp
Fogarty-Chin extrusion balloon
   catheter
Fogarty embolectomy, transfemoral
Fogarty forceps
Fogarty Hydragrip clamp
Fogarty occlusion catheter
Fogarty venous thrombectomy catheter
Foix-Alajouanine syndrome
fold
   epicanthic
   pericardial
   Rindfleisch
   ventriculoinfundibular
folic acid deficiency anemia
follow-up duplex study
follow-up examination
fomites
Fontan anastomosis of atrial
   appendage to pulmonary artery
Fontan baffle
Fontan circuit
Fontan conversion to an extracardiac
   conduit procedure
Fontan conversion to a lateral tunnel
   procedure
Fontan-Kreutzer repair, modified
Fontan modification of Norwood
   procedure for hypoplastic left-sided
   heart syndrome
Fontan operation for tricuspid atresia
   and pulmonary stenosis
Fontan operation, takedown of
Fontan repair
foot cradle
foot, trash (embolization of small
   vessels in feet)

foramen of Morgagni
foramen ovale
foramen ovale, patent
foramen, restrictive bulboventricular
foramen secundum
Forbes disease
force
   contractile
   lateral anterior
   reciprocal
   reserve
   rest
   stroke
Force balloon dilatation catheter
forced exhalation
forced expiratory flow (FEF)
forced expiratory volume (FEV)
forced expiratory volume in 1 second
   (FEV_1)
forced expiratory volume in 3 seconds
   (FEV_3)
forced inspiratory oxygen (FiO_2)
forced midexpiratory flow
   ($FEF_{25-75\%}$)
forced vital capacity (FVC)
force-frequency relation
forceful heartbeat
forcefully wedged
forceful parasternal motion
force-length relation
force of contraction
forceps
   Adson
   alligator
   Allis
   artery
   Babcock
   Bailey aortic valve cutting
   bayonet bipolar
   Bengolea artery
   biopsy
   biopsy cup

forceps *(cont.)*
   BiPal biopsy
   Bloodwell
   blunt
   Boettcher artery
   bone-cutting
   bottle nose
   bronchus
   Brown-Adson
   Brunschwig artery
   bulldog
   Carmalt artery
   Castroviejo-Colibri
   cone nose
   Cooley-Baumgarten aortic
   Cooley vascular
   Crile
   cupped
   curved Kelly
   curved mosquito
   Cushing
   Dale
   Davis
   DeBakey
   DeBakey arterial
   DeBakey Autraugrip
   DeBakey-Diethrich vascular
   DeBakey dissecting
   DeBakey-Semb
   DeBakey tissue
   DeBakey vascular
   Doyen
   duckbill
   Duval-Crile lung
   Duval lung
   Effler-Groves
   Ferguson
   Finochietto
   Fitzgerald aortic aneurysm
   Foerster
   Foerster sponge
   Fogarty

forceps *(cont.)*
   Foss
   Gemini thoracic
   Gerald
   Gerbode
   grasping
   Halsted
   Halsted hemostatic mosquito
   Harrington-Mixter thoracic
   Harrington thoracic
   Hartmann hemostatic mosquito
   Hayes Martin
   Heiss artery
   hemoclip-applying
   hemostatic
   Hopkins aortic
   Jacobson hemostatic
   Jawz endomyocardial biopsy
   jeweler's
   Johns Hopkins
   Johnson thoracic
   Jones IMA
   Julian thoracic
   Karp aortic punch
   Kocher
   Koeberlé
   Lahey thoracic
   Laurer
   Lees artery
   Lejeune thoracic
   Lillehei valve
   Mayo-Péan
   Mazzariello-Caprini
   McKernan-Adson
   McKernan-Potts
   Meeker
   micro
   Mixter
   mosquito
   Multibite biopsy
   NIH mitral valve
   Ochsner

forceps *(cont.)*
   O'Shaughnessy artery
   Overholt thoracic
   Péan
   Pennington
   Phaneuf artery
   Pilling Weck Y-stent
   Potts bronchus
   Potts bulldog
   Potts-Smith tissue
   Potts thumb
   Potts vascular
   Price-Thomas bronchial
   Quadripolar cutting
   Randall stone
   Rochester-Mixter artery
   Ruel
   Rumel thoracic
   Russian tissue
   Samuels
   Sarot artery
   Seitzinger tripolar cutting
   Selman tissue
   Semb
   Singley
   Snowden-Pencer
   sponge
   spoon
   straight biopsy cup
   straight-end cup
   Take-apart scissors and
   Thomas-Allis
   thumb
   tissue
   tonsillar
   toothed Adson tissue
   torsion
   Tuttle thoracic
   up-biting biopsy cup
   Vickers ring tip
   Westphal
   Yasargil artery

force-velocity relation
forcipressure
Foregger ventilator
foreign-body aspiration
foreign body extractor, in-time
    vascular
foreign body in respiratory
    passages
foreign body reaction
foreign body upper airway obstruction
ForeRunner automatic external
    defibrillator device
foreshortening, anular
forestall
form, wave
format
    hemodynamic
    slice
    three-dimensional
    two-dimensional
formation
    arteriovenous fistula
    eddy
    exuberant atheroma
    honeycomb
    thrombus
formation of blood clots within leg
    veins
forme fruste (pl. formes frustes)
forme tardive
formidable risk
formula (see also *equation*, *method*)
    Bazett
    Boyd
    Cannon
    Fick
    Ganz coronary sinus flow
    Gorlin
    Gorlin valve area
    Hakki
    Hamilton-Stewart
    Yeager

Forney syndrome
Forrester syndrome
Forrester Therapeutic Class
40-joule rescue shock
45° position
forward failure
forward flow
forward flow velocity
forward heart failure
forward triangle method
forward velocity (on Doppler)
fossa
    antecubital
    cardiac
    oval (of heart)
    popliteal
fossa ovalis
fossa ovalis cordis
fossae ovalis, limbus
Foss forceps
foul-tasting sputum
Fountain catheter
four-beat run
four-chamber apical view
four-chamber plane on echocardi-
    ography
Four Corners virus
Fourier analysis of electrocardiogram
Fourier transform
fourth intercostal space
fourth left interspace
foveated chest
Fowler position
Fox green dye
FPA (fibrinopeptide A)
F point of cardiac apex pulse
fraction (see also *ejection fraction*)
    beta lipoprotein
    blood plasma
    depressed ejection
    ejection
    left ventricular shortening

fraction *(cont.)*
  MB
  plasma
  regurgitant
  shortening
fractional area
fractional inspired oxygen concentration)
fractional myocardial shortening
fractional shortening (of left ventricle)
fraction of expired carbon dioxide ($FeCO_2$)
fracture
  anular
  laryngeal
  lead
  pacing lead
  plaque
  stent
fractured ribs
fracturing, plaque
fragility, capillary hereditary
fragmentation
fragments, Fab
Framingham criteria for heart failure
Framingham data
frank blood
Frank capillary toxicosis
frank cyanosis from hypoxemia
frank edema
Frank EKG lead system placement
frank hemorrhage
Frank lead
frank pulmonary edema
frank rigors
Frank sign
Frank-Starling law of the heart
Frank-Starling mechanism or principle
Frank-Starling relationship
Frank vectorcardiogram (VCG)
Frank XYZ orthogonal lead system
Fräntzel murmur

frappage
Frater annuloplasty
Frater stitch or suture
fraught with error
fraying of the edges
Frazier suction tip or tube
FRC (functional residual capacity)
freckling, myxoma syndrome with facial
Fredrickson and Lees classification of hyperlipoproteinemia (type I-V)
free air passage
free air under the diaphragm
free end of electrode
free-flap reconstruction (anastomotic technique)
free-floating electrode
free-GEPA graft
freehand aortic valve homograft
free induction decay
freeing up of adhesions
freely movable mass
free pericardial space
Freer elevator
free tie
free wall
  posterior
  ventricular
free wall tract
Freeway PTCA catheter
Freezor cryocatheter
fremitus (see also *bruit*, *murmur*, *rale*, *sound*)
  bronchial
  friction
  pectoral
  pericardial
  pleural
  rhonchal
  tactile
  tussive
  vocal (VF)

French MBIH catheter
French scale for caliber of catheter
frequency
    angina with recent increase in
    resonant
    respiratory
frequency analysis of Doppler signal
frequent sneezing
frequent ventricular ectopy
fresh frozen plasma (FFP)
fresh frozen plasma infusion
Freund anomaly
FR4 guiding catheter
friability
friable ductus
friable lesion
friable mass
friable mucosa
friable thickened degenerated intima
friable tumor
friable vegetations
friable wall
friction between pleural and
    pericardial surfaces
friction fremitus
friction rub
    coarse
    creaking
    faint
    grating
    harsh
    loud
    pericardial
    pleural
    saddle leather
    scratchy
    shuffling
    soft
Friedel Pick syndrome
Friedländer bacillus
Friedländer disease
Friedländer pneumonia

Friedländer endarteritis obliterans
    disease
Friedreich ataxia
Friedreich ataxic cardiomyopathy
Friedreich phenomenon
Friedreich sign
Friend catheter
Frimodt-Moller syndrome
frog breathing
frond-like appearance
frontal plane loop
frontal plane on EKG
frontotemporal muscle
Frostline linear cryoablation system
frothy fluid
frothy mixture
frothy sputum
Frouin, quadrangulation of
Frouin technique
FRP (functional refractory period)
    atrial
    ventricular
FSV (forward stroke volume)
fucosidosis
fugax, amaurosis
Fujinon NAP-F nasopharyngoscope
Fulcrum catheter
Fulcrum distal filter device
Fulcrum distal occlusion device
Fulcrum guidewire
Fulcrum stent
fulcrum, left ventricular
fulguration during electrophysiologic
    study
fulguration, endocavitary
full anticoagulation
full-blown cardiac tamponade
full bypass
full fill-full empty mode (VAD or
    pump)
fullness, periorbital
full pause

full respiratory excursions
full-thickness button of aortic wall
full-thickness Carrel button
full-thickness infarction of ventricular
  septum
full-thickness mass into the atrial wall
full-to-empty mode (VAD or heart
  pump)
full-volume loop spirometry
fully implanted ventricular assist device
fulminant course of disease
fulminant pulmonary edema
fulminant tuberculosis
fumes
  metal
  polytetrafluoroethylene
  Teflon-Fluon
  toxic
function
  baseline pulmonary
  compromised ventricular
  contralateral pulmonary
  depressed right ventricular
    contractile
  exercise LV
  global left ventricular
  global systolic left ventricular
  global ventricular
  left atrial (LA)
  left ventricular (LV)
  left ventricular systolic/diastolic
  left ventricular systolic pump
  myocardial contractile
  preserved left ventricular
  regional left ventricular
  regional ventricular
  reserve cardiac
  rest LV (left ventricular)
  rest RV (right ventricular)
  right atrial (RA)
  right ventricular (RV)
  right ventricular systolic/diastolic
  ventricular contractility (VCF)

functional aerobic impairment (FAI)
functional asymmetry
functional classification of congestive
  heart failure
functional dyspnea
functional heart murmur
functional impairment
functional intact fibrinogen (FiF) test
functional reentry
functional refractory period (FRP)
functional residual capacity (FRC)
funduscopic
funduscopy
fungal endocarditis
fungal hyphae and spores
fungal infections of the lungs
fungal myocarditis
fungal pericarditis
fungal pneumonia
fungal smear
fungus, filamentous
fungus-laden straw
funic souffle
funicular souffle
funnel chest syndrome
Fürbringer sign (Fuerbringer)
furosemide inhalation
furrier's lung
fused commissures
fused papillary muscle
fusiform aneurysm
fusiform bronchiectasis
fusiform dilatation
fusiform narrowing of arteries
fusiform shadow
fusion
  commissural
  leaflet
fusion beat
fusion QRS complex
fuzzy echo
FVC (forced vital capacity)
f wave of jugular venous pulse

G, g

gadolinium-diethylenetriamine-
    pentaacetic acid (Gd-DTPA)
gadolinium-enhanced subtracted MR
    angiography, 3-D
gadopentetate dimeglumine
gadoteridol
gadoversetamide
GAGs (glycosaminoglycans)
Gailliard syndrome
Gairdner disease
Gaisböck syndrome
galactose
galactose-based ultrasound contrast
    medium
galactose; palmitic acid
galactose ultrasound contrast medium
galactosidase deficiency, alpha-
Galaxy pacemaker
Gallavardin dissociation
Gallavardin murmur
Gallavardin phenomenon
Gallavardin syndrome
gallium scan
gallium-68 (^{68}gallium)
gallop
    atrial
    diastolic

gallop *(cont.)*
    early diastolic
    late diastolic
    low-frequency
    mid diastolic
    presystolic
    presystolic atrial
    prominent ventricular diastolic
    protodiastolic
    S_3 (third heart sound)
    S_4 (fourth heart sound)
    summation (S_3 and S_4)
    systolic
    ventricular
    ventricular diastolic
gallop, murmur, or rub (GMR)
gallop rhythm
gallop sound
gamma camera
ganglion (pl. ganglia)
ganglion blocker
ganglionectomy, left stellate
gangrene
    atherosclerotic
    embolic
    lung
    presenile

gangrene *(cont.)*
    pulmonary
    Raynaud
    static
    thrombotic
    venous
gangrenous emphysema
gangrenous lung tissue
gannister disease
Ganz-Edwards coronary infusion
    catheter
Ganz formula for coronary sinus flow
gap, auscultatory
Garcia aortic clamp
Gardner-Diamond syndrome
gargle, Dyclone
gargoylism
Garland triangle
garment
    Flowtron intermittent compression
    Jobst
    pneumatic antishock (PASG)
    pneumatic foot compression
Garrett dilator
Garrett retractor
Garrett vascular dilator
Gärtner (Gaertner) phenomenon
gas, gases
    alveolar
    arterial blood (ABG)
    expired
    hypoxic-hypercapnic
    inspired
gas accumulation under serous tunic
    of intestine
gas chromatography
gas endarterectomy
gas exchange, pulmonary
gas nitrogen embolism
gasping for breath
gasping respirations

gastric contents, pulmonary aspiration
    of
gastric window
gastrinoma, malignant
gastritis, hemorrhagic
gastrocardiac syndrome
gastrocnemius muscle
gastroenteritis, primary eosinophilic
gastroepiploic artery
gastroepiploic artery (GEPA) graft
gastrohepatic omentum
gas volumes, thoracic
GATA3 gene mutation
gated blood (pool) cardiac wall motion
    study
gated blood-pool study (GBPS)
gated blood pool ventriculogram
gated cardiac blood pool imaging
gated equilibrium blood pool scanning
gated inflow technique
gated magnetic resonance imaging
gated radionuclide ventriculography
gated view (in MUGA, multiple gated
    acquisition scan)
gate, respiratory
GateWay Y-adapter rotating hemo-
    static valve
gating
    echocardiographic
    respiratory
gating of heartbeats
Gaucher disease
gauge, strain
gauze (see *dressing*)
GCVF (great cardiac vein flow)
GEA (gastroepiploic artery) graft
gel
    Carra Sorb M wound
    DuoDerm hydroactive
    EKG
    electrode

gel *(cont.)*
   Lectron II electrode
   SoloSite wound
gelatin compression boot
gelatinous debris
gelatinous mottled sputum
gelatin-resorcinol-formol biological
   glue injection
gelatin sponge slurry
Gelfilm
Gelfoam
Gelfoam soaked in thrombin
Gelfoam, thrombin-soaked
Gelofusine (4% succinylated gelatin)
   hemostatic agent
Gelpi retractor
Gem DR implantable defibrillator
Gemini DDD pacemaker
Gemini thoracic forceps
GEM II DR/VR implantable
   cardioverter-defibrillator
GEM III AT implantable cardioverter-
   defibrillator
gene
   FBN1 (implicated in Marfan
      syndrome)
   fibrillin
   GATA3
   microfibrillar protein fibrillin
gene mutation, fibrillin
General Electric pacemaker
General Electric Pass-C echocardiograph machine
generalized alveolitis
generalized arteriosclerosis
generalized capillary leak
generalized emphysema
generalized pulmonary edema
generation, cardiac electromotive force
generator (see also *pacemaker*)
   asynchronous
   Aurora pulse

generator *(cont.)*
   bipolar
   Chardack-Greatbatch implantable
      cardiac pulse
   Cosmos pulse
   Cyberlith multi-programmable
      pulse
   fixed rate
   implantable pulse
   Infinity pulse
   intrapleural pulse
   Jewel pulse
   lithium-powered pulse
   Medtronic demand pulse
   multiprogrammable pulse
   Pacesetter Trilogy DR+ pulse
   PCD pulse
   Philos DR-T pulse
   physiologic
   Programalith III pulse
   pulse
   Regency SR+ single-chamber,
      rate-responsive pulse
   Spectrax SXT pulse
   subpectoral pulse
   Telectronics PASAR antitachy-
      cardia pulse
   unipolar programmable rate-
      responsive
   Ventak PRX pulse
   Ventak P2 pulse
   Ventak pulse
   ventricular demand
   ventricular inhibited pulse
   Ventritex Cadence
   Versatrax pulse
   VNUS Closure radiofrequency
GenESA pharmacological stress test
genetic dyslipidemia, familial
Gengraf (cyclosporine capsules
   modified)
Genisis pacemaker

Gensini cardiac device
Gensini catheter
Gensini scoring of coronary artery
   disease
GenStent biologic therapy
Gentle-Flo suction catheter
GentleLASE Plus
geometrical asymmetry
geometry, ventricular cavity
GEPA (gastroepiploic artery) graft
Gerald forceps
Gerbode dilator
Gerbode forceps
Gerbode mitral valvulotome
Gerbode patent ductus clamp
Gerbode valve dilator
Gerhardt sign
Gerhardt triangle
German measles
Gerota fascia
GE single-photon emission computer-
   ized tomography
GE Starcam single-crystal tomograph-
   ic scintillation camera
Gey solution
GFR (glomerular filtration rate)
GFX coronary stent
Ghajar guide for intraventricular
   catheter placement
Ghon complex
Ghon lesion
Ghon tubercle
ghosts, alveolar cell
giant A waves
giant bullous emphysema
giant capillary hemangioma with
   thrombocytopenia and purpura
giant cavernous hemangioma
giant cell aortitis
giant cell arteritis
giant cell carcinoma
giant cell interstitial pneumonia (GIP)

giant cell myocarditis
giant cells
   Langhans
   multinucleate
giant edema
giant left atrium
giant platelets
Gianturco embolization coils
Gianturco occlusion coils
Gianturco-Roehm Bird's Nest vena
   caval filter
Gianturco-Roubin flexible coil stent
Gianturco wool-tufted wire coil stent
Gibbon and Landis test for peripheral
   circulation
Gibson murmur
Giertz rongeur
gigantism of pulmonary acini
Gigli saw
Gill-Jonas modification of Norwood
   procedure
GIP (giant cell interstitial pneumonia)
giving up/given up syndrome
gland
   alveolar
   paramediastinal
   thymus
Glanzmann disease
Glasgow sign
glass blower's emphysema
Glassman clamp used in thoracoscopy
Glenn anastomosis
Glenn operation for congenital
   cyanotic heart disease
Glenn procedure
   bidirectional
   classic
Glenn shunt
GLH (Green Lane Hospital)
GLH insertion method
GLH syndrome
Glidecath catheter

Glidecath dilator
Glidecath entry needle
Glidecath sheath
Glidecath torque device
Glidewire, long taper/stiff shaft
Glidewire guidewire
gliding and rotatory movements
global cardiac disease
global cerebral hypoperfusion
global ejection fraction
global hypokinesis
global left ventricular dysfunction
globally depressed ejection fraction
global myocardial ischemia
global systolic left ventricular dysfunc-
    tion
global ventricular dysfunction
global ventricular function
global wall motion abnormality
globoid heart
globular chest
globular sputum
globulin
    antihemophilic (AHG)
    antithymocyte
    rabbit antithymocyte (RATG)
globus hystericus
globus sensation
Glofil-125 (iothalamate sodium
    I 125)
glomectomy, carotid
glomerular filtration rate (GFR)
glomiform arteriolovenular anastomosis
glomus jugulare
glossopharyngeal breathing
glossopharyngeal neuralgia
glossopharyngeal syncope
glottis
gloved finger signs
Glover coarctation clamp
Glover patent ductus clamp
Glover vascular clamp

Gluck rib shears
glucocerebrosidase deficiency
glucocorticoid, exogenous
glucocorticoid-remediable hyper-
    aldosteronism
glue (see *adhesive; medications*)
glutamic oxaloacetic transaminase
    (GOT)
glutaraldehyde-stabilized human
    umbilical cord vein graft
glutaraldehyde-tanned bovine carotid
    artery graft
glutaraldehyde-tanned bovine collagen
    tubes for grafts
glutaraldehyde-tanned bovine valve
    prosthesis
glutaraldehyde-tanned porcine heart
    valve
glutaraldehyde-tanned umbilical vein
    graft
glycogen storage disease
glycogenosis, cardiac
glycolipid deposit
glycolysis
Glycoprene hemostatic agent
Glycoprene mesh
Glycoprene surgical clip
Glycoprene surgical staples
Glycoprene suture
Glycoprene suture anchor
Glycoprene tissue adhesive
Glycoprene vascular occlusion device
glycoproteinosis
glycosides, cardiac
glycosphingolipid metabolism
glycosaminoglycans (GAGs)
glycyrrhetinic acid
GMR (gallop, murmur, or rub)
goblet cells
Goethlin test
Goetz cardiac device
Golaski knitted Dacron graft

gold-195m radionuclide
Goldblatt clamp to produce hyperten-
  sion experimentally
Goldblatt hypertension
Goldblatt phenomenon
Goldenhar syndrome
Goldman cardiac risk index score
Goldman class or score
Gold Probe bipolar hemostasis
  catheter
gonococcal endocarditis
gonococcal pericarditis
Gonzales blood group
Goodale-Lubin cardiac catheter
good caliber
good cholesterol
Goodpasture syndrome
Goodtec disposable catheter
goose flesh
Goosen aortotomy
gooseneck deformity of outflow tract
  (on x-ray)
Gore-Tex bifurcated vascular graft
Gore-Tex cardiovascular patch
Gore-Tex catheter
Gore-Tex, extruded
Gore-Tex FEP-Ringed vascular graft
Gore-Tex limb
Gore-Tex Propaten vascular graft
Gore-Tex shunt
Gore-Tex soft tissue patch
Gore-Tex surgical membrane
Gore-Tex vascular graft
gore vascular graft
Gorlin catheter
Gorlin formula for aortic valve area
Gorlin hydraulic formula for mitral
  valve area
Gorlin method for cardiac output
Gorlin pacing catheter
Gorlin syndrome
Gosling pulsatility index

Gott shunt
Gott shunt/butterfly heart valve
Gould PentaCath 5-lumen thermodilution catheter
Gould Statham pressure transducer
Gouley syndrome
Gowers syndrome
gracile habitus
gracilis, habitus
grade 2/6 systolic ejection murmur
grade 2-3/6 ("grade two to three over
  six") (or II-III/VI) murmur
gradient
  A-a (alveolar-arterial)
  alveolar-arterial oxygen tension
  aortic outflow
  aortic valve (AVG)
  aortic valve peak instantaneous
  arteriovenous pressure
  brain-core
  coronary perfusion
  diastolic
  elevated
  end-diastolic aortic–left ventricular
    pressure
  holosystolic
  instantaneous
  left ventricular outflow pressure
  maximal estimated
  mean mitral valve
  mean systolic
  mitral valve
  negligible pressure
  outflow tract
  peak diastolic
  peak instantaneous
  peak pressure
  peak right ventricular–right atrial
    systolic
  peak systolic (PSG)
  peak-to-peak pressure
  pressure-flow

gradient *(cont.)*
 pulmonary artery diastolic and
  wedge pressure (PADP-PAWP)
 pulmonary artery to right ventricle
  diastolic
 pulmonary outflow
 pulmonic valve
 residual
 right ventricular to main pulmonary
  artery pressure
 stenotic
 subvalvular
 systolic
 transaortic systolic
 translesional
 transmitral
 transmitral diastolic
 transpulmonary pressure
 transpulmonic
 transstenotic pressure
 transtricuspid valve diastolic
 transvalvar
 transvalvular
 transvalvular pressure
 tricuspid valve
 ventricular
gradient across valve
gradient-echo imaging sequence
gradient-echo pulse sequence
gradient-echo sequence imaging
graduated exercises
graft
 AFBG (aortofemoral bypass graft)
 albumin-coated vascular
 albuminized woven Dacron tube
 allograft
 Ancure vascular
 AneuRx
 AneuRx tube
 Angiotech vascular
 Aorfix stent
 Aorfix vascular

graft *(cont.)*
 aorta to left anterior descending
  saphenous vein bypass
 aortic allograft
 aortic bifurcation
 aortic homograft
 aortic stent
 aortic tube
 aortobifemoral bypass
 aortobiprofunda bypass
 aortocoronary bypass
 aortocoronary saphenous vein
  bypass
 aortocoronary snake
 aortofemoral
 aortofemoral bypass (AFBG)
 Aria coronary artery bypass
 ascending aorta–abdominal aorta
  bypass
 autogenous
 autogenous saphenous vein
 autologous
 autologous fat
 autologous patch
 autologous reversed vein
 AV (atrioventricular)
 axillary-axillary bypass
 axillary-femorofemoral bypass
 axillobifemoral bypass
 axillofemoral bypass
 below-knee popliteal to distal
  peroneal reversed vein
 bifurcated
 bifurcated vascular
 bifurcation
 Biograft
 BioPolyMeric
 Björk-Shiley
 bovine allograft
 bovine heterograft
 brachial artery to axillary vein
  dialysis

graft *(cont.)*
  brachioaxillary interposition
    bypass
  Cabrol I tube
  Cabrol-II interposition coronary
    prosthetic
  cardiac allograft
  CardioPass vascular
  carotid-carotid venous bypass
  CBAS stent-grant
  CBAS vascular
  collagen-impregnated knitted
    Dacron velour
  composite
  composite valve
  composite vein
  compressed Ivalon patch
  conduit
  Cooley woven Dacron
  coronary artery bypass (CABG)
  Cragg endoluminal
  Credent artificial vascular access
  crossover
  cryopreserved human aortic
    allograft
  cryopreserved vein (CPVG)
  Dacron knitted
  Dacron onlay patch
  Dacron outflow
  Dacron patch
  Dacron preclotted
  Dacron tightly woven
  Dacron tube (or tubular)
  Dacron velour
  Dacron velour tube
  de-aired
  deploy the
  diamond-shaped sequential vein
  Diastat vascular access
  discordant cellular xenograft
  Distaflo bypass
  double velour knitted

graft *(cont.)*
  DTAFA (descending thoracic
    aorta-to-femoral artery) bypass
  E-CABG (endoscopic coronary
    artery bypass)
  Edwards woven Teflon aortic
    bifurcation
  endoscopic coronary artery bypass
    (E-CABG)
  endothelialization of vascular
  endothelialized vascular
  endovascular stented
  expanded polytetrafluoroethylene
    (ePTFE) vascular
  expanded reinforced polytetra-
    fluoroethylene (ER-PTFE)
    vascular
  extracardiac
  extracavitary prosthetic arterial
  extracavitary-infected
  extrathoracic carotid subclavian
    bypass
  extruded Gore-Tex
  Exxcel ePTFE soft vascular
  femoral-distal popliteal bypass
  femoral-distal vein
  femoral-femoral bypass
  femoral-peroneal in situ vein
    bypass
  femorofemoral subcutaneous
    suprapubic
  femoroperoneal bypass
  femorotibial bypass
  Fluency
  Fluency XX stent
  free-GEPA
  gastroepiploic artery (GEPA)
  GEA (gastroepiploic artery)
  glutaraldehyde-stabilized human
    umbilical cord vein
  glutaraldehyde-tanned bovine
    carotid artery

graft *(cont.)*
  glutaraldehyde-tanned bovine
    collagen tubes for vascular
  glutaraldehyde-tanned porcine
    heart valve
  glutaraldehyde-tanned umbilical
    vein
  Golaski
  Gore-Tex
  Gore-Tex bifurcated vascular
  Gore-Tex FEP-Ringed vascular
  Gore-Tex jump
  Gore-Tex Propaten vascular
  Guidant EVT (Endovascular
    Technologies) tube
  Hancock pericardial valve
  Hancock vascular
  HeartHope coronary artery bypass
  HeartHope vascular
  Hemashield
  Hemashield Gold branch
  Hemashield Gold Microvel knitted
    double velour
  Hemashield Vantage vascular
  Hemobahn nitinol stent-graft
  hepatorenal bypass
  hepatorenal saphenous vein bypass
  heterograft
  heterologous
  homograft
  horseshoe tubular
  HUV (human umbilical vein)
    bypass
  IEA (inferior epigastric artery)
  iliac-renal bypass
  ilioprofunda bypass
  IMA (internal mammary artery)
  infected
  infrainguinal vein bypass
  infrapopliteal arterial bypass
  infrarenal aortobifemoral bypass
  in situ

graft *(cont.)*
  in situ vein
  interatrial
  internal mammary artery (IMA)
  internal saphenous vein
  internal thoracic artery (ITA)
  interposition
  interposition vein
  Ionescu-Shiley pericardial valve
  Ionescu-Shiley vascular
  ITA (internal thoracic artery)
  jawed conduit
  jump
  kinking of
  knitted
  knitted Dacron
  knitted Dacron arterial
  knitted double velour Dacron patch
  LIMA (left internal mammary
    artery)
  Lifespan ePTFE vascular
  Litespeed synthetic vascular
  Meadox Microvel
  Microvel double velour
  mitral valve homograft
  modified human umbilical vein
    (HUV)
  noncavitary prosthetic
  nonreversed saphenous vein
  nonvalved
  Ochsner
  occluded
  OmniFlow vascular
  onlay
  outflow
  patch
  patent
  Perma-Flow coronary bypass
  Plasma TFE vascular
  polyfluorotetraethylene (PTFE)
  popliteal-blind peroneal
  popliteal-distal bypass

graft *(cont.)*
    porcine xenograft
    postage-stamp-type skin
    preclotted
    preclotted patch
    Preclude pericardial membrane
    prosthetic patch
    PTFE (polytetrafluoroethylene)
    pulmonary autograft
    radial artery
    Rapidgraft
    saphenous vein (SVG) bypass
    Sauvage
    sequential
    sequential bypass
    snake
    splenorenal arterial bypass
    St. Jude composite valve
    stabilized human umbilical vein
    straight
    straight tubular
    supraceliac aorta-femoral artery
        bypass
    supraceliac aorta-visceral artery
        bypass
    supraceliac aortic bypass
    supraceliac aortofemoral bypass
    synthetic
    Talent LPS endoluminal stent-graft
    Teflon
    thoracic aorta-femoral artery
        bypass
    Thoralon biomaterial used in
    thrombosed
    Tiason stent
    Tiason vascular
    transluminal endovascular graft
        placement
    transluminally placed endovascular
        (TPEG)
    transluminally placed stented
    tube

graft *(cont.)*
    tube endograft
    tubular
    umbilical vein
    unilateral aortofemoral
    valved
    Vascu-Guard
    vascular
    VascuLink vascular access
    Vascutek Gelseal knitted and
        woven vascular
    Vascutek Gelsoft
    Vectra vascular access (VAG)
    vein patch
    Venaflow vascular
    ventriculoarterial
    W. L. Gore vascular
    woven Dacron
    woven Dacron tube
    wraparound
    XL-Endograft
    Y
    Y-shaped
    Zenith AAA endovascular
graftable
graft ACE fixed-wire balloon catheter
GraftAssist vein and graft holder
graft connector
    Jocath
    Jography
    Joguide
graft dependent
graft endocarditis
graft-enteric erosion
graft-enteric fistula
graft entrapment
graft erosion into bowel lumen
graft excision
grafting (see *graft*)
graft insertion site
graft-into-graft deployment
graft material, synthetic (see
        prosthesis)

graft occlusion
graft occlusive disease
graft-patch
Graftpatch
graft patency
graft preservation
   complete
   partial
graft replacement of descending aorta
graft seeding technique
graft-seeking catheter
graft shrinkage
graft stenosis
graft trimmed on the bias
graft versus host disease (GVHD)
graft versus host reaction
Graham-Burford-Mayer syndrome
Graham Steell heart murmur
grain-handler's disease
grain-handler's lung
gram-negative bacterial endotoxins
gram-negative cocci
gram-negative sepsis
gram-positive cocci
Gram stain
Grancher sign
Grancher triad
Grant aneurysm clamp
granular cell tumor of the heart
granular pharyngitis
granulated
granulation stenosis
granulation tissue
granules
   aggregated eosinophil
   Much ("mook")
granulocytic leukemia
granuloma
   coccidioidal
   eosinophilic
   extravascular
   lethal midline

granuloma *(cont.)*
   noncaseating
   tuberculous
granulomatosis
   allergic
   allergic angiitis and
   bronchocentric
   Langerhans cell
   necrotizing respiratory
   organic
   Wegener
granulomatous and necrotizing replacement of bronchial epithelium
granulomatous disease, allergic
   myocardial
granulomatous inflammation of
   bronchi
granulomatous myocarditis
granulomatous pneumonitis
granulomatous reaction
granulomatous rhinitis
grapelike appearance in pulmonary
   tuberculosis
grapes appearance in pulmonary
   tuberculosis
graphite fibrosis of lung
grasper, En Garde
grasping forceps
grass
   June
   Timothy
GRASS (gradient recalled acquisition
   in steady state)
grating bruit
grating friction rub
Graupner method
grave prognosis
gravido-puerperal cardiomyopathy
gravitational edema
gray hepatization of lung
grayish sputum

great arteries, complete transposition
    of the
great artery disease
great artery, overriding
great cardiac vein
great cardiac vein flow
great coronary vein
greater saphenous vein reflux
great saphenous vein
great vessel, orientation of
great vessels transposition
greater cardiac vein
greater saphenous system
greater saphenous vein
Green retractor
green sputum
Greene sign
Greenfield filter
Greenfield IVC (inferior vena cava)
    filter
Greenfield vena caval filter
Gregg-type cannula
Gregoire's blue leg syndrome
Gregory baby profunda clamp
Gregory carotid bulldog clamp
Gregory external clamp
Gregory forceps
Gregory stay suture
Greyhound surgical spring clip (for
    temporary vessel occlusion)
grim prognosis
Grinfeld cannula
GRIP torque device
grippe
Gripper needle
grippy feeling
Grocco sign of pleural effusion
Grocco triangular dullness
groin area
groin complications
groin wound
Grollman catheter

Grollman pigtail catheter
groove
    anterior interventricular
    AV (atrioventricular)
    deltopectoral
    interatrial
    interventricular
    posterior interventricular
    Waterston
Groshong double-lumen catheter
Gross coarctation occlusion clamp
grossly audible wheezing
Grossman scale for regurgitation
Grossman sign
ground-glass appearance of lungs
ground-glass infiltrates in lungs
ground-glass opacities
ground plate
grounding lead
Grover clamp
growth factor, platelet-derived
growth retardation
Gruentzig (Grüntzig)
grumose (or grumous) material
grumous debris
grunting
    expiratory
    minimal expiratory
    respiratory distress with
grunting and retractions
grunting expiration
grunting murmur
grunting respirations
Grüntzig (Gruentzig)
Grüntzig angioplasty technique
Grüntzig balloon catheter angioplasty
Grüntzig technique for PTCA
Gsell-Erdheim syndrome
G suit (for syncope)
G syndrome
Guangzhou GD-1 prosthetic valve
guanine nucleotide binding protein

guanine nucleotide regulatory proteins
guarded condition
guarded prognosis
Guardian AICD (automatic implant-
   able cardioverter-defibrillator)
Guardian ICD (implantable cardio-
   verter-defibrillator)
Guardian pacemaker
guarding
GuardWire angioplasty system
guidance
   color-flow Doppler sonographic
   fluoroscopic
   under fluoroscopic
Guidant EVT (Endovascular
   Technologies) tube graft
Guidant introducer
Guidant Multi-Link Tetra coronary
   stent system
Guidant sheath
Guidant TRIAD three-electrode
   energy defibrillation system
guide
   ACS LIMA
   Amplatz tube
   Arani
   Cor-Flex wire
   FL4
   Flexguide intubation
   McGuire suture
   Muller catheter
   Pilotip catheter
   PTFE-coated spring-wire
   spring-wire
   steerable wire
guidewire
   ACS (Advanced Catheter Systems)
   ACS Hi-Torque Balance middle-
     weight
   Amplatz Super Stiff
   angiographic
   atherolytic

guidewire *(cont.)*
   atherolytic reperfusion
   Athlete coronary
   Bentson floppy-tip
   Blue Scout
   Cerebrence
   Chameleon
   Cinch QR steerable
   Commander
   Constant
   Control Wire
   Cordis Stabilizer steerable
   Cordis Wizdom steerable
   Critikon
   Driver
   Easy Twist steerable
   Emerald diagnostic
   Endeavor
   Extra Sport coronary
   FasTrac
   FilterWire
   FilterWire EX
   Flex
   flexible
   flexible J
   floppy
   floppy-tipped
   FloWire Doppler
   Fulcrum
   GlideCath
   Hemo-Cath
   Heprotec vascular
   High Performance Detach
   high torque
   high-torque floppy
   Hi-Per Flex
   Hi-Torque Flex-T
   Hi-Torque Floppy (HTF)
   Hi-Torque Intermediate
   Hi-Torque Standard
   hydrophilic
   Hyperflex

guidewire *(cont.)*
  Iguana
  Innovante
  InQwire
  Intercept Vascular
  J
  Jocath
  Jography
  Joguide
  J tip
  J-tipped exchange
  J-tipped spring
  Linx exchange
  long taper/stiff shaft Glidewire
  Lumina
  Magnum
  Manx
  Medrad
  Microvasive Glidewire
  Microvasive stiff piano wire
  Mirage Guidewire
  Mustang steerable
  Navius
  Opta
  Outcomes by Design steerable
  PDT
  preformed
  Prima laser
  QuickSilver hydrophilic-coated
  Radiofocus Glidewire
  Rapid-Trak
  Redifocus
  Reflex steerable
  Roadrunner
  Rosen
  RotaWire Floppy Gold
  Schwarten LP
  Sensor PTFE-nitinol guidewire
    with hydrophilic tip
  shapeable
  Shinobi Plus
  Shinobi steerable

guidewire *(cont.)*
  Silk
  SilverSpeed
  Sof-T
  soft-tipped
  Sones
  SOS
  SR
  Stabilizer Plus steerable
  Stabilizer steerable
  Stabilizer XS steerable
  steerable
  stiff
  Storq steerable
  straight
  Symbiant
  TAD
  Teflon-coated
  TherOx 0.014 infusion
  Tomcat
  Tomcat Fighter
  transluminal angioplasty
  USCI
  WaveWire high-performance
    angioplasty
  Wholey ("wooley")
  Wholey Hi-Torque Floppy
  Wholey Hi-Torque Modified J
  Wholey Hi-Torque Standard
  Wizdom and Wizdom ST steerable
guidewire exchanged
guiding catheter
guiding shots
guillotine, rib
Gunn crossing sign
gusset, woven Dacron
Gutgeman clamp
guy suture
guy-wire support for mitral valve
  leaflet
GVHD (graft versus host disease)

H, h

habitus
   asthenic
   body
   gracile
   large
habitus gracilis
hacking cough
Haemaccel (polygeline)
haematobium, Schistosoma
Haemonetics Cell Saver I autotransfusion system
Haemonetics Cell Saver III autotransfusion system
Haemonetics Cell Saver IV autotransfusion system
Haemonetics Cell Saver Plus autotransfusion system
Haemonetics Haemolite autotransfusion system
Haemophilus infection
Haemophilus influenzae (*H. influenzae*)
Haemophilus influenzae bronchitis
Haemophilus influenzae laryngitis
Haemophilus influenzae pneumonia
Hagar probe
Hageman blood coagulation factor
Hageman factor

Hageman factor activation
Hagner disease
Haight-Finochietto rib retractor
Haight rasp
Haight rib spreader
Haimovici arteriotomy scissors
hair growth
   decreased lower leg
   distribution of
hair loss
Hakki formula
Haldane-Priestley tube
Hale syndrome
half-hitch knots
Hall cutter
Hall Easy-Fit prosthetic heart valve
Hall-effect position sensor
Hall-Kaster mitral valve prosthesis
Hall-Kaster tilting-disk valve prosthesis
Hall prosthetic heart valve
Hall sign
Hall sternal saw
Hall valve disruption
Hall valvulotome
Halo catheter
halothane

261

Halsted hemostatic mosquito forceps
hamartoma
   benign vascular
   cardiac
   chondromatous
Hamburg classification of congenital
   vascular defect
Hamilton-Stewart formula for
   measuring cardiac output
Hamman crunch
Hamman disease
Hamman murmur
Hamman pneumopericardium sign
Hamman-Rich syndrome
hammocking of leaflet
hammocking of mitral valve
hammock mitral valve
hammock valve
Hampton hump
Hanafee catheter
Hancock aortic bioprosthesis
Hancock aortic punch
Hancock bioprosthesis
Hancock bioprosthetic valve
Hancock conduit
Hancock mitral valve prosthesis
Hancock M.O. II porcine bioprosthesis
Hancock obturator
Hancock pericardial prosthetic valve
Hancock porcine heterograft valve
Hancock porcine prosthetic heart valve
Hancock II tissue valve
Hancock trocar
Hancock trocar blade
Hancock valved conduit
Hancock valve prosthesis
Hancock vascular graft
hand-agitated contrast medium
hand-agitated solution with micro-
   bubbles
hand-bagging of oxygen
handgrip exercise test

H&H (hemoglobin and hematocrit)
hand-heart syndrome
handheld mapping probe
handheld nebulizer (HHN)
handheld retractor
hand injection
hand-made injection
hand-shaped bend
Hands Off balloon pacing catheter
Hands-Off thermal dilution catheter
   with Twist-Lock Cath-Gard
Hands Off thermodilution (TD)
   catheter
hand turgor
HANE (hereditary angioneurotic
   edema)
hanging drop test for pneumoperitoneum
hangout interval
hangout of dicrotic notch in
   pulmonary arterial pressure
Hank balanced salt solution
Hantavirus pulmonary syndrome
HAP (hepatic arterial-dominant phase)
   images (CT scan)
HAPE (high-altitude pulmonary
   edema)
HAR (hyperacute rejection)
Harbitz syndrome
hardening of arteries
hard metal disease
hard, pitting edema
hardware disease
Harkavy syndrome
Harken auricle clamp
Harken prosthetic valve
Harken rib spreader
Harley paroxysmal hemoglobinuria
Harmonic Scalpel
harmonious aortic root
Harrell Y stent
Harrington-Mayo thoracic scissors

Harrington-Mixter thoracic forceps
Harrington retractor
Harrington thoracic forceps
Harrison groove
Harris syndrome
harsh cough
harsh friction rub
harsh murmur
harsh systolic murmur
Hartmann hemostatic mosquito
    forceps (straight/curved)
Hartzler ACX-II or RX-014 balloon
    catheter
Hartzler angioplasty balloon
Hartzler LPS dilatation catheter
Hartzler Micro II balloon
Hartzler Micro XT dilatation catheter
Hartzler rib retractor
Harvard ventilator
harvest a vein
harvest of donor organs for
    transplantation
harvested vein
harvester lung
harvesting, vein
harvesting vein, tissue, or organ from
    donor for transplantation
Hatle method to calculate mitral valve
    area
Hattler respiratory support catheter
    (artificial lung device)
Hayem-Widal acquired hemolytic
    anemia
Hayem-Widal syndrome
Hayes Martin forceps
hay fever
Haynes 25 material for prosthetic
    valve construction
haze
    hilar
    perihilar edema
HBE (His bundle electrogram)

HBO (hyperbaric oxygen)
HBP (high blood pressure)
HC or HCM (hypertrophic cardio–
    myopathy)
HCT or Hct (hematocrit)
HCTZ (hydrochlorothiazide)
HCVD (hypertensive cardiovascular
    disease)
H-DCSA (His bundle-distal coronary
    sinus atrial) depolarization
HDI 1000 ultrasound system
HDL (high-density lipoproteins)
HDM (house dust mites)
HDM bronchial provocation test
HDM challenge
headache after cocaine use
head-down tilt test
headhunter catheter
head-up tilt test
healing infarct
Healthdyne apnea monitor
Heart Failure Knowledge Test
Health Failure Self-Care Behavior
    Scale, revised
HealthShield antimicrobial mediastinal
    wound drainage catheter
heart
    abdominal
    air-driven artificial
    Akutsu total artificial
    alcoholic
    ALVAD (intra-abdominal left
        ventricular assist device)
    artificial
    angiosarcoma of
    armored
    artificial
    athlete's
    athletic
    axis of
    balloon-shaped
    Baylor total artificial

heart *(cont.)*
  beer
  beriberi
  boat-shaped
  bony
  booster
  boot-shaped (on x-ray)
  bovine
  bread-and-butter
  bulb of
  cardiogenic shock
  cervical
  chaotic
  conical
  crisscross
  dome-shaped
  donor
  drop
  dynamite
  electrical axis of
  electromechanical artificial
  electromechanically quiescent
  elongated
  empty
  encased
  enlarged
  extracorporeal
  extracorporeal artificial
  failing
  fat
  fatty
  fibroid
  fibroma of
  flabby
  flask-shaped
  frosted (frosting; icing)
  globoid
  hairy
  hanging (suspended)
  holiday
  Holmes
  horizontal

heart *(cont.)*
  hyperdynamic
  hyperkinetic
  hyperthyroid
  hypertrophied
  hypoplastic
  hypoplastic left
  hypothermic
  icing (frosting)
  intermediate
  intracorporeal artificial
  irritable
  ischemic
  Jarvik 7 or 8 artificial
  Jarvik 7-70 artificial
  left (atrium and ventricle)
  Liotta total artificial (TAH)
  luxus
  lymphosarcoma of
  malposition of the
  massively enlarged
  mean electrical axis of
  mechanical
  mildly enlarged
  movable
  myxedema
  myxoma of
  nervous
  nonshocked
  normothermic fibrillating
  nutrition
  one-ventricle
  orthotopic biventricular artificial
  orthotopic univentricular artificial
  ovoid
  ox
  paracorporeal
  parchment
  pear-shaped
  pectoral
  pendulous
  Penn State total artificial

heart *(cont.)*
    permanent artificial
    Phoenix total artificial
    pulmonary
    Quain fatty
    recipient
    resting
    rhabdomyoma of
    right (atrium and ventricle)
    round
    sabot
    semihorizontal
    semivertical
    single-outlet
    skin (peripheral blood vessels)
    snowman (on x-ray)
    soft
    soldier's
    spastic
    stiff
    stone
    superoinferior
    suspended
    Symbion J-7 70 mL total artificial
    Symbion Jarvik-7 artificial
    systemic
    tabby cat
    teardrop
    temporary artificial
    three-chambered
    thrush breast
    tiger
    tiger lily
    tobacco
    total artificial (TAH)
    transplanted
    transverse
    Traube
    triatrial
    trilocular
    univentricular
    University of Akron artificial

heart *(cont.)*
    upstairs-downstairs
    Utah artificial
    Utah TAH (total artificial heart)
    venous
    venting of
    vertical
    wandering
    water-bottle
    wooden shoe
Heart Aid 80 defibrillator
heart and great vessels
heart and hand syndrome
heart and lung transplantation
heart apex
heart assist system
heart attack (myocardial infarction)
HeartBar Orange Drink dietary
    supplement
heartbeat (see also *beat*)
    coupling
    dropped
    fascicular
    fluttering
    forceful
    irregular
    irregularly irregular
    pounding
    racing
    rapid
    regular
    regularly irregular
    skipping
heart block (see *block*)
    atrioventricular
    bifascicular
    bundle branch
    complete
    complete atrioventricular
    complete congenital
    congenital
    deceleration-dependent

heart *(cont.)*
   diffuse
   entrance
   exit
   first-degree atrioventricular (AV)
   incomplete atrioventricular (AV)
   intraventricular
   Mobitz type I
   Mobitz type II
   myofibrillar intraventricular
   peri-infarction
   secondary atrioventricular
   sinoatrial
   sinoauricular
   surgically induced complete
   trifascicular
   2:1 atrioventricular
   Wenckebach's incomplete
     atrioventricular (AV)
heartburn (pyrosis; water brash)
heartburn type of pain
HeartCard
heart catheterization (see *catheterization*)
heart contraction
   isometric
   isotonic
heart decortication
heart disease
   amyloid
   atherosclerotic
   cyanotic congenital
   neonatal
   nutritional
heart failure
   acute
   backward
   chronic
   compensated congestive
   congestive
   decompensated congestive
   diastolic

heart *(cont.)*
   donor
   fetal
   forward
   Framingham criteria for
   high-output
   intrauterine
   left-sided
   low-output
   refractory
   right-sided
   systolic
heart failure cells
heart failure from thiamine deficiency
heart forward failure
heart-hand II syndrome
HeartHope coronary artery bypass
   graft
HeartHope vascular graft
HeartHope ventricular assist device
heart in sinus rhythm
Heart Laser for TMR (transmyocardial
   revascularization)
heart-lung bloc
heart-lung machine
   Cobe-Stockert
   Crafoord-Senning
   Cobe CPS
   Mayo-Gibbon
   Sarns 5000 Console
   Sarns 7000 MDX
   Sarns 9000
   Sorin
heart-lung transplant (transplantation)
heart massage
HeartMate air-driven implantable left
   ventricular assist system (LVAS)
HeartMate battery-operated portable
   system
HeartMate implantable left ventricular
   assist device (LVAD)

HeartMate implantable ventricular assist device
HeartMate vented electric LVAS (left ventricular assist system)
heart murmur (see *murmur*)
heart overload
Heartport Endoclamp aortic catheter
Heartport Port-Access system
heart power failure
heart prosthesis
heart pump (see *pump*)
HeartQuest device
heart rate (see also *monitor*; *rate*)
   intrinsic
   maximum predicted
   natural
   percent of predicted maximum
   resting
   slowing of
   target
heart rate reserve mechanism
heart rate response
heart rhythm, dual
heart remnant
heart sac
HeartSaver VAD (ventricular assist system)
Heartscan heart attack prediction test
heart-shaped baffle
heart sound (see *sound*)
heart stabilization device, acrobat
Heartstream ForeRunner automatic external defibrillator
Heartstring proximal seal system
heart tamponade
heart tones (sounds)
heart transplant or transplantation
   heterotopic
   orthotopic
heart transplant rejection
heart valve (see *valve*; *prosthesis*)
HeartView CT cardiac imaging

heart wall at risk for injury from infarction
heartwire, bipolar temporary
heat-expandable stent
heated humidified oxygen
Heath-Edwards classification of pulmonary vascular disease
Heath-Edwards criteria
heating, nonablative
heat intolerance
heave
   left lower parasternal
   parasternal
   substernal
   sustained left ventricular
heave and lift
heaviness, chest
heaving of chest wall
heaving precordial motion
heavy chain, myosin
heavy steel wires
Heberden angina pectoris disease
Heberden sign
Heberden syndrome
Heckathorn disease
Heckathorn factor VIII deficiency
hectic flush
heelstick hematocrit in neonates
Hegar dilator
Hegglin syndrome
Heifitz clip
Heim-Kreysig sign
Heimlich tube
Heineke-Mikulicz maneuver
Heineke-Mikulicz procedure
Heinz body
Heiss artery forceps
helical coil stent
helical-tip Halo catheter
Helios diagnostic imaging system
Helisal rapid blood test
helium-filled balloon catheter

Helistat absorbable collagen hemostatic sponge
Helitene absorbable collagen
hemostatic agent
Heller-Döhle (Doehle)
Heller-Döhle syphilitic aortitis disease
Heller esophagocardiomyotomy
HELLP (hemolysis, elevated liver
enzymes, and low platelets)
syndrome
Helminthosporium
helplessness
Hemaflex PTCA sheath with obturator
Hemaflex sheath collagen
hemangioendothelioma, malignant
hemangiolymphangioma
hemangioma
bulky
cardiac
cavernous
deep
extremity
familial intracranial
fibrofatty
giant cavernous
intramuscular
lung
problematic
proliferative
proliferative phase
subcutaneous
verrucous
hemangioma-thrombocytopenia
syndrome
hemangiomatosis, pulmonary capillary
hemangioma with platelet trapping
hemangiopericytoma
Hemaquet catheter introducer
Hemaquet PTCA sheath with
obturator
Hemaquet sheath
Hemaquet sheath introducer

Hemaseel HMN biological tissue glue
Hemashield Gold branch graft
Hemashield Gold Microvel knitted
double velour graft
Hemashield graft
Hemashield Vantage vascular graft
Hemashield woven vascular graft
HemAssist artificial blood
HemaStrip-HIV 1/2 whole blood test
Hemasure r/LS red blood cell
filtration system
hematemesis
Hematest positive, trace
hematocrit (HCT)
dilutional
heelstick
Wintrobe
hematogenous dissemination from
lungs
hematogenous metastasis
hematogenous pulmonary involvement
hematoma
acute intramural
aneurysmal
dissecting aortic
infected
intramural
intrarenal
mural
pericardial
perirenal
pulsating
retroperitoneal
subcapsular
hematoma cap
azygos
left pleural apical
hematopoiesis
hematopoietic cells
hematoporphyrin derivative (HPD)
Hemex prosthetic valve
hemianesthesia

hemiarch
hemiaxial view (x-ray)
hemiazygos vein
hemiblock (left or right)
    anterior
    anterior-posterior
    bundle branch
    left anterior-superior (LASH)
    left posterior (LPH)
hemicardium
hemic calculus
hemicranial pain
hemidiaphragmatic paresis
hemidiaphragm, attenuation by
hemidiaphragm depression
hemi-Fontan operation
hemihypertrophy
hemilaryngectomy
hemi-Mustard pericardial baffle
hemiparesis
    contralateral
    ipsilateral
hemithorax (pl. hemithoraces)
hemithymectomy
hemitruncus
hemitruncus repair
hemoaccess
Hemobahn endovascular prosthesis
    (nitinol stent-graft)
Hemo-Cath catheter
Hemo-Cath dilator
Hemo-Cath guidewire
Hemo-Cath introducer needle
Hemo-Cath scalpel
hemochromatosis, idiopathic
Hemochron Response whole blood
    coagulation
hemoclip, Samuels
hemoconcentration
HemoCue photometer for hemoglobin
    determination
hemodialysis, continuous venovenous
    (CVVHD)

hemodilution, intentional transopera-
    tive
hemodynamically unstable
hemodynamically unstable ventricular
    tachycardia
hemodynamic abnormalities
hemodynamic assessment
hemodynamic changes
hemodynamic collapse
hemodynamic data
hemodynamic depression
hemodynamic dysfunction
hemodynamic effect
hemodynamic embarrassment
hemodynamic factors
hemodynamic findings
hemodynamic format
hemodynamic impairment
hemodynamic instability
hemodynamic monitoring, continuous
hemodynamic overload
    acute
    chronic
hemodynamic pathogenesis of
    vascular-bone syndromes
hemodynamic pattern
hemodynamic picture
hemodynamic profile
hemodynamic results
hemodynamic significance
hemodynamic stress
hemodynamic support
hemodynamically significant findings
hemodynamically significant lesion
hemodynamically stable
hemodynamics, cardiovascular
hemofiltration
hemoglobin (Hb, Hgb)
    abnormal
    glycosylated
    low
    normal

hemoglobin *(cont.)*
    pyridoxalated stroma-free (SFHb)
      (also pyridoxylated)
    recombinant (rHb1.1)
    stroma free (SFHb)
hemoglobin A
hemoglobin and hematocrit (H&H)
hemoglobin C
hemoglobin C–thalassemia disease
hemoglobin electrophoresis
hemoglobin E–thalassemia disease
hemoglobinopathy (pl. hemoglobin-
    opathies)
hemoglobin S (sickle hemoglobin)
Hemolink red blood cell substitute
hemolysis
hemolytic anemia
hemolytic disease of the newborn
    (HDN)
Hemopad absorbable collagen
hemoperfusion
hemopericardium
hemophilia
    classical
    vascular
hemophilia A (factor VIII deficiency)
hemophilia B (factor IX deficiency)
Hemophilus (see *Haemophilus*)
hemopleuropneumonia syndrome
hemopneumothorax
hemoptysis
Hemopump, Nimbus
Hemopure (hemoglobin glutamer-250)
hemorrhage
    anastomotic
    arterial
    capillary
    chronic parenchymal
    diffuse subarachnoid
    Duret
    exsanguinating (into pleural space)
    external

hemorrhage *(cont.)*
    extrapleural
    familial intracranial
    focal endocardial
    frank
    internal
    intracranial
    intramural arterial
    intraplaque (IPH)
    intrapleural
    intrapulmonary
    intraventricular (IVH)
    life-threatening
    massive exsanguinating
    meningeal
    nontraumatic epidural
    parenchymal
    peribronchiolar
    postoperative mediastinal
    pulmonary
    salmon-patch
    splinter
    subarachnoid (SAH)
    venous
hemorrhage in plaque
hemorrhage into atheromatous plaque
hemorrhage per rhexin
hemorrhagic bronchitis
hemorrhagic bronchopneumonia
hemorrhagic consolidation
hemorrhagic diathesis
hemorrhagic disease of the newborn
hemorrhagic disorder
hemorrhagic duodenitis
hemorrhagic fluid
hemorrhagic gastritis
hemorrhagic pericarditis
hemorrhagic pleurisy
hemorrhagic shock
hemorrhagic telangiectasia, hereditary
hemorrhagic zone, pyramidal
hemosiderin deposit

hemosiderin, phagocytized
hemosiderosis
   idiopathic pulmonary
   pulmonary idiopathic
   transfusional
Hemosonic hemodynamic monitor and
   probe
Hemosplit catheter
hemostasis was achieved
hemostat (see also *forceps; hemostatic*
   material or sponge)
   Crile
   Kelly
   Kocher
   Mayo
   mosquito
   Woodward
hemostatic material or sponge (see
   also *collagen*; *hemostat*;
   medications)
   Avitene topical
   collagen hemostatic
   Collastat
   Endo-Avitene
   4% succinylated gelatin
   Gelofusine
   Glycoprene
   Haemaccel
   Helistat absorbable collagen
   Helitene absorbable
   Hemopad absorbable collagen
   Hemotene absorbable collagen
   Instat MCH collagen absorbable
   microfibrillar
   polygeline colloid
   polygeline gelatin sponge
   SuperStat
   Surgical Nu-Knit
   Tissucol fibrin-collagen
Hemo-Stream dialysis catheter
Hemo-Stream vascular catheter
Hemotene absorbable collagen

hemothorax
Henle-Coenen test
Henle elastic membrane
Henle fenestrated membrane
Henle loop
Henle membrane
Henley dilator
Henley vascular clamp
Henoch-Schönlein purpura
Hepacoat coating for medical devices
Hepamed-coated Wiktor stent
heparin
   low-dose
   neutralize the effects of
heparin administration
heparin anticoagulation, systemic
heparin anticoagulation therapy
heparinization
   adequate
   post-PTCA
   systemic
   total body
heparinized blood
heparinized saline flush
heparinized saline solution
heparin lock for administering
   medication
heparin lock introducer
heparin neutralized thrombin time
   (HNTT)
heparin neutralized with protamine
   sulfate
heparinoid compound
heparin rebound
heparin not reversed
heparin reversed with protamine
hepatic arterial-dominant phase (HAP)
   images (CT scan)
hepatic arteriovenous fistula
hepatic congestion
hepatic necrosis
hepatic vein pulsation

hepatic vein thrombosis
hepatic veno-occlusive disease
hepatization
　gray
　red
hepatoclavicular view
hepatojugular reflux
hepatomegaly, pulsating
hepatopleural fistula
hepatorenal bypass graft
hepatorenal saphenous vein bypass
　graft
Hep-Lock (heparin sodium)
Hep-Lock PF (heparin sodium)
Hep-Lock U/P (heparin sodium)
Heprotec vascular filter
Heprotec vascular guidewire
Herbst appliance, removable
Herbst corpuscles
Hercules power injector
hereditary angioedema
hereditary angioneurotic edema
　(HANE)
hereditary capillary fragility
hereditary hemolytic anemia
hereditary hemorrhagic diathesis
hereditary hemorrhagic telangiectasia
hereditary lymphedema
hereditary ovalocytosis
hereditary pseudohemophilia
hereditary sideroblastic anemia
hereditary spherocytosis
Hering-Breuer inverted oculocardiac
　reflex
Hering, nerve of
Hering phenomenon
hermetically sealed standby pacemaker
hernia
　diaphragmatic
　inguinal
　intrapericardial diaphragmatic
　mediastinal
　umbilical

Hershey left ventricular assist device
Hespan (hetastarch) plasma volume
　expander
Hess capillary test
hetastarch (Hespan)
heterogeneity, temporal
heterogeneous appearance
heterograft (see also *graft*)
　bovine
　porcine
　xenograft
heterologous graft
heterologous surfactant
heterophile antibodies
heterotaxy
　abdominal
　visceral
heterotaxy syndrome
heterotopic heart transplantation
Hetzel forward triangle method for
　cardiac output
Heubner disease
Hewlett-Packard color flow imager
Hewlett-Packard defibrillator
Hewlett-Packard transducer
Hewlett-Packard ultrasound unit
Hexabrix (ioxaglate meglumine;
　ioxaglate sodium)
hexaxial reference system
HFD40 (duration of terminal QRS
　high frequency signal)
HFJV (high-frequency jet ventilation)
HFLA duration
HFOV (high-frequency oscillating
　ventilator)
HFQRSD (duration of high frequency
　QRS)
HFRMS (voltage of terminal QRS
　high frequency signal)
HFV (high-frequency ventilation)
Hgb (hemoglobin)
HHD (hypertensive heart disease)

HH' interval
HHN (handheld nebulizer)
hiatus, tendinous
hibernation, myocardial
Hickman indwelling right atrial
  catheter
Hidalgo catheter
Hiebert vascular dilator
Hieshima Taper Select catheter
high-altitude pulmonary edema
  (HAPE)
high-amplitude impulse
high arched palate
high blood pressure (HBP)
high defect in atrial septum
high-density lipoprotein (HDL)
high-dose hypofractionated IGRT
high-dose thrombin time (HiTT)
high-fidelity pressure transducer
high filling pressure
high-flow, low-resistance pattern
high-flow oxygen
high-fluid shear stresses
high-frequency nebulizer
high-frequency jet ventilation (HFJV)
high-frequency oscillating ventilator
  (HFOV)
high-frequency ventilation (HFV)
high-grade lesion
high-grade obstructive lesion
high-grade stenosis
high interstitial pressure
high lateral wall myocardial infarction
high left main diagonal artery
high ligation of varicose veins
high-low (see *Hi-Lo*)
high minute ventilation
high-osmolar imaging agent
high-output circulatory failure
high-output heart failure
high pacing thresholds
High Performance Detach embolization coil

High Performance Detach guidewire
high-pitched ejection murmur
high-pitched opening snap
high-pitched rhonchi
high-pitched signal
high-power field
high-rate detect interval
high-rate pacing
high-rate ventricular response, atrial
  fibrillation with
high reflectivity
high-resolution computed tomography
  scan
high-resolution computed tomography
high-resolution magnification
high-resolution storage phosphor
  managing
high right atrium
high right atrium electrode
high risk for cardiovascular disease
high-risk situation
high shear blood flow
high-speed bur
high-speed rotational atherectomy
  (RA)
high-speed rotation dynamic
  angioplasty catheter
high take-off of left coronary artery
high torque (see *Hi-Torque*)
high-velocity jet
high-voltage pulsed galvanic
  stimulator
hila (plural of *hilum*)
hilar adenopathy
hilar area
hilar artery
hilar haze
hilar lymphadenopathy
hilar lymph node enlargement
hilar mass
hilar prominence
hilar shadows (on x-ray)

Hill sign
Hi-Lo Jet tracheal tube
hilum (pl. *hila*)
hilum of lung
hilus (hilum)
hilus tuberculosis
Himmelstein sternal retractor
Himmelstein valvulotome
Hines and Brown test
H. influenzae organism
hip claudication
Hi-Per cardiac device
Hi-Per Flex guidewire
Hippel-Lindau syndrome
hippocratic sound
hirudin (recombinant)
His bundle ablation
His bundle deflection
His bundle electrogram, electrography
    (HBE)
His, bundle of
Hislop-Reid syndrome
His-Purkinje conducting system
His-Purkinje system (HPS)
His-Purkinje system fibrosis
histamine acid phosphatase
histamine challenge
histamine concentration
histamine control
histamine flush
histamine receptors
His-Tawara atrioventricular bundle
His-Tawara atrioventricular node
histiocytoid cardiomyopathy
histiocytosis X
histocompatibility antigen
histogram, plasma
histologic examination
histomorphometric analysis of biopsy
    specimen
Histoplasma myocarditis
histoplasmosis

histoplasmotic endocarditis
history
    antecedent
    family
    pack-a-day smoking
    pack-year smoking
    remote
    salient
Hi-Torque Flex-T guidewire
Hi-Torque Floppy (HTF) guidewire
Hi-Torque Intermediate guidewire
Hi-Torque Standard guidewire
HiTT (high-dose thrombin time)
HIV (human immunodeficiency virus)
HIV infection
HK-Cardiosol organ preservation
    solution
HLA-B27 antigen
HLA-DR (histocompatibility antigen-
    DR) marker protein
HLA typing
HLHS (hypoplastic left heart
    syndrome)
HLP (hyperlipoproteinemia)
H-MCSA (His bundle-middle coro-
    nary sinus atrial) depolarization
HMG CoA reductase inhibitor
H-mode echocardiography
HNTT (heparin neutralized thrombin
    time)
HOC or HOCM (hypertrophic
    obstructive cardiomyopathy)
hockey-stick appearance of catheter tip
hockey-stick deformity of cusp (on
    echocardiogram)
hockey-stick deformity of tricuspid
    valve
hockey-stick incision, midline
Hodgkin disease
Hodgkin-Key murmur
Hodgson aneurysmal dilatation of the
    aorta

Hodgson aortic disease
Hodgson disease
Hoen nerve hook
Hohn central venous catheter
  double-lumen
  single-lumen
Hohn vessel dilator
holder
  needle
  prosthetic valve
  valve
  wire needle
Holger-Nielsen artificial respirations
holiday heart syndrome
Holinger dissector
hollow chest syndrome
hollow cough
hollow tunneler
Holmes heart
Holmes syndrome
holmium laser
holmium yttrium aluminum garnet
  (Ho:YAG) laser
holmium:YAG laser for angioplasty
holoprosencephaly, alobar
holosystolic mitral valve prolapse
holosystolic murmur
Holter monitor
Holter monitoring, continuous
Holter shunt
Holter tubing
Holter valve
Holt-Oram atriodigital dysplasia
Holt-Oram syndrome
Holzknecht space
Homans sign
Hombach lead placement system
home ambulatory inotropic therapy
HomeTrak Plus compact cardiac event
  recorder
HomMed Monitoring System
homoartery

homocystinuria, congenital
homocystinuria syndrome
homogeneity
homogeneous appearance
homogeneous echo
homogeneous material
homogeneous perfusion
homogeneous thallium distribution
homograft
  cryopreserved
  denatured
  freehand aortic valve
  mitral valve
homograft conduit
homograft reaction
homograft root replacement
homologous blood transfusion
homonymous hemianopia
homotransplantation
honeycomb formation
honeycombing (cysts), fibrotic
honeycomb lung
honk
  late systolic
  precordial
honking murmur
hood forceps
hooding, interchordal
hood of graft
hood punch
hook
  Adson
  fishhook
  Hoen nerve
  Krayenbuehl vessel
  nerve
  Selverstone cardiotomy
  Smithwick
  tracheal
  valve
hook scissors
hook wire localization, CT-directed

Hoover sign
hopelessness
Hope murmur
Hope sign
Hopkins aortic clamp
Hopkins forceps
Horizon AutoAdjust CPAP system
horizontal axis
horizontal chin cleft
horizontal fissure of lung
horizontal long-axis slice
horizontal mattress suture
horizontal plane loop
horizontal ST segment depression
hormone
    adrenocorticotropic
    antidiuretic
    somatotropin-releasing
Horner syndrome
horseshoe configuration on thallium
    imaging
horseshoe-shaped syncytium
horseshoe tubular graft
Horton disease
Horton giant cell arteritis
hose, support (see *stockings*)
hostile neck
host, nonimmunocompromised
hot spots (on technetium pyrophos-
    phate scan)
hourglass deformity
hourglass-shaped lesion
house dust mite
housing and pusher plate
Howell coronary scissors
Howell-Jolly body
Howell test for hemoglobin
Ho:YAG (holmium yttrium aluminum
    garnet) laser
HPD (hematoporphyrin derivative)
H-PCSA (His bundle-proximal coro-
    nary sinus atrial depolarization)

h peak of jugular venous pulse
H'P interval
h plateau of jugular venous pulse
HPS (His-Purkinje system)
HP (Hewlett-Packard) SONOS 5500
    ultrasound imaging system
HPV (human papillomavirus)
H-Q interval
H-QRS interval
HR (heart rate) (beats/min)
HRA (high right atrium)
HRF (hypercapnic respiratory failure)
H spike and H' spike
HTN or Htn (hypertension)
hub of balloon lumen
hub of needle
Huchard continued arterial
    hypertension
Huchard disease
Huchard essential hypertension
Huchard sign
hue, violaceous
Hufnagel aortic clamp
Hufnagel prosthetic valve
Hughes-Stovin syndrome
hum
    buzzing venous
    cervical venous
    venous
human albumin microspheres
human amniotic fluid derived
    surfactant
human fibroblast growth factor-I
    (FGF-I)
human immunodeficiency virus (HIV)
human leukocyte antigen B27
human papillomavirus (HPV)
Humby excisional knife
HumidAire heated humidifier
humidifier lung
humming rhonchi
humoral response

hump, Hampton
hunger, air
Hunter canal
Hunter operation for correction of
    aneurysm
Hunter-Sessions balloon
Hunter-Sessions inferior vena cava
    balloon occluder
Hunter syndrome
Hunter tendon rod insertion for deep
    venous insufficiency (DVI)
Hurler-Scheie syndrome
Hurler syndrome
Hürthle cell tumor
Hurwitz thoracic trocar
Hutchinson-Gilford progeria syndrome
Hutinel disease
Hutinel-Pick syndrome
HUV (human umbilical vein) bypass
    graft
H-V (His-ventricular) interval
HV-1 patch lead
h wave of jugular venous pulse
H waves
Hx (history)
hyalin nodules
hyaline cartilage
hyaline change
hyaline degeneration
hyaline membrane disease
hyaline necrosis
hyaline thrombi
hyalinization
    arteriolar
    subendothelial
hyaluronidase
hybrid open-endoluminal technique
hydatid cysts
hydatid disease
    alveolar
    unilocular

hydatidosis
HydraCross TLC catheter
hydrate, hydrated
hydration
hydrochlorothiazide (HCTZ)
Hydrocoil XT vascular embolization
    device
hydrocyanic acid release
Hydrofiber wound packing material
hydrogen density
Hydro-Glide coating for guidewires
Hydrolyser microcatheter
hydropericardium
hydrophilic guidewire
hydropic degeneration
HydroPlus coating material for stent
hydropneumothorax
hydrops
    nonimmune fetal
    nonimmunologic fetal
hydrops fetalis (fetal hydrops)
hydrostatic pressure of the blood
hydrothorax
hydroxyl radical
hydroxylase deficiency
hydroxyurea
Hypaque Meglumine 60%
    (diatrizoate meglumine 60%)
Hypaque-76 (diatrizoate meglumine
    66% and diatrizoate sodium 10%)
Hypaque Sodium 50% (diatrizoate
    meglumine 50%)
hyparterial bronchi
hyperabduction maneuver
hyperactive carotid sinus reflex
hyperactive sympathetic tone
hyperacute rejection (HAR)
hyperadrenergic orthostatic
    hypotension
hyperaeration, cystlike foci of

hyperaldosteronism
  glucocorticoid-remediable
  idiopathic
  indeterminate
hyperalphalipoproteinemia
hyperamylasemia
hyperbaric chamber
hyperbaric oxygen
hyperbasemia
hyperbetalipoproteinemia, familial
hyperbilirubinemia
hypercalcemia-supravalvular aortic
  stenosis
hypercalcemic face
hypercapnia
  progressive
  well-compensated
hypercapnic acute asthma
hypercapnic respiratory failure (HRF)
hypercarbia (hypercapnia)
hypercholesterolemia
  familial
  polygenic
hyperchylomicronemia, familial
hypercoagulability
hypercoagulable state
hypercyanotic angina
hypercyanotic episode
hypercyanotic spell
hyperdynamic apical impulse
hyperdynamic AV fistulae
hyperdynamic heart syndrome
hyperdynamic impulse
hyperdynamic PMI
hyperdynamic right ventricular
  impulse
hyperdynamic state
hyperechoicity
hyperemia
  active
  arterial
  collateral
  diffuse

hyperemia *(cont.)*
  fluxionary
  passive
  reactive
  venous
hyperemia of mucous membranes
hypereosinophilic syndrome, idiopathic
hyperestrogenemia
hyperextensibility
hyperextension of neck
Hyperflex guidewire
Hyperflex steerable wire
hyperfunction, adrenal gland
hypergammaglobulinemia
hyperhidrosis
hyperimmunoglobulinemia E
  syndrome
hyperinflation, dynamic pulmonary
hyperinsulinemia
hyperintense
hyperkalemia
hyperkalemic crystalloid cardioplegic
  solution for heart-lung machine
hyperkinesia, compensatory
hyperkinetic circulation
hyperkinetic heart disease
hyperkinetic heart syndrome
hyperkinetic hypertension
hyperkinetic PMI (point of maximal
  impulse)
hyperkinetic segmental wall motion
hyperlipidemia
  carbohydrate-inducible
  combined
  familial
  familial combined
  mixed
  multiple lipoprotein-type
  remnant
hyperlipoproteinemia (HLP), Fredrickson and Lees classification of
  (type I-V)
hyperlucency

hyperlucent lung
hyperlucent lung syndrome
hypermagnesemia
hypernephroma, metastatic to heart
hyperosmotic solution
hyperostosis associated with venous
  malformation
hyperoxaluria
hyperoxia
hyperparathyroidism, primary
hyperpermeability, capillary
hyperpiesia
hyperpiesis
  adrenocortical
  arterial fibromuscular
  congenital adrenal
  congenital segmental renal
  fibrous
  intimal
  medial
  neointimal
hyperplasia
  adenomatous
  adrenal, congenital
  adrenocortical
  arterial fibromuscular
  atypical adenomatous (AAH)
  congenital adrenal
  congenital segmental renal
  fibrous
  intimal
  medial
  multicentric angiofollicular
    (MAFH)
  neointimal
  plantar
hyperplastic lesion
hyperpnea
  paroxysmal
  unloaded
hyperreactivity to isocyanate vapor
hyperreninemia

hyperresonance
hyperresonant percussion note
hyperresponsiveness
  airway
  allergen-induced bronchial
  persistent bronchial
hypersecretion
  ACTH
  mucus
hypersensitive carotid sinus syndrome
hypersensitive xiphoid syndrome
hypersensitivity angiitis
hypersensitivity
  carotid sinus (CSH)
  paraaminosalicylic acid
hypersensitivity pneumonia
hypersensitivity pneumonitis
hypersensitivity reaction
hypersensitivity vasculitis
hypertelorism-hypospadias syndrome
hypertension (HTN, Htn)
  accelerated
  acquired
  adrenal
  aortic coarctation-related
  arterial (AHT)
  Baumgarten portal
  benign
  borderline
  chronic thromboembolic
  chronic thromboembolic pulmonary
  complicated
  continued arterial
  disproportionate femoral systolic
  endolymphatic
  essential
  familial pulmonary
  glucocorticoid-induced
  Goldblatt
  Huchard essential
  hyperkinetic
  hypoxic pulmonary

hypertension *(cont.)*
  idiopathic
  intermittent
  intracranial
  labile
  long-standing
  low-renin
  low-renin essential
  malignant
  mineralocorticoid-induced
  obesity-related
  occult
  oral contraceptive-induced
  pale
  paroxysmal
  poorly controlled
  portal
  posterior fossa
  precapillary pulmonary
  pregnancy-induced
  pregnancy-related
  primary
  primary pulmonary (PPH)
  profound
  proximal
  pulmonary (PHTN)
  pulmonary arterial
  pulmonary thromboembolic
  pulmonary venous
  red
  refractory
  renal
  renin-dependent
  renovascular
  secondary
  surgically curable
  sustained
  symptomatic
  systemic
  systemic venous
  systolic

hypertension *(cont.)*
  thromboembolic pulmonary
  untreated
  vascular
  venous
  volume-dependent
  white-coat (fear of doctors)
hypertension exacerbated by dialysis
hypertension secondary to excessive
  licorice ingestion
hypertension variant, Baumgarten
  portal
hypertensive cardiomegaly
hypertensive cardiopathy
hypertensive cardiovascular disease
  (HCVD)
hypertensive crisis
hypertensive diathesis
hypertensive emergency
hypertensive encephalopathy
hypertensive heart disease
hypertensive ischemic ulcer
hypertensive left ventricular
  hypertrophy
hypertensive paroxysmal crisis
hypertensive renal disease
hypertensive retinopathy
hypertensive vascular degeneration
hypertensive vascular disease
hyperthyroidism
hyperthyroidism-induced atrial
  fibrillation
hypertonic airways
hypertonic saline challenge
hypertonicity
hypertrichosis of skin
hypertriglyceridemia
  carbohydrate-induced
  endogenous
  familial
  sporadic

hypertrophic cardiomyopathy (HC)
hypertrophic obstructive cardio-
    myopathy (HOC or HOCM)
hypertrophic pulmonary osteo-
    arthropathy
hypertrophic rhinitis
hypertrophic subaortic stenosis
hypertrophied arterioles
hypertrophied heart
hypertrophied intima
hypertrophied myocardium
hypertrophy
    adaptive
    asymmetric septal (ASH)
    biatrial
    biventricular
    cardiac
    concentric left ventricular
    eccentric
    eccentric left ventricular
    four-chamber
    hypertrophic
    left atrial
    left ventricular (LVH)
    lipomatous (of the interatrial
        septum)
    myocardial cellular
    panchamber
    right atrial
    right ventricular (RVH)
    scalenus anticus muscle
    type A (B or C) right ventricular
    unilateral
    ventricular
    Wigle scale for ventricular
hypertrophy of bone
hypertrophy of cardiac muscle fibers
hypertrophy of muscle
hypertrophy of myocardium
hyperuricemia
hypervagotonia

hypervascular arterialization
hyperventilation
    coughing
    eucapnic voluntary
    psychophysiologic
hypervolemia
hyphae
hypoadrenergic orthostatic hypotension
hypoaeration
hypoalbuminemia
hypoaldosteronism, hyporeninemic
hypobarism-acute mountain sickness
hypobasemia
hypocalcemia
hypocapnia
hypocapnic
hypocarbia (hypocapnia)
    alveolar
    arterial
hypochromic anemia
hypochromic microcytic anemia
hypocontractile
hypocontractility
hypoechogenic
hypoechoic layer
hypoechoic mantle
hypofunction, adrenal gland
hypogastric artery
hypogastric system
hypogenetic lung syndrome
hypoglossus
hypoglycemia
hypointense
hypokalemia, iatrogenic
hypokalemia-induced arrhythmia
hypokinesia, hypokinesis
    apical
    cardiac
    diffuse
    diffuse ventricular
    global

hypokinesia *(cont.)*
  hypokinetic
  inferior wall
  regional
  septal
hypokinetic left ventricle
hypokinetic segmental wall motion
hypolucency of lung
hypomagnesemia
hyponatremia
  dilutional
  essential
hypo-osmolality, cellular
hypoparathyroidism
hypoperfusion
  acute alveolar
  apical
  global cerebral
  peripheral
  pulmonary
  resting regional myocardial
  septal
  systemic
hypopharynx
hypophosphatemia
hypoplasia
  alveolar
  anular
  aortic arch
  aortic tract complex
  arterial
  ascending aorta
  congenital isolated
  deep venous
  diffuse
  left ventricle
  left ventricular
  pulmonary artery
  right ventricular
  transverse aortic arch
  ventricular
hypoplasia of aortic anulus

hypoplasia of aortic isthmus
hypoplasia of artery
hypoplasia of vein
hypoplastic aorta syndrome
hypoplastic aortic arch
hypoplastic emphysema
hypoplastic heart
hypoplastic heart ventricle
hypoplastic horizontal ribs
hypoplastic left (or left-sided) heart
  syndrome (HLHS)
hypoplastic left ventricle syndrome
hypoplastic right heart
hypoplastic subpulmonic outflow
hypoplastic tricuspid orifice
hypoplastic valve
hypopnea, obstructive
hypopotassemia
hypoproteinemia
hypoprothrombinemia
hyporeninemic hypoaldosteronism
hyporeninism
hyposensitive carotid sinus syndrome
hyposensitization
hypostatic bronchopneumonia
hypostatic congestion
hypostatic pneumonia
hypostatic pulmonary insufficiency
hypotension
  chronic orthostatic
  drug-induced orthostatic
  exercise-induced
  exertional
  hyperadrenergic orthostatic
  hypoadrenergic orthostatic
  idiopathic orthostatic
  orthostatic
  orthostatic primary
  permanent idiopathic
  postural
  stress-induced
  sympathicotonic orthostatic
  vascular

hypotension unresponsive to volume
   administration
hypotensive response to saralasin
hypothermia
   deep
   endogenous
   local
   mild whole body
   moderate whole body
   myocardial
   profound
   surface-induced deep
   systemic and topical
   topical
   total body
hypothermia blanket
hypothermic arrest
hypothermic cardioplegic arrest
hypothermic cardiopulmonary bypass
hypothermic circulatory arrest,
   profound (PHCA)
hypothermic fibrillating heart
hypothermic perfusion
hypothermic, profoundly
hypothyroidism
hypotonicity
hypotonic syndrome
hypoventilation
   alveolar
   central
   congenital central
   idiopathic
   primary alveolar

hypovolemia
hypovolemic shock
hypoxanthine
hypoxemia
   arterial
   episodic
   refractory
hypoxemia at rest
hypoxemic respiratory failure
hypoxemic spell
hypoxia
   arterial
   cerebral
   chronic
   myocardial
   relative
hypoxia-ischemia
hypoxia without acidosis
hypoxic apnea
hypoxic drive
hypoxic-hypercapnic gas
hypoxic pulmonary hypertension
hypoxic pulmonary vasoconstriction
hypoxic spell
hysteresis
   AV (atrioventricular) delay
   (AVDH)
   rate
hysterical syncope
hystericus, globus

I, i

IAB (intra-aortic balloon) catheter
IABP (intra-aortic balloon pump)
IART (intra-atrial reentrant tachy-cardia)
IAS (interatrial septum)
iatrogenic avulsion
iatrogenic complications
iatrogenic hypokalemia
iatrogenic pseudoaneurysms
iatrogenic puncture
IAVB (incomplete atrioventricular block)
IAVD (incomplete atrioventricular dissociation)
ICA (internal carotid artery)
ICAM-1 (intercellular adhesions molecule-1) marker protein
ICCF (intermittent cross-clamp fibrillation)
ICD (internal cardioverter-defibrillator) inappropriate activation of tiered-therapy
ICD-ATP (implantable cardioverter-defibrillator/atrial tachycardia pacing) device
ICD data log
ICD interrogation, transtelephonic

ICE (intracardiac echocardiography)
I-cell disease
ice-pick view on M-mode echocardio-gram
ice, topical
ICEG or ICEGM (intracardiac electrogram)
ICEUS (intracaval endovascular ultra-sonography)
ICG-Pulsion cardiac output monitor
ICHD pacemaker code
ichorous pleurisy
ICRT (intracoronary radiation therapy), postangioplasty
ICS (intracellular-like, calcium-bearing crystalloid solution)
icteric sputum
ICU (intensive care unit)
ICUK (intracoronary urokinase)
ICUS (intracoronary ultrasound)
IDC (idiopathic dilated cardio-myopathy)
Ideal cardiac device
idiojunctional rhythm
idiopathic benign pericarditis
idiopathic bradycardia
idiopathic cardiomegaly

idiopathic cardiomyopathy
idiopathic dilated cardiomyopathy
idiopathic eosinophilic lung disease
idiopathic familial eosinophilia
idiopathic fibrosing alveolitis
idiopathic fibrosis, pulmonary
　interstitial
idiopathic hemochromatosis
idiopathic hyperaldosteronism (IHA)
idiopathic hypereosinophilic syndrome
idiopathic hypertrophic cardiomyopathy
idiopathic hypertrophic subaortic
　stenosis (IHSS)
idiopathic hypoventilation
idiopathic mural endomyocardial
　disease
idiopathic obstructive sleep apnea
idiopathic orthostatic hypotension
idiopathic pleural calcification
idiopathic pulmonary arteriosclerosis
　(IPA)
idiopathic pulmonary fibrosis
idiopathic pulmonary hemosiderosis
　(IPH)
idiopathic regressing arteriopathy
idiopathic respiratory distress
　syndrome (IRDS)
idiopathic restrictive cardiomyopathy
idiopathic thrombocytopenic purpura
idiopathic unilobar emphysema
idiopathic ventricular fibrillation
idiopathic ventricular tachycardia
idioventricular rhythm (IVR),
　accelerated
IDIS (intraoperative digital subtrac-
　tion) angiography system
IDL (intermediate density lipoprotein)
IDM (immediate diastolic murmur)
ID-OD, ID/OD (internal diameter-
　outside diameter) ratio
IDSA (intraoperative digital subtrac-
　tion angiography)

IEA (inferior epigastric artery) graft
I-E ("I to E") (inspiratory–expiratory)
　ratio
^{125}I (I 125) fibrinogen scan
IgE level
IGRT (image-guided radiotherapy),
　high-dose hypofractionated
Iguana guidewire
IHA (idiopathic hyperaldosteronism)
IHSS (idiopathic hypertrophic
　subaortic stenosis)
intra-atrial conduction delay
IJ (internal jugular) vein
IJV (internal jugular vein)
ILBBB (incomplete left bundle branch
　block)
iliac artery aneurysm
iliac artery angioplasty
iliac artery system
iliac atherosclerotic occlusive disease
iliac fossa
iliac-renal bypass graft
iliac stenosis, external
iliac vessel
iliocaval compression syndrome
iliocaval junction
iliocaval tree
iliofemoral bypass
iliofemoral thrombophlebitis
iliofemoral vein thrombosis
iliopopliteal bypass
ilioprofunda bypass graft
ill-defined chest pain
ill-defined mass
illness, flu-like
Illumen-8 guiding catheter
IMA (inferior mesenteric artery)
IMA (internal mammary artery)
IMA graft
IMA pedicle
IMA retractor

image, images (see also *imaging*)
    artifact
    attenuated
    bull's eye
    coronal
    cross-sectional
    delayed
    initial
    intermediate
    multi-echo
    sagittal
    silhouette
    tomographic
    T1-weighted
    T2-weighted
    transaxial
    ultrasonic tomographic
image-guided radiotherapy (IGRT)
image quality degradation
Imagent US (perflexane)
imaging (see also *image, scan*)
    Acuson computed sonography
    Advantx LC+ cardiovascular
    A-FAIR (arrhythmia-insensitive
        flow-sensitive alternating
        inversion recovery)
    Altaire open MR
    antifibrin antibody
    Biad SPECT
    cardiac blood pool
    cardiac scan
    CathScanner ultrasound
    C-11 (^{11}C) acetate
    Ceretec technetium 99m (^{99}m)
    chest tomograms
    color flow
    Convergent color Doppler
    CT-Linac (computed tomography
        with linear accelerator)
    CVIS
    digital vascular (DVI)
    dipyridamole thallium

imaging *(cont.)*
    DirectView CR 900
    Discovery LS
    dobutamine stress echocardiog-
        raphy (DSE)
    Doppler color flow
    Doppler tissue (DTI)
    duplex
    dynamic helical scan
    dynamic single photon emission
        tomography
    echo-contrast variability
    EchoEye 3-D ultrasound
    echo-planar
    ED (end-diastolic)
    electronic portal images (EPI)
    EnSite 3000
    exercise
    FluoroPlus Cardiac
    four-hour delayed thallium
    gallium scan
    gated blood-pool study (GBPS)
    gated cardiac blood pool
    gradient-echo sequence
    HeartView CT cardiac
    high-resolution computed
        tomography
    IGRT (image-guided radiotherapy)
    image-guided radiotherapy (IGRT)
    indium-111 (^{111}In) antimyosin
    infarct avid
    Isocam SPECT
    isotropic thin slice CT
    light reflection rheography
    linacography
    magnetic resonance (MRI)
    megavoltage x-rays
    moving-bed infusion-tracking MRA
        method for imaging
    multiple gated acquisition (MUGA)
        cardiac blood pool
    myocardial perfusion

imaging *(cont.)*
 MyoSight cardiology
 native tissue harmonic (NTHI)
 Nicolet Elite Doppler ultrasound
 PASTA (polarity-altered spectral
  selective acquisition)
 perfusion scintigraphy
 portal venous-dominant phase
  (PVP) images (CT scan)
 POSICAM medical
 postexercise
 pulse inversion harmonic
 radioisotope
 real-time
 redistribution myocardial
 redistribution thallium-201
 regional ejection fraction (REFI)
 rest
 rest myocardial perfusion
 rest thallium-201 myocardial
 Reveal XVI PET/CT
 rubidium-82
 resting
 sequential CT imaging
 sestamibi scan
 SieScape ultrasound
 SonoCT (real-time spatial
  compound imaging)
 steady-state projection imaging
  with dynamic echo-train readout
  (SPIDER)
 stress
 stress thallium-201 myocardial
 Subtraction Ictal SPECT Co-registered to MRI (SISCOM)
 Synthetic Aperture Focusing
  Technique (SAFT) in intravascular ultrasound imaging
 99mTc sestamibi
 technetium (Tc 99m) myocardial
 technetium (Tc 99m) pyrophosphate myocardial

imaging *(cont.)*
 thallium myocardial perfusion
 thallium-201 myocardial
 3DE (three-dimensional echocardiography)
 timed
 transesophageal Doppler color flow
 transesophageal echocardiography
  (TEE)
 transthoracic 3DE
 ultracardiography
 ultrafast
 venography
 VersaLab ultrasonic medical device
 Virtuoso portable three-dimensional
 VisCath fiberoptic
 VScore with AutoGate cardiac
 Xplorer digital radiography
imaging agent (see also *medications*)
 Adenoscan
 Albunex (sonicated human
  albumin)
 angio contrast
 Angiovist 370
 carbonated saline solution
 carbon-11 (^{11}C)
 carbon-11-labeled fatty acids
 carbon-11-labeled tracer
 carbon-11 palmitic acid radioactive
  tracer
 Cardio-Green (indocyanine green)
 Cardiolite (technetium Tc 99m
  sestamibi) (^{99m}Tc)
 CardioTec or Cardiotec teboroxime
  (technetium Tc 99m) (^{99m}Tc)
 CEA-Tc 99m
 Conray (iothalamate meglumine)
 Conray 30 (iothalamate meglumine
  30%)
 Conray 43 (iothalamate meglumine
  43%)
 Definity (perflutren)

imaging *(cont.)*
  depreotide
  diatrizoate meglumine
  diatrizoate sodium
  EchoGen (perflenapent;
    perflisopent)
  Echovist 200 (d-galactose)
  ^{18}FDG (fludeoxyglucose F 18)
  Fibrimage technetium Tc 99m
  gadodiamide
  gadolinium-diethylenetriamine-
    pentaacetic acid (Gd-DTPA)
  gadopentetate dimeglumine
  gadoteridol
  gadoversetamide
  galactose-based ultrasound contrast
    medium
  galactose; palmitic acid
  gallium-68 (^{68}gallium)
  Glofil-125 (iothalamate sodium
    I 125)
  gold-195m
  hand-agitated
  Hexabrix (ioxaglate meglumine;
    ioxaglate sodium)
  high osmolar
  human albumin microspheres
  Hypaque Meglumine 60%
    (diatrizoate meglumine 60%)
  Hypaque-76 (diatrizoate meglumine
    66% and diatrizoate sodium
    10%)
  Hypaque Sodium 50% (diatrizoate
    meglumine 50%)
  Imagent US (perflexane)
  imciromab pentetate
  indium 111 (^{111}In)
    ^{111}In imciromab pentetate
    ^{111}In-labeled antimyosin
    ^{111}In murine monoclonal
      antibody Fab to myosin
    ^{111}In pentetreotide
    ^{111}In radioisotope

imaging *(cont.)*
  indocyanine green
  iobenguane sulfate (I-131)
  iodine 123, 125, or 131
    (^{123}I, ^{125}I, ^{131}I)
    ^{123}I heptadecanoic acid radio-
      isotope
    ^{123}I phenyl-pentadecanoic acid
      (IPPA) radioisotope
    ^{123}I b-methyl-phenyl-penta-
      decanoic acid (BMIPP,
      BMIPPA)
    ^{125}I radioisotope
    ^{131}I radioisotope
  iodixanol
  iohexol
  ionic
  iopamidol
  Iopamiron 310; 370
  iopromide
  iothalamate meglumine
  iothalamate sodium ^{125}I
  ioversol
  ioxaglate meglumine
  ioxaglate sodium
  Isopaque (metrizoate sodium)
  Isovue-200 (iopamidol)
  Isovue-250 (iopamidol)
  Isovue-300 (iopamidol)
  Isovue-370 (iopamidol)
  Levovist (d-galactose; palmitic
    acid)
  low-osmolar nonionic
  Magnevist (gadopentetate
    dimeglumine)
  MD-76 R (diatrizoate meglumine;
    diatrizoate sodium 10%)
  meglumine
    amidotrizoate
    diatrizoate
    iothalamate
    ioxaglate

imaging *(cont.)*
  metaiodobenzylguanidine sulfate
    (now iobenguane sulfate ^{131}I)
  metrizamide
  metrizoate sodium; also sodium
    metrizoate
  Myoscint (imciromab pentetate)
  Myoview (technetium ^{99m}Tc
    tetrofosmin)
  NeoTect (technetium ^{99m}Tc
    depreotide)
  nofetumomab merpentan
  nonionic
  OctreoScan (oxidronate sodium)
  Omnipaque (iohexol)
  Omniscan (gadodiamide)
  OncoTrac (technetium ^{99m}Tc
    antimelanoma murine)
  OptiMARK (gadoversetamide)
  Optiray 160 (ioversol 34%)
  Optiray 240 (ioversol 51%)
  Optiray 300 (ioversol 64%)
  Optiray 320 (ioversol 68%)
  Optiray 350 (ioversol 74%)
  Optison (human albumin
    microspheres)
  oxidronate sodium
  oxygen-15
  oxygen-15 labeled water
  oxygen-15 water
  ^{31}P
  palmitic acid
  perflenapent
  perflexane
  perflisopent
  perflutren
  potassium-43 (^{43}K)
  ProHance (gadoteridol)
  RenoCal 76 (diatrizoate meglumine
    66% and diatrizoate sodium
    10%)
  Reno-Dip (diatrizoate meglumine
    30%)

imaging *(cont.)*
  Renografin-60 (diatrizoate meglu-
    mine 52%, diatrizoate sodium
    8%)
  Reno-60 (diatrizoate meglumine
    60%)
  rubidium chloride Rb 82 (^{82}Rb)
  rubidium-82 radioisotope (^{82}Rb)
  sestamibi, technetium ^{99m}Tc
  sodium metrizoate; also metrizoate
    sodium
  Sonazoid (perfluorobutane micro-
    bubbles) ultrasound
  sonicated meglumine sodium
  teboroxime, technetium ^{99m}Tc
  TechneScan MAA (technetium
    ^{99m}Tc macroaggregated
    albumin)
  TechneScan PYP (technetium ^{99m}Tc
    pyrophosphate)
  technetated (^{99m}Tc) aggregated
    albumin, human
  technetium bound to DTPA
  technetium bound to serum
    albumin
  technetium bound to sulfur colloid
  technetium-99m-labeled fibrinogen
  technetium-99m-labeled red blood
    cells
  technetium Tc 99m albumin
    aggregated
  technetium Tc 99m biciromab
  technetium Tc 99m DTPA
  technetium Tc 99m furifosmin
  technetium Tc 99m macro-
    aggregated albumin
  technetium Tc 99m pentetate
  technetium Tc 99m pyrophosphate
  technetium Tc 99m sestamibi
  technetium Tc 99m sodium
    pertechnetate
  technetium Tc 99m teboroxime

imaging *(cont.)*
  technetium Tc 99m tetrofosmin
  technetium-99m-tin-pyrophosphate
  thallium-201 (^{201}Tl)
  thallous chloride
  Ultravist 300 (iopromide)
  Ultravist 370 (iopromide)
  Urografin-76 (meglumine amido-
    trizoate)
  Urovist-Angiografin (meglumine
    amidotrizoate)
  Verluma (nofetumomab merpentan)
  Visipaque 270 (iodixanol)
  Visipaque 320 (iodixanol)
IMax, IMAX (slang for internal
  maxillary artery)
imbalance
  acid-base
  electrolyte
  ventilation-perfusion (V/Q)
  ventilatory capacity-demand
imciromab pentetate
IMI (inferior myocardial infarction)
immediate diastolic murmur (IDM)
immediate intervention
imminent death
imminent demise
immobilization
immobilized
immotile cilia syndrome
immune complex, circulating (CIC)
immunoassay (see *assay*)
immunoblastoid lymphocytes
immunoblot assay, three-antigen
  recombinant (see also *assay*)
immunocytologic monitoring (also
  cytoimmunologic monitoring)
immunodeficiency with thrombocytopenia and eczema
immunohemolytic anemia
immunohistochemical analysis
immunohistochemistry

immunologic deficiencies
immunologic derangement
immunologic injury
immunologic markers
immunomodulate
immunoscintigraphy
immunosuppress
immunosuppression
immunosuppressive agent
immunosuppressive drug
immunosuppressive induction
immunosuppressive therapy
immunotherapy
immunothrombocytopenic purpura
impaction, mucoid (in bronchi)
impaired consciousness
impaired exercise capacity
impaired filling pressures
impaired oxygen diffusion
impaired venous return
impaired ventilation-perfusion
impairment
  circulatory
  functional
  inspiratory muscle function
  motor
  renal function
  sensory
impairment of contractility
impedance
  acoustic
  aortic
  electrical
  lead
  pacemaker lead
  pulmonary arterial input
  pulmonary vascular bed
  vascular
impedance electrodes
impedance phlebography
impedance plethysmography (IPG)
impede filling

impediment
Impella intracardiac pump
impending closure
impending doom, feeling of
impending infarction
impending myocardial infarction
imperfecta, osteogenesis
imperforate aneurysm
impinges
impinging
implant (see *implantation*)
implant threshold
implantable automatic atrial cardioverter-defibrillator
implantable cardioverter-defibrillator
    (ICD)
  Cadence
  Cadence biphasic
  PCD
implantable circulatory support device
implantable system
implantation
  Angiotech
  CardioSEAL septal occluder
  cardioverter-defibrillator
  Contigen Bard collagen
  epicardial
  intrapleural pulse generator
  Myomate
  pacemaker
  percutaneous
  permanent pacemaker
  subcoronary aortic valve
  subpectoral pulse generator
  subxiphoid
  ThermoRod
  transluminal stent-graft
  transvenous
implantation of atrioventricular
  sequential pacemaker
implantation response
implanted pacemaker

impotence
Impra Carboflo vascular prosthesis
Impragraft
impulse
  absent apical
  apical
  atrial filling
  bifid precordial
  cardiac
  cardiac apex
  double systolic apical
  downward displacement of apical
  ectopic
  episternal
  fibrillatory
  high-amplitude
  hyperdynamic
  hyperdynamic apical
  hyperdynamic right ventricular
  jugular venous
  juxta-apical
  late systolic
  left parasternal
  left ventricular
  mild systolic
  palpable apical
  paradoxic apical
  point of maximal (PMI)
  precordial
  prolonged left ventricular
  prominent systolic venous
  right parasternal
  sustained apical
  systolic
  undulant
impulse-conducting system of heart
impulse oscillometry
IMT (intima-media thickness)
IMV (intermittent mandatory
  ventilation)
IMV-Bird ventilator
inactive mode

inactivity, electrical
inadequate cardiac output
inadequate numbers of platelets
inadequate oxygenation of blood
inadequate runoff
inadequate visualization
inappropriate activation of ICD
inappropriate discharges
inappropriately elevated plasma renin
    activity
inaudible
incentive spirometer
incentive spirometry
incessant tachycardia
incision
    anterolateral
    bayonet-type
    cervical extension
    chevron
    clamshell
    collar
    commissural
    copiously irrigated
    cruciate
    curvilinear
    deltopectoral
    Denis Browne abdominal
    flank
    inguinal crease
    intercostal
    lazy H
    lazy Z
    left paramedian
    longitudinal
    L-shaped
    median sternotomy
    midline hockey-stick
    midline sternotomy
    muscle-splitting
    oblique abdominal
    oblique subcostal
    parasternal

incision *(cont.)*
    periosteal
    pleuropericardial
    posterior parietal peritoneal
    posterolateral
    posterolateral thoracotomy
    pterional
    quasitransmural endocardial
    rib-resecting
    smile
    smiling
    stab wound
    stepladder
    sternotomy
    submammary
    subxiphoid
    suprasternal notch
    tangential
    T-d
    thoracicoabdominal
    thoracoabdominal
    thoracotomy
    transverse
    transverse anterior thoracotomy
    transverse submammary
    trap-door
    visceral rotation
    watchband incision for endoscopic
        radial artery harvesting
    xiphoid to os pubis
    xiphopubic midline
incisional macroreentrant atrial tachy-
    cardia
incision of aorta
incisura
    aortic
    pulmonary artery
incisura apicis cordis
incisura of carotid arterial pulse
inciting event
inciting factors
inclination of the treadmill

indolent ulcer
indomethacin
induced thrombosis of aortic aneurysm
inducibility basal state
inducibility, VT (ventricular tachycardia)
inducible
induction
   immunosuppressive
   sputum
induction anesthesia
induction chemotherapy
indurated mass
indurated tissue
induration
   brawny
   brown pulmonary
   erythema without
indurative mediastinitis
indurative pleurisy
induratum, Bazin erythema
inefficiency, ventilatory
inelastic pericardium
inequality, ventilation-perfusion
inexorable progression
In-Exsufflator cough machine
in extremis
Inf (infarction)
Infamyst aerosol spray device
Infant Flow nasal CPAP system
infantile cardiomyopathy
infantile histiocytoid cardiomyopathy
infantile lobar emphysema
infantile pneumonia
infantile respiratory distress
infantile syndrome
infantile thoracic dystrophy
infant, profoundly obtunded
Infant Star ventilator
infarct (see also *infarction*)
   anemic
   bland

infarct *(cont.)*
   bleeding into the
   embolic
   focal skin
   healing
   hemorrhagic
   livedo reticularis-digital
   red
   thrombotic
   transmural
   transmural myocardial
   uninfected
infarct avid imaging (hot spot scan,
   technetium pyrophosphate scan)
infarct expansion
infarctectomy
infarcted heart muscle
infarcted lung segment
infarcted segment of lung
infarction (see also *infarct*)
   acute myocardial (AMI)
   age indeterminate
   anterior myocardial (AMI)
   anterior-wall myocardial
   anteroinferior myocardial
   anterolateral myocardial
   anteroseptal myocardial
   apical myocardial
   arrhythmic myocardial
   atherothrombotic
   atherothrombotic brain
   atrial
   Battey-avium complex
   cardiac
   cerebral
   concomitant
   diaphragmatic myocardial (DMI)
   evolving myocardial
   extensive anterior myocardial
   full-thickness
   high lateral myocardial
   hyperacute myocardial

infarction *(cont.)*
  impending
  impending myocardial
  inferior myocardial (IMI)
  inferolateral myocardial
  inferoposterolateral myocardial
  intestinal
  intraoperative myocardial
  lacunar
  lateral myocardial
  lung tissue
  mesenteric
  myocardial (MI)
  myocardial (see *myocardial*
    infarction)
  non-Q wave myocardial
  nonarrhythmic myocardial
  nonfatal myocardial
  nontransmural myocardial
  old myocardial
  papillary muscle
  posterior myocardial
  posteroinferior myocardial
  postmyocardial
  postmyocardiotomy
  pulmonary
  Q-wave myocardial
  recent myocardial
  right ventricular
  segmental bowel
  septal myocardial
  septic pulmonary
  severe
  silent myocardial
  sinoatrial node
  subacute myocardial
  subendocardial (SEI)
  subendocardial myocardial
  transmural myocardial
infarctionlike
infarction of the lung
infarctoid cardiopathy

infarct size limitation
Infatabs
infected abscess
infected hematoma
infected lead
infected pseudoaneurysms
infected thrombosed graft
infection
  anaerobic lung
  Ancylostoma braziliense
  Ancylostoma duodenale
  Ascaris lumbricoides
  Ascaris suum
  aspergillosis
  atypical tuberculosis
  bacterial
  bronchial nocardiosis
  Brugia malayi
  chronic indolent bacterial
  Clonorchis sinensis
  clostridial
  complicating
  concurrent
  Corynebacterium pseudo-
    tuberculosis
  cytomegalovirus
  Dirofilaria immitis
  Echinococcus granulosus
  endovascular
  Enterobacteriaceae
  enterococcal
  enteroviral
  Epstein-Barr virus
  Haemophilus
  HIV
  intestinal parasitic
  Kingella
  Legionella pneumophila
  mediastinal
  meningococcal
  Mycobacterium avium-intracellulare
    (MAI)

infection *(cont.)*
  Mycobacterium avium complex
    (MAC)
  Mycobacterium simiae
  mycobacterial
  Mycoplasma pneumoniae
  Necator americanus
  Neisseria
  nocardiosis
  nonarterial groin
  nosocomial lung
  nosocomial opportunistic
  opisthorchiasis
  opportunistic
  Paragonimus westermani
  parasitic
  polymicrobial
  primary prosthetic graft
  Pseudomonas aeruginosa
  Rickettsia burnetii
  Schistosoma
  secondary bacterial
  self-limited (limiting) respiratory
  sinopulmonary
  spirochetal
  Staphylococcus aureus
  Strongyloides stercoralis
  superimposed bronchial
  suppurative pulmonary
  suppurative pulmonary
  Toxocara
  Treponema pallidum
  Trichinella spiralis
  tubercular
  tuberculosis
  viral
  viridans streptococcal
  Wuchereria bancrofti
  Yersinia
infectious disease
infectious insult
infective aneurysmal endocarditis

infective embolism
infective endocarditis, marantic
infective myocarditis
infective pericarditis
infective rhinitis
infective silicosis
infective thrombosis or thrombus
inferior basal segment
inferior border of heart
inferior border of lung
inferior border of rib
inferior bronchi
inferior lead
inferior ligaments
inferior lobe of lung
inferior margin of superior rib
inferior mediastinum
inferior mesenteric artery
inferior pulmonary ligament
inferior pulmonary vein
inferior thyroid vein
inferior tip of the scapula
inferior vena cava (IVC)
inferior vena cava orifice
inferior vena cava syndrome
inferior vena cava to left atrium
  conduit
inferior wall akinesis
inferior wall hypokinesis
inferior wall MI (myocardial
  infarction)
inferoapical
inferobasal
inferolateral displacement of apical
  beat
inferolaterally
inferolateral wall myocardial infarction
inferomedially
inferoposterior wall myocardial
  infarction
inferoposterolateral
inferoseptal infarction

infestation
  metazoal
  parasitic
  Plasmodium falciparum
  protozoal
  roundworm
  Toxocara canis
infiltrate, infiltration
  aggressive interstitial
  aggressive perivascular
  apical
  basilar
  basilar zone
  bilateral interstitial pulmonary
  bilateral upper lobe cavitary
  bronchocentric inflammatory
  butterfly pattern of
  cavitary
  consolidated
  diffuse
  diffuse aggressive polymorphous
  diffuse alveolar interstitial
  diffuse bilateral alveolar
  diffuse interstitial
  diffuse perivascular
  diffuse reticulonodular
  eosinophilic
  fluffy
  focal interstitial
  focal perivascular
  ground glass
  interstitial
  interstitial nonlobar
  invasive angiomatous interstitial
  lung
  lymphocytic
  massive
  micronodular
  migratory
  mononuclear
  multifocal aggressive
  mural

infiltrate *(cont.)*
  patchy, migratory
  peripheral
  pulmonary
  pulmonary eosinophilic
  pulmonary parenchymal
  reticulonodular
  retrocardiac
  strandy
  sulfasalazine-induced pulmonary
  transient
infiltration of pulmonary parenchyma
infiltrative cardiomyopathy
infiltrative disease
infiltrative interstitial disease
Infiniti catheter from Cordis
Infinity pulse generator
inflamed edematous medium-sized
  bronchi
inflamed left upper lobe
inflamed main stem bronchial mucosa
inflamed pleura
inflamed throat
inflammation
  airway
  allergic airway
  alveolar septal
  fibrinous
  granulomatous (of bronchi)
  mucosal
  patchy
inflammation and fibrosis, periaortic
inflammation of a vein
inflammation of cardiac muscle
inflammation of heart muscle
inflammatory adhesions
inflammatory aortoarteritis,
  nonspecific
inflammatory exudate
inflammatory granulomatous reaction
inflammatory myocarditis
inflammatory polypoid mass

inflammatory reaction
inflammatory response syndrome,
    systemic
inflammatory response, whole body
inflated to 300 mm Hg, tourniquet
inflation
    sequential balloon
    simultaneous balloon
inflow cuff
inflow disease progression
inflow tract of left ventricle
influenza
influenzal myocarditis
infra-apical
infra-auricular
infracardiac type total anomalous
    venous return
infraclavicular
infraclavicular pocket
infracolic midline
infracristal ventricular defect
infracristal ventricular septal defect
infradiaphragmatic vein
infragenicular popliteal artery
infragenicular position
infrageniculate artery
infrainguinal bypass stenosis
infrainguinal revascularization
infrainguinal vein bypass graft
infrainguinal vein graft
inframammary crease
inframammary syndrome
inframyocardial
infrapopliteal arterial bypass grafts
infrapopliteal disease
infrapopliteal vessel
infrapulmonary position
infrarenal abdominal aorta
infrarenal aortic disease
infrarenal aortic repair
infrarenal aortobifemoral bypass graft
infrarenal stenosis

infrasternal angle
infundibular atresia
infundibular chamber
infundibular dissection
infundibular pulmonary stenosis
infundibular resection
infundibular septum, parietal extension
    of
infundibular stenosis, subpulmonic
infundibular subpulmonic stenosis
infundibulectomy, right ventricular
infundibuloventricular crest
infundibulum, right ventricular
Infuse-A-Cath catheter
infusion
    antegrade
    continuous
    fresh frozen plasma
    intermittent
    isoproterenol
    packed red blood cells
    prostaglandin
    retrograde coronary sinus
    saralasin
    volume
    whole blood
infusion line, peripheral intravenous
ingestion
    chronic excessive licorice
    chronic salicylate
    salicylate
inguinal crease incision
inguinal region
inhalation
    furosemide
    methacholine chloride
    smoke
    toxic gas
    toxic vapor
inhalation aerosol, pirbuterol acetate
inhalation aspirin challenge
inhalation bronchial challenge testing

inhalation by slow inspiration
inhalation challenge, methacholine
inhalation of beryllium dust
inhalation of dust particles
inhalation of environmental dusts
inhalation of radioactive xenon gas
inhalation pneumonia
inhalation tuberculosis
inhaled bronchodilator
inhaled corticosteroids
inhaler (see *drug delivery devices*)
inherent asymmetry
inherently unstable condition
inhibited respiration
inhibition
    lipoprotein plasminogen
    myopotential
    prostaglandin synthesis
inhibitor
    HMG-CoA reductase
    monoamine oxidase (MAO)
    phosphodiesterase
    serine proteinase
    thrombus
inhibitor of platelet aggregation
inhibitory effect
initial shock
injection
    bolus
    double
    hand
    intra-amniotic
    intra-arterial
    intramuscular (I.M.)
    intramuscular fetal
    intraperitoneal fetal
    intravascular
    intravascular sonotherapy
    intravenous (I.V.)
    intravenous bolus
    intravenous fetal
    manual

injection *(cont.)*
    opacifying
    power
    sclerosing
    selective
    serial
    sonographically guided human
        thrombin
    straight AP pelvic
    thrombin (into false aneurysm)
    ultrasound-guided percutaneous
        thrombin
injection at peak exercise
injection port
injection test for pneumoperitoneum
injector
    Hercules power
    Medrad power angiographic
    pressure
injury
    blunt
    brachial plexus
    concomitant tracheal
    crushing
    decelerative
    immunologic
    intercostal nerve
    obstetrical
    penetrating lung
    postcatheterization
    pulmonary parenchymal
    radial vascular thermal
    rapid deceleration
    subendocardial
    thoracic duct
    thoracic great vessel
    through-and-through
injury pattern
Injury Scale, Abbreviated
Injury Severity Score (ISS)
inner bright layer
innermost intercostal muscles

InnerVasc sheath
innocent heart murmur
innocuous
innominate (*not* innominant)
innominate artery arteritis
innominate artery buckling
innominate artery kinking
innominate artery, penetrating injury to
innominate artery stenosis
innominate (brachiocephalic) veins
Innovante balloon
Innovante catheter
Innovante dilator
Innovante filter
Innovante guidewire
Innovante introducer
Innovante occluder
Innovante retrieval device
Innovante sheath
Innovante stent
Innovator Holter system
inoperable disease
inotropes
inotropic activity of drug
inotropic activity of the heart,
    increased
inotropic agent
inotropic effect
inotropic state
inotropic stimulation
inotropic support
inotropic therapy
Inoue balloon
Inoue balloon catheter
InQwire guidewire
INR (international normalized ratio)
insertion
    chordal
    percutaneous (via femoral vein)
insidious onset
insidious progression
in situ bypass

in situ graft
in situ grafting
in situ vein graft
inspiration, inhalation by slow
inspiration phase
inspiration-to-expiration asymmetry
Inspirator
inspiratory and expiratory times
    (Ti, Te)
inspiratory augmentation of A_2-P_2
    interval (heart sounds)
inspiratory crepitation
inspiratory dyspnea
inspiratory-expiratory breath sounds
inspiratory-expiratory (I-E) ratio
inspiratory flow rates, rapid
inspiratory flow-volume, tidal
inspiratory increase in venous pressure
inspiratory maneuvers, repetitive
    maximal (against closed shutter)
inspiratory muscle function impairment
inspiratory phase
inspiratory positive airway pressure
    (IPAP)
inspiratory prolongation of interval
inspiratory rales
inspiratory reserve volume (IRV)
inspiratory retraction
inspiratory rhonchi, post-tussive
inspiratory spasm
inspiratory vital capacity (IVC)
inspiratory wheeze
InspirEase device
inspired air
inspissated mucus
instability
    hemodynamic
    ischemic
    ventricular electrical
instantaneous gradient
Instat MCH (microfibrillar
    hemostat)

in-stent balloon redilation
InStent CarotidCoil stent
in-stent restenosis (ISR)
InStent self-expanding and balloon
   expandable stent
instrument, tunneling
instrumentation
insufficiency
   acute cerebrovascular
   acute coronary
   aortic (AI)
   aortic valve
   arterial
   autonomic
   basilar artery
   brachial-basilar
   cardiac
   cardiopulmonary
   chronic venous
   congenital pulmonary valve
   coronary
   hypostatic pulmonary
   mitral (MI)
   myocardial (MI)
   nonischemic mitral valve
   nonocclusive mesenteric arterial
   nonrheumatic aortic
   postirradiation vascular
   post-traumatic pulmonary
   pulmonary (PI)
   pulmonary valve
   renal
   respiratory
   Sternberg myocardial
   transient ischemic carotid
   tricuspid (TI)
   valvular
   valvular aortic
   venous
   vertebrobasilar arterial
insufficiency of aortic valve
insufficient pulmonary arterial flow

insulating pad to retard premature
   rewarming
insult
   aortic
   infectious
   toxic
InSync implantable cardioverter-
   defibrillator
InSync multisite cardiac stimulator
Insyte-N Autoguard shielded IV
   catheter
intact Medtronic xenograft valve
intact valve cusp
intact ventricular septum
Intact xenograft prosthetic valve
intake, restricted fluid
Intec implantable defibrillator
integral
   aortic flow velocity
   pulmonary flow velocity
integral hemostasis valve
integrated bipolar sensing
Integrity AFx AutoCapture pacing
   system
Integrity AFx pacemaker
integrity of the suture line violated
Intelli-Clamp vascular occlusion clamp
Intelli-Clip vascular occlusion clip
Intelligent dressing
IntelliSystem 25 disposable inflation
   syringe
intense disabling cramping
intense pulsed light source (IPLS)
intensity
   angina with recent increase in
   decreased
   equal in
   maximal
   signal
   variable
intensity of heart sounds
intensive anticoagulation

intensive care unit (ICU)
intentional transoperative hemodilution
interatrial baffle
interatrial baffle leak
interatrial communication
interatrial groove
interatrial septal defect
interatrial septum, lipomatous hypertrophy of the
interatrial transposition of venous return
interbronchial mass
intercalated disks
intercellular edema
intercellular space
Intercept Vascular guidewire
interchondral joint
interchordal hooding
interchordal space fenestration
intercommunicating channels
intercoronary anastomosis
intercoronary collateral flow
intercoronary steal syndrome
intercostal artery
intercostal bundle fibers
intercostal incision
intercostal lymph nodes
intercostal muscle
intercostal muscle flap
intercostal nerve block
intercostal nerve injury
intercostal neuromuscular bundle
intercostal retraction on inspiration
intercostal space
   left fifth
   ninth
   right first
   right second
intercostal vein
intercostal vessels
interdiction
interdigitating coil stent

interface
   air (on x-ray)
   catheter-skin
   media-adventitia
interference dissociation
interferon level
interfibrosis
interlobar empyema
interlobar fissure
interlobar pleurisy
interlobar septa
interlobular emphysema
interlobular pleurisy
interlobular septa
interlobular vessels
intermedia, angina
intermediate artery
intermediate coronary syndrome
intermediate-density lipoprotein
intermediate heart
intermediate images
intermediate tuberculin test
Intermedics epicardial pacing lead
Intermedics patch leads
Intermedics Quantum pacemaker
intermedius, bronchus
intermittent apneic episodes
intermittent cannon A waves on jugular venous pulse tracing
intermittent claudication
intermittent cross-clamp fibrillation (ICCF)
intermittent infusion (of cardioplegia)
intermittent junctional bradycardia
intermittently nonconducted P waves
intermittent mandatory ventilation (IMV)
intermittent occlusion
intermittent positive pressure breathing (IPPB)
intermittent shortness of breath
intermittent venous claudication

internal caliber
internal capsule intracerebral hemorrhage
internal carotid artery
internal clot
internal diameter-outside diameter
  (ID-OD) ratio
internal elastic lamina
internal intercostal membrane
internal intercostal muscles
internal jugular acute hemodialysis
  catheter
internal jugular approach for cardiac
  catheterization
internal jugular bulb
internal jugular triangle
internal jugular vein
internal jugular venous cannula
internal mammary artery (IMA)
internal maxillary artery (IMax,
  IMAX)
internal pacemaker
internal saphenous vein grafting
internal thoracic artery
internal thoracic artery (ITA) graft
internal thoracic vein
internodal pathway
internodal tract
interpleural analgesia
interpleural space
interpolated ventricular premature
  complex
interposition graft
interposition vein graft
interrenal stenosis
interrogation
  color-duplex
  pulse Doppler
  transtelephonic ICD
interrupted aortic arch
interrupted pledgeted sutures
interruption, aortic arch

interscalene space
interscapulovertebral arterial bruit
interspace
  fifth left
  fourth left
  second left
  third left
interstitial arteriosclerotic nephritis
interstitial diffuse pulmonary fibrosis
interstitial edema
interstitial emphysema
interstitial fibrosis
interstitial fluid
interstitial infiltrate
  diffuse alveolar
  invasive angiomatous
interstitial lung disease (ILD),
  rheumatoid-arthritis-associated
interstitial markings, increased
interstitial nonlobar infiltrates
interstitial plasma cell pneumonia
interstitial pneumonia air leak
interstitial pneumonia, lymphoid
interstitial prematurity fibrosis
interstitial pulmonary edema
interstitial pulmonary fibrosis
interstitial scarring
interstitial space
interstitial structures, coarse
  thickening of
interstitial tissues
interstitium
Intertach pacemaker
interval
  A-A
  A_1-A_2
  abbreviated
  absolute QT
  A-C
  acquired prolonged Q-T
  Ae-H
  A-H

interval *(cont.)*
    A_2 incisural
    A_2/MVO (aortic valve closure to
        mitral valve opening)
    A_2 to opening snap
    atrial escape (AEI)
    atrioventricular
    AV (atrioventricular)
    AV delay (AVDI)
    cardioarterial
    confidence
    coupling
    escape
    fixed coupling
    flutter R
    H-Ae
    hangout
    H-H'
    H1-H2
    H'P
    H-Q
    H-QRS
    H-V
    inspiratory prolongation
    interectopic
    isoelectric
    long Q-T
    lower rate
    P-A
    pacemaker escape
    P-H
    P-P
    P-R
    preejection
    prolongation of QRS
    prolonged
    prolonged P-R
    prolonged Q-T
    Q to first sound
    Q-T
    Q-H
    QRS

interval *(cont.)*
    QRST
    Q-S_1
    Q-S_2
    Q-T
    Q-Tc
    Q-U
    right ventricular systolic time
        (RVSTI)
    R-P
    R-R
    S-QRS
    S_1-S_2
    S_1-S_3
    S_2OS (second sound to opening
        snap)
    short P-Q
    short P-R
    spike-Q
    ST
    systolic time (STI)
    upper rate
    V-A
    varying P-R
    V-H
interval development (on x-ray)
interval intra-atrial conduction
intervention
    catheter-based
    immediate
    surgical
    therapeutic
    transcatheter
interventional EP (electrophysiology)
interventional equipment
interventional procedure
interventricular (IV)
interventricular conduction delay
interventricular groove
    anterior
    posterior
interventricular septal defect

interventricular septum
interventricular sulcus, posterior
interventricular vein, posterior
intestinal emphysema
intestinal parasitic infection
intima
    diffuse thickening of arterial
    friable thickened degenerated
    hypertrophied
    tunica
intimal atherosclerotic disease
intimal debris
intimal dissection
intimal fibroplasia
intimal flap
intimal hyperplasia
intimal irregularity
intimal-medial dissection
intima-media thickness (IMT)
intimal plaque
intimal proliferation
intimal tear
intimal thickening
intimate attachment of diseased vessel
intimomedial thickness
intolerance
    exercise
    heat
in toto
intoxication, potassium
intra-abdominal arterial bypass graft
intra-acinar pulmonary arteries
intra-adrenal pheochromocytoma
intra-alveolar fibrosis
intra-amniotic injection
intra-aortic balloon assist
intra-aortic balloon counterpulsation
intra-aortic balloon double-lumen
    catheter
intra-aortic balloon pump (IABP)
    AutoCat (AutoCAT) with AutoPilot
    cutdown

intra-aortic *(cont.)*
    Datascope
    Datascope System 83
    Datascope System 90
    Datascope System 90T
    KAAT II Plus
    Kontron KAAT
    Kontron KAAT II+
    postcardiotomy
    St. Jude Aries 700
    TransAct
intra-arterial filling defects
intra-arterially
intra-arterial filtration system
intra-arterial thrombus
intra-articular ligament
intra-atrial baffle
intra-atrial baffle operation
intra-atrial conduction defect
intra-atrial conduction interval
intra-atrial electrogram
intra-atrial filling defect
intra-atrial reentrant tachycardia
intra-atrial reentry
intra-atrial thrombi
intrabronchial casts
intracardiac air
intracardiac baffle
intracardiac calcium
intracardiac echocardiography (ICE)
intracardiac electrogram
intracardiac mass
intracardiac pressure in Doppler
    echocardiogram
intracardiac repair
intracardiac right-to-left shunt
intracardiac shunt
intracardiac shunting
intracardiac thrombus
Intracath catheter
intracaval conduit

intracaval endovascular ultrasonography (ICEUS)
intracavitary clot formation
intracavitary electrogram
intracavitary extension of tumor
intracavitary filling defect
intracavitary mass
intracavitary pressure-electrogram dissociation
intracavitary thrombus
intracellular acidosis
intracerebral hemorrhage
  basilar
  bulbar
  cerebellar
  cerebral
  cerebromeningeal
  cortical
  internal capsule
  intrapontine
  pontine
  subcortical
  ventricular
IntraCoil self-expanding nitinol stent
intracoronary artery radiation
intracoronary Doppler flow wire
intracoronary ethanol ablation
intracoronary stent placement
intracoronary stenting
intracoronary thrombolytic therapy
intracoronary ultrasound (ICUS)
intracoronary urokinase (ICUK)
intracranial berry aneurysm
intracranial hemorrhage
intracranial hypertension
intracranial pressure, increased
intracranial tuberculoma
intractable heart failure
intractable bleeding disorder
intradiaphragmatic aortic segment
intraerythrocytic *Babesia*
intra-Hisian (or intrahisian) AV block

intra-Hisian (or intrahisian) delay
intraluminal defect
intraluminal dimension
intraluminal filling defect
intraluminal flap
intraluminal flow, turbulent
intraluminal sutureless prosthesis
intraluminal thrombus, laminated
intramural arterial hemorrhage
intramural coronary artery aneurysm
intramural hematoma, acute
intramuscular aortic segment
intramuscular fetal injection
intramuscular hemangioma
intramuscular ketamine
intramyocardial electrocardiography during sleep
intramyocardially
intranodal block
Intra-Op autotransfusion
intraoperative arteriography
intraoperative autologous transfusion (IOAT)
intraoperative digital subtraction angiography (IDSA)
intraoperative hypotension
intraoperative laser ablation
intraoperative laser photocoagulation of ventricular tachycardia
intraoperative myocardial infarction
intraoperative testing
intraoperative transmyocardial revascularization (ITMR)
intraosseous vascular malformations
intrapericardial bleeding
intrapericardial dissection
intrapericardial ligation
intrapericardial patch lead placement
intrapericardial poudrage
intrapericardial pressure
intraperitoneal exposure
intraperitoneal fetal injection

intraperitoneal migration of pacemaker
intrapleural hemorrhage
intrapleural implantation of pulse
  generator
intrapleurally
intrapleural pressure
intrapontine intracerebral hemorrhage
intrapulmonary arteriovenous malformation
intrapulmonary artery baffle
intrapulmonary baffle
intrapulmonary disease
intrapulmonary hemorrhage
intrapulmonary metastasis
intrapulmonary pressure
intrapulmonary shunt (or shunting)
intrarenal hematoma
intraretinal microangiopathy (IRMA)
IntraStent DoubleStrut LD stent
intrathoracic airway obstruction
intrathoracic airway pressure
intrathoracic dimension
intrathoracic Kaposi sarcoma
intrathoracic pressure
intrathoracic upper airway obstruction
intrauterine cardiac failure
intrauterine growth retardation (IUGR)
intrauterine heart failure
intravascular clotting process
intravascular coagulation, disseminated
intravascular coagulation of blood
intravascular contents, secondary
  extravasation of
intravascular filling defect
intravascular fragmentation of red
  blood cells
intravascular mass
intravascular MRI technique
intravascular oxygenator (IVOX)
  artificial lung
intravascular polymorphonuclear
  leukocytosis

intravascular pressure
intravascular prosthesis
intravascular red light therapy (IRLT)
intravascular sickling, lung
intravascular signal intensity in MR
  angiography
intravascular sonotherapy
intravascular space
intravascular stenting
intravascular thrombosis
intravascular ultrasound (IVUS)
intravascular volume depletion
intravascular volume status
intravascularly volume depleted
intravenous (I.V. or IV)
intravenous bolus
intravenous bolus injection
intravenous coronary thrombolysis
intravenous fetal injection
intravenous fluorescein angiography
  (IVFA)
intravenous infusion line, peripheral
intravenous leiomyomatosis with
  intracardiac extension
intravenous line
intravenous pyelogram, pyelography
  (IVP)
  excretory
  rapid-sequence
intravenous TKO (to keep open [the
  vein, needle, or catheter])
intraventricular aberration
intraventricular block, conduction
  delay
intraventricular conduction abnormality
intraventricular conduction defect
intraventricular conduction delay
  (IVCD)
intraventricular hemorrhage (IVH)
intraventricular rerouting
intraventricular right ventricular
  obstruction

intraventricular systolic tension
intraventricular tunnel repair
Intrepid PTCA catheter
intrinsic asthma
intrinsic deflection
intrinsic disease
intrinsic heart rate
intrinsic positive end-expiratory
   pressure
intrinsic pulmonary disease
intrinsic sensing
intrinsic sick sinus syndrome
intrinsic stenotic lesions
intrinsic vein graft lesion
intrinsic vein graft stenosis
intrinsicoid deflection
introduced, catheter
introducer
   Angioport angiographic vascular
   Arrow-Flex percutaneous sheath
   Avanti angiographic catheter
   AVA HF
   AVA 3XI
   BD Introsyte-N Autoguard shielded
   Becton-Dickinson
   BriteMax sheath
   Cath-Lock
   Check-Flo
   Ciaglia percutaneous tracheostomy
   Cook
   Desilets-Hoffman catheter
   electrode
   Excalibur
   Guidant
   Hemaquet catheter
   Hemaquet sheath
   heparin lock
   Innovante
   Littleford-Spector
   LPS Peel-Away
   Mullins catheter

introducer *(cont.)*
   Outcomes by Design sheath
   Pacesetter
   peel-away
   percutaneous lead
   permanent lead
   Prelude vascular
   Razi cannula
   Swartz SL Series Fast-Cath
   Tuohy-Borst
introducer sheath
Introsyte-N Autoguard shielded
   introducer
intubate
intubated
intubation
   blind nasal
   direct vision nasal
   direct vision orotracheal
   endotracheal
   orotracheal
Intuitive surgical telemanipulation
   system
intussusception of vein
in utero exposure
invaginate
invagination
invariability of cardiac dullness during
   phases of respiration
invariable
invasion
   chest wall
   exogenous
   mediastinal
invasive angiomatous interstitial
   infiltration
invasive cardiology
invasive pulmonary aspergillosis
invasive pulmonary mycosis
inverse inspiratory/expiratory time
   ratio

inversion
  diffuse T-wave
  isolated ventricular
  T-wave
  U-wave
  ventricular
inversus
  situs
  situs viscerum
inversus totalis, situs
inverted P wave
inverted T partial upper re-sternotomy
  for aortic valve replacement (AVR)
inverted T waves in V_1 and V_3
inverted terminal T wave
inverted U wave
inverted Y configuration
in vivo balloon pressure
involvement of lingula
INX stainless steel stent
IOAT (intraoperative autologous
  transfusion)
Ioban prep
iobenguane sulfate (I-131)
iodine (see also *imaging agent*)
iodine 123 (^{123}I) heptadecanoic acid
  radioisotope
iodine 123 (^{123}I) phenyl pentadecanoic
  acid (IPPA) radioisotope
iodine 123 (^{123}I) b-methyl-phenyl
  pentadecanoic acid (BMIPP,
  BMIPPA)
iodine 125 (^{125}I) radioisotope
iodine 131 (^{131}I) radioisotope
iodixanol
Iodoflex absorptive dressing
iodoform gauze
iodophor-impregnated adhesive drape
Iodosorb absorptive dressing
iohexol
Ionescu-Shiley bioprosthetic valve
Ionescu-Shiley bovine pericardial valve

Ionescu-Shiley heart valve
Ionescu-Shiley low-profile prosthetic
  valve
Ionescu-Shiley pericardial xenograft
  valve
Ionescu-Shiley standard pericardial
  prosthetic valve
Ionescu-Shiley valve prosthesis
Ionescu-Shiley vascular graft
Ionescu tri-leaflet valve
ionic potassium
Iopamiron 310; 370
iopromide
iothalamate meglumine
iothalamate sodium ^{125}I
ioversol
ioxaglate meglumine
ioxaglate sodium
IPA (idiopathic pulmonary arteriosclerosis)
IPAP (inspiratory positive airway
  pressure)
IPC (ischemic preconditioning)
IPF (idiopathic pulmonary fibrosis)
IPG (impedance plethysmography)
IPH (idiopathic pulmonary hemosiderosis)
IPH (intraplaque hemorrhage)
IPLS (intense pulsed light source)
IPPA (iodine-123 phenylpentadecanoic
  acid)
IPPB (intermittent positive pressure
  breathing)
ipsilateral hemispheric carotid TIA
  (transient ischemic attack)
ipsilateral nonreversed greater
  saphenous vein bypass
IRBBB (incomplete right bundle
  branch block)
IRDS (idiopathic respiratory distress
  syndrome)
Iressa (gefitinib)

Irex Exemplar ultrasound
IRIS coronary stent
IRLT (intravascular red light therapy)
IRMA (intraretinal microangiopathy)
iron-deficiency anemia
iron overloading
iron storage disease
irradiation, nodal
irradiation pneumonia
irregular hazy luminal contour
irregular heartbeat
irregular mass, polypoid calcified
irregular rhythm, sinusoidal
irregularity
    diffuse
    intimal
    luminal
    pulse
irregularly irregular cardiac rhythm
irreversible airways obstruction
irreversible ischemia
irreversible narrowing of the
    bronchioles
irreversible organ failure
irrigated, copiously
irrigation
    continuous
    continuous-flow
    continuous saline
    saline
irrigator, Vozzle Vacu-Irrigator
irritability
    atrial
    copious
    myocardial
    ventricular
irritable heart
irritant-induced asthma
irritants
    exposure to
    nonspecific
    respiratory

irritants to respiratory system
    air pollution
    fumes from burning wood
    gas fumes
    tobacco smoke
irritation, bronchial
Irukandji syndrome
IRV (inspiratory reserve volume)
Isch (ischemia)
ischemia
    brachiocephalic
    cardiac
    carotid artery
    cerebral
    coronary
    exercise-induced
    exercise-induced myocardial
    exercise-induced transient
      myocardial
    global myocardial
    hypoxia-
    irreversible
    limb
    limb-threatening
    myocardial
    nonlocalized
    peri-infarction
    peri-infarctional
    provocable
    regional myocardial
    regional transmural
    remote
    reversible
    segmental
    silent
    silent myocardial
    subendocardial
    transient cerebral
    transient myocardial
    vertebral-basilar
    vertebrobasilar
    zone of

ischemic cardiomyopathy
ischemic changes, persistence of
ischemic congestive cardiomyopathy
ischemic contracture
ischemic decompensation
ischemic disease
ischemic episode
ischemic event
ischemic heart disease (IHD)
ischemic heart disease syndrome
ischemic instability
ischemic necrosis
ischemic preconditioning (IPC)
ischemic-reperfusion injury
ischemic rest pain
ischemic segment (on echocardiogram)
ischemic stimuli
ischemic ST segment changes
ischemic time
ischemic ulcer, hypertensive
ischemic viable myocardium
ischemic zone
ischemically mediated mitral
   regurgitation
Isocam SPECT imaging system
isocapnic hyperventilation-induced
   bronchoconstriction
isocenter
isoelectric at J point
isoelectric line
isoelectric period
isoelectric ST segment
isoenzyme
   cardiac
   CK
   CK-BB (CK$_1$)
   CK-MB
   CK-MM (CK$_3$)
   CPK
   CPK-MB (CK$_2$)
   LDH$_1$ (LDH1)
   LDH$_2$ (LDH2)

isoenzyme *(cont.)*
   Regan
   serial cardiac
isolated angiitis
isolated diffuse myocarditis
isolated heat perfusion of an extremity
isolated ventricular inversion
isolation, respiratory
isomerism, atrial
isometric exercise stress test
isometric heart contraction
isometrics
Isopaque (metrizoate sodium)
Isovue-200 (iopamidol)
Isovue-250 (iopamidol)
Isovue-300 (iopamidol)
Isovue-370 (iopamidol)
isoproterenol infusion
isorhythmic AV (atrioventricular)
   dissociation
isotonic exercise
isotonic heart contraction
isotope (see *imaging agent*)
isotropic lung scan
isotropic thin slice CT
isovolumetric contraction
isovolumetric period
isovolumic contraction time
isovolumic period
isovolumic relaxation
ISS (Injury Severity Score)
isthmic coarctation, congenital
isthmus
   aortic
   stenotic
isthmus aneurysm
isthmus of aorta
isthmus of Vieussens
Isuprel drip
ITA (internal thoracic artery) graft
ITC balloon catheter

ITMR (intraoperative transmyocardial revascularization)
Itrel 3 spinal cord stimulation system
IUGR (intrauterine growth retardation)
I.V. or IV (intravenous)
  I.V. bolus
  I.V. drip
  I.V. TKO (to keep open)
Ivalon prosthesis
IVB (intraventricular block)
IVC (inferior vena cava)
IVC (inspiratory vital capacity)
IVCD (intraventricular conduction delay)
IVC filter
  percutaneous
  prophylactic
Ivemark syndrome

iVent ventilator
IVFA (intravenous fluorescein angiography)
IVH (intraventricular hemorrhage)
IVM electrode
IVM vascular occluder
IVOX (intravascular oxygenator)
IVOX (intravascular oxygenator) artificial lung
IVP (intravenous pyelogram)
IVR (idioventricular rhythm)
IVS (interventricular septum)
IVSD (interventricular septal defect)
IVST (interventricular septal thickness)
IVUS (intravascular ultrasound)
Ivy bleeding time
Ixodes dammini

J, j

J (joule)
JA (jet area)
Jaccoud arthritis
Jaccoud sign
jacket, Medtronic cardiac cooling
Jackman orthogonal catheter
Jackson bronchoscope
Jackson-Olympus bronchoscope
Jackson sign
Jacobson hemostatic forceps
Jacobson-Potts clamp
Jade II SSI pacemaker
Jaffé rate reaction, creatinine
    estimated using
Jahnke anastomosis clamp
Jako anterior commissure scope
James atrionodal bypass tract
James bundles or fibers
James intranodal bypass tract
Janeway lesion in infective
    endocarditis
Janeway skin lesion in bacterial
    endocarditis
Jannetta dissector
Janus syndrome
Jarcho-Levin syndrome
Jarvik-7 (and 8) artificial heart
Jarvik 7-70 total artificial heart
Jarvik 2000 ventricular assist device
Jatene arterial switch procedure
Jatene-Macchi prosthetic valve
Jatene operation for transposition of
    great arteries
Javid carotid artery clamp
Javid endarterectomy shunt
jawed conduit
jawed conduit graft
Jawz endomyocardial biopsy forceps
Jelco intravenous catheter
Jelco needle
jeopardize
jeopardy, myocardial
Jerome Kay technique
Jervell and Lange-Nielsen syndrome
jet
    central
    high-velocity
    mitral insufficiency
    regurgitant
jet area (JA)
jet length (JL)
jet lesion
jet nebulizer
Jet-Tip (for a catheter)

315

Jeune syndrome
Jeune-Tommasi syndrome
Jewel AF implantable defibrillator
jeweler's forceps
Jewel pulse generator
J guide, Teflon
J guidewire
JL (jet length)
JL4 (Judkins left 4) catheter
JL5 (Judkins left 5) catheter
J loop technique on catheterization
Jobst compression stockings
Jobst garment
Jobst stockings
Jobst-Stride (or Stridette) support
    stockings
Jocath coronary balloon catheter
Jocath diagnostic catheter
Jocath graft connector
Jocath guidewire
Jocath stent
Jocath stent-graft
Jocath suture
Jocath ventricular assist device
Joe's hoe (retractor)
Jography angiographic catheter
Jography balloon catheter
Jography diagnostic catheter
Jography graft connector
Jography guidewire
Jography stent
Jography stent-graft
Jography suture
Jography ventricular assist device
Joguide balloon catheter
Joguide coronary guiding catheter
Joguide diagnostic catheter
Joguide graft connector
Joguide guidewire
Joguide stent
Joguide stent-graft
Joguide suture

Joguide ventricular assist device
Johns Hopkins coarctation clamp
Johns Hopkins forceps
Johnson-Stevens disease
Johnson thoracic forceps
joint
    costochondral
    costotransverse
    costovertebral
    interchondral
    manubriosternal
    secondary cartilaginous
    sternal
    sternoclavicular
    sternocostal
    xiphisternal
joint hyperextensibility
joint of thorax
Jonas modification of Norwood
    procedure
Jones criteria for acute rheumatic
    fever
Jones IMA forceps
Jones thoracic clamp
J orthogonal electrode
joule (pl. joules) (J)
joule shocks
J (junction) point on EKG tracing
J tip wire
J-tipped exchange guidewire
J-shaped lead
J-shaped tube
J-tipped spring guidewire
judicious vasodilation
Judkins 4 diagnostic catheter
Judkins cardiac catheterization
Judkins coronary angiography
Judkins coronary arteriography
Judkins coronary catheter
Judkins femoral catheterization
Judkins left 4 coronary catheter (JL4)
Judkins right 4 coronary catheter
    (JR4)

Judkins selective coronary
    arteriography
Judkins USCI catheter
jugular bulb, internal
jugular pulse tracing
jugular triangle, internal
jugular vein
    anterior
    external
jugular vein distention (JVD)
jugular veins filled from above
jugular veins filled from below
jugular venous distention (JVD)
jugular venous excursions
jugular venous impulse
jugular venous pressure (JVP)
jugular venous pressure collapse
jugular venous pulsation (pulse)
jugulovenous distention (JVD)
Julian thoracic forceps
jump vein graft
jump-graft
Junct (junctional)
junction
    aortic sinotubular
    atriocaval
    atrioventricular
    cardiophrenic
    caval-atrial
    chondrosternal
    costochondral
    iliocaval
    J
    mucocutaneous
    QRS-ST
    saphenofemoral
    sinotubular
    sternoclavicular
    subclavian
junctional bradycardia

junctional defect
junctional escape beats, atrio-
    ventricular
junctional escape rhythm
junctional extrasystole
junctional focus
junctional (nodal) rhythm
junctional impulse
junctional premature complex
junctional premature contraction,
    atrioventricular (AV)
junctional rhythm
junctional tachycardia
junction between AV node and bundle
    of His
June grass
Jürgensen sign
juvenile laryngoscope
juvenile sulfatidosis
juxta-anastomotic stenoses
juxta-apical impulse
juxta-arterial ventricular septal defect
juxtacapillary J receptors
juxtacrural
juxtaductal
juxtaductal coarctation of aorta
juxtaglomerular cell tumor
juxtaposed leftward
juxtaposed rightward
juxtaposition
juxtarenal aortic aneurysm
juxtarenal aortic atherosclerosis
juxtarenal cava
juxtatricuspid ventricular septal defect
JVD (jugulovenous or jugular venous
    distention)
JVP (jugular venous pressure)
J wave on EKG
J wire

K, k

KAAT II Plus intra-aortic balloon pump
K (vitamin) antagonist therapy
Kabuki make-up syndrome
Kairos pacemaker
Kairos rate-adaptive single and dual chamber pacemakers
kaliuretic effect of licorice
kallikrein-kinin system
Kalos pacemaker
Kaltostat wound packing material
kangaroo care
Kangaroo pump
Kantrowitz vascular scissors
Kaplan-Meier life-table
Kaposi sarcoma
   endobronchial
   epicardial
   intrathoracic
   myocardial infiltration by
   pulmonary
Kaposi-Besnier-Libman-Sacks syndrome
Kappa 400 Series pacemaker
Kapp-Beck-Thomson clamp
Karl Storz bronchoscope
Karmody venous scissors

Karp aortic punch forceps
Karplus sign of pleural effusion
Kartagener syndrome
Kartagener triad
karyolysis
karyorrhexis
Kasabach-Merritt phenomenon
Kasabach-Merritt syndrome
Kast syndrome
Kaster mitral valve prosthesis
Katayama snails
Katayama syndrome
Kattus treadmill exercise protocol
Katz-Wachtel phenomenon or sign
Kaufman-McKusick syndrome
Kawai bioptome
Kawasaki disease or syndrome
Kawashima technique
Kayexalate enema
Kayexalate via nasogastric tube
Kaye tamponade balloon catheter
Kay-Reed-Wooler anuloplasty
Kay-Shiley disk valve prosthesis
Kay-Shiley mitral valve
Kay-Suzuki disk prosthetic valve
Kay tricuspid valvuloplasty
kDa (kilodalton)

kDa antigen
kDa band
kDa profile
Kearns-Sayre syndrome
keeled chest
keel excision
keel, laryngeal
keel-like ridge
Keith bundle of fibers in heart
Keith-Flack sinoatrial node
Keith-Wagener-Barker classification of arteriolosclerosis, based on retinal changes, group 1-4
Kell blood antibody type
Kell blood group
Kellock sign of pleural effusion
Kelly forceps, curved
Kelly hemostat
Kelly retractor
Kelvin Sensor pacemaker
Kemp-Elliot-Gorlin syndrome
Kempner rice diet
Kendall Sequential Compression Device
Kennedy area-length method
Kennedy method for calculating ejection fraction
Kensey atherectomy catheter
Kensey catheter
Kent atrioventricular bundle in the heart
Kent bundle
Kent fibers
Kerckring nodule
Kerley A, B, or C lines
Kerra Boot
Kerrison rongeur
Keshan disease
ketamine, intramuscular
ketotifen
kick, atrial (AK)
Kidd blood antibody type

kidney arteriovenous fistula
kidney transplantation
Kifa catheter
Killip classification (I through IV) of heart disease
Killip classification of pump failure
Killip-Kimball classification of heart failure
Killip wire to give heart shock during cardiac arrest
Kim-Ray Greenfield caval filter
Kim-Ray Greenfield inferior vena caval filter
Kindt carotid artery occlusion clamp
KinetiX ventilation monitor
kinetocardiogram
King bioptome
King cardiac device
King-Mills procedure
King multipurpose coronary graft catheter
King syndrome
Kingella infection
kinked innominate artery
kinking
    carotid artery
    catheter
    innominate artery
kinking carotid artery
kinking of blood vessel
kinking of catheter
kinking of graft
kinking of patch
kinking of vessels secondary to shift of intrathoracic structures
Kinsey atherectomy catheter
Kirklin atrial retractor
Kirklin fence
kissing atherectomy technique
kissing balloon catheters
kissing balloon technique
Klauder syndrome

Klebsiella pneumoniae
Klebsiella rhinoscleromatis
Kleihauer-Betke test
Klein-Waardenburg syndrome
Klippel-Feil sequence
Klippel-Feil syndrome
Klippel-Trénaunay syndrome
Klippel-Trénaunay-Weber syndrome
knee-chest position
knife
    Bailey-Glover-O'Neill commis–
      surotomy
    Bard-Parker
    Beaver
    Brock commissurotomy
    cautery
    commissurotomy
    CyberKnife Express
    Derra commissurotomy
    Humby excisional
    intimectomy
    Lebsche sternal
    Lorenz PC/TC scissors ultrasharp
    UltraCision ultrasonic
    Visitec circular
    Visitec crescent
knitted Dacron graft
knitted double velour Dacron patch
  graft
knitted tantalum
knob
  aortic
  blurring of aortic
knock, pericardial
knots, half-hitch
knuckle sign
Kobert test for hemoglobin
Kocher grasping forceps
Kocher hemostats
Kocher maneuver
Koch reaction
Koch sinoatrial node

Koch triangle, apex of
Koch reaction
Koch sinoatrial node
KoGENate blood factor VIII product
Kohn, pores of
Kommerell diverticulum
Konno bioptome
Konno operation for aortic stenosis
Konno procedure for patch enlarge-
  ment of ascending aorta
Kontron balloon catheter
Kontron intra-aortic balloon
Kontron KAAT intra-aortic balloon
  pump
Kontron KAAT II+ intra-aortic
  balloon pump
"koo sur koo" (coup sur coup)
Korányi-Grocco sign
Korányi-Grocco triangle
Korányi sign of pleural effusion
Korotkoff method in Doppler
  cerebrovascular examination
Korotkoff sounds (in blood pressure
  determination by cuff method)
Korotkoff test for collateral circulation
Kostmann syndrome
Kouchoukos method
Kousseff syndrome
Krayenbuehl vessel hook
Krishaber disease
Kronecker puncture
Krovetz and Gessner equation
Kugel anastomosis
Kugel artery
Kugel collaterals
Kugelberg-Welander syndrome
Kurtz-Sprague-White syndrome
Kussmaul breathing
Kussmaul-Maier disease
Kussmaul-Maier variant
Kussmaul respiration
Kussmaul syndrome

Kussmaul venous sign

Kveim test

KVO (keep vein open) rate

kyphoscoliotic heart disease

kyphosis, loss of thoracic

L, l

LA (left atrium)
LAA (left atrial appendage)
LAA (left auricular appendage)
LA-Ao (left atrial to aortic [root] ratio)
LA-AR (left atrium/aortic root) ratio
LABA (laser-assisted balloon angioplasty)
Labbé syndrome
labeling, radioactive
labile blood pressure
labile hypertension
laboratory
    cardiac catheterization
    EP (electrophysiology)
labored breathing
labored respirations
LACD (left apexcardiogram, calibrated displacement)
lactate dehydrogenase (LDH)
lactate, elevated plasma
lactic acid accumulation
lactic acidosis
lactic dehydrogenase
Lactoprene mesh
Lactoprene surgical clip

Lactoprene surgical staple
Lactoprene suture
Lactoprene suture anchor
Lactoprene vascular occlusion device
lacunae, bluish nail
lacunar infarct
LAD (left anterior descending) coronary artery
LAD (left axis deviation)
LAD saphenous vein graft angioplasty
LAD wraps around the apex
Ladder diagram
LAE (left atrial enlargement)
Laënnec pearls
Laënnec sign
Laerdal resuscitator
LAFB (left anterior fascicular block)
Lahey bag
Lahey thoracic forceps
LAID (left anterior internal diameter)
LAIS excimer laser for coronary angioplasty
lake, lipid
Laks method
LAM (lymphangioleiomyomatosis)
LAMA (laser-assisted microanastomosis)

LAMA (laser-assisted microvascular
   anastomosis)
LAMB (lentigines, atrial myxoma,
   blue nevi) syndrome
Lambda pacemaker
Lambert aortic clamp
Lambert-Eaton syndrome
Lambert-Kay vascular clamp
Lambl excrescences
lamellar body density (LBD) count
lamina
   elastic
   internal elastic
lamina propria
laminated clot
laminar flow
laminated intraluminal thrombus
laminography, cardiac
Landis-Gibbon test
Lancisi muscle
Lancisi sign
landmark, bony
Landolfi sign
Landouzy-Dejerine dystrophy
Langerhans cell granulomatosis
Langhans giant cells
LAO (left anterior oblique)
LAO position
LAO projection
LAP (left atrial pressure)
LaparoSonic coagulating shears for
   autograft harvesting
laparotomy, median xiphopubic
Laplace effect
Laplace law
Laplace mechanism
large-bore slotted aspirating needle
large-caliber tube
large-cell carcinoma
large cell neuroendocrine carcinoma of
   the lung
large defibrillating patch

large obtuse marginal branch
large patch lead
large Q waves
large thymus shadow obscuring
   cardiac silhouette
large undifferentiated cells (LUCs)
large vein pulsation
large venous tributaries
Larsen syndrome
laryngeal cartilage
laryngeal edema
laryngeal epilepsy
laryngeal fistulectomy
laryngeal fracture
laryngeal keel
laryngeal nerve, recurrent
laryngeal nodule
laryngeal papillomatosis
laryngeal rales
laryngeal vertigo
laryngeal vestibule
laryngeal web
laryngectomy, radical
laryngis, pachyderma
laryngismus stridulus
laryngitis
   acute
   catarrhal
   Haemophilus influenzae
   hypertrophic
laryngitis sicca
laryngogram, contrast
laryngopharyngectomy
laryngoplegia
laryngoscope
   juvenile
   pediatric
laryngoscopy
laryngospasm
laryngostomy
laryngotracheal bronchitis
laryngotracheal fistulectomy

laryngotracheitis
laryngotracheobronchitis
larynx, artificial
laser
   AccuLase excimer
   ARC (argon beam electro-
      coagulator)
   argon
   Candela 405-nm pulsed dye
   ClearView CO_2
   CO_2 (carbon dioxide)
   DermaLase
   Eclipse TMR
   Eclipse TMR holmium
   erbium:YAG
   excimer
   GentleLASE Plus
   Heart Laser for TMR (trans-
      myocardial revascularization)
   helium-neon
   Ho:YAG (holmium:yttrium
      aluminum garnet)
   holmium
   infrared-pulsed
   ion
   Lastec System angioplasty
   microsecond pulsed flashlamp
      pumped dye
   Nd:YAG (neodymium:yttrium-
      aluminum-garnet)
   PhotoGenica V-Star pulsed-dye
   Polaris 1.32 Nd:YAG
   SLS (Spectranetics laser sheath)
   Visulas Nd:YAG
   XeCl
laser ablation
laser angioplasty
laser-assisted balloon angioplasty
   (LABA)
laser-assisted microanastomosis
   (LAMA)
laser-assisted microvascular
   anastomosis (LAMA)

laser balloon angioplasty (LBA)
laser desiccation of thrombus
Laserdish electrode
Laserdish pacing lead
Laserflo blood perfusion monitor
   (BPM)
laser-light vaporization of intimal
   plaque material
laser photocoagulation, intraoperative
   (for ventricular tachycardia)
laser photocoagulation of capillary
   malformation (CM)
Laserprobe-PLR Plus
laser recanalization
laser thermal coronary angioplasty
LASH (left anterior-superior hemiblock)
lasing techniques
Laslett-Short syndrome
Lastac System angioplasty laser
late asthmatic response
late diastolic murmur
late false aneurysm
late graft occlusion
late inspiratory crackles
late-onset asthma
late phase
late potential activity, ventricular
late potentials (after-potentials)
lateral basal bronchi
lateral bronchi
lateral costotransverse ligament
lateral decubitus position
lateral hemispheric asymmetry (in
   heart rate modulation)
lateral leaflet obliteration
lateral precordial leads
lateral precordium
lateral thoracic vein periphlebitis
lateral thrombus
lateral webs
late systolic bulge

late systolic click
late systolic honk
late systolic impulse
late systolic murmur (LSM)
late systolic posterior displacement on
  echocardiogram
late systolic retraction
late systolic whoop
latex, two-layer
latissimus dorsi muscle
Laubry-Pezzi syndrome
Laubry-Soulle syndrome
Laurence-Moon-Biedl-Bardet
  syndrome
Laurer forceps
lavage
  bronchoalveolar (BAL)
  bronchopulmonary
  bronchoscopy
  continuous pericardial
  pleural
  pulsatile
  pulsed
  saline
  tracheal-bronchial
  tracheobronchial
  whole-lung (WLL)
law
  Einthoven
  Laplace
  Starling
laxa, cutis
layer
  bright
  circumferential echodense
  echodense
  echo-free
  hypoechoic
  inner bright
  musculofascial
  parietal
  platysma

layer *(cont.)*
  sonolucent
  subcuticular
  visceral
lazy H incision
lazy leukocyte syndrome
lazy Z incision
LBA (laser balloon angioplasty)
LBBB (left bundle branch block)
LBCD (left border of cardiac dullness)
LCA (left coronary artery)
L-Cath single-lumen polyurethane
  peripherally inserted central
  catheter
LCF or LCX (left circumflex)
  coronary artery
LCL (Levinthal-Coles-Lillie) bodies
LD or LDH (lactate dehydrogenase)
LD_1 or LDH_1 isoenzyme
LD_2 or LDH_2 isoenzyme
LDH_1, LDH_2, flipped
LDH_1 or LDH_2 isoenzyme
LDH_1-LDH_2 ratio
LDL (low-density lipoprotein)
lead (see also *electrode*)
  Accufix bipolar
  Accufix pacemaker
  Accufix pacing
  active fixation
  Aescula left ventricular (LV)
    cardiac
  AngeFlex
  anterior precordial
  anterolateral
  anteroseptal
  atrial
  atrial J
  augmented bipolar limb
  augmented limb: aVR, aVL, aVF
  barb-tip
  bifurcated J-shaped tined atrial
    pacing and defibrillation

lead *(cont.)*
  bipolar
  bipolar endocardial
  bipolar limb
  bipolar precordial
  braided
  break in insulation of
  Cadence TVL nonthoracotomy
  CapSure
  Cardifix EZ pacing
  cathodal
  chest
  CM5
  cobra-head epicardial
  Cordis pacing
  coronary sinus
  CPI Sweet Tip
  CPI ventricular
  deep limb
  DF (defibrillation, Telectronics
    endocardial)
  dislodgement of
  EKG
  electrode
  Encor pacing
  endocardial
  Endotak C
  Endotak Picotip cardiac
    defibrillation
  Endotak Reliance
  ensiform cartilage: V_E
  epicardial
  epicardial pacemaker
  esophageal: E_{15}, E_{24}, E_{50}, etc.
  finned pacemaker
  fishhook
  Flextend pacing
  Frank
  Frank XYZ orthogonal
  grounding
  Hombach placement of
  impedance

lead *(cont.)*
  infected
  inferior
  inferior precordial
  inferolateral
  J-shaped
  Laserdish pacing
  lateral
  lateral precordial
  left precordial
  Lewis
  limb
  Mason-Likar placement of EKG
  Medtronic Sprint Quattro Secure
  monitor
  myocardial screw-in rate-sensing
  nonthoracotomy
  I ("one") (right arm, left arm)
  orthogonal Frank XYZ EKG
  Oscor pacing
  pacemaker
  pacing
  pacing/sensing
  passive fixation
  Polyrox fractal active fixation
  Possis epicardial pacing
  precordial: V_1 through V_9
  rate-sensing
  Retrox fractal active fixation
  reversed arm
  right precordial: V_{3R}, V_{4R}, etc.
  right ventricular endocardial
    sensing lead
  right-sided chest
  scalar
  screw-in
  screw-in straight atrial
  screw-on
  screw-on epicardial pacemaker
  screw-on epimyocardial
  screw-tipped
  sew-on

lead *(cont.)*
 shock(ing)
 side-wire pacing
 silicone
 Sprint Quattro Secure
 SRT (segmented ring tripolar)
 standard (bipolar): I, II, III
 standard limb
 steroid-eluting
 steroid-eluting active fixation
 superior vena cava
 sutureless electrode
 Telectronics endocardial
  defibrillation (DF)
 Telectronics pacing
 temporary pacemaker
 Tendril DX implantable pacing
 Tendril SDX pacing
 third interspace: $3V_1$, $3V_2$, etc.
 III ("three") (left arm, left leg)
 ThinLine EZ bipolar cardiac
  pacing
 three-turn epicardial
 tined
 tined atrial J pacing/defibrillation
 tined J
 Transvene
 transvenous ventricular sensing
 tripolar tined endocardial
 II ("two") (right arm, left leg)
 two-turn epicardial
 unipolar
 unipolar limb
 unipolar precordial
 urethane
 vector
 ventricular
 V_1 through V_6
 Wilson central terminal on EKG
 XYZ Frank EKG
lead configuration
 bidirectional
 unidirectional

lead dislodgement
lead electrode malfunction
lead fracture
lead impedance
lead insulation break
lead malfunction
lead migration
lead placement, chronic
lead resistance
lead reversal
lead system, Transvene
lead threshold
leaflet, leaflets
 anterior
 anterior mitral (AML)
 anterior mitral valve
 anterior motion of posterior mitral
  valve
 anterior tricuspid (ATL)
 aortic valve
 apposition
 arching of mitral valve
 ballooning of
 bileaflet
 billowing mitral (BML)
 bowing of mitral valve
 calcified
 cleft
 coaptation of
 commissural
 conjoined
 degenerated
 doming of
 doughnut-shaped prolapsing
 flail mitral
 floating
 fluttering of valvular
 fused
 hammocking of
 incompetent
 mitral valve
 mural
 myxomatous valve

leaflet *(cont.)*
  nodularity of
  noncalcified mitral
  noncoronary
  paradoxical motion of
  poorly mobile
  posterior
  posterior mitral (PML)
  posterior mitral valve
  posterior tricuspid (PTL)
  prolapse of
  prolapsed
  pseudomitral
  redundant aortic
  redundant mitral valve
  sail-like anterior
  septal
  thickened
  tricuspid valve
  trileaflet
  valve
leaflet cleft
leaflet fusion
leaflet incompetence
leaflet motion
leaflet prolapse
  anterior
  posterior
leaflet tip
leak, leakage
  air
  aortic paravalvular
  baffle
  blood
  capillary
  chyle
  current
  endoleak
  generalized capillary
  interatrial baffle
  mitral
  paraprosthetic

leak *(cont.)*
  paravalvular
  periprosthetic
  perivalvular
leaking vein
leaky valve
leather valve cutter
leather venous valvulotome
Lebsche sternal knife
LeCompte maneuver
LeCompte modification of arterial
  switch operation
Lectron II electrode gel
ledge, eccentric
Lee bronchus clamp
Lee microvascular clamp
Lees artery forceps
Lee-White whole blood clotting time
  method
left accessory pathways
left anterior chest wall
left anterior descending (LAD) artery,
  superdominant
left anterior descending coronary
  artery takeoff
left anterior descending occlusion
left anterior fascicular heart block
left anterior hemiblock
left anterior oblique projection
left atrial active emptying fraction
left atrial active emptying volume
left atrial appendage
left atrial cannulation
left atrial chamber
left atrial contraction
left atrial diameter
left atrial end-diastolic pressure
left atrial enlargement
left atrial maximal volume
left atrial myxoma
left atrial pressure (LAP)
left atrial tension

left atrial thrombosis
left atrial to aortic (root) ratio
  (LA/Ao, LA-Ao)
left atrial vent
left atriotomy for mitral valve surgery
left atrium, giant
left auricle
left auricular appendage (LAA)
left axis deviation
left border of heart
left bundle branch block (LBBB)
left bundle branch hemiblock
left circumflex (LCX) coronary artery
left common femoral artery
left coronary artery arising from
  pulmonary artery
left coronary artery, dominant
left coronary cusp
left coronary plexus (of heart)
left fibrous trigone
left fifth intercostal space
left free-wall pathway
left-handedness, ventricular
left heart catheter
left heart failure
left heart pressure
left iliac system
left internal mammary artery (LIMA)
  graft
left Judkins catheter
left lower lobe
left lower lobe collapse
left lower parasternal heave
left lung collapsed
left lung retracted under a laparotomy
  pad
left main coronary artery (LMCA)
left main stem bronchus
left paramedian incision
left pleural apical hematoma cap
left pleural cap
left posterior fascicular heart block

left posterior hemiblock
left posterolateral thoracotomy
left precordial Q waves
left pulmonary artery
left pulmonary cusp
left-right asymmetry
left semilunar valve
left-sided heart failure
left sinoatrial node, vestigial
left sternal border
left subcostal approach
left to right shunt of blood
left to right ventricular pressure ratio
left to right ventricular shunt
left upper lobe, emphysematous
  expansion of
left ventricle
  double-inlet
  hypoplastic
  morphologic
left ventricle hypoplasia
left ventricle to aorta baffle
left ventricle to pulmonary artery
  conduit
left ventricular afterload
left ventricular apical to aorta
  (LV-Ao) conduit
left ventricular assist device (LVAD)
  (see *ventricular assist device*)
left ventricular assist system (LVAS)
left ventricular bypass pump
left ventricular cavity pressure
left ventricular chamber
left ventricular contractility, deranged
left ventricular dysfunction, exercise-
  induced
left ventricular ejection fraction by
  acoustic quantification
left ventricular ejection time, increased
left ventricular end-diastolic pressure
  (LVEDP)
left ventricular end-diastolic volume

left ventricular end-systolic volume
left ventricular filling
left ventricular heave, sustained
left ventricular hypertrophy (LVH)
left ventricular hypoplasia
left ventricular impulse, prolonged
left ventricular lift
left ventricular loading
left ventricular maximal volume
left ventricular outflow tract
    obstruction (LVOTO)
left ventricular papillary muscle
left ventricular patch placed over
    diaphragmatic surface of the left
    ventricle
left ventricular preload
left ventricular preponderance
left ventricular pressure
left ventricular reconditioning
left ventricular reduction myoplasty
left ventricular regional wall motion
    abnormality
left ventricular retraining
left ventricular segmental contraction
left ventricular shortening fraction
left ventricular stenotic pulmonary
    artery
left ventricular stroke work (LVSW)
left ventricular stroke work index
    (LVSWI)
left ventricular systolic pump function
left ventricular systolic time interval
    ratio
left ventricular thrombosis
left ventricular thrust
left ventricular to descending aorta
    (LV-DAo) conduit
left ventricular vent
left ventricular volume
left ventriculogram
left ventriculography
left vocal cord

leg claudication
leg edema
leg fatigue
leg pain at rest
leg, postphlebitic
Legend pacemaker
Legionella pneumophila infection
legionnaires' disease
Lehman cardiac device
Lehman ventriculography catheter
Leiden factor
Leigh syndrome
leiomyomatosis of heart
leiomyosarcoma of the heart
leiomyosarcoma, right atrial extension
    of uterine
Leios pacemaker
Leitner syndrome
Lejeune thoracic forceps
Leland-Jones vascular clamp
Lemmon intimal dissector
Lemmon sternal approximator
Lemmon sternal spreader
Lenègre acquired complete heart block
Lenègre disease or syndrome
length
    basic cycle (BCL)
    basic drive (BDL)
    basic drive cycle (BDCL)
    chordal
    drive cycle
    paced cycle (PCL)
    sinus cycle
    VA block cycle
    wave
lentigines, multiple
lentiginosis
    cardiomyopathic
    diffuse
    progressive cardiomyopathic
lentis, ectopia
Lenz syndrome

LEOPARD (lentigines, electrocardiographic abnormalities, ocular
hypertelorism, pulmonary valve
stenosis, abnormalities of genitalia,
retardation of growth, and deaf-
ness) syndrome
Leptos pacemaker
leptospirosis
Leriche syndrome
Lermans-Means scratch
Lermans-Means systolic grating sound
lesion
  acanthotic
  accessible
  acquired
  angulated
  aortic arch
  atherosclerotic
  bifurcation
  Blumenthal
  Bracht-Wachter
  calcified
  central
  circular cherry-red
  coin
  complex
  concentric
  constrictive
  coronary artery
  coronary branch ostial
  critical
  cryosurgical
  culprit
  de novo
  Dieulafoy's gastric
  diffuse
  discrete
  eccentric
  eccentric restenosis
  endobronchial
  extrinsic
  flow-compromising

lesion *(cont.)*
  flow-limiting
  focal
  friable
  hemodynamically significant
  high-grade
  high-grade obstructive
  hourglass-shaped
  hyperplastic
  intrinsic stenotic
  Janeway
  jet
  lesions
  mixed
  multifocal
  multiverrucous friable
  noninfective endocardial
  occlusive
  occult
  ostial
  oval cherry-red raised
  partial
  regurgitant
  rheumatic
  secondary
  segmental
  serial
  space-occupying
  spherical
  stenotic
  subtotal
  tandem
  target
  telangiectatic
  tight
  total
  transmural linear
  tubular
  type A, B, or C
  ulcerated
  unstable
  valvular regurgitant
  vegetative

lesser saphenous vein
lesser saphenous vein in situ bypass
less-than-full pause
lethal arrhythmias
lethal consequences
lethal midline granuloma
lethal multiple pterygium syndrome
lethal myocardial injury
lethal tachyarrhythmia
lethargy
Letterer-Siwe disease
leukemia
    chronic myeloid (CML)
    chronic myelomonocytic (CMML)
    eosinophilic
    granulocytic
    null cell lymphoblastic
leukocyte-depleted terminal blood
    cardioplegic solution
leukocyte-poor red blood cells
leukocyte reduction filter
leukocytes, polymorphonuclear
leukocytic infiltration of submucosa
leukocytic trapping of bacteria
leukocytoblastic vasculitis
leukocytosis
    intravascular polymorphonuclear
    polymorphonuclear
LeukoNet filter
leukopenia, drug-induced
leukoplakia
leuko-poor red blood cells
Leukos pacemaker
Leukotrap RC (red cell) storage
    system
leukotrienes
Lev acquired complete heart block
Lev classification of complete AV
    block
Lev disease or syndrome
LeVeen plaque-cracker

level
    air-fluid
    baseline (of drugs or lab values)
    beta thromboglobulin plasma
    $beta_2$-microglobulin
    complement
    cotinine
    elevated serum lactate
    fluid
    IgE
    interferon gamma
    peak and trough (of drug)
    ring shadows with air-fluid
    serum phosphorus
    subtherapeutic
    theophylline
    thiocyanate blood
    threshold
level of first division of main stem
    bronchus
Levine-Harvey classification of heart
    murmur
Levine sign or test
Levinthal-Coles-Lillie (LCL) bodies
levocardia
levoposition
levorotatory
levotransposition (L-transposition)
levoversion
Levovist (d-galactose; palmitic acid)
Lewis and Pickering test for
    peripheral circulation
Lewis angle
Lewis lead
Lewis upper limb cardiovascular
    disease
LGL (Lown-Ganong-Levine)
    syndrome
LGL variant syndrome
LHMT (low-range heparin manage-
    ment test)

Lian-Siguier-Welti venous thrombosis
   syndrome
liberation of thromboplastic material
   into circulation
Libman-Sacks endocarditis disease
Libman-Sacks syndrome
licorice ingestion, chronic excessive
licorice ingestion-related hypertension
licorice, kaliuretic effect of
LICS (left intercostal space)
Liddle aortic clamp
Liddle syndrome
Lido-Pen Auto-Injector
lidocaine, aerosolized
lidocaine drip
lidocaine neurotoxicity
lidocaine spray, topical
Liebermann-Burchard reaction
Liebermann-Burchard test
Liebow and Carrington classification
   for pulmonary eosinophilia
lifelong anticoagulation
lifelong smoker
Life-Pack 5 cardiac monitor
life-saver or doughnut of Teflon felt
Lifespan ePTFE vascular graft
Lifestream coronary dilatation catheter
Lifestream personal cholesterol
   monitor
lifestyle changes
lifestyle, sedentary
life-table
   Kaplan-Meier
   Mantel-Haenszel
life-threatening hemorrhage
life-threatening pneumothorax
life-threatening respiratory distress
life-threatening ventricular arrhythmias
LifeVest WCD 3000 external
   cardioverter-defibrillator
LifeVest wearable cardiac defibrillator

lift
   aneurysmal
   ectopic
   late systolic parasternal
   left ventricular
   parasternal
   parasternal systolic
   pulmonary artery
   right ventricular
   sternal
   substernal
   sustained right ventricular
Ligaclip
ligament
   conus
   Cooper
   costoxiphoid
   inferior pulmonary
   intra-articular
   lateral costotransverse
   Poupart
   pulmonary
   radiate
   sternopericardial
   superior costotransverse
ligament of Treitz
ligamentum arteriosum
ligamentum teres cardiopexy
ligate
ligation
   intrapericardial
   PDA (patent ductus arteriosus)
   selective vascular
ligation of communicating veins
ligation of perforators
ligature
   popliteal veins
   rubber band
   silk
   stump
   suture
   tape

light chain, myosin
lightheaded
lightheadedness
light reflection rheography
Lilienthal rib spreader
Lillehei-Cruz-Kaster prosthesis
Lillehei-Hardy-Hunter operation
Lillehei-Kaster mitral valve
   prosthesis
Lillehei-Kaster pivoting-disk
   prosthetic valve
Lillehei valve forceps
LIMA (left internal mammary artery)
   graft
LIMA-Lift procedure
limb
   decreased inspiratory
   Gore-Tex
limb asymmetry
limb-girdle dystrophy
limb ischemia
limb of artery
limb of bifurcation graft
limb of vein
limb salvage
limb-shaking TIA (transient ischemic
   attack)
limb-threatening ischemia
limb-threatening thrombosis
limbus fossae ovalis
limbus of Vieussens
limited respiratory chest excursion
limited thoracotomy
limulus amebocyte lysate assay
linacography
Lincoln-Metzenbaum scissors
Lindesmith operation
Lindholm tracheal tube
line
   A (arterial)
   Aldrich-Mees
   anterior axillary

line *(cont.)*
   aortic
   arterial
   axillary
   central venous
   central venous pressure (CVP)
   commissural
   Correra
   demarcation
   Eberth
   Ellis
   Ellis-Garland
   intravenous
   isoelectric
   Kerley A, B, C
   Linton
   lower lung
   Mees
   midaxillary
   midclavicular (MCL)
   midscapular
   midsternal
   monitoring
   peripheral intravenous infusion
   posterior axillary
   radial arterial
   radial artery
   subpleural curvilinear
   suture
   Swan-Ganz radial artery pressure
      monitoring
   transcutaneous drive
   triple-lumen
   venous
   Z
   Zahn
linea alba
linear artifact
linear atelectasis
linear scar in lungs
linear shadow
linear tear

linea semicircularis
lingula involvement
lingula, right middle lobe
lingular artery
lingular bronchus
    inferior
    superior
lingular orifice
Linton line
Linton open subfascial division tech-
    nique in treatment of varicose veins
Linton treatment of varicose veins
Linx exchange guidewire
LINX-EZ cardiac device
LionHeart left ventricular assist device
Liotta-BioImplant LPB prosthetic
    valve
Liotta TAH (total artificial heart)
LIP (lymphocytic interstitial pneu-
    monitis)
lipemia retinalis
lipid
    plasma
    serum levels of
lipid deposits
lipid-laden plaque
lipid lake
lipid-lowering therapy
lipid-rich material
lipid tests
lipid zone
lipofuscin
lipofuscinosis
    ceroid
    neuronal ceroid
lipogranulomatosis, Farber's
lipoid material
lipoid pneumonia or pneumonitis
lipoma, cardiac
lipomatous hypertrophy of the
    interatrial septum
lipophilic anticancer compounds

lipopolysaccharide
lipoprotein
    high-density (HDL)
    intermediate density (IDL)
    low-density (LDL)
    plasma
    very-low-density (VLDL)
lipoprotein electrophoresis
lipoprotein lipase deficiency
lipoprotein plasminogen inhibition
lipoproteins
liposarcoma of the heart
Liposorber LA-15 system
liquefactive emphysema
LiquiVent liquid intrapulmonary
    ventilating agent
LITE (low-intensity treadmill
    exercise) protocol
liters per minute per meter squared
    (L/min./m^2)
Litespeed catheter
Litespeed endovascular grafting
    system
Litespeed stent
Litespeed synthetic vascular graft
Litespeed wire
lithium pacemaker
Litten diaphragm phenomenon
Littleford-Spector introducer
Littman defibrillation pad
Litwak cannula
Litwak left atrial-aortic bypass
Litwak mitral valve scissors
livedo reticularis-digital infarct
livedo vasculitis
liver cirrhosis
liver function
liver-jugular sign
liverlike lung
livid
Livierato sign
Livierato reflex

living related transplant (LRT)
L-loop heart
L-looping
L-loop ventricular situs
Lloyd-Davies scissors
L-malposition of aorta
LMCA (left main coronary artery)
L/min./m² (liters per minute per
    meter squared)
loading dose
loading wire cut at tip and
    withdrawn, leaving two nylon
    strands holding device
loads
    combination flow and pressure
    predominantly flow
    pure pressure
lobar agenesis (of lung)
lobar bronchus (pl. bronchi)
lobar cavitation
lobar consolidation
lobar emphysema, congenital
lobar lung atrophy
lobar pneumonia
lobe, lobes
    accessory
    azygos
    left lower
    left middle
    left upper
    right lower
    right middle
    right upper
    sequestered (lung)
lobe collapse, left lower
lobectomy
    en masse
    right middle
    SIS (simultaneous individual
        stapling)
lobe of azygos vein
lobulated filling defect

lobulated saccular appearance
lobules
local blood oximetry
localization
    CT-directed hook wire
    percutaneous (of pulmonary
        nodules using suture-ligated
        microcoils)
localized mass effect
localized obstructive emphysema
localized stabbing pain
local thrombolytic therapy
location, precordial impulse
locked lung syndrome
lock-tip connector
lock washer configuration
locoregional recurrence of metastases
loculated collections of old clotted
    blood
loculated fluid collection
Loeffler (Löffler)
Loeffler disease
Loeffler endocarditis
Loeffler endomyocardial syndrome
Loeffler eosinophilia
Loeffler fibroblastic endocarditis
Loeffler parietal fibroplastic endo-
    carditis
Loeffler pneumonia
Loeffler syndrome
Loeffler variant
Loehr-Kindberg syndrome
Löffler (Loeffler)
Löfgren syndrome
log, episode
Logocath electrophysiology catheter
long ACE fixed-wire balloon catheter
long-acting bronchodilator
long-acting drugs
long axial oblique view
long axis
long-axis parasternal view

long-axis view
long chain acyl-CoA dehydrogenase
Longdwel Teflon catheter
longitudinal aortotomy
longitudinal arteriography
longitudinal arteriotomy
longitudinal incision
longitudinally
longitudinal muscles
longitudinal narrowing
long Péan clamp
long Q-T interval
long Q-T syndrome
long segment narrowing
Long Skinny over-the-wire balloon
    catheter
long taper/stiff shaft Glidewire
long-term anticoagulation
long thoracic nerve
loop
    capillary
    counterclockwise superiorly
        oriented frontal QRS
    endarterectomy
    flow-volume
    Gerdy interauricular
    J (on catheterization)
    P (on vectorcardiography)
    QRS
    reentrant
    rubber vessel
    silastic
    subclavian
    T (on vectorcardiography)
    vector
    ventricular
    vessel
    Vieussens
loop diuretics
loops, Retract-O-Tape surgical vessel
loose cough
Lo-Por tracheal tube

Lo-Por vascular graft prosthesis
Lo-Profile and Lo-Profile II balloon
    catheter
Lo-Profile steerable dilatation catheter
Lorenz PC/TC scissors ultrasharp
    knife
loss of AV synchrony
loss of capture of pacemaker
loss of lung elasticity
loss of postural tone
loss of sensing of pacemaker
loss of thoracic kyphosis
Lotensin (benazepril HCl)
Lotrel (amlodipine besylate,
    benazepril HCl)
loud friction rub
loud murmur (high-grade)
loud pulmonic component of second
    heart sound
loud pulmonic second sound
Louis, sternal angle of
Lovén reflex
low-amplitude P wave
low cardiac output syndrome
low-cholesterol diet
low-density lipoprotein (LDL)
low-dose heparin prophylaxis
lower left sternal border
lower lobe lung mass
lower lung line
lower rate interval
lower respiratory tract disease
Lower rings (Richard Lower)
Lower-Shumway cardiac orthotopic
    transplant technique
lower sternal pulsation
Lower tubercle (Richard Lower)
low-fat diet
low-flow syndrome
low-frequency diastolic murmur
low-frequency positive-pressure
    ventilation

low-grade fever
low-intensity systolic click
low-level contamination
low-level treadmill
low-lying bifurcation
low moderate rejection
Lown and Graboys classification of
ventricular arrhythmias
Lown classification of ventricular premature beats
Lown-Ganong-Levine syndrome
(LGL) syndrome
Lown modified grading system for
ventricular arrhythmia
low-osmolar nonionic contrast agent
low-output heart failure
low-output syndrome
low oxygen saturation
low-pitched rhonchi
low-pitched, rumbling apical
diastolic murmur
low-pressure cardiac tamponade
low-profile balloon cannula
low profile balloon feeding device
low-profile bioprosthesis
low-range heparin management test
(LHMT)
low-renin essential hypertension
syndrome
low-salt diet
low-salt syndrome
low septal right atrium
low-sodium diet
low-speed rotational angioplasty
catheter
low wedge pressure
Lp(a) (apolipoprotein)
LPA (left pulmonary artery)
LPFB (left posterior fascicular block)
LPH (left posterior hemiblock)
LPS balloon catheter
LPS Peel-Away introducer

LPV (left pulmonary vein)
LQTS (long QT syndrome)
LRA (low right atrium)
LRT (living related transplant)
LSB (lower sternal border)
LSCVP (left subclavian central venous
pressure)
L-shaped incision
L-shaped trocar
LSM (late systolic murmur)
L-transposition (levotransposition)
L-transposition of great arteries
LubriCath catheter
Lubri-Sil catheter
Lucas-Champonnière disease
Lucchese mitral valve dilator
LUCs (large undifferentiated cells)
Ludovici angle
Ludwig angina
Ludwig angle
Luer fitting
Luer-Lok connector
luer-locked
Luer-Lok ports
Luer-Lok syringe
Luer-Slip connector
Luer-Slip IAB catheter
lues myocarditis
luetic aortic aneurysm
luetic aortitis
luetic arteritis
Lugol fixative solution
Lukens collector
Lukens trap
Lumaguide catheter
lumbotomy
lumen (pl. lumens, lumina)
    aortic
    arterial
    bronchial
    cloverleaf-shaped
    crescentic

lumen *(cont.)*
    D-shaped vessel
    double-barrel
    eccentrically placed
    elliptical
    false
    fistula
    slit-shaped vessel
    slitlike
    star-shaped vessel
    true
    vascular
lumen diameter, minimal
lumen-intimal interface
lumen of the fistula
lumenogram
Lumina guidewire
luminal area
luminal caliber
luminal configuration, scalloped
luminal contour, irregular hazy
luminal cross-sectional area
luminal diameter
luminal dimension
luminal encroachment
luminal irregularity
luminal narrowing
luminal plaquing
luminal silhouette
luminal stenosis
luminal thrombosis
Luminexx biliary stent and stent
    delivery system
Lumiscan 150 scanner
lump in the throat
lumpy appearance of lung
lung
    accessory
    acquired unilateral hyperlucent
    air-conditioner
    airless
    aluminosis of

lung *(cont.)*
    arc welder's
    artificial
    bauxite
    bird breeder's
    bird fancier's
    bird handler's
    black
    brown
    bubbly
    budgerigar-fancier's
    cardiac
    cheese handler's
    cheese washer's
    coal miner's
    coal worker's
    coffee worker's
    collapsed
    consolidated
    cork handler's
    cork worker's
    corundum smelter's
    dark and mottled
    drowned
    dynamic
    empty collapsed
    eosinophilic
    farmer's
    fibroid
    fish-meal worker's
    fresh
    furrier's
    gangrene of
    grain handler's
    hardened
    harvester's
    hen worker's
    honeycomb
    humidifier
    hyperlucent
    hypogenetic
    light pink

lung *(cont.)*
  liverlike
  malt worker's
  maple bark-stripper's
  mason's
  meat wrapper's
  miller's
  miner's
  mottled gray
  mushroom worker's
  pigeon-breeder's
  pigeon-fancier's
  premature infant's
  pump
  pseudocysts of
  rheumatoid
  septic
  shock
  silicotic
  silo-filler's
  silver finisher's
  silver polisher's
  static
  stiff noncompliant
  stretched
  subsegment of
  thatched roof worker's
  thresher's
  tropical eosinophilic
  underventilated
  unilateral hyperlucent
  vanishing
  wedge resection of
  welder's
  wet
  white
lung abscess
  nonputrid
  putrid
lung agenesis
lung airspace
lung allograft

lung apex (pl. apices)
lung architecture
lung biopsy
lung calculus
lung carcinoma
lung cirrhosis
lung collapse
  massive
  postoperative acute massive
lung compliance, decreased
lung consolidation
lung decortication
lung diffusion test
lung disease
  idiopathic eosinophilic
  interstitial
lung disease and associated secretory
  problems
lunger disease
lunger pulmonary adenomatosis
lung expansion
lung fever
lung field, collapsed
lung fissure
lung fluke disease
lung hemangioma
lung hepatization
lung hypoplasia
lung infiltrates (infiltration)
lung inflammation
lung injury, penetrating
lung lobule
lung mass
lung mass with mediastinal invasion
lung necrosis
lung overinflation
lung parenchyma consolidation
lung periphery
lung reexpansion
lung resection
lung scan, perfusion and ventilation

lungs clear to A & P (auscultation and percussion)
lung segment, infarcted
lung sounds, adventitious
lung stiffness
lung transplantation
lung tumor resection
lung volume
   diminished
   end-expiratory
lung volume asymmetry (on x-ray)
lung volume determination
   FRC (functional residual capacity)
   RV (residual volume)
   TLC (total lung capacity)
   VC (vital capacity)
lung volume reduction surgery (LVRS), unilateral
lung washout
lungworm
lunula (pl. lunulae)
lupus erythematosus
   neonatal
   systemic
lupus-like syndrome
Luschka muscle
lusoria, dysphagia
Lutembacher complex
Lutembacher syndrome
Lu-Tex (lutetium texaphyrin)
Lutheran blood group
Lutz-Splendore-Almeida disease
Lutz-Splendore-Almeida paracoccidioidomycosis
luxury perfusion
LV (left ventricular) function
   pressure
LV (left ventricular) function wall motion
LVAD (left ventricular assist device), HeartMate
LVAS (left ventricular assist system) implantable pump

LVd (left ventricular diastolic dimension)
LVD (left ventricular dysfunction)
LVEDD (left ventricular end-diastolic dimension)
LVEDI (left ventricular end-diastolic volume index)
LVEDP (left ventricular end diastolic pressure)
LVEF (left ventricular ejection fraction)
LVESD (left ventricular end-systolic dimension)
LVESVI (left ventricular end-systolic volume index)
LVET (left ventricular ejection time)
LVFS (left ventricular functional shortening)
LVFW (left ventricular free wall)
LVG (left ventriculogram)
LVH (left ventricular hypertrophy)
LVH with strain
LVID (left ventricular internal diameter or dimension)
LVIDD (left ventricular internal diastolic dimension)
LVIEd (left ventricular internal dimension at end-diastole)
LVIEs (left ventricular internal dimension at end-systole)
LVIV (left ventricular inflow volume)
LVM (left ventricular mass)
LVMI (left ventricular mass index)
LVOT (left ventricular outflow tract)
LVOTO (left ventricular outflow tract obstruction)
LVOV (left ventricular outflow volume)
LVP (left ventricular pressure)
LVP1 and LVP2 (left ventricular pressure on apex cardiogram)

LVPW (left ventricular posterior wall)
LVRS (lung volume reduction surgery)
LVS (left ventricular support) system
LVs (left ventricular systolic)
   dimension
LVS (left ventricular systolic)
   pressure
LVSW (left ventricular stroke work)
LVSWI (left ventricular stroke work
   index)
LVW (left ventricular wall)
Lyme carditis
Lyme disease
lymphadenopathy
   hilar
   mediastinal
   paratracheal
lymph and emulsified fat
lymphangiectasis, pulmonary cystic
lymphangioleiomyomatosis (LAM)
lymphangioma, cardiac
lymphangioma circumscriptum
lymphangioma diffusum
lymphangioma of the heart
lymphangitic pulmonary spread
lymphapheresis
lymphatic channels
lymphatic drainage of heart
lymphatic drainage of lungs
lymphatic duct
lymphatic malformation (LM)
lymphatic system
lymphatic vessels
lymphaticovenous malformation
   (LVM)
lymphatics, prominent septal
lymph capillaries
lymphedema
   acquired
   hereditary
   Meige
   Nonne-Milroy
   praecox

lymph node
   axillary
   brachiocephalic
   bronchopulmonary
   diaphragmatic
   hilar
   intercostal
   medial supraclavicular
   mediastinal
   parasternal
   peribronchial
   posterior mediastinal
   supraclavicular
   tracheobronchial
lymph node enlargement, hilar
lymph node metastases
lymph node syndrome, mucocutaneous
lymphocytes
   B (bone-marrow)
   circulating
   immunoblastoid
   peripheral blood
   T (thymus-dependent)
lymphocytic infiltrate
lymphocytic interstitial pneumonitis
   (LIP)
lymphocytic splenomegaly, postcardiotomy
lymphogenous dissemination
lymphogenous metastasis
lymphography
lymphoid alveolitis
lymphoid interstitial pneumonia
lymphoma, multifocal
lymphoreticular malignant disease
lymphosarcoma of heart
lymph vessels of thymus
lyophilized allergen extract
lyophilized DPT (house dust mites)
lysis of adhesions
lysis of clot
lysophospholipid

lysosomal alpha-1,4-glucosidase
  deficiency
lysosomal enzymes

lysosomal storage disorders
lysosomes, myocytic
lytic intervention

M, m

m (meter)
m (murmur)
mA (milliampere)
MAC (minimal alveolar concentration)
MAC (mitral anular calcium)
MAC (monitored anesthesia care)
MAC (*Mycobacterium avium* complex)
MAC (multi-lumen access) catheter
MacCallum patch
machinery (or machinery-like) murmur
Macleod syndrome
macroangiopathy
macrocytic anemia
Macrodex
macrofistulous AV (arteriovenous)
    communications
macrophage, macrophages
    alveolar
    pigmented
macrophage reaction
macroreentrant tachycardia
macroreentry
macroscopically evident tumor
MAD2 nebulizer
Maddahi method of calculating right
    ventricular ejection fraction
Maestro pacemaker

Maffucci syndrome
MAFH (multicentric angiofollicular
    hyperplasia)
Magic Wallstent
magna
    anastomotica
    arteria
    radicularis
MAGneedle controllers
magnesium plasma concentration
magnesium, serum
magnet application over pulse
    generator
magnet, doughnut
Magnetic Controlled Suturing (MCS)
magnetic field gradient
magnetic moment
magnetic resonance angiography
    (MRA)
magnetic resonance imaging
    gated
    velocity-encoded
magnetic resonance signal
magnetic resonance spectroscopy
    (MRS)
magnetic resonance spin incoherence
magnetic resonance, tagging cine

magnification
  high-resolution
  signal
magnetization prepared three-dimensional gradient-echo (MP-RAGE)
  sequences
magnet mode
magnet rate
magnet response
magnitude
magnum guidewire
Magnum guidewire used in coronary
  angioplasty
Magovern-Cromie ball-cage prosthetic
  valve
Mahaim and James fibers
Mahaim bundles (in the heart)
Mahaim fibers (in the heart)
Mahler sign
mahogany flush
MAI (*Mycobacterium avium-intracellulare*)
MAI infection
main bronchus
main pulmonary artery
main stem bronchial cartilage
main stem bronchial mucosa
main stem bronchus
main stem carina
maintenance dose
MAIPA (monoclonal antibody-specific
  immobilization of platelet antigens)
  assay
Majestik shielded angiography needle
Majocchi disease
Majocchi purpura anularis telangiectodes
major crossmatch
majus, erythema multiforme
Mal de Meleda syndrome
maladie de Roger (Roger disease)
malaise

malaligned atrioventricular septal
  defects
malar flush
malarial pneumonitis
maldevelopment
maldistribution of ventilation and
  perfusion
malformation
  adenomatoid
  angiographically occult vascular
    (AOVM)
  Arnold-Chiari
  arterial (AM)
  arteriovenous (AVM)
  capillary (CM)
  capillary-lymphatic (CLM)
  Chiari I
  congenital cardiac
  congenital vascular
  conotruncal
  coronary artery
  costosternal
  cystic adenomatoid
  Ebstein
  embolization of vascular
  endocardial cushion
  extracardiac
  fast-flow
  hyperostosis associated with
    venous
  intraosseous vascular
  intrapulmonary arteriovenous
  laser photocoagulation of capillary
    (CM)
  lymphatic (LM)
  lymphaticovenous (LVM)
  septal
  slow-flow
  submucosal arterial
  Taussig-Bing congenital
  truncular venous
  valve

malformation *(cont.)*
   vascular
   venous (VM)
malformed phlebectasias in the calf
malfunction, lead electrode
malignant airway obstruction
malignant arrhythmia
malignant endocarditis
malignant gastrinoma
malignant hemangioendothelioma
malignant hypertension
malignant lymphoma of the heart
malignant melanoma metastatic to
   heart
malignant mesothelioma
malignant pheochromocytoma
malignant pleural effusion
malignant pleural implants
malignant teratoma of the heart
malignant vasovagal syncope
malignant ventricular arrhythmias
malignant ventricular dysrhythmias
malignant ventricular tachyarrhythmias
Malin anemia
Malin syndrome
malleable ribbon retractors
Mallinckrodt angiographic catheter
Mallory-Weiss tear in the mucosa at
   the cardioesophageal junction
malperfused
malperfusion
malposition of the heart
malt worker's lung
mammary pedicle
mammary souffle murmur
mammary-coronary artery bypass
mandibular advancement device,
   Herbst
maneuver, maneuvers
   Adson
   costoclavicular
   de-airing

maneuver *(cont.)*
   flushing
   Heineke-Mikulicz
   hyperabduction
   Kocher
   Müller (Mueller) cardiac
     auscultation
   Osler
   Rivero-Carvallo
   scalene
   squatting
   transabdominal left lateral
   retroperitoneal
   Valsalva
manganese pneumonitis
manifest
manifestation of overt clinical disease
manifold, Morse
Mannkopf sign
mannosidosis
manometer
   Riva-Rocci
   strain gauge
manometer-tipped cardiac catheters
Mansfield Atri-Pace catheter
Mansfield balloon
Mansfield catheter
Mansfield orthogonal electrode
   catheter
Mansfield Scientific dilatation balloon
   catheter
Manson schistosomiasis-pulmonary
   artery obstruction syndrome
Mantel-Haenszel life-table
mantle
   anechoic
   hypoechoic
Mantoux test
manual compression of lungs
manual pressure over carotid sinus
manual resuscitation bag
manual subtraction films

manubriosternal joint
manubriosternal syndrome
manubrium
Manx guidewire
MAO (monoamine oxidase)
MAO inhibitor
MA-1 ventilator
MAP (mean arterial pressure)
map, acceleration
MapCath catheter
MAP digital inflation system
map-guided partial endocardial
   ventriculotomy
maple bark disease
maple bark stripper's disease
   (pneumonitis)
maple bark stripper's lung
maple bark worker's suberosis
mapping
   activation-sequence
   body surface
   body surface potential
   catheter
   Doppler color flow
   electrophysiologic
   endocardial activation
   endocardial catheter
   epicardial
   ice
   intramural
   pace
   phase-shift velocity
   precordial
   retrograde atrial activation
   sinus rhythm
mapping probe, handheld
Marable syndrome
marantic clot
marantic infective endocarditis
marantic thrombus
marasmus
Marathon guiding catheter

Marchiafava-Micheli paroxysmal
   nocturnal hemoglobinuria
Marchiafava-Micheli syndrome
marching paresthesia
Mardis firm stent with HydroPlus
   coating
Marfan syndrome
marfanoid hypermobility syndrome
margin
   cardiac
   costal
   obtuse
marginal artery, Drummond
marginal branch
marginal candidate
marginal circumflex bypass
marginal rales
marginal vein
margin of error
Marie-Bamberger syndrome
marked asymmetry
markedly accentuated pulmonic
   component
marked respiratory distress
marked wheezes
marker
   gold
   immunologic
   radioactive string
   unreliable
marker-channel diagram
marker channel of pacemaker
marker protein
   HLA-DR (histocompatibility
      antigen-DR)
   ICAM-1 (intercellular adhesions
      molecule-1)
markings
   bronchovascular
   coarse bronchovascular
   increased pulmonary vascular
   pulmonary vascular
   vascular

Marlex methylmethacrylate sandwich
Marlow Primus instrument collection
Maroteaux-Lamy syndrome
Marquest Respirgard II nebulizer
Marquette Holter monitor
Marquette 3-channel laser holder
Marquis stopcock
marrow, sternal
Marshall, vein of
marsupialization of laryngeal cyst
Martin-Gruber anastomosis
Martini and Melamed, criteria of
Martorell aortic arch syndrome
Martorell-Fabre syndrome
Martorell hypertensive ulcer
Mary Allen Engle ventricle
MAS (Morgagni-Adams-Stokes)
    syndrome
mask
    Aerochamber face
    BLB
    Maxima Forté blood oxygen by
    meter
    Mirage nasal ventilation
    nonrebreather
    nonrebreathing
    oxygen by nonrebreather
    partial rebreather
    particle
    rebreathing
    Respironics nasal
    ventilation
    Ventimask
    venturi
    Viasys resuscitation
mask anesthesia
masking
mask ventilation
Mason-Likar 12-lead ECG system
mason's lung
Mason vascular clamp

mass
    airless
    cavitary
    cavitary lung
    cordlike
    doughy
    echogenic
    firm
    fixed
    fluid-filled
    freely movable
    friable
    full thickness
    hilar
    ill-defined
    indurated
    inflammatory polypoid
    interbronchial
    intracardiac
    intracavitary
    intracavity
    intraventricular
    left ventricular (LVM)
    lower lobe lung
    lung
    movable
    mushy
    nonpulsatile
    nonpulsatile abdominal
    paracardiac
    parenchymal tumor
    polypoid calcified irregular
    pulsatile
    pulsatile abdominal
    right ventricular (RVM)
    rubbery
    saccular
    solid
    solitary
    spherical
    stony
    ventricular
    woody

massage
  carotid sinus
  external cardiac
  heart
  manual
  open cardiac
  vapor
  vigorous manual cardiac
mass effect
massive aortic regurgitation
massive ascites
massive blood transfusion
massive edema
massive effusion
massive embolism (embolization)
massive exsanguinating hemorrhage
massive gastrointestinal bleeding
massive heart attack
massive infiltration
massive left hemothorax
massive lung collapse
mass ligation in lung resection
Masson body in pulmonary alveoli
mast cell inhibitors
mast cell mediator
MAST (Medical Anti-Shock Trousers)
Master Flow Pumpette
Master syndrome
Master two-step exercise stress test for
  coronary insufficiency
mastocytosis syndrome
MAT (multifocal atrial tachycardia)
Matas aneurysmoplasty
matched V/Q defect
match test
material
  atheromatous
  contrast
  Dacron synthetic ligament
  hemostatic
  lipoid
  PAS-positive proteinaceous
  purulent

maternal hypotension syndrome
maternal rubella syndrome
Matson-Alexander rib elevator
Matson rib elevator
Matson stripper
matter, pulverized plaque particulate
Mattox aortic clamp
mattress suture
mattress-type suture
maturation, disparity of
mature fistula
Maugeri syndrome
Maverick Monorail balloon catheter
Maverick over-the-wire balloon
  catheter
Maverick PTCA catheter
Maverick XL PTCA catheter
Maverick2 Monorail catheter
Maxair Autohaler
Max Force balloon catheter
maxillary sinusitis
Maxima Forté blood oxygenator
maximal capacity for work
maximal exercise test
maximal expiratory flow at 25% vital
  capacity (V25)
maximal expiratory flow at 50% vital
  capacity (V50)
maximal expiratory flow at 75% vital
  capacity (V75)
maximal inspiratory effort
maximal intensity
  point of
  site of
maximal midexpiratory flow (MMEF)
maximal respiratory pressure
maximal voluntary ventilation (MVV)
maximal volume (of left atrium)
maximal voluntary ventilation (MVV)
maximum blood pressure
maximum diameter to minimum
  diameter ratio

maximum electrical activity
maximum midexpiratory flow
maximum predicted heart rate
　(MPHR)
maximum velocity of the jet
maximum voluntary ventilation
　(MVV)
Maxon suture
Maxorb alginate wound dressing
Max-Prene mesh
Max-Prene surgical clip
Max-Prene surgical staple
Max-Prene suture anchor
Max-Prene tissue adhesive
Max-Prene vascular occlusion device
May-Hegglin anomaly
Mayo curved scissors
Mayo exercise treadmill protocol
Mayo-Gibbon heart-lung machine
Mayo-Gibbon pump oxygenator
Mayo Hegar needle holder
Mayo hemostat
Mayo ligature carrier
Mayo Péan forceps
Mayo straight scissors
Mayo vein stripper
maze operation in atrial fibrillation
maze procedure, Cox
Mazzariello-Caprini forceps
Mb (myoglobin)
MB band or fraction
MBF (myocardial blood flow)
MB fraction
MBIH catheter
MB isoenzyme of CK (CK-MB)
MBTS (modified Blalock-Taussig
　shunt)
MCA (middle cerebral artery)
McArdle syndrome
MCAT (myocardial contrast appear-
　ance time)
McDowall oculovagal reflex

MCE (myocardial contrast echocardi-
　ography)
MCFSR (mean circumferential fiber
　shortening rate)
McGinn-White sign
McGoon coronary perfusion catheter
McGoon method of avoiding heart
　block
McGoon ratio
McGovern nipple (airway)
McHenry treadmill exercise protocol
mCi (millicurie)
McIntosh double-lumen catheter
McKernan-Adson forceps
McKernan-Potts forceps
McKinley EpM infusion pump
McKusick-Kaufman syndrome
MCL (midclavicular line)
McLeod blood phenotype
MCLS (mucocutaneous lymph node
　syndrome), acute febrile
MCS (middle coronary sinus)
MDI (metered dose inhaler)
MDR-TB (multidrug-resistant
　tuberculosis)
meadow fescue
Meadows syndrome
Meadox biograft
Meadox Microvel arterial graft
Meadox woven velour prosthesis
mean airway pressure (MAP)
mean aortic pressure
mean arterial pressure (MAP)
mean atrial pressure
mean blood pressure
mean cardiac vector
mean circulatory filling pressure
mean circumferential fiber shortening
　rate (MCFSR)
mean corpuscular red cell volume
mean electrical axis of heart
mean left atrial pressure

mean maximal expiratory flow
(MMEF)
mean mitral valve gradient
mean platelet volume (MVP)
mean pulmonary artery (MPA)
pressure
mean pulmonary capillary pressure
(MPCP)
mean pulmonary transit time
mean rate of circumferential shortening
mean right atrial pressure
mean vectors
mean venous pulsation
Means-Lermans scratch
measles, German
measure, prophylactic
measurement
cardiac output
occlusion
ventilometric
meat wrapper's asthma
meat wrapper's lung
mechanical augmentation
mechanical circulatory support
mechanical cough
mechanical counterpulsation
mechanical dottering effect
mechanical insufflation
mechanical obstruction of respiratory
tract
mechanical respiratory assist
mechanical rotational atherectomy
(MRA)
mechanical saw
mechanical stress
mechanical valve
mechanical ventilation
mechanical ventilatory support
mechanism
compensatory
Frank Starling
heart rate reserve

mechanism *(cont.)*
Laplace
reserve
sensing
Starling
triggering
ventricular escape
Medallion syringe
Medcor pacemaker
MEDDARS analysis system for
cardiac catheterization
media (pl. of medium)
fibrotic and scarred
tunica
media-adventitia interface
medial arteriosclerosis
medial basal bronchi
medial bronchi
medial calcified sclerosis
medial disruption
medial extension
medial fibroplasia
medial hyperplasia
medial incision
medialis, ramus
medial necrosis, cystic
medial papillary muscle
medial plantar artery
medial rotation of viscera to the right
of midline
medial supraclavicular lymph nodes
medial surface of lung
median arcuate ligament of diaphragm
median percent shortening
median sternotomy
primary
secondary
median sternotomy approach (incision)
medianus, ramus
median xiphopubic laparotomy
mediastinal adenopathy
mediastinal border

mediastinal compression
mediastinal contamination
mediastinal drainage fluid
mediastinal emphysema
mediastinal exploration
mediastinal fat
mediastinal fistula
mediastinal flutter
mediastinal hernia
mediastinal idiopathic fibrosis
mediastinal infection
mediastinal invasion
mediastinalis, pleura
mediastinal lymph nodes
mediastinal lymphadenopathy
mediastinal neoplasm
mediastinal node
mediastinal part of medial surface
    of lung
mediastinal pleura
mediastinal pleurisy
mediastinal prominence
mediastinal shift
mediastinal structures
mediastinal surface of lung
mediastinal tracheostomy
mediastinal tumor
mediastinal widening
mediastinitis
    fibrous
    indurative
    sclerosing
    silicotic
mediastinodiaphragmatic pleural
    reflection
mediastinopericarditis
mediastinoscope
mediastinoscopy
mediastinotomy
mediastinum
    anterior
    deviated
    inferior

mediastinum *(cont.)*
    middle
    posterior
    superior
    widened
mediastinum displacement
mediator, mast cell
medical cardiac tamponade
medications—a quick-reference list of
    pharmaceuticals, including chemi-
    cals, chemotherapy drugs and proto-
    cols, investigational drugs, natural
    substances, prescription and over-
    the-counter drugs, and radioiso-
    topes. See also *drug delivery de-
    vices*; *drug-related terms*; *imaging
    agents.*
AccuNeb (albuterol sulfate)
Accupril (quinapril HCl)
ACE (angiotensin-converting
    enzyme) inhibitor
Adalat CC (nifedipine)
Adalat XL
Advair Diskus (fluticasone
    propionate and salmeterol
    inhalation powder)
AeroDose inhaler
Agrylin (anagrelide HCl)
Airozin
Aldurazyme (laronidase)
Altace (ramipril)
anisoylated plasminogen strepto-
    kinase activator complex
    (APSAC)
Antrin (motexafin lutetium)
Apo-Atenol (atenolol)
Apo-Furosemide (furosemide)
Apo-Hydro (hydrochlorothiazide)
Apo-Metoprolol L (metoprolol)
Apo-Salvent (salbutamol)
aprikalim
arbutamine
Arixtra (fondaparinux sodium)

medications *(cont.)*
  atenolol
  Atrovent (ipratropium bromide)
  Azmacort (triamcinolone acetonide)
  bacillus Calmette-Guérin (BCG)
    vaccine
  BeneFix hemophilia B blood
    clotting factor drug
  Body Glue
  bucrylate
  Cafcit (caffeine citrate)
  caffeine
  calcium channel blockers
  calcium entry blockers
  captopril
  carbon dioxide (CO_2)
  Cardiolite
  Cardizem
  Cardizem CD (diltiazem HCl)
  Cardizem LA (diltiazem HCl)
  Cardizem SR (diltiazem HCl)
  Cardura (doxazosin mesylate)
  Cartia XT (diltiazem HCl)
  cefazolin and dextrose
  Celsior organ preservation solution
  Ceresine
  Chloraprep One-Step (chlorhexi-
    dine gluconate; isopropyl
    alcohol)
  Cholestagel (colesevelam
    hydrochloride)
  ciclesonide
  Clarinex (desloratadine)
  clonidine
  Coagulin-B
  colesevelam
  collagen hemostatic material for
    wounds
  Combivent (ipratropium bromide)
  CoQ10; Co-Q10 (coenzyme Q10)
  Coumadin (warfarin sodium)
  Cozaar (losartan potassium)

medications *(cont.)*
  Curosurf (poractant alfa)
  digoxin
  Dilatrend (carvedilol)
  Diovan (valsartan)
  Diovan HCT (valsartan, hydro-
    chlorothiazide)
  eicosapentaenoic acid (EPA)
  EPA (eicosapentaenoic acid)
  eplerenone
  eptifibatide
  E2F Decoy solution
  Exosurf (lung surfactant)
  Factive (gemifloxacin)
  Fiblast (trafermin)
  FluMist influenza virus vaccine
  furosemide
  gelatin sponge slurry
  Gengraf (cyclosporine capsules
    modified)
  Haemaccel (polygeline)
  HCTZ (hydrochlorothiazide)
  Hemopure (hemoglobin glutamer-
    250)
  Hep-Lock (heparin sodium)
  Hep-Lock PF (heparin sodium)
  Hep-Lock U/P (heparin sodium)
  hirudin (recombinant)
  HK-Cardiosol organ preservation
    solution
  hydrochlorothiazide (HCTZ)
  Iressa (gefitinib)
  Kayexalate
  ketotifen
  LiquiVent
  Lotensin (benazepril HCl)
  Lotrel (amlodipine besylate,
    benazepril HCl)
  Lugol fixative solution
  Lu-Tex (lutetium texaphyrin)
  MEPIG (mucoid exopolysaccharide
    Pseudomonas hyperimmune
    globulin)

medications *(cont.)*
- metoprolol tartrate
- Micardis (telmisartan)
- mixed respiratory vaccine (MRV)
- Monopril (fosinopril sodium)
- Mono-Vacc Test
- Monsel's hemostatic solution
- morphine sulfate (MS)
- mucoid exopolysaccharide, *Pseudomonas* (hyper)immune globulin (MEPIG)
- Myers solution
- nitric oxide
- nitro (slang for nitroglycerin)
- Nitro-Dur (nitroglycerin)
- nitroglycerin (NTG)
- Nitrol ointment
- "nitro paste" (nitroglycerin ointment)
- NitroQuick (nitroglycerin) sublingual tablets
- Norvasc (amlodipine)
- No Sting barrier film
- Novo-Hydrazide (hydrochlorothiazide)
- Novo-Salmol (salbutamol)
- Novo-Semide (furosemide)
- NPA (novel plasminogen activator)
- NTS (nitroglycerin transdermal system)
- Nutrim dietary fat substitute
- Orapred
- Panafil enzymatic debriding agent
- Panafil White ointment
- pentaerythritol tetranitrate (PETN)
- pexelizumab
- Picovir (pleconaril)
- Plasmalyte A cardioplegic solution
- Plavix (clopidogrel bisulfate)
- Pneumovax
- povidone-iodine solution
- Pravigard PAC (buffered aspirin and pravastatin sodium)

medications *(cont.)*
- Prinivil (lisinopril)
- Procardia XL (nifedipine)
- Prodec-DM drops
- propranolol HCl
- protamine
- Proventil HFA (albuterol)
- Pulmicort Turbuhaler (budesonide)
- Puri-Clens wound cleanser
- QVAR (beclomethasone dipropionate)
- R-albuterol
- Ranexa (ranolazine)
- recombinant tissue plasminogen activator (rt-PA)
- Remodulin (treprostinil sodium)
- Rythmol (propafenone)
- Saf-Clens chronic wound cleanser
- Salbutamol Nebuamp (salbutamol sulfate)
- Sclavo PPD solution (tuberculin purified protein derivative)
- Sclavo Test-PPD (tuberculin purified protein derivative)
- Sea-Clens wound cleanser
- Serevent (salmeterol xinafoate)
- 7-valent vaccine
- Shur-Clens wound cleanser
- Singulair (montelukast sodium)
- sivelestat
- Sonazoid ultrasound contrast agent
- Spectracef (cefditoren pivoxil)
- Spiriva (tiotropium)
- spironolactone
- streptokinase (SK)
- superoxide dismutase (SOD), recombinant human
- surface active extract of saline lavage of bovine lungs
- surfactant, human amniotic fluid-derived
- surfactant TA (modified bovine lung surfactant extract)

medications *(cont.)*
   Surgi–Prep (Betadine, povidone-
      iodine)
   Survanta
   tecadenoson
   Techni-Care surgical scrub
   terazosin HCl
   theophylline (sustained-release
      form)
   ThromboSol
   thromboxanes (TxA1 and TxB2)
   tissue plasminogen activator (t-PA)
   TNKase (tenecteplase)
   Toprol XL (metoprolol succinate)
   Total-Lo
   t-PA, tPA (tissue plasminogen
      activator)
   Tracleer (bosentan)
   triamterene/hydrochlorothiazide
   Tricor (micronized fenofibrate)
   UltraKlenz wound cleanser
   Uniprost (prostacyclin)
   Vanlev (omapatrilat)
   Vasotec (enalaprilat maleate)
   Veletri (tezosentan)
   Venofer (iron sucrose)
   verapamil HCl (sustained-release
      form)
   warfarin sodium
   Welchol (colesevelam hydro-
      chloride)
   Xolair (omalizumab)
   Zaditen (ketotifen)
   Zemaira (alpha$_1$ proteinase
      inhibitor, human)
   Zestoretic (hydrochlorothiazide,
      lisinopril)
   Zestril (lisinopril)
   Zetia (ezetimibe)
   Ziac (hydrochlorothiazide,
      bisoprolol fumarate)
   Zyvox (linezolid)

Medicon instruments for vascular and
   cardiac surgery
Medicon rib spreader
Medicon vascular and cardiac surgery
   instruments
Medifil collagen hemostatic wound
   dressing
Medigraphics analyzer
Medinvent stent
mediolysis
medionecrosis
   cystic
   Erdheim cystic
Medipore Dress-it precut surgical
   dressing
MediPort implanted vascular access
   device
Medi-Quet surgical tourniquet
Medi-Tech steerable system
Mediterranean anemia
medium crackles
medneb (slang for medication
   nebulizer)
MEDOS/HIA ventricular assist device
Medrad contrast medium injector
Medrad guidewire
Medtel pacemaker
Medtronic anuloplasty ring
Medtronic aortic punch
Medtronic AVE BeStent with Discrete
   Technology over-the-wire coronary
   stent delivery system
Medtronic balloon catheter
Medtronic/Bio-Medicus 520
   centrifugal pump system
Medtronic/Bio-Medicus 540
   centrifugal pump system
Medtronic bipolar electrode
Medtronic cardiac cooling jacket
Medtronic Cardioverter
Medtronic DDD pacemaker
Medtronic demand pulse generator

Medtronic electrode
Medtronic endocardial defibrillation lead
Medtronic endocardial defibrillation-sensing/pacing lead
Medtronic External Tachyarrhythmia Control Device (ETCD)
Medtronic Gem automatic implantable defibrillator
Medtronic GEM implantable cardio-verter-defibrillator
Medtronic-Hall monocuspid tilting-disk valve
Medtronic-Hall prosthetic heart valve
Medtronic Hall rotatable aortic valved collagen-impregnated conduit
Medtronic-Hall valve prosthesis
Medtronic-Hancock device
Medtronic Hemopump cardiac assist device
Medtronic InSync implantable cardioverter-defibrillator
Medtronic Interactive Tachycardia Terminating System
Medtronic Jewel AF implantable arrhythmia management device
Medtronic Micro Jewel II implantable defibrillator
Medtronic Minix
Medtronic Octopus stabilizing device
Medtronic Octopus tissue stabilizing system
Medtronic pacemaker
Medtronic pacemaker generator
Medtronic patch leads
Medtronic PCD (programmable cardioverter-defibrillator)
Medtronic Physio-Control automatic and semiautomatic defibrillators
Medtronic prosthetic valve
Medtronic Pulsor Intrasound pain reliever

Medtronic Radio-Frequency (RF) Receiver
Medtronic SPO pacemaker
Medtronic Sprint lead for cardioverter-defibrillator
Medtronic subcutaneous patch lead
Medtronic Symbios pacemaker
Medtronic temporary pacemaker
Medtronic Transvene electrode
Medtronic tremor control therapy device
medulla, adrenal
Meeker dissecting forceps
Meeker grasping forceps
Mee protocol
Mees lines
Mee technique
$MEF_{50\% \, VC}$ (mid-expiratory flow at 50% vital capacity)
megahertz (MHz)
megavoltage x-rays
Meige lymphedema
Meigs capillaries
Meigs-Cass syndrome
Meigs syndrome
melanoma metastatic to heart, malignant
melanoma, pedunculated
Melrose solution
Meltzer sign
membranacea, pars
membrane
    alveolar-capillary
    asphyxial
    basement
    Bichat
    diphtheritic
    Dorhas
    fenestrated
    Gore-Tex surgical
    Henle
    Henle elastic

membrane *(cont.)*
  Henle fenestrated
  hyaline
  pleuropericardial
  smooth glistening
  supramitral
  vernix
membrane oxygenator contamination
membrane potential
membranous bronchitis
membranous croup
membranous septum
membranous subvalvular aortic stenosis
membranous ventricular septal defect
MemoryTrace AT ambulatory cardiac
  monitor
Memotherm nitinol self-expanding
  stent
Mendelson syndrome
Ménière syndrome
meningeal hemorrhage
meningitis, complicating
meningococcal endocarditis
meningococcal infection
meningococcal myocarditis
meningococcal pericarditis
meningococcus
meniscus (crescent) of contrast-saline
  mixture
meniscus of saline test for pneumoperitoneum
MEPIG (mucoid exopolysaccharide
  Pseudomonas hyperimmune
  globulin)
Mepitel contact-layer wound dressing
Mepore absorptive dressing
mercurial diuretics
mercury-in-Silastic strain gauge for
  blood flow determination
Meridian echocardiography
Merit Medical stent inflation kit

Meritrans disposable blood pressure
  transducer
Mersilene braided nonabsorbable
  suture
Mersilene suture
Mersilk braided silk suture
"Mer-suh" (MRSA)
MES (multi-electrode surgical) device
Mesalt dressing
mesenchymal connective tissue
mesenchymal tissue migration
mesenteric angiography
mesenteric arterial thrombosis
mesenteric artery occlusion, acute
mesenteric artery, superior
mesenteric infarction
mesenteric venous thrombosis
mesh (see also *dressing*)
  Bard SpermaTex preshaped
  Composix E/X
  Dexon
  Glycoprene
  Lactoprene
  Max-Prene
  Osteoprene
  PermaMesh suture
  SpermaTex preshaped
mesh-wrapping of aortic aneurysm,
  subtotal
mesocardia
mesocaval anastomosis
mesothelioma, atrioventricular (AV)
  node
mesothelium, pleural
mesoversion of heart
Mester test for rheumatic disease
MET (measurement of oxygen
  consumption/kilogram/minute)
metabolic aberration
metabolic acidemia
metabolic acidosis
metabolic alkalosis

metabolic cardiomyopathy
metabolic disorders affecting heart
    function
metabolic equivalents (mets)
metabolism
    glycosphingolipid
    myocardial
metaiodobenzylguanidine scintigraphy
Meta DDDR pacemaker
metal fume fever
metal needle
metallic clips
metallic cough
metallic rales
metal stent
Meta MV pacemaker
metanephrine, urinary
MetaPF pulmonary function monitor
metaplasia, squamous
metapneumonic empyema
metapneumonic pleurisy
Meta rate responsive pacemaker
metastasectomy
    lung
    pulmonary
metastasis (pl. metastases)
    distant
    systemic
    unresectable pulmonary
    intrapulmonary
metastasis to mediastinum
metastatic abscess
metastatic bronchogenic carcinoma
metastatic hypernephroma to heart
metastatic myocardial tumor
metasynchronous tumor
metazoal infestation
metazoal myocarditis
meter (m), peak flow
meter per second (m/sec) velocity
metered-dose aerosol
metered-dose inhaler (MDI)

meter mask
methacholine bronchial provocation
    test
methacholine challenge, inhaled
methacholine chloride challenge
methacholine chloride inhalation
methemoglobin reductase deficiency
methemoglobinemia
methimazole
method (see also *formula, operation,
    procedure, technique*)
    Anel
    Antyllus
    Barbero-Marcial
    Brasdor
    Brisbane
    Brisbane aortic valve and ascending
        aorta replacement
    Carpentier
    Clauss modified method of plasma
        fibrinogen measurement
    Danielson
    direct Fick
    Dodge area-length
    Douglas bag (for determining
        cardiac output)
    downstream sampling
    EliSpot
    Ellman
    empty beating heart
    Fick
    forward triangle
    GLH (Green Lane Hospital)
        insertion
    Graupner
    Hatle valve area
    Hetzel forward triangle
    indicator-dilution (for determining
        cardiac output)
    indocyanine green dye (cardiac
        output measurement)
    Kennedy ejection fraction

method *(cont.)*
  Kouchoukos
  Laks
  Lee-White
  McGoon
  metrizamide contrast medium
  Narula
  Orsi-Grocco
  Pachon
  polarographic oxygen (for deter-
    mining cardiac output)
  Purmann
  pyramid ventricular volume
  Quick
  Sahli
  Scarpa
  Shimazaki area-length
  Stoney
  Strauss
  Theden
  thermodilution (cardiac output
    measurement)
  trapdoor flap (for ALCAPA)
  upstream sampling
  Valdes-Cruz
  van den Bergh
  Wardrop
  Westergren
methyl methacrylate repair of
  aneurysm
meticulous dissection
metoprolol tartrate
Metricath catheter and transducer
Metrix atrial defibrillation system
metrizoate acid contrast material
metrizamide contrast material
mets (metabolic equivalents)
Metzenbaum curved scissors
Metzenbaum straight scissors
Meyer vein stripper
MFAT (multifocal atrial tachycardia)
MHz (megahertz)

MI (mitral insufficiency)
MI (myocardial infarction)
MI (myocardial ischemia)
Micardis (telmisartan)
Michel aortic clamp
microaneurysm
microangiopathic anemia
microangiopathic hemolytic anemia
microangiopathy
  intraretinal (IRMA)
  thrombotic
microbubbles
  carbon dioxide
  hydrogen peroxide
  oxygen
microcavitation
microcirculation, pulmonary
microcoils, suture-ligated embolization
microcytic anemia
Micro-Driver balloon catheter
Micro-Driver stent
Micro-Driver stent delivery system
microembolization, cholesterol
microfibrillar hemostat (Instat MCH)
microfibrillar protein fibrillin gene
microfilariae
microfistulous AV (arteriovenous)
  communications
microfistulous AV (arteriovenous)
  shunt
micro forceps
MicroKlenz wound cleanser
MicroMed DeBakey ventricular assist
  device
MicroMewi multiple sidehole infusion
  catheter
MicroMewi occlusion/infusion
  catheter
Micro Minix pacemaker
Micron Res-Q implantable cardioverter-defibrillator
Microny K SR pacemaker

Microny II SR+ pulse generator
  pacemaker
microsomal triglyceride transfer
  protein (MTP)
MicroStent II over-the-wire PTCA
  stent
MicroTrach
microvascular anastomotic coupler
  system
microvascular angiopathy (MVA)
microvascular disease
Microvasive Glidewire
Microvasive stiff piano wire guidewire
microwave atrial ablation
microwave cardiac ablation system
MIDCAB (minimally invasive direct
  coronary artery bypass) procedure
middle cerebral artery (MCA)
midlung field
migration, stent
milia
miliaria
Millenia balloon catheter
Miller syndrome
mill-house murmur
mill-wheel murmur
Miltex surgical instruments
MINI Crown stent
minimal lumen diameter (MLD)
minimally invasive direct coronary
  artery bypass (MIDCAB) operation
minocycline-rifampin-impregnated
  catheter
minor crossmatch
minute volume
Mirage Guidewire
Mirage nasal ventilation mask system
Miser tube device
Mistique catheter
mist stick
mitral click syndrome
mitral click-murmur syndrome

mitral configuration of cardiac shadow
  on x-ray
mitral deceleration slope
mitral inflow velocities
mitral insufficiency
mitral insufficiency jet
mitral leaflets, noncalcified
mitral leak
mitral orifice
mitral regurgitant murmur
mitral regurgitant signal area
mitral regurgitation
  congenital
  pansystolic
mitral regurgitation artifact (cineangiography)
mitral regurgitation-chordal elongation
  syndrome
mitral ring calcification
mitral stenosis (see *stenosis*)
mitral valve (see *valve*)
  billowing
  cleft
  flail
  floppy
  hammock
  hammocking of
  parachute
  thickened
mitral valve abnormalities
mitral valve atresia
mitral valve calcification
mitral valve commissures
mitral valve configuration, fishmouth
mitral valve echogram
mitral valve homograft
mitral valve leaflet tip
mitral valve myxomatous degeneration
mitral valve obstruction
mitral valve prolapse (MVP),
  holosystolic
mitral valve prolapse murmur

mitral valve prolapse syndrome
mitral valve regurgitation
mitral valve regurgitation without
 prolapse
mitral valve replacement
mitral valve septal separation
mitral valve stenosis (MVS)
mitral valvulitis
Mitroflow pericardial prosthetic valve
Mitroflow Synergy PC stented pericardial bioprosthesis
Mitsubishi angioscope
Mitsubishi angioscopic catheter
mixed angina
mixed apnea
mixed connective tissue disease
mixed grass pollen
mixed lesion
mixed respiratory vaccine (MRV)
mixed restrictive-obstructive lung
 disease
mixed venous saturation
Mixter clamp
Mixter dissecting forceps
Mixter grasping forceps
Mixter right-angle clamp
MLD (minimal luminal diameter)
MM band
MM coronary syringe
MMEF (maximal midexpiratory flow)
MMEF (mean maximal expiratory
 flow)
MM fraction
mm Hg (millimeters of mercury)
M-mode Doppler echocardiography
M-mode echocardiogram
M-mode echocardiogram in utero
M-mode echophonocardiography
M-mode transducer
MO (mitral orifice)
MoAb (monoclonal antibodies)
mobile pedunculated left atrial tumor

mobile thrombus
mobilize pulmonary secretions
mobilization
Mobin-Uddin embolus trap
Mobin-Uddin umbrella filter
Mobin-Uddin vena caval filter
Mobitz classification (type I or II) of
 atrioventricular (AV) heart block
Mobitz heart block type 1
Mobitz heart block type 2
Mobitz I second-degree block
Mobitz II second-degree block
Mobitz type I on Wenckebach heart
 block
Mobius artificial heart valve
Mobius open heart pump
Mobius vascular prosthesis
Mobius vascular stent
moccasin feet
modality
 alternative
 diagnostic
 pacing
 standard
 therapeutic
mode
 A-mode (on echocardiogram)
 AAI (noncompetitive atrial
  demand)
 AAI rate-responsive
 active
 atrial triggered and ventricular
  inhibited
 atrial-burst
 atrioventricular dual-demand
 B-mode (on ultrasound)
 bipolar pacing
 committed
 DDD pacing
 dual-demand pacing
 DVI
 ECG asynchronous

mode *(cont.)*
  ECG synchronous
  ECG triggered
  fixed rate
  full fill-full empty heart pump
  full fill-full empty VAD
    (ventricular assist pump)
  full-to-empty heart pump
  full-to-empty VAD (ventricular
    access device)
  inactive
  inhibited pacing
  M-mode (on echocardiogram)
  noncommitted
  pacing
  semicommitted
  sequential
  stimulation
  synchronous pacemaker
  triggered pacing
  underdrive
  unipolar pacing
  untriggered
  VVI (noncompetitive demand
    ventricular)
mode abandonment
model
  figure-of-eight
  leading circle
  ring
moderate acidosis
moderate growth of normal
    respiratory flora
moderate respiratory acidemia
moderate respiratory distress
moderate wheezing
moderate whole body hypothermia
moderator band
modification
  Bentall procedure, Cabrol II
  Carpentier repair
  Dor

modification *(cont.)*
  Lecompte
  Quaegebeur
  slow-pathway
modified Bentall button technique
modified Blalock-Taussig shunt
    (MBTS)
modified Bruce protocol
modified endoventricular circularplasty
modified pericardium-baffle recon-
    struction
modulation, respiratory
Moenckeberg ((Mönckeberg)
MOF (multiple organ failure)
Mohr syndrome
moist atelectatic rales
moist mucous membranes
moist rales
moisture vapor permeability (MVP)
MOL (middle of life)
molding, atheroma
Molina needle-catheter
moment, magnetic
Monaghan 300 ventilator
Monarch digital inflation device
Mönckeberg (Moenckeberg)
Mönckeberg arteriosclerosis
Mönckeberg calcification
Mönckeberg degeneration
Mönckeberg medial sclerosis
Monday fever syndrome
Mondor phlebitis disease
Mondor syndrome
Mondor thrombophlebitis
M1 (marginal branch #1)
M_1 heart sound (mitral valve closure)
Monge disease or syndrome
Mongoose PTCA catheter
monilial endocarditis
monitor (see also *monitoring*)
  Accucap CO_2/O_2
  Accucom cardiac output

monitor *(cont.)*
  Accutorr
  Acuson V5M multiplanar TEE (transesophageal echocardio-graphic)
  ambulatory Holter
  Androflo
  Androsonix biological sound
  AquaSens irrigation fluid
  Arrhythmia Net arrhythmia
  Avea
  Bear NUM-1 tidal volume
  Belos VR-T ICD home monitoring system
  CA (cardiac-apnea)
  cardiac
  cardiac-apnea (CA)
  CardioDiary heart
  Chronicle implantable hemo-dynamic
  Commucor A+V Patient
  continuous Holter
  Dinamap blood pressure
  Discovery portable
  DynaPulse 5000A ambulatory blood pressure
  electrocardiograph
  endotracheal cardiac output (ECOM)
  event
  Healthdyne apnea
  Hemosonic hemodynamic
  Holter
  ICG-Pulsion cardiac output
  KinetiX ventilation
  Lifestream personal cholesterol
  MetaPF pulmonary function
  Ohmeda CO_2
  Polar Vantage XL heart rate
  Physio-Control bedside
  Propaq Encore vital signs
  Pulse Pro heart rate

monitor *(cont.)*
  Reveal insertable loop recorder
  Reveal Plus insertable loop recorder implantable heart
  Selection AFm (atrial fibrillation)
  Smart-Inflate heart
  Vasotrax blood pressure
  VentCheck
  Vigilance CCO/SvO2/CEDV
  Vitatron Selection AFm (atrial fibrillation)
  WinABP ambulatory blood pressure
  VEST ambulatory function
monitor bed
monitored anesthesia care (MAC)
monitoring (see also *monitor*)
  ambulatory blood pressure (ABPM)
  bedside
  continuous Holter
  continuous (of myocardial ischemia)
  cytoimmunologic
  hemodynamic
  Nellcor Symphony blood pressure
  Neotrend blood gas
  Physios CTM 01 noninvasive cardiac transplant
monitoring line
Monneret bradycardia
Monneret pulse
monoamine oxidase (MAO) inhibitor
monobacteria
monoclonal antibody
  OKT3
  whole blood
monoclonal antibody-based enzyme immunoassay
monoclonal antibody-specific immobi-lization of platelet antigens (MAIPA) assay
monocrotic pulse

Monocryl suture (polyglecaprone 25)
monocusp valve
monofilament absorbable suture
monofilament nylon suture
monofilament polypropylene sutures
Monolyth oxygenator
monomorphic premature ventricular
    contractions (PVCs)
monomorphic VT (ventricular tachy-
    cardia)
mononeuritis multiplex
mononuclear cell, pleomorphic
mononuclear infiltrate
monoparesis
monophasic contour of QRS complex
monophasic shock waveforms
monophasic waveforms, truncated
    exponential simultaneous
Monorail angioplasty catheter
Monorail balloon catheter
Monorail catheter system
Monostrut cardiac valve prosthesis
Mono-Vacc Test
Monovial infusion delivery system
Monsel's hemostatic solution
"mooks" (see *Much's granules*)
moon facies
morbid event
morbidity and mortality
morbid thinking
morbus cordis
More-Flow double-lumen hemo-
    dialysis catheter
Morgagni-Adams-Stokes (MAS)
    attacks
Morgagni-Adams-Stokes syndrome
Morgagni, foramen of
moribund
morphine
morphine sulfate (MS)
morphologically
morphologic features

morphologic left ventricle
morphology
    dominant left ventricular
    turning point (TMP)
    ventricle
    ventricularized
Morquio syndrome
Morris aortic clamp
Morse manifold
Morse sternal spreader
Morton Salt Substitute
mosaic-jet signals
mosaic perfusion
Mosaic porcine bioprosthesis
Mosaic valve
Moschcowitz disease
Moschcowitz sign (of arterial occlu-
    sive disease)
Moschcowitz syndrome
Moschcowitz test for arteriosclerosis
Moschcowitz thrombotic thrombo-
    cytopenic purpura
mosquito clamp
moss-agate sputum
motion
    akinetic segmental wall
    anterior wall
    apical wall
    brisk wall
    catheter tip
    cusp
    discernible venous
    dyskinetic segmental wall
    dyskinetic wall
    forceful parasternal
    heaving precordial
    hyperkinetic segmental wall
    hypokinetic segmental wall
    hypokinetic wall
    inferior wall
    leaflet
    left ventricular regional wall

motion *(cont.)*
  palpable anterior
  paradoxical leaflet
  paradoxical (of chest wall)
  paradoxical septal
  posterior wall
  posterolateral wall
  regional hypokinetic wall
  regional wall
  rocking precordial
  segmental wall
  septal wall
  sustained anterior parasternal
  systolic anterior (SAM)
  trifid precordial motion
  ventricular wall
  visible anterior
motion artifact
motion cough
motor impairment
MOTT (*Mycobacterium* other than
  tuberculosis)
mottled density
mottled extremities
mottled gray lung
mottled thickening
mottling
Mounier-Kuhn syndrome
mountain sickness
  acute
  chronic
  chronic emphysematous
  chronic erythremic
  subacute
mouth-to-mouth respirations
movement
  basal (on x-ray)
  circus
  paradoxical
moving-bed infusion-tracking MRA
  method for imaging

moxibustion
moyamoya ("puff of smoke")
moyamoya cerebrovascular disease
Moynahan syndrome
MPA (main pulmonary artery)
MPAP (mean pulmonary artery
  pressure)
M pattern on right atrial waveform
MPF catheter
MPHR (maximum predicted heart
  rate)
MPIF-1 (myeloid progenitor inhibitory
  factor-1)
MPM hydrogel dressing
MPR (multiplanar reformation)
MPR (myocardial perfusion reserve)
MP-RAGE (magnetization prepared
  three-dimensional gradient-echo)
  sequences
MR (mitral regurgitation)
MRA (magnetic resonance
  angiography)
MRA (mechanical rotational atherec-
  tomy)
MRA gated inflow technique
MRI (magnetic resonance imaging)
  ECG-gated multislice technique
  ECG-gated spin-echo MR image
  echo-planar imaging
  FLASH (fast low-angle shot)
  free induction decay
  gradient-echo sequence imaging
  GRASS (gradient recalled acquisi-
    tion in steady state) cardiac MRI
  hydrogen density
  magnetic moment
  magnetic resonance signal
  MPR (multiplanar reformation)
  MP-RAGE (magnetization
    prepared three-dimensional
    gradient-echo) sequences

MRI *(cont.)*
  MSCTA (multislice computed
    tomographic angiography)
  multi-echo images
  multinuclear MRI
  multiphasic multislice technique
  paramagnetic substances
  proton density
  proton MRI
  proton spectroscopy
  relaxation
  relaxation times
  resonant frequency
  short-axis plane
  spin density
  spin-echo imaging sequence
  surface coils
  TE (echo delay time)
  tesla
  T1 relaxation time
  T1-weighted image
  T2 relaxation time
  T2-weighted image
  TR (repetition time)
  transverse plane
  voxel
  XY plane
  ZY plane
MR imaging without MT, triple-dose
  gadolinium-enhanced
MRS (magnetic resonance spectroscopy)
MRSA (pronounced "mer-suh")
  (methicillin-resistant *Staphylococcus*
  aureus)
MRV (mixed respiratory vaccine)
ms (milliseconds)
MS (mitral stenosis)
MS (morphine sulfate)
MSA (multiple system atrophy)
  syndrome
MS Classique catheter

msec (millisecond)
M-shaped pattern of mitral valve
MSLT (multiple sleep latency test)
MSOF (multisystem organ failure)
MTD (*Mycobacterium tuberculosis*
  direct) test
MTP (microsomal triglyceride transfer
  protein)
MTEs (main timing events)
MTT (mean pulmonary transit time)
Much's ("mooks") granules in sputa
  of patients with tuberculosis
mucocele
mucociliary transport
mucoid exopolysaccharide,
  Pseudomonas (hyper)immune
  globulin (MEPIG)
mucoid plugging of airways
mucocutaneous junction
mucocutaneous lymph node syndrome
mucoid degeneration, cardiac valve
mucoid exopolysaccharide, *Pseudo-*
  monas (hyper)immune globulin
  (MEPIG)
mucoid impaction in bronchi
mucoid medial degeneration
mucoid plugging of airways
mucoid plugs
mucolipidosis
mucopolysaccharidoses (plural)
mucopolysaccharidosis cardiomyopathy
mucoproteins
mucopurulent bronchitis
mucopurulent exudate
mucopurulent secretions
mucopurulent sputum
mucosa
  bronchial
  endobronchial
  friable
  main stem bronchial
mucosal inflammation

mucosectomy, endoscopic aspiration
mucous membranes
   dry
   moist
mucous rales
mucoviscidosis
mucus
   bloody nasal
   inspissated
   tenacious
mucus hypersecretion
mucus plug or plugging
Mueller (Müller)
muffled breath sounds
muffled heart sounds
MUGA (multiple-gated acquisition)
MUGA blood pool radionuclide scan
MUGA scan, preoperative resting
mulibrey nanism
Müller (Mueller)
Müller catheter guide
Müller maneuver (cardiac auscultation)
Müller sign (aortic regurgitation)
Mullins blade technique for dilatation
   of patent foramen ovale
Mullins catheter introducer
Mullins cardiac device
Mullins modification of transseptal
   catheterization
Mullins sheath
Mullins sheath in transseptal catheteri-
   zation
Mullins transseptal blade and balloon
   atrial septostomy
Mullins transseptal catheter
Mullins transseptal sheath
multiadjustable fitting device
Multibite biopsy forceps
multicapture burst
Multicath catheter
multicentric angiofollicular hyperplasia
   (MAFH)

multichannel ECG (EKG)
Multicor Gamma pacemaker
Multicor II pacemaker
multicrystal gamma camera
Multidex wound-filling material
multidrug resistance
multidrug resistance-associated protein
   (MRP)-positive tumor cells
multidrug-resistant tuberculosis
   (MDR-TB)
multidrug therapy
multi-echo images
multifactorial
MultiFEV spirometer
multifiber catheter
multifocal aggressive infiltrate
multifocal atrial tachycardia with
   aberrancy
multifocal lesions
multifocal lymphoma
multifocal PVCs (premature ventricular
   contractions)
multifocal short stenoses
multiforme, erythema
multiform PVC
multiform ventricular complexes
multi-infarct dementia
multilaminar bodies
multilead electrode
multilesion angioplasty
multilineage dysplasia
Multilink Duet noncoated coronary
   stent
Multilith pacemaker
Multilink Penta coronary stent system
Multilink Tetra coronary stent system
Multi-Med triple-lumen infusion
   catheter
multinuclear MRI
multinucleate giant cells
multiorgan failure
Multipad absorptive dressing

multiphasic multislice MRI technique
multiplanar reformation (MPR)
multiple blood transfusions
multiple chord, center line technique
    in echocardiogram
multiple drug resistance
multiple endocrine neoplasia
multiple extrastimuli
multiple-gated acquisition (MUGA)
multiple lentigines
multiple logistic regression
multiple mural dilatations
multiple organ failure (MOF)
multiple-puncture tuberculin test
multiple sleep latency test (MSLT)
multiple sulfatase deficiency
multiple system atrophy (MSA)
    syndrome
multiple-system disease
multiple unidentified respiratory flora
    (MURF)
multiplex, mononeuritis
multipolar electrode catheter
multiprogrammable pulse generator
multipurpose catheter
Multipurpose-SM catheter
multi-sideport infusion catheter
multislice computed tomographic
    angiography (MSCTA)
multislice multiphase spin-echo
    imaging technique
multislice spin-echo technique
multisystem organ failure (MSOF)
multivalvular disease
multiverrucous friable lesions
multivessel angioplasty
multivessel disease
multivessel stenting
mural aneurysm
mural architecture
mural degeneration
mural endomyocardial fibrosis

mural infiltration
mural leaflet of mitral valve
mural thrombosis
mural thrombus (pl. thrombi)
mural thrombus formation
MURF (multiple unidentified respira-
    tory flora)
mu rhythm (mu, twelfth Greek letter)
murmur (see also *sound*)
    accidental
    acquired heart
    amphoric
    anemic
    aneurysmal
    aortic diastolic
    aortic insufficiency
    aortic systolic
    apex
    apical
    apical diastolic
    arterial
    atrial systolic (ASM)
    atriosystolic
    attrition
    Austin Flint
    basal
    basal diastolic
    basal systolic
    basilar carotid
    bellows (blowing)
    blood
    blowing
    blowing pansystolic
    blubbery diastolic
    brachiocephalic systolic
    brain
    bronchial
    buzzing
    Cabot-Locke
    cardiac
    cardiopulmonary
    cardiorespiratory

murmur *(cont.)*
  Carey Coombs (no hyphen)
  click
  coarse
  Cole-Cecil
  congenital heart
  continuous (CM)
  continuous mammary souffle
  continuous rumbling
  cooing
  cooing-dove
  Coombs
  crescendo
  crescendo-decrescendo
  crescendo-decrescendo configura-
    tion
  crescendo presystolic
  Cruveilhier-Baumgarten
  decrescendo
  decrescendo holosystolic
  delayed diastolic (DDM)
  diamond-shaped
  diastolic (graded from 1 to 4)
  diastolic flow
  diastolic rumbling
  diffusely radiating
  diminuendo
  Docke
  Docke diastolic
  Duroziez
  dynamic
  early diastolic
  early systolic
  ejection
  ejection systolic (ESM)
  ejectionlike systolic
  endocardial
  even
  extracardiac
  extracardiac systolic arterial
  Flint
  Fräntzel

murmur *(cont.)*
  friction
  functional
  functional heart
  Gallavardin
  Gibson
  goose honk
  grade 1/6 or I/VI
    2/6 or II/VI
    1-2/6 or I-II/VI
    1 to 6 or I to VI
  Graham Steell heart
  groaning
  grunting
  Hamman
  harsh
  harsh systolic
  heart
  hemic
  high
  high-frequency
  high-pitched
  high-pitched ejection
  Hodgkin-Key
  holodiastolic
  holosystolic
  holosystolic ejection
  honking
  Hope
  hourglass
  humming
  humming-top
  immediate diastolic (IDM)
  incidental
  innocent heart
  innocent systolic
  inorganic
  late apical systolic
  late diastolic
  late-peaking systolic
  late systolic (LSM)
  left ventricular outflow

murmur *(cont.)*
   Levine Harvey grading system for
   loud (high-grade)
   low-frequency
   low-frequency diastolic
   low-pitched
   low-pitched, rumbling apical
      diastolic
   machine-like
   machinery
   machinery-like
   mammary souffle
   mid-diastolic
   mid-diastolic flow
   mid-diastolic mitral
   midsystolic
   mid-to-late diastolic
   mill-house
   mill-wheel
   mitral
   mitral click
   mitral regurgitant
   mitral valve prolapse
   muscle-splitting incision
   musical
   nun's venous hum
   obstructive
   organic
   outflow
   outflow midsystolic
   pansystolic (PSM)
   parasternal
   parasternal systolic
   pathologic
   pericardial
   peripheral pulmonic systolic
   plateau
   pleuropericardial
   prediastolic
   presystolic (PSM)
   presystolic Austin Flint
   presystolic crescendo

murmur *(cont.)*
   protodiastolic
   prototypical holosystolic
   pulmonary outflow
   pulmonary trunk
   pulmonary valve flow
   pulmonic radiating
   pulmonic systolic
   rasping
   regurgitant
   Roger
   rough
   rumbling
   rumbling diastolic
   Sansom rhythmical
   scratchy
   seagull
   seesaw (to-and-fro)
   Smith
   soft (low grade)
   squeaking
   Steell
   stenosal
   Still early systolic
   subclavicular
   supraclavicular
   supraclavicular systolic
   systolic (graded from 1 to 6)
   systolic ejection
   systolic mammary souffle
   to-and-fro (seesaw)
   Traube
   tricuspid
   tricuspid diastolic
   uneven
   unknown type
   valvular pulmonic stenosis
   variable
   vascular
   venous
   vibratory systolic
   waterwheel
   whooping

murmur abolished by digital pressure
murmur at the apex and left sternal
  border
murmur augmented by vigorous
  coughing
murmur grades: I to VI; 1 to 6
murmur increased during inspiration
murmur increased in intensity on
  Valsalva
murmur obliterated by digital pressure
murmur of long duration
murmur of short duration
murmur or gallop
murmur radiating into suprasternal
  notch
murmur radiating to apex of heart
murmur radiating to axilla
murmur radiating to base of neck
murmur radiating to neck
murmur radiating to sternal border
murmur, rub, or gallop
murmurs, clicks, or gallops
murmur transmitted to apex of heart
murmur transmitted to axilla
murmur transmitted to base of heart
murmur transmitted to carotids
murmur transmitted to neck
murmur with/without radiation
muscle, muscles
  accessory (of respiration)
  adductor magnus
  circular
  conal papillary
  electrically conditioned and driven
    skeletal
  fused papillary
  gastrocnemius
  intercostal
  Lancisi
  latissimus dorsi
  left ventricular
  longitudinal

muscle *(cont.)*
  Luschka
  medial papillary
  omohyoid
  papillary
  pectoralis major
  pectoralis minor
  peroneal
  plantaris
  platysma
  rhomboideus major
  sacrospinalis
  serratus anterior
  soleus
  sternocleidomastoid
  sternohyoid
  sternothyroid
  strap
  subaortic
  trapezius
  vastus medialis
  vocalis
muscle artifact
muscle cramps
muscle flap
muscle-splitting incision
muscle training, ventilatory
muscular atrioventricular septum
muscular bridging
muscular crus of diaphragm
muscular dystrophy
  Becker
  Duchenne
  Emery-Dreifuss
muscular subaortic stenosis
muscular venous pump
musculi pectinati
musculofascial layer
musculofascial pedicle
musculophrenic artery
musculophrenic branch
musculoskeletal pain

musculotendinous covering
mushroom picker's disease
mushroom worker's lung
mushroom worker's disease
mushy edema
mushy mass
musical murmur
musical rales
musical rhonchi
musical whoop
Musset sign (aortic aneurysm)
Mustang steerable guidewire
Mustard atrial baffle repair
Mustard baffle
Mustard baffle takedown
Mustard correction of transposition
 of great vessels
mutation
 fibrillin gene
 GATA3 gene
 Z
mutism, akinetic
mV (millivolt)
MV (mitral valve)
MVA (microvascular angiopathy)
MVA (mitral valve area)
MVD (mitral valve dysfunction)
MVO (maximum venous outflow)
MVO (mitral valve opening or orifice)
MVO$_2$ (myocardial oxygen consumption)
MVP (mean platelet volume)
MVP (mitral valve prolapse)
MVP (moisture vapor permeability)
MVP over-the-wire balloon catheter
MVR (mitral valve replacement)
MVS (mitral valve stenosis)
MVV (maximal voluntary ventilation)
MWT (maximum walking time)
myalgias and arthralgias
MycoAKT latex bead agglutination
 test

mycobacterial infection
mycobacteria, nontuberculous
mycobacteria susceptibility testing
Mycobacterium abscessus
Mycobacterium alvei
Mycobacterium avium complex
 (MAC)
Mycobacterium avium-intracellulare
 (MAI) infection
Mycobacterium fortuitum
Mycobacterium gordonae
Mycobacterium intracellulare
Mycobacterium kansasii
Mycobacterium, nonchromogenicum
Mycobacterium other than *tuberculosis*
 (MOTT)
Mycobacterium tuberculosis
Mycobacterium simiae infection
Mycobacterium tuberculosis
Mycoplasma antibody titer
mycoplasmal pneumonia
Mycoplasma pneumoniae infection
mycosis
 fatal systemic
 invasive pulmonary
 Posadas
mycotic aneurysm of pulmonary artery
mycotic suprarenal aneurysm
mydriasis
myectomy
myeloid progenitor inhibitory factor-1
 (MPIF-1)
Myers solution
MYHIIA (nonmuscle myosin heavy
 chain IIa) mutations
Myler catheter
myocardial adrenergic signaling
myocardial blood flow (MBF)
myocardial blush
myocardial bridging
myocardial cell necrosis
myocardial contractile function

myocardial contractility
myocardial contraction
myocardial contracture
myocardial contrast appearance time
  (MCAT)
myocardial contusion
myocardial degeneration
myocardial depression
myocardial dysfunction
myocardial fibers degeneration
myocardial fibrosis
myocardial granulomatous disease,
  allergic
myocardial hibernation
myocardial hypoperfusion, resting
  regional
myocardial hypothermia
myocardial hypoxia
myocardial incompetency
myocardial infarction (see also
    infarction)
  anterior
  anterior wall
  anteroapical wall
  anterobasal
  anterolateral wall
  anteroseptal wall
  apical
  apical-lateral wall
  basal-lateral wall
  diaphragmatic wall
  esophageal spasm mimicking
  high lateral wall
  impending
  inferior (diaphragmatic)
  inferolateral wall
  inferoposterior wall
  intraoperative
  nontransmural
  perioperative
  posterior wall
  posterobasal wall

myocardial *(cont.)*
  posteroinferior
  posterolateral wall
  posteroseptal
  stuttering
  subendocardial
  transmural
  true posterior wall
  uncomplicated, non-Q-wave
  uncomplicated Q-wave
myocardial infiltration by Kaposi
  sarcoma
myocardial injury
  lethal
  nonlethal
myocardial insufficiency, Sternberg
myocardial irritability
myocardial ischemia, exercise-induced
  transient
myocardial lactate extraction
myocardial muscle
myocardial necrosis
myocardial oxygen consumption
myocardial oxygen demand
myocardial performance
myocardial perfusion
myocardial perfusion defect
myocardial perfusion imaging
myocardial perfusion imaging agent
  (see *medications*)
myocardial perfusion scan
myocardial perfusion tomography
myocardial preservation
myocardial protection
myocardial recovery
myocardial remodeling
myocardial reperfusion injury
myocardial revascularization
myocardial rupture
myocardial scan
myocardial screw-in rate-sensing lead
myocardial shortening, fractional

myocardial-specific marker
myocardial stiffness
myocardial straining
myocardial stunning
myocardial tagging
myocardial tissue viability
myocardial tumor, metastatic
myocardial uptake of thallium
myocardial work
myocardiopathy (see *cardiomyopathy*)
  dilated
  postpartum
  primary
  puerperium
  secondary
myocardiorrhaphy
myocarditic
myocarditis
  acute bacterial
  acute interstitial
  acute isolated
  acute rheumatic
  aseptic (of newborn)
  bacterial
  chronic
  chronic hypertrophic
  chronic interstitial
  chronic pernicious
  coxsackievirus
  diphtheritic
  eosinophilic
  fibroid
  fibrous
  Fiedler
  fragmentation
  fungal
  giant cell
  granulomatous
  Histoplasma
  hypersensitivity
  idiopathic
  infectious

myocarditis *(cont.)*
  infective
  inflammatory
  influenzal
  interstitial
  isolated diffuse
  lues
  lymphocytic
  meningococcal
  metazoal
  neutrophilic
  nonspecific granulomatous
  parenchymatous
  peripartum
  pernicious
  pneumococcal
  protozoal
  rheumatic
  rickettsial
  senile
  septic
  spirochetal
  staphylococcal
  subepicardial
  syphilitic
  toxic
  toxoplasmotic
  Trichinella
  tuberculoid
  tuberculous
  viral
myocardium
  ablation of
  asynergic
  calcification of
  dilated
  hibernating
  hypertrophied
  hypertrophy of
  ischemic reperfused
  ischemic viable
  jeopardized

myocardium *(cont.)*
  noninfarcted
  nonperfused
  perfused
  perfusion of
  reperfused
  rupture of
  stunned
  ventricular
  viable
myocardosis
myocellular area
myocyte necrosis
myocyte
  Anichkov (or Anitschkow)
  atrial
myocytic lysosomes
myocytolysis, focal (of the heart)
myoendocarditis
  acute
  subacute
myofibrillar area
myofibrillar intraventricular heart
  block
myofibril volume fraction
myoglobin (Mb) concentration, serum
Myolift heart positioning device
Myomate implant
myopathy
  myotubular
  nemaline
myopericarditis
myoplasty
  Batista
  left ventricular reduction
  sartorius

myopotential inhibition
MyoSight cardiology imaging system
myosin heavy chain
myosin light chain
Myo-Star injection catheter for endocardial drug delivery
Myotherm XP cardioplegia delivery
  system
myotonia atrophica cardiomyopathy
myotonia congenita
myotonic dystrophy
myotubular myopathy
myovascular
myriad
Mystic Mongoose PTCA catheter
myxedema
myxoid degeneration
myxoma
  atrial
  biatrial
  cardiac
  familial (of the heart)
  heart
  left atrial
  pedunculated
  vascular
  ventricular
myxoma syndrome, with facial freckling
myxomatous degeneration of mitral
  valve
myxomatous degeneration of
  myocardium
myxomatous degeneration of valve

N, n

Nabatoff vein stripper
N-acetyl-p-aminophenol (NAPA) level
nadir of lung function
nadir of QRS complex
nadir, protodiastolic
NAET (Nambudripad's Allergy
   Elimination Technique)
nail bed, clubbing of
nail bed color
nail bed cyanosis
nailing graft in place
nail-patella syndrome
nail the graft in place
nail-to-nailbed angle (clubbing)
Nakata index
Nambudripad's Allergy Elimination
   Technique (NAET)
NAME (nevi, atrial myxoma, myxoid
   neurofibroma, ephelides) syndrome
nanism, mulibrey
N-ANP (N-terminal fragment atrial
   natriuretic peptide)
NAPA (N-acetyl-p-aminophenol) level
napkin-ring stenosis
Narcomatic flowmeter
narcosis, carbon dioxide
naris (pl. nares), anteverted

narrow anteroposterior diameter
narrowed bronchi
narrow expiratory splitting
NarrowFlex intra-aortic balloon
   catheter
NarrowFlex prewrapped double-lumen
   IAB catheter
narrow inspiratory splitting
narrow QRS complex
narrowed pulse pressure
narrowed S_1 splitting
narrowed S_2 splitting
narrowing
   arterial
   atherosclerotic
   diffuse
   focal
   high-grade
   luminal
   residual luminal
   subcritical
narrowing in large airway
narrowing of bronchiolar passages
Narula method
nasal airway resistance
nasal antigen challenge
nasal brush T-cells

nasal cannula
nasal CPAP (continuous positive
    airway pressure)
nasal dosimetry
nasal flaring
nasal intermittent pressure ventilation
    (NIPPV)
nasogastric tube
nasopharyngeal temperature probe
nasopharyngeal secretions
nasopharyngitis
nasopharyngoscope (see *endoscope*)
nasotracheal suction
nasotracheal tube
Nathan pacemaker
National Heart, Lung, and Blood
    Registry guidelines
National Institute for Allergy and
    Infectious Diseases (NIAID)
National Institutes of Health (NIH)
    catheter
native aortic valve, preservation of
native atherosclerosis
native coronary artery
native tissue harmonic imaging
    (NTHI)
native valve endocarditis
native ventricle
native vessel
natriuresis
natriuretic peptide, atrial
natural (intrinsic) heart rate
natural surfactant in the lungs
nature, evanescent
Naughton-Balke treadmill protocol,
    modified
Naughton cardiac exercise treadmill
    test
Naughton treadmill protocol, modified
navigating coronary structures
navigating heart structures
Navi-Star diagnostic/ablation deflec-
    table tip catheter

Navi-Star mapping catheter
Navius catheter
Navius guidewire
Navius stent
NBIH cardiac device
NBTE (nonbacterial thrombotic endo-
    carditis)
NB200 vascular access device
NC Ranger PTCA catheter
NC Raptor PTCA dilatation catheter
Nd:YAG (neodymium:yttrium-
    aluminum-garnet) laser
near field
near-infrared spectroscopy
near-loss of consciousness
near-syncopal episode
near-syncope
nebulization therapy, continuous
    (CNT)
nebulize
nebulized bronchodilator
nebulized isoproterenol
nebulizer (see also *inhaler*)
    Acorn
    Aero Tech II
    AERx electronic inhaler
    air-powered
    Avea
    DeVilbiss ultrasound
    Fisoneb
    handheld
    high-frequency
    jet
    MAD2
    Marquest Respirgard II
    Portasonic
    Pulmo-Aide
    Pulmosonic
    Respirgard II
    Small Particle Aerosol
    Twin Jet
    Ultravent

nebulizer *(cont.)*
   Varic ultrasound
   Wright
   ultrasonic (USN)
NEC (nonejection click)
Necator americanus infection
neck
   hostile
   hyperextension
neck breathers
neck emphysema
neck of the aneurysm
neck rotation
neck vein distention
neck veins
   distended
   elevated
   flat
   fullness of
neck vessel engorgement
necrosed the vein
necrosis
   acute tubular
   alveolar
   alveolar septa
   idiopathic (of aorta)
   arteriolar
   caseous
   cheesy
   coagulation
   contraction band
   cystic medial
   embolic
   Erdheim cystic medial (of aorta)
   fibrinoid
   heart muscle
   hepatic
   hyaline
   ischemic
   lung
   myocardial
   myocyte

necrosis *(cont.)*
   perioperative myocardial
   skin (due to distal steal)
   subendocardial
   ventricular muscle
necrosis of lung
necrotic angiitis
necrotic cells
necrotic debris
necrotic fibrinoid vegetation
necrotic flap
necrotizing angiitis
necrotizing arterial disease
necrotizing arteriolitis
necrotizing arteritis
necrotizing bronchitis
necrotizing emphysema
necrotizing granulomatous angiitis
   involving lungs
necrotizing pneumonia
necrotizing respiratory granulomatosis
necrotizing thrombosis
necrotizing vasculitis
NED (no evidence of disease)
needle
   Abrams
   Aldrete
   AMC
   aortic root perfusion
   aspirating
   Atraloc
   Becton Dickinson Teflon-sheathed
   Bengash-type
   beveled thin-walled
   Brockenbrough
   Brockenbrough transseptal
   BV-2
   Caldwell
   Captiva (for vascular access)
   cardioplegic
   Cardiopoint
   Control-Release pop-off

needle *(cont.)*
  Cope biopsy
  Cournand
  cutting
  DLP cardioplegic
  Dos Santos
  Echo-Coat ultrasound biopsy
  Ethalloy TruTaper cardiovascular
  eXcel-DR pneumo
  GlideCath entry
  Gripper
  Hemo-Cath introducer
  Jelco
  large-bore slotted aspirating
  MAGneedle controllers
  Majestik shielded angiography
  metal
  non-coring
  Nordenstrom (Rotex II) biopsy
  olive-tipped
  PercuCut cut-biopsy
  percutaneous cutting
  pericardiocentesis
  pleural biopsy
  Potts
  Potts-Cournand
  Protect Point
  Riza-Ribe
  root
  Rotex II biopsy
  Sabreloc spatula
  Seldinger
  self-aspirating cut-biopsy
  Sensi-Touch anesthesia
  side-cutting spatulated
  slotted
  spinal
  Stifcore aspiration
  swaged-on
  THI
  thoracentesis
  T12

needle *(cont.)*
  UMI
  venting aortic Bengash-type
needle biopsy, CT-scan directed
needle holder
  Barraquer
  Berry sternal
  Castroviejo
  Crile-Wood
  Vital Cooley microvascular
  Vital Ryder microvascular
  Webster
needle hub
needleless injection cannula
needle, sponge, and instrument counts
NEFA (non-esterified fatty acid)
  scintigraphy
negative chronotropic effect
negative deflection on EKG
Nefertiti sniff position
negative image of pulmonary edema
negative pressure at the airway
  opening during expiration
negligible pressure gradient
Neisseria infection
Nellcor Symphony blood pressure
  monitoring system
Nelson scissors
Nelson thoracic trocar
nemaline myopathy
neoadjuvant therapy
neoaorta
neoaortic valve
neodymium:yttrium-aluminum-garnet
  (Nd:YAG) laser
neointimal hyperplasia
neointimal proliferation
neonatal apnea
neonatal asphyxia
neonatal cystic pulmonary emphysema
neonatal lupus erythematosus
neonatal thyrotoxicosis

neonate
neonatorum, edema
Neon tip (for a catheter)
Neo PICC neonatal peripherally
    inserted central catheter
neoplasia, multiple endocrine
neoplasm
    endobronchial
    mediastinal
    primary lung
neoplastic pericarditis
Neos M pacemaker
NeoSpect diagnostic imaging agent
Neostar vascular access catheter
neostigmine test
NeoTect (technetium Tc 99m
    depreotide) imaging agent
Neotrend blood gas monitoring system
neovascularity, stump-related
nephritis
    arteriolar
    interstitial arteriosclerotic
    radiation
    vascular
nephritis repens
nephroblastoma
nephropathy, radiocontrast-induced
nephrosclerosis
nephrotic edema
Nernst equation in cardiac action
    potential (resting phase)
nerve
    Hering
    Kuntz
    long thoracic
    phrenic
    recurrent laryngeal
    supraclavicular
    vagus
nervous heart syndrome
nervous system, parasympathetic
NESC (nonejection systolic click)

NESP (Novel erythropoiesis stimulat-
    ing protein)
neural crest origin, tumor of
neuralgia, glossopharyngeal
neurally mediated syncope
neurectomy, periaortic
neurocardiogenic syncope
neurocirculatory asthenia
neuroepithelium
neurofibroma of the heart
neurofibromatosis
neurogenic pulmonary edema
neurogenic sarcoma of the heart
neurologic signs, focal
neuromuscular blockade
neuronal ceroid lipofuscinosis
neuropathy, autonomic
neuroregulatory asthenia
neuroregulatory syncope
Neuroshield cerebral protection device
neurosis, postphlebitic
neurotoxicity, lidocaine
neurovascular bundle
neutral fat (triglyceride)
neutropenia
neutrophil alveolitis
neutrophil concentration
neutrophil elastase
neutrophilia, absolute
NEV (noninvasive extrathoracic venti-
    lator) (see *Porta-Lung*)
nevus (pl. nevi)
    senile
    spider
    stellar
nevus araneus
Nevyas drape retractor arched frame
New Leaf cardiopulmonary perform-
    ance testing device
Newman-Keuls test
New York Heart Association (NYHA)
NexStent carotid stent

Nexus 2 linear ablation catheter
NF-ATc (NFAT-3) proteins
NH region of AV (atrioventricular) node
NI-NR (no infection—no rejection)
niacin test for *Mycobacterium tuberculosis*
Niagara dialysis catheter
NIAID (National Institute for Allergy and Infectious Diseases)
NIAV (noninvasive assisted ventilation)
Nicoladoni-Branham sign
nicking, AV (arteriovenous)
Nicks procedure
nicotinic acid
NIDCM (nonischemic dilated cardiomyopathy)
nidus, thrombus
Niemann-Pick disease
NIF-negative inspiratory force
night sweats
NIH (National Institutes of Health)
NIH cardiac device
NIH cardiomarker catheter
NIH left ventriculography catheter
NIH mitral valve forceps
Nikaidoh-Bex technique
Nikaidoh translocation of aorta
Nikolsky sign
nil blood loss
Nimbus Hemopump
Ninja FX PTCA dilatation catheter
nipple, blind
nipple sign, aortic
NIPPV (nasal intermittent pressure ventilation)
NIPPV (noninvasive positive pressure ventilation)
NIPS (noninvasive programmed stimulation)
NIR ON stent
NIR premounted stent delivery system

NIR Prince (or NIR pRINce) stent
NIR stent
NIR with SOX over-the-wire coronary stent system
NIRflex coronary stent
NIRoyal Elite Monorail coronary stent system
NIRS (near-infrared spectroscopy)
nitinol (nickel/titanium alloy) thermal memory stent
nitrates, long-acting
nitric oxide
nitro (slang for nitroglycerin)
Nitro-Dur (nitroglycerin)
nitroglycerin (NTG)
nitroglycerin paste
nitroglycerin transdermal system (NTS)
Nitrol ointment
"nitro paste" (nitroglycerin ointment)
NitroQuick (nitroglycerin) sublingual tablets
nitrogen, blood urea (BUN)
nitrogen-13 ammonia radioactive tracer
nitrogen washout
nitroglycerin (NTG)
   sublingual (SL)
   topical
   transdermal
   translingual
   transmucosal
nitroglycerin drip
nitroprusside
NitroQuick (nitroglycerin) sublingual tablets
nitrous oxide
N, nl, nml (normal)
no CPR status
Nocardia fungus
nocardial infection of the bronchi
nocardiosis, bronchial

nocardiotic pericarditis
nociceptive
nocturia times two
nocturnal angina
nocturnal asthma
nocturnal cough
nocturnal polyuria
nocturnal worsening of asthma
nodal conduction
nodal contractions
nodal escape
nodal impulse
nodal irradiation
nodal rhythm
nodal premature contraction
nodal rhythm disorder
node, nodes (see also *nodules,*
　　nodulus)
　aortic window
　Aschoff
　Aschoff-Tawara
　atrioventricular (AV, AVN)
　axillary lymph
　cardiac
　Flack sinoatrial
　hilar
　Keith-Flack sinoatrial
　Koch sinoatrial
　lymph
　mediastinal lymph
　NH region of AV (atrioventricular)
　nonverrucous
　Osler
　periaortic
　pericardial lymph
　SA (sinoatrial)
　sentinel
　shotty lymph
　sick sinus
　singer's
　sinoatrial (SAN)
　sinoauricular

node *(cont.)*
　sinus
　supraclavicular lymph
　Tawara atrioventricular
　vestigial left sinoatrial
no discernible findings
no evidence of disease (NED)
nodo-Hisian (nodohisian)
nodo-Hisian bypass
nodo-Hisian bypass tract
nodosa
　chorditis
　panarteritis
　periarteritis
　polyarteritis
nodosum, erythema
nodoventricular bypass fiber
nodoventricular bypass tract
nodoventricular pathway
nodoventricular tachycardia
nodular aneurysm
nodular fibrosis
nodularity
　coarse
　valve leaflet
　vein
nodule, nodules (see also *node,*
　　nodulus)
　Albini
　aortic valve
　Arantius
　Aschoff
　Bianchi
　Cruveilhier
　hyalin
　Kerckring
　laryngeal
　Morgagni
　noncavitary
　ossific
　rheumatic
　rheumatoid

nodule *(cont.)*
  silicotic
  singer's
  solitary lung
  solitary pulmonary
nodules of pulmonary trunk valves
nodulus Arantii (pl. noduli Arantii)
  (nodule of Arantius)
nodus arcus venae azygos
noise, respiratory
nonablative heating
nonaeruginosa pseudomonads
nonallergenic factors
nonallergic asthma
nonapneic snorer
nonarrhythmic
nonarrhythmogenic
nonarterial groin infection
nonasbestos pneumoconiosis
nonatopic
nonazotemic
nonbacterial endocarditis
nonbacterial thrombotic endocarditis
  (NBTE)
nonbacterial verrucous endocarditis
nonballoon therapies (stents,
  atherectomy, and excimer laser
  angioplasty)
noncalcific subacute constrictive
  pericarditis
noncalcified mitral leaflets
noncardiac basis
noncardiac chest pain
noncardiac death
noncardiac dyspnea
noncardiac etiology
noncardiac pulmonary edema
noncardiogenic pulmonary edema
noncardiogenic shock
noncaseating granuloma
noncaseating tubercles
noncavitary nodules

noncavitary prosthetic graft
nonchromogenicum *Mycobacterium*
noncircularity degree
noncoaxial catheter tip position
noncollagenous pneumoconiosis
noncompensatory pause
noncompliant plaque
noncontractile scar tissue
noncoplanar multiple static port
non-coring needle
noncoronary anulus
noncoronary cardiomyopathy
noncoronary cusp
noncoronary seating of the valve
noncoronary sinus
noncritical coronary artery disease
noncrushing vascular clamps
nondecremental
nondiaphoretic
nondistensible pericardium
nondominant vessel
nondrinker, nonsmoker
non-ejection click (NEC)
non-ejection systolic click (NESC)
non-everting suture
nonexpansional dyspnea
nonfenestrated Fontan procedure
nonfilarial chylocele
nonfilling venous segment
nonforeshortened angiographic view
nonhypertension-related disease
nonhypertension syndrome
nonimaging probe
nonimmune fetal hydrops
nonimmunocompromised host
nonimmunologic fetal hydrops
noninducible tachycardia
noninfarcted segment
noninfectious reactions of lung
noninfective endocardial lesion
noninfective verrucous endocarditis
noninflammatory fluid accumulation
  in pleural cavity

noninvasive assessment
noninvasive assisted ventilation (NIAV)
noninvasive extrathoracic ventilator
(NEV)
noninvasive mechanical ventilation
noninvasive positive pressure ventilation (NIPPV)
noninvasive technique
noninvasive testing
noninvasive treatment
noninvasive vascular imaging
technique
nonionic contrast material
nonischemic dilated cardiomyopathy
(NIDCM)
nonischemic mitral valve insufficiency
nonlethal arrhythmias
nonlethal myocardial ischemic injury
non-lifestyle-limiting lower extremity
claudication
nonlingular branches of upper lobe
bronchus
nonmuscle myosin heavy chain IIa
(MYHIIA) mutations
Nonne-Milroy lymphedema
non-nodular fibrosis
non-nodular silicosis
nonobstructive cardiomyopathy
(NOCM)
nonocclusive mesenteric arterial
insufficiency
nonoperable disease
nonoperative
nonoxygenated blood
nonpalpable pulses
nonparoxysmal atrioventricular
junctional tachycardia
nonparoxysmal automatic atrial
tachycardia
nonparoxysmal AV (atrioventricular)
nodal tachycardia
nonpenetrating trauma to heart

nonpleuritic precordial pain
nonpneumoconiotic
nonproductive cough
nonproductive dry cough
nonpulsatile abdominal mass
nonpulsatile mass
nonpulsatile ventricular assist device
nonpurulent pericarditis
nonpurulent pulmonary secretions
nonpyogenic thrombosis
non-Q wave
non-Q-wave myocardial infarction
(NQWMI)
nonrebreather mask
nonrebreathing mask
nonreversed saphenous vein graft
nonreversed translocated vein bypass
nonrheumatic aortic stenosis
nonrheumatic endocarditis
nonrheumatic valvular aortic stenosis
nonsegmental areas of opacification
nonselective beta blocker
nonshocked heart
non-small cell carcinoma of lung
non-small cell lung cancer (NSCLC)
nonsmoker, nondrinker
nonspecific changes
nonspecific granulomatous myocarditis
nonspecific inflammatory aortoarteritis
nonspecific irritants
nonspecific scooping (on EKG)
nonspecific ST and T-wave changes
(NSTTWC)
nonspecific ST-segment changes
nonspecific ST-segment and T-wave
changes
nonspecific T-wave aberration
nonspecific T-wave abnormality
nonspecific T-wave changes
nonsteroidal anti-inflammatory drugs
(NSAID)
nonstress test (NST)

nonsustained ventricular tachycardia
(NSVT)
nonsustained monomorphic ventricular
tachycardia
nonsustained polymorphic ventricular
tachycardia
nonthoracotomy cardioverter-
defibrillator
nonthoracotomy endocardial lead
systems
CPI Endotak
Medtronic Transvene
Telectronics
nonthoracotomy lead (NTL)
nontrabeculated atrium
nontransmural myocardial infarction
nontraumatic epidural hemorrhage
nontraumatizing catheter
nontuberculous mycobacteria
nonuniform rotational defect (NURD)
nonunion of operated sternum
nonvalved conduit
nonverrucous node
nonviable scar from myocardial infarction
Noonan AV (arteriovenous) fistula
clamp
Noonan syndrome
noosed down
noose occluder
NoProfile balloon catheter
Nordenstrom biopsy needle
no-reflow phenomenon
norepinephrine
normal (N, nl, nml)
normal-appearing bronchi
normal flora
normalization of inverted T waves
normal QRS axis
normal QRS complex
normal S_1 and S_2 (heart sounds)
normal sinus rhythm (NSR)

normetanephrine
Normigel hydrogel dressing
normocapnic
normochromic anemia
normocytic anemia
normokalemic reperfusion
normotensive
normothermia
normothermic cardiopulmonary bypass
normothermic fibrillating heart
normothermic temperature
normovolemia
normovolemic
normoxia
Northern blot analysis or test
Norvasc (amlodipine)
Norwood operation for hypoplastic
left-sided heart syndrome
Fontan modification of
Gill-Jonas modification of
Jonas modification of
Sade modification of
NOS (not otherwise specified)
nose cone
nosocomial infection
nosocomial infective endocarditis
nosocomial lung infection
nosocomial opportunistic infection
nosocomial pneumonia
nosocomial TB (tuberculosis) transmission
No Sting barrier film
nostril symptoms
not a candidate for cardiac surgery
not a candidate for transplant surgery
notch
anacrotic
aortic
dicrotic
sternal
suprasternal
notched aortic knob on chest x-ray

notched P wave
notching of pulmonic valve on
  echocardiogram
notching, rib
note
  drumlike percussion
  dull percussion
  flat percussion
  hyperresonant percussion
  percussion
  resonant percussion
  tympanitic percussion
no therapy zone
Nothnagel paresthesia
Nothnagel syndrome
No Torque Right coronary angiography catheter
no-touch technique in vascular anastomosis
not-so-sudden cardiac death
NovaCath multi-lumen infusion
  catheter
Novacor DiaSys cardiac device
Novacor implantable left ventricular
  assist device (LVAD)
Novacor LVAS (left ventricular assist
  system)
Novacor ventricular assist device
  (VAD)
Nova MR pacemaker
Nova II pacemaker
Novel erythropoiesis stimulating
  protein (NESP)
novel plasminogen activator (NPA)
Novofil suture
Novo-Hydrazide (hydrochlorothiazide)
Novo-Salmol (salbutamol)
Novo-Semide (furosemide)
no-wrap technique
noxious agent
noxious inhalants

noxious stimuli
NPA (novel plasminogen activator)
NPC (nodal premature contraction)
NPJT (nonparoxysmal AV [atrioven-
  tricular] junctional tachycardia)
NPRJT (nonparoxysmal reciprocating
  junctional tachycardia)
NQWMI (non-Q-wave myocardial
  infarction)
NSAID (nonsteroidal anti-inflamma-
  tory drugs)
NSAID-precipitated asthma
NSCLO (non-small cell lung cancer)
NSR (normal sinus rhythm)
NSTTWC (nonspecific ST and
  T-wave changes)
NSVT (nonsustained ventricular tachy-
  cardia)
NTG (nitroglycerin)
N-13 ammonia uptake on PET scan
NTHI (native tissue harmonic imaging)
NTL (nonthoracotomy lead)
NTP (noninvasive temporary pacemaker)
NT-proBNP immunoassay, also
  Elecsys proBNP Immunoassay
NTS (nitroglycerin transdermal
  system)
nuchal rigidity
nuclear gated blood pool testing
nuclear-tagged red blood cell bleeding
  study
Nu-Derm hydrocolloid dressing
  material
null cell lymphoblastic leukemia
null point
numb extremities
number of puffs of bronchodilator
number of puffs of corticosteroids
numbness
nummular sputum

nun's murmur (venous hum)
NURD (nonuniform rotational defect)
Nurolon suture
Nu-Salt salt substitute
Nu-Tip disposable scissor tip
nutrient cardioplegia
Nutrim dietary fat substitute
nutrition heart syndrome
nutritional anemia
nutritional macrocytic anemia
Nycore angiography catheter

Nycore cardiac device
Nydex catheter
NYHA (New York Heart Association)
NYHA classification of angina
NYHA classification of congestive
  heart failure
NYHA classification of heart block
  (types I-IV)
nylon paracostal sutures
nylon sutures
Nyquist limit

O, o

O_2 saturation
Oasis thrombectomy system
oat bran
oat cell carcinoma
oat-shaped cell
obesity, cardiopulmonary
obesity-related hypertension
objective symptoms
obligatory admixture of systemic
  venous and pulmonary venous
  blood
oblique abdominal incision
oblique fissure of lung
oblique pericardial sinus
oblique sinus
oblique subcostal incision
oblique vein of left atrium
obliquity
obliterans
  arteriosclerosis
  bronchiolitis
  endarteritis
  thromboangiitis
obliterate
obliterating phlebitis

obliteration
  lateral leaflet
  omental flap
obliteration of the costophrenic angle
obliterative arteriolitis, pulmonary
obliterative arteriosclerosis
obliterative arteritis
obliterative bronchiolitis
obliterative cardiomyopathy
obliterative pericarditis
obliterative phlebitis
obscuration of hilum
obscure cardiomyopathy of Africa
obscured coronary anatomy
obstructed pulmonary artery
obstructing bronchogenic carcinoma
obstructing embolus
obstruction
  airway
  aortic arch
  aortic outflow
  aortoiliac
  bronchial
  chronic airways
  congenital left-sided outflow

obstruction *(cont.)*
  congenital subpulmonic
  cowl-shaped
  endobronchial
  fixed airway
  fixed coronary
  foreign body upper airway
  increased pulmonary
  intrathoracic airway
  intrathoracic upper airway
  intraventricular right ventricular
  irreversible airways
  malignant airway
  preocclusive
  pulmonary artery
  pulmonary outflow
  pulmonary vascular
  pulmonary venous
  respiratory tract, mechanical
  right ventricular outflow
  subpulmonic
  subvalvular aortic
  subvalvular diffuse muscular
  superior caval
  superior vena caval
  upper airway
  vascular
  venous
  ventricular outflow
  ventricular outflow tract
obstructive apnea
obstructive atelectasis
obstructive cardiomyopathy,
  hypertrophic
obstructive emphysema
obstructive hypertrophic cardiomyopathy
obstructive hypopnea
obstructive mitral valve murmur
obstructive murmur
obstructive pneumonia
obstructive pneumonitis

obstructive pulmonary disease (OPD)
obstructive pulmonary overinflation
obstructive rhinitis
obstructive shock
obstructive sleep apnea, idiopathic
obstructive small airways disease
obstructive thrombus within the lumen
obstructive ventilatory defect
obtainment
obtunded infant, profoundly
obturating embolus
obturator
  AVA HF
  AVA 3XI
  Hancock
obtuse marginal (OM) coronary artery
obtuse marginal branch (OMB)
obtuse marginal bypass
obtuse marginal, first
obviate the morbidity
obviate the mortality
obviate the need for surgery
occipital vessels
occlude
occluded graft
occluder
  Amplatzer ductal
  CardioSEAL septal
  Clamshell
  Flo-Rester vessel
  Hunter-Sessions balloon
  Innovante
  IVM vascular
  noose
  occluding noose
  radiolucent plastic
  Rashkind
  Rashkind double-disk
  Sarns 5000
  Sarns 7000
  Stockert/Shiley venous

occluder button component folded and introduced into sheath
occluder delivered into left atrium under fluoroscopic control
occluder equals button
occluding noose occluders
occluding spring emboli
occluding thrombus
occlusion
    acute mesenteric artery
    anterior descending (artery)
    ASD transcatheter (with button device)
    balloon
    coil
    complete
    coronary
    coronary artery
    coronary orifices
    ductus arteriosus
    embolic
    fenestration
    graft
    intermittent
    late graft
    left anterior descending
    pressure-controlled intermittent coronary
    renal artery
    side branch
    snowplow
    subtotal
    tapering
    total
    vein graft
    vessel (atraumatic)
occlusion measurement
occlusion of blood supply
occlusion of internal carotid arteries above the clinoids
occlusive arterial thrombus
occlusive dressing

occlusive impedance phlebography
occlusive lesion
occlusive vascular disease
occult circulatory abnormalities
occult constrictive pericarditis
occult disease
occult hypertension
occult lesion
occult pericardial constriction
occupational asthma
occupational disease
occupational stress
Ochsner forceps
Ochsner graft
Ochsner retractor
O_2 crystalloid cardioplegia
octapolar catheter
Octopus retractor
Octopus stabilizing device
Octopus 3 tissue stabilizing system
ocular cardiac reflex syncope
ocular pneumoplethysmography (OPG)
oculoplethysmography/carotid phonoangiography (OPG/CPA)
oculopneumoplethysmography
ODAM defibrillator
Oehler symptoms
Oertel treatment
offending organism
offending pericardial fluid, evacuation of
off-pump aneurysmectomy
off-pump beating heart revascularization
off-pump coronary artery bypass (OPCAB)
off-pump coronary artery bypass graft (OPCABG)
OHD (organic heart disease)
Ohio 560 ventilator
ohm (pl. ohms)
Ohmeda 6200 CO_2 monitor

oil embolism
OKT3 monoclonal antibody
OKT3 prophylaxis
Olbert catheter
oligemia
oligemic
oligonucleotide probes
OligoNucleotides, Respiratory Anti-
Sense (RASON)
oliguria, postoperative
Oliver-Cardarelli sign
Oliver-Rosalki method of testing
serum CPK
olive-tipped needle
Olympus angioscope
Olympus BF P-10 bronchoscope
Olympus BF 4B2 bronchoscope
Olympus BF 3C4 bronchoscope
Olympus BF-10 bronchoscope
Olympus BF-160 video bronchoscope
Olympus BF-1T10 bronchoscope
Olympus BF-1T160 video broncho-
scope
Olympus BF-1T20 bronchoscope
Olympus BF-1T200 bronchoscope
Olympus BF-1T20D bronchoscope
Olympus BF-1T240 video broncho-
scope
Olympus BF-20 bronchoscope
Olympus BF-20D bronchoscope
Olympus BF-240 video bronchoscope
Olympus BF-3C160 video broncho-
scope
Olympus BF-3C20 bronchoscope
Olympus BF-3C40 fiber bronchoscope
Olympus BF-40 bronchoscope
Olympus BF-N20 bronchoscope
Olympus BF-P 200 bronchoscope
Olympus BF-P10 bronchoscope
Olympus BF-P160 video broncho-
scope
Olympus BF-P200 bronchoscope

Olympus BF-P20D bronchoscope
Olympus BF-P240 bronchoscope
Olympus BF-P240 video broncho-
scope
Olympus BF-P40 fiber bronchoscope
Olympus BF-XP40 fiber broncho-
scope
Olympus BF-XT40 bronchoscope
Olympus BF1T40 fiber bronchoscope
Olympus bioptome
Olympus bronchoscope
Olympus Evis Exera video broncho-
scope
Olympus fiberoptic bronchoscope
Olympus LF-DP portable intubation
fiberscope
Olympus LF-GP portable intubation
fiberscope
Olympus LF-TP portable intubation
fiberscope
OM (obtuse marginal) artery
OMB (obtuse marginal branch)
OMB1 (obtuse marginal branch #1)
Omed bulldog vascular clamp
Omega-NV balloon
omega-3 fatty acids
omental flap obliteration of the chest
cavity
omentum
gastrohepatic
sigmoid
ominous chest discomfort
ominous findings
ominous prognosis
ominous sign
Omnicarbon prosthetic heart valve
Omnicarbon prosthetic valve
OmniCath atherectomy catheter
Omnicor pacemaker
OmniFilter
Omniflex balloon catheter
OmniFlow vascular graft

Omni Flush shape Accu-Vu catheter
OmniMesh ablation catheter
OmniMesh bidirectional catheter
OmniMesh braided-tip catheter
Omni-Orthocor II pacemaker
Omnir stent
Omni retractor
Omniscience prosthetic heart valve
Omniscience single leaflet cardiac
　　valve prosthesis
Omniscience tilting-disk valve
　　prosthesis
Omniscience valve device
Omni-Stanicor pacemaker
OmniStent
Omni-Theta pacemaker
Omni-Tract adjustable wishbone
　　retractor
Omni-Tract retractor system
omohyoid muscle
Ondine's curse
one-second forced expiratory volume
　　(FEV_1)
one-shot anastomotic instrument
one-stage clotting test
one-stage prothrombin time test
one-way valve (of catheter)
onionskin configuration of collagenous
　　fibers
onlay graft
OnLineABG monitoring system
onset
　　acute
　　early
　　insidious
onset of atrial systole
On-X aortic prosthetic heart valve
Onyx finger pulse oximeter
OPA (oropharyngeal airway)
opacification
　　nonsegmental areas of
　　pedal artery

opacities, patchy alveolar
opacity (pl. opacities), ground-glass
opalescent sputum
OPCAB (off-pump coronary artery
　　bypass)
OPCABG (off-pump coronary artery
　　bypass graft)
OPD (obstructive pulmonary disease)
open cardiac massage
open endarterectomy
open-heart CPR
open-heart endocardial radiofrequency
　　ablation
opening
　　amplitude of valve
　　buttonhole
　　slitlike
　　valvular
opening pressure, airway
opening snap (OS)
　　high-pitched
　　palpable
open lung biopsy
open pneumothorax
OpenSail balloon catheter
open subfascial division technique in
　　treatment of varicose veins
open tuberculosis
open valvotomy
operation (see also *method, procedure,*
　　technique)
　　ablation of bundle of His
　　acute intraoperative
　　arterial elongation
　　Alfieri mitral valve repair
　　Alfieri-plasty (bow-tie repair;
　　　double orifice repair)
　　aneurysmectomy
　　antegrade transseptal approach
　　　in valvuloplasty
　　anterograde percutaneous aortic
　　　valvotomy

operation *(cont.)*
  anuloplasty
  aorticopulmonary window
  aortic-pulmonary shunt
  aortic root replacement
  aortic valve repair
  aortic valve replacement
  aortic valve re-replacement
    (AVreR)
  aortic valve resuspension
  aortic valvuloplasty
  aortofemoral bypass
  aortopulmonary window
  aortotomy
  arterial switch
  arteriotomy
  atherectomy
  atrial baffle
  atrial switch
  atrioventricular valve replacement
  AV (aortic valve) repair
  Babcock
  balloon atrial septostomy
  balloon mitral valvuloplasty
  balloon tuboplasty
  balloon valvuloplasty
  banding of pulmonary artery
  Batista left ventriculectomy
  Batista myoplasty
  beating-heart surgery
  Bentall inclusion technique
  bidirectional Glenn
  BIMA (bilateral internal mammary
    artery) reconstruction
  blade and balloon atrial septostomy
  Blalock-Hanlon atrial septectomy
  Blalock-Hanlon cardiac
  Blalock-Taussig anastomosis
  Blalock-Taussig cardiac
  bow-tie repair
  Brockenbrough commissurotomy
  Brock transventricular closed
    valvotomy

operation *(cont.)*
  Brom repair (aortic stenosis)
  bronchopulmonary lavage
  CABS (coronary artery bypass
    surgery)
  cardiomyoplasty
  carotid angioplasty with stenting
  carotid endarterectomy
  Carpentier anuloplasty
  Carpentier tricuspid valvuloplasty
  catheter ablation of bundle of His
  catheter balloon valvuloplasty
    (CBV)
  classic Glenn procedure
  coarctectomy
  commissurotomy
  commissurotomy of pulmonary
    valve
  computer-enhanced telemetric
    mitral valve repair
  conotruncal repair
  contralateral lung volume reduction
  Cooley anastomosis
  coronary atherectomy
  corridor
  costectomy
  cryosurgery
  cryosurgical interruption of AV
    (atrioventricular) bypass tract
  cryosurgical interruption of AV
    (atrioventricular) node
  Damus-Kaye-Stansel (DKS)
  David
  decortication of lung
  De Vega tricuspid anuloplasty
  directional coronary angioplasty
    (DCA)
  directional coronary atherectomy
    (DCA)
  division of accessory bundle of
    Kent
  Dor remodeling ventriculoplasty

operation *(cont.)*

    double-orifice repair of mitral
regurgitation in Barlow disease

    ELAS (endoluminal laser ablation
of the greater saphenous vein)

    ELCA (excimer laser coronary
angioplasty)

    electrode catheter ablation

    encircling endocardial ventricu-
lotomy

    endocardial ablation

    endocardial resection

    endocardial to epicardial resection

    endoscopic aspiration mucosectomy

    endoscopic mitral valve repair

    endoventricular circular patchplasty

    end-to-side portocaval anastomosis

    excimer laser coronary angioplasty
(ELCA)

    extended vertical transseptal
approach in mitral valve
surgery

    extracardiac conduit Fontan

    femorodistal bypass

    femoropopliteal bypass

    fenestrated Fontan

    first-stage Norwood

    flap tracheostomy

    Fontan-Kreutzer repair

    Fontan tricuspid atresia

    Glenn

    heart transplant

    heart-lung transplant

    Heller esophagocardiomyotomy

    hemi-Fontan

    high-speed rotational atherectomy
(RA)

    Hunter

    infarctectomy

    inferior vena cava interruption

    infundibular resection

    internal saphenous vein grafting

operation *(cont.)*

    intra-atrial baffle

    inverted T partial upper
re-sternotomy for aortic valve
replacement (AVR)

    Jatene arterial switch

    Jatene transposition of great
arteries

    Kay tricuspid valvuloplasty

    King-Mills procedure

    Konno patch enlargement of aorta

    laser recanalization

    left atriotomy for mitral valve
surgery

    left ventricular reduction myoplasty

    ligamentum teres cardiopexy
fundoplication

    ligature of popliteal veins

    Lillehei-Hardy-Hunter

    LIMA-Lift

    limited thoracotomy

    Lindesmith

    Linton treatment of varicose veins

    Lower-Shumway heart transplant

    lung volume reduction surgery
(LVRS)

    Matas aneurysmoplasty

    maze

    mediastinal exploration

    median sternotomy

    MIDCAB (minimally invasive
direct coronary artery bypass)

    mitral valve replacement

    modified endoventricular
circularplasty

    modified pericardium-baffle
reconstruction

    moving-bed infusion-tracking MRA
method for imaging

    Mullins blade and balloon
septostomy

operation *(cont.)*
   Mullins transseptal atrial
      septostomy
   Mustard atrial baffle repair
   Mustard correction of transposition
      of great vessels
   Nicks
   nonfenestrated Fontan procedure
   Norwood hypoplastic left-sided
      heart
   Norwood univentricular heart
   off-pump coronary artery bypass
      graft (OPCABG)
   OPCAB (off-pump coronary artery
      bypass)
   open heart
   open mitral commissurotomy
   orthotopic cardiac transplant
   pacemaker implantation
   palliative
   palliative arterial switch
   Park blade and balloon atrial
      septostomy
   partial encircling endocardial
      ventriculotomy
   partial left ventriculectomy (PLV)
   patent ductus arteriosus (PDA)
      ligation
   percutaneous aortic balloon
      valvuloplasty (PABV)
   percutaneous aortic valvuloplasty
      (PAV)
   percutaneous balloon mitral
      valvuloplasty
   percutaneous dilational tracheos-
      tomy (PDT)
   percutaneous coronary rotational
      atherectomy (PCRA)
   percutaneous mitral balloon
      valvotomy (PMBV)
   percutaneous transluminal
      angioplasty (PTA)

operation *(cont.)*
   percutaneous transluminal balloon
      dilatation (PTBD)
   percutaneous transluminal coronary
      angioplasty (PTCA)
   percutaneous transluminal septal
      myocardial ablation
   percutaneous transvenous mitral
      commissurotomy (PTMC)
   pericardial window
   pericardiectomy
   peripheral artery bypass
   peripheral laser angioplasty (PLA)
   peripheral excimer laser angio-
      plasty (PELA)
   phlebectomy
   photoablation, laser
   photoangioplasty
   plastic
   plication repair of flail leaflet
   pneumonectomy
   port access CABG (PACAB)
   Port-Access minimally invasive
      cardiac surgery
   post balloon angioplasty restenosis
   postcardiotomy intra-aortic balloon
      pumping
   Potts anastomosis between
      descending aorta and left
      pulmonary artery
   Potts-Smith side-to-side anastomosis
   profunda Dacron patchplasty
   profundaplasty
   pulmonary artery banding
   pulmonary balloon valvuloplasty
   pulmonary valvotomy
   pulmonary valvuloplasty
   punch aortotomy
   Rashkind balloon atrial septotomy
   Rashkind-Miller atrial septostomy
   Rastelli
   recanalization

operation *(cont.)*
  recanalization of total coronary
    occlusion
  redirection of inferior vena cava
  Reed ventriculorrhaphy
  re-sternotomy (resternotomy)
  Ross aortic valve replacement
  Ross switch procedure
  rotational atherectomy (RA)
  Sade modification of Norwood
  saloon door approach in MIDCAB
    (minimally invasive direct
    coronary artery bypass)
  sandwich patch closure
  Schede thoracoplasty
  selective subendocardial resection
  Senning atrial baffle repair
  Senning transposition
  septectomy
  septostomy
  SIMA (single internal mammary
    artery) reconstruction
  Simpson atherectomy
  sleeve pneumonectomy
  STAE (subsegmental transcatheter
    arterial embolization)
  Starnes
  stellectomy
  subcoronary aortic valve
    implantation
  subfascial endoscopic perforating
    vein surgery (SEPS)
  Sucquet-Hoyer anastomosis
  sympathectomy, regional cardiac
  synthetic patch angioplasty
  systemic to pulmonary artery
    anastomosis
  Takeuchi repair
  Tanner
  TASH (transcoronary ablation of
    septal hypertrophy)

operation *(cont.)*
  thoracoabdominal aortic aneurysm
    (TAAA) surgery
  thoracophrenolaparotomy
  thromboendarterectomy
  thrombolysis, intracoronary
  totally endoscopic coronary artery
    bypass (TECAB)
  transcarotid balloon valvuloplasty
  transcatheter anterograde
    valvotomy
  transcatheter arterial chemo-
    embolization (TACE)
  transcatheter arterial embolization
    (TAE)
  transcatheter closure of atrial septal
    defect
  transcatheter patent ductus
    arteriosus closure
  transcoronary ablation of septal
    hypertrophy (TASH)
  transfemoral liver biopsy
  transmural resection
  transseptal extended atriotomy
  transvenous cryoablation of
    supraventricular tachycardia
  Trendelenburg excision of varicose
    veins
  triangular resection of leaflet
  tricuspid valve anuloplasty
  TriVex transilluminated powered
    phlebectomy procedure for
    varicose vein removal
  tunnel
  unifocalization
  unilateral lung volume reduction
    surgery
  valved venous transplant
  valvotomy
  valvuloplasty
  valvulotomy

operation *(cont.)*
    VCAB (ventriculocoronary artery
      bypass)
    VCAB (ventricle-to-coronary artery
      bypass)
    VCAB revascularization
    vein patch angioplasty
    vein stripping
    venotomy
    ventricular endoaneurysmorrhaphy
    ventricular exclusion
    ventriculorrhaphy
    ventriculotomy
    video-assisted thoracic surgery
      (videothoracoscopy)
    video-assisted thoracoscopic lung
      metastasectomy
    video-assisted thoracoscopic lung
      volume reduction surgery
    video-assisted thoracoscopy of lung
    Vineberg cardiac revascularization
    Vineberg implantation of internal
      mammary artery into
      myocardium
    Waterston anastomosis for
      congenital pulmonary stenosis
    Waterston extrapericardial
      anastomosis
    wedge-shaped sleeve aneurysm
      resection
    Wooler-plasty
    wrapping of abdominal aortic
      aneurysm
OPG/CPA (oculoplethysmography/
  carotid phonoangiography)
ophthalmic retractor
opisthorchiasis
Opisthorchis infestation
Opitz disease
Opitz-Frias syndrome
Opitz thrombophlebitic splenomegaly
O point of cardiac apex pulse

opportunistic fungal pneumonia
opportunistic infection
opportunistic organism
opposing pleural surfaces
OpSite dressing
OpSite Flexigrid transparent adhesive
  film dressing
Opta catheter
Opta guidewire
Optease permanent vena cava filter
Opti-Clear cannula
optic loupe
Opti-Flow angiography catheter
Opti-Flow dialysis catheter
OptiForm mitral valve
OptiHaler
Optima MP pacemaker
Optima MPT Series III pacemaker
Optima MPT Series III pulse
  generator
Optima SPT pacemaker
Opti-Plast XT balloon catheter
Optipore wound-cleaning sponge
Optiscope catheter
Optison contrast agent
Optiva intravenous catheter
Opus cardiac troponin I assay
Oracle Focus PTCA catheter
Oracle Megasonics PTCA catheter
Oracle Micro catheter
Oracle Micro Plus PTCA catheter
Orapred
oral airway
oral anticoagulation
oral aspirin provocation
oral contraceptive-induced hyper-
  tension
oral drugs
oral steroid contraceptives are
  contraindicated
orbit, artifacts due to body contour
Orbiter PV catheter

orders or status
  Do Not Attempt Resuscitation
    (DNAR)
  Do Not Resuscitate (DNR)
organ, extrapleural
organic dust toxic syndrome
organic granulomatosis
organism (see *pathogen*)
  causative
  H. influenzae
  offending
  opportunistic
  pleuropneumonia-like (PPLO)
organizing thrombus
orifice (see also *ostium*)
  aortic
  atriotomy
  atrioventricular
  cardiac
  coronary
  coronary sinus
  double coronary
  hypoplastic tricuspid
  inferior vena cava
  lingular
  mitral
  narrowed
  pulmonary
  regurgitant
  segmental
  slitlike
  tricuspid
  valve
orifice-to-anulus ratio
origin, anomalous
origin of artery
origin of vessel
Orion balloon dilatation catheter
Orion pacemaker
Ormond syndrome
oroendotracheal tube
oropharynx

oropharyngeal airway (OPA)
orotracheal direct vision intubation
orotracheal intubation
Orqis pump
Orsi-Grocco method
ORT (orthodromic reciprocating tachycardia)
Orthoclone
Orthocor II pacemaker
orthodromic atrioventricular (AV)
  reciprocating tachycardia
orthodromic reciprocating tachycardia
  (ORT)
orthodromic tachycardia
orthogonal angiographic projection
orthogonal lead arrangement for EKG
orthogonal view on angiography
orthopnea
  three-pillow
  two-pillow
orthopnea position
orthopneic position
orthostasis
orthostatic blood pressure
orthostatic dyspnea
orthostatic hypotension, hyperadrenergic
orthostatic hypotension variant
orthostatic primary hypotension
orthostatic syncope
orthostatism, vasovagal
orthotopic cardiac transplantation
orthotopic heart transplantation
orthotopic total heart replacement
Ortner syndrome
OS (opening snap)
os, coronary sinus
Osborn wave (hypothermia)
Osborn wave on EKG
Osciflator balloon inflation syringe
oscillation, pressure
oscillatory

oscillography
oscillometry, impulse
oscilloscope, Tektronix
Oscor active fixation leads
Oscor pacing lead
O'Shaughnessy artery forceps
Osler (see *Weber-Osler-Rendu
    syndrome*)
Osler disease
Osler hereditary hemorrhagic telangi-
    ectasia
Osler-Libman-Sacks syndrome
Osler maneuver
Osler nodes in subacute bacterial
    endocarditis
Osler polycythemia vera
Osler sign
Osler triad
OsmoCyte pillow wound dressing
osmotic diuretics
osmotic edema
osmotic effect
osmotic pressure, plasma colloid
ossific nodule
osteoarthropathy
    hypertrophic pulmonary
    pulmonary
osteogenesis imperfecta syndrome
osteomyelitis of sternum
Osteoprene mesh
Osteoprene surgical clip
Osteoprene surgical staple
Osteoprene tissue adhesive
Osteoprene vascular occlusion device
osteosarcoma of heart
osteosclerotic anemia
ostia
ostial cannulation
ostial lesion
ostial reimplantation, coronary
ostial revascularization, coronary
ostial segment

ostial stenosis
ostium (pl. ostia) (see also *orifice*)
    aortic
    artery
    atrioventricular
    coronary
    coronary sinus
ostium atrioventriculare commune
ostium primum defect
ostium secundum defect
outcome, portend a poor
Outcomes by Design balloon
Outcomes by Design catheter
Outcomes by Design sheath introducer
Outcomes by Design steerable
    guidewire
Outcomes by Design stent
outflow
    hypoplastic subpulmonic
    maximum venous (MVO)
    subpulmonic
outflow anastomosis
outflow disease progression
outflow midsystolic murmur
outflow tract
outflow tract prosthesis
outlet chamber, rudimentary
outlet, widened thoracic
out of synchrony
outpouching of portion of wall of
    artery
output
    adequate cardiac
    augmented cardiac
    cardiac (CO)
    Dow method for cardiac
    Fick method for cardiac
    Gorlin method for cardiac
    Hetzel forward triangle method for
        cardiac
    inadequate cardiac
    low cardiac

output *(cont.)*
　pulmonic
　reduced systemic cardiac
　Stewart-Hamilton technique for
　　cardiac
　stroke
　systemic
　thermodilution cardiac
　ventricular
output amplitude
oval cherry-red raised lesion
ovalis, anulus
ovalocytosis, hereditary
ovarian carcinoma metastatic to heart
ovarian hyperstimulation syndrome
　over-and-over stitch or suture
overdistention
overdistention of alveolar spaces in
　lungs
overdistention of lung tissue
overdistention, pulmonary
overdrive pacing
overdrive suppression
overexpansion, pulmonary
Overholt thoracic forceps
overinflation
　lung
　unilateral
overlapping structures, angiographic-
　ally
overload, overloading
　acute hemodynamic
　cardiac
　chronic hemodynamic
　diastolic
　fluid
　pressure
　right ventricular
　systolic ventricular
　volume
overlying epicardial fat
over-read (noun)

over-responsive programming
overriding great artery
overriding great vessel
overriding of anulus
overriding of aorta
overriding of tricuspid valve
overriding ventricular septum of aorta
oversensing, pacemaker
overt clinical disease, manifestation of
over-the-wire balloon catheter
overventilation
　alveolar
　total
overwhelming sepsis
ovoid heart
Owren disease
Owren factor V deficiency
oxalosis
ox heart (cor bovinum)
oxidative phosphorylation
oximeter
　American Optical
　ear
　finger
　Hewlett-Packard ear
　intracardiac
　Onyx finger pulse
　Oxytrak pulse
　pulse
oximetry
　ear
　exercise
　finger
　pulse
　reflectance
Oxycel
oxygen (O_2)
　arterial blood gases on 100%
　heated humidified
　increased
　supplemental
oxygenated blood

oxygenated cardioplegic solution
oxygenated perfluorocarbon blood
   substitute
oxygenation, extracorporeal membrane
oxygenation of blood, inadequate
oxygenator
   Bentley
   bubble
   Capiox-E bypass system
   disk
   film
   Maxima Forté blood oxygen
     by mask
   membrane
   Monolyth
   pump
   rotating disk
   SciMed membrane
   screen
   Shiley
oxygen-binding capacity
oxygen by nasal cannula
oxygen by nasal catheter
oxygen by nasal prong
oxygen by nonrebreather mask
oxygen-carrying capacity
oxygen capacity
oxygen consumption index
oxygen content

oxygen debt, severe
oxygen deficit
oxygen delivery
oxygen delivery index
oxygen-dependent emphysema
oxygen difference, arteriovenous
oxygen extraction index
oxygen extraction ratio
oxygen saturation
   aortic
   low
   PA (pulmonary artery)
   RA (right atrium)
oxygen step-up (or stepup)
oxygen tension gradient, alveolar-
   arterial
oxygen tent
oxygen toxicity
oxygen unsaturation
oxygen utilization capacity
oxygen via nasal cannula
oxygenation
oxygenator
oxyhemoglobin (HbO_2)
oxyhemoglobin dissociation curve
oxyhemoglobin saturation
Oxy-Hood
Oxytrak pulse oximeter
ozena

P, p

P (posterior)
PA (pulmonary artery)
PA oxygen saturation
PA pressure
PAB (premature atrial beat)
PABP (pulmonary artery balloon
    pump)
PABV (percutaneous aortic balloon
    valvuloplasty)
PAC (premature atrial complex)
PAC (premature atrial contraction)
PACAB (Port-Access coronary artery
    bypass) graft
Pace bipolar pacing catheter
paced beat
paced impulse
paced ventricular evoked response
    (PVER)
Pacefinder pacemaker lead placement
    system
pacemaker (see also *generator*)
    AAI (atrial demand inhibited)
    AAIR
    AAT (atrial demand triggered)
    Accufix
    Acculith
    Activitrax

pacemaker *(cont.)*
    Activitrax II single-chamber VVI
    Activitrax variable rate
    activity sensing
    AddVent atrioventricular
    Aequitron
    AFP
    AICD
    AID-B
    antitachycardia
    AOO (atrial asynchronous)
    Arco
    Arcolithium
    artificial
    Arzco
    Astra
    ASVIP (atrial synchronous,
        ventricular inhibited)
    asynchronous (atrial or ventricular)
        mode
    atrial asynchronous
    atrial demand inhibited
    atrial demand triggered
    atrial synchronous ventricular
    atrial synchronous, ventricular-
        inhibited (ASVIP)
    atrial tracking

pacemaker *(cont.)*
    atrial triggered, ventricular-
        inhibited
    Atricor
    atrioventricular junctional
    atrioventricular sequential
    Aurora dual-chamber
    Autima II dual-chamber cardiac
        automatic
    AV (atrioventricular) junctional
    AV (atrioventricular) sequential
    Avius sequential
    Basix
    Biorate
    Biotronik
    bipolar
    Brio
    burst
    Byrel SX
    Byrel-SX/Versatrax
    Cardio-Pace Medical Durapulse
    Chardack-Greatbatch implantable
        cardiac pulse generator
    Chorus
    Chorus dual-chamber
    Chorus II dual-chamber
    Chorus RM rate-responsive dual-
        chamber
    Chronocor IV external
    Circadia dual-chamber rate-adaptive
    Classix
    Command PS
    committed mode
    Cook
    Cordis
    Cordis Gemini
    Cordis Sequicor
    Cosmos 283 DDD
    Cosmos II DDD
    Cosmos pulse generator
    CPI (Cardiac Pacemakers, Inc.)
    CPI Astra

pacemaker *(cont.)*
    CPI DDD
    CPI 910 ULTRA II
    cross-talk
    Cyberlith
    Cybertach automatic-burst atrial
    Cybertach 60
    Daig ESI-II or DSI-III screw-in
        lead
    Dash rate-adaptive
    Dash single-chamber rate-adaptic
        cardiac
    DDD (fully automatic sequential)
    DDDR mode
    DDI mode
    Delta
    demand
    Devices, Ltd.
    diaphragmatic
    Diplos M
    downward displacement of
    Dromos
    dual-chamber
    dual chamber Medtronic.Kappa
        400
    Durapulse
    DVI (AV sequential)
    Ectocor
    ectopic atrial
    Ela
    Electrodyne
    Elema-Schonander
    Elevath
    Elgiloy
    Elite dual-chamber rate-responsive
    Encor
    endless loop, dual-chamber
    Enertrax
    Entity
    Ergos O_2
    escape
    external transthoracic

pacemaker *(cont.)*
  externally controlled noninvasive
    programmed stimulation
  Fast-Pass lead
  fixed-rate, asynchronous atrial
  fixed-rate, asynchronous ventricular
  fixed-rate permanent
  fully automatic, atrioventricular
    universal dual-channel
  Galaxy
  Gemini 415 DDD
  General Electric
  Genisis *(not* Genesis)
  Guardian
  hermetically sealed standby
  implantation of atrioventricular
    sequential
  implanted
  Integrity AFx
  Intermedics
  Intermedics Quantum
  internal
  Intertach
  intraperitoneal migration of
  Jade II SSI
  junctional
  Kairos
  Kalos
  Kappa 400 Series
  Kelvin 500 Sensor
  Lambda
  latent
  Legend
  Leios
  Leptos-01
  Leukos
  lithium
  Maestro
  Medcor
  Medtel
  Medtronic
  Medtronic DDD

pacemaker *(cont.)*
  Medtronic RF 5998
  Medtronic SPO 502
  Medtronic Symbios
  Medtronic temporary
  Meta DDDR
  Meta MV
  META rate responsive
  Micro Minix
  Microlith P
  Microny K SR
  Microny II SR+ (SR Plus) pulse
    generator
  Midros
  Minix
  Minix ST
  Microthin P2
  Multicor Gamma
  Multicor II
  Multilith
  multiprogrammable
  Nathan
  natural
  Neos M
  noncompetitive atrial demand
  noncompetitive atrial synchronous
  noncompetitive atrial triggered
  noncompetitive demand ventricular
  noncompetitive ventricular
    synchronous
  noncompetitive ventricular
    triggered
  noninvasive temporary (NTP)
  Nova MR
  Omnicor
  Omni-Orthocor
  Omni-Stanicor
  Omni-Theta
  Optima MP; MPT; SPT
  Optima MPI Series III pulse
    generator
  Orion

pacemaker *(cont.)*
    Orthocor II
    oversensing
    Pacefinder
    Pacesetter
    Pacesetter AFP
    Pacesetter Synchrony
    Pacesetter systems
    PASAR (permanent scanning anti-
        tachycardia)
    PASAR tachycardia reversion
    Pasys
    PDx pacing and diagnostic
    permanent
    permanent rate-responsive
    permanent rate-responsive dual-
        chamber
    permanent ventricular
    Permathane Pacesetter lead
    Philos DR
    Phoenix single-chamber
    Phymos 3D (foreign)
    Pinnacle
    PolyFlex lead
    Prima
    Prism-CL
    Programalith
    programmable
    Prolith
    Pulsar NI
    P-wave triggered ventricular
    QT interval sensing
    QT sensing
    Quantum
    radiofrequency
    rate responsive
    Regency SR+ single-chamber,
        rate-responsive pulse generator
    Relay
    rescuing
    respiratory-dependent
    RS4

pacemaker *(cont.)*
    runaway
    SAVVI
    screw-in lead
    secondary
    Seecor
    Sensolog
    Sensor Kelvin
    Sequicor
    shifting
    Siemens-Elema
    Siemens-Pacesetter
    single-chamber
    sinus node
    Sorin
    Spectraflex
    Spectrax programmable Medtronic
    Spectrax SXT
    standby
    Stanicor
    Starr-Edwards
    supraventricular ectopic
    Swing DR1 DDDR
    Symbios
    synchronous mode
    Synergyst DDD
    tachycardia-terminating
    Tachylog
    Telectronics
    Talent
    temperature-sensing
    temporary
    temporary transvenous
    Thermos
    tined lead
    Topaz II SSIR
    transcutaneous
    transthoracic
    transvenous
    Trilogy DC+
    Trilogy SR+ single-chamber
    Trios M

pacemaker *(cont.)*
  Triumph VR
  troubleshooting of
  undersensing malfunction of
  Unilith
  unipolar
  Unity-C
  universal
  variable rate
  VAT (atrial synchronous
    ventricular)
  VDD (atrial synchronous
    ventricular inhibited)
  Ventak AICD
  Ventricor
  ventricular
  ventricular asynchronous
  ventricular demand inhibited (VVI)
  ventricular demand triggered
    (VVT)
  Versatrax and Versatrax II
  Vicor
  Vista
  Vitatrax II
  Vitatron
  Vitatron Diamond
  Vitatron Diamond II
  VOO (ventricular asynchronous)
  VVD mode
  VVI (ventricular demand inhibited)
  VVI/AAI
  VVIR mode
  VVT (ventricular demand
    triggered)
  wandering
  wandering atrial (WAP)
  Xyrel
  Zitron
  Zoll NTP (noninvasive temporary)
pacemaker adaptive rate
pacemaker afterpotential
pacemaker amplifier refractory period

pacemaker amplifier sensitivity
pacemaker artifact
pacemaker AV disable mechanism
pacemaker battery
pacemaker battery failure
pacemaker battery status
pacemaker burst pacing
pacemaker capability
pacemaker capture
  erratic
  lack of
pacemaker cell
pacemaker classifications
pacemaker code system
pacemaker complication
pacemaker crosstalk
pacemaker-defibrillator
pacemaker demand
pacemaker electrode
pacemaker escape interval
pacemaker failure
pacemaker generator pouch
pacemaker hysteresis
pacemaker implantation
pacemaker insertion
  transarterial
  transvenous
pacemaker introducer
pacemaker lead
pacemaker lead impedance
pacemaker loss of capture
pacemaker loss of sensing
pacemaker malfunction
pacemaker marker channel
pacemaker-mediated tachycardia
pacemaker mode (see *pacemaker*)
  AOO
  AAI
  DDD
  DDDR
  DDI
  DVI

pacemaker *(cont.)*
  universal
  VOO
  VDD
  VVD
  VVI
  VVIR
  VVT
pacemaker oversensing
pacemaker pacing mode
pacemaker pocket
pacemaker potential
pacemaker programmability
pacemaker programmed settings
pacemaker rate
pacemaker reprogramming
pacemaker self-inhibition
pacemaker sensing
pacemaker sensitivity
pacemaker spike
pacemaker stimulus output amplitude
pacemaker syndrome
pacemaker system analyzer
pacemaker tester system
pacemaker threshold
pacemaker twiddler's syndrome
pacemaker undersensing
pace mapping
Paceport catheter
pacer-dependent
pacer spike
Pacesetter AFP pacemaker
Pacesetter APS pacemaker
  programmer
Pacesetter cardiac pacemaker
Pacesetter introducer
Pacesetter Synchrony pacemaker
Pacesetter systems pacemaker
Pacesetter Trilogy DR+ pulse
  generator
pace-termination

Pacewedge dual-pressure bipolar
  pacing catheter
Pachon method
Pachon test of collateral circulation in
  aneurysm
pachyderma laryngis
pachypleuritis
Pacifico venous cannula
pacing (see also *pacemaker*)
  activity sensor modulated atrial rate
  adaptive
  adaptive burst
  antitachycardia
  asynchronous
  asynchronous atrioventricular
    sequential
  atrial
  atrial overdrive
  atrial rate adaptive
  atrial synchronous ventricular
  autodecremental
  AV sequential
  backup bradycardia
  bipolar atrial
  biventricular pacing
  burst
  burst-overdrive
  cardiac
  committed
  competitive
  constant rate atrial
  continuous rapid atrial
  coronary sinus
  coupled
  decremental
  demand
  double ventricular
  dual-chamber
  endocardial
  epicardial
  external

pacing *(cont.)*
  external cardiac
  extrastimulus
  fixed-rate
  incremental
  incremental atrial
  noncommitted
  overdrive
  paired
  permanent
  phrenic nerve
  physiologic
  prophylactic
  P synchronous
  P triggered ventricular
  ramp
  ramp atrial
  ramp overdrive
  rapid atrial
  rapid ventricular
  rate adaptive
  rate-modulated
  rate responsive (RRP)
  scan
  scanning
  semicommitted
  sequential
  single-chamber
  synchronous
  temporary cardiac
  temporary transvenous
  transcutaneous
  transesophageal
  transesophageal atrial
  transesophageal cardiac
  transthoracic cardiac
  transvenous
  triggered
  ultrafast train
  ultrarapid
  underdrive
  unipolar

pacing *(cont.)*
  ventricular
  ventricular burst
  ventricular cardiac
  ventricular demand
  ventricular overdrive
  ventricular triggered
  vibration based
pacing analyzer
pacing cable, alligator
pacing electrode catheter, bipolar
pacing-induced termination of
    arrhythmia
pacing lead (see *lead*)
pacing lead fracture
pacing mode (see *pacemaker*)
pacing/sensing lead
pacing stimulus
pacing system
  Integrity AFx AutoCapture
  Rx5000 cardiac
  Vitatron Activity (ACT) sensor
  Vitatron Diamond II DDR
  Vitatron Jade II SSI
  Vitatron QT sensor
  Vitatron Ruby II DDD
  Vitatron Topaz II SSIR
pacing system analyzer (PSA)
pacing threshold
pacing wire, pacing wires
pacing wire fracture
pack, moist laparotomy (lap)
pack-a-day smoking history
packed red blood cells (PRBCs)
pack-year smoking history
pack-years of cigarette smoking
$PaCO_2$ (arterial partial pressure of
    CO_2) (mm Hg)
pad, pads
  defibrillator
  epicardial fat
  insulating

pad *(cont.)*
   laparotomy (lap)
   Littmann defibrillation
   R2 defibrillator
   Telfa
PAD (public access defibrillation)
PAD (pulmonary artery diastolic)
   pressure
PAD (pulsatile assist device)
paddle
   defibrillatory
   pediatric defibrillator
PA diastolic pressure
Padogram device
PADP-PAWP (pulmonary artery
   diastolic and wedge pressure)
   gradient
pad sign of aortic insufficiency
PAEC (Parodi anti-embolization
   catheter)
PAEDP (pulmonary artery end-
   diastolic pressure)
PAF (paroxysmal atrial fibrillation)
PAFD (percutaneous abscess and fluid
   drainage)
Page episodic hypertension with
   tachycardia
Page syndrome
Paget-Schroetter (Schrötter) syndrome
Paget-Schroetter venous thrombosis of
   axillary vein
Paget-von Schroetter syndrome
PAI (plasminogen activator inhibitor)
pain (see also *angina*)
   acme
   anginal chest
   anomalous
   atypical chest
   boring
   burning
   calf
   cardiaclike chest

pain *(cont.)*
   chest
   chest wall
   concomitant chest
   crushing
   crushing chest
   deep visceral
   dull
   esophageal
   evanescent chest
   excruciating
   exertional
   exertional chest
   exquisite
   focal
   heartburn type of
   hemicranial
   ischemic rest
   localized stabbing
   musculoskeletal
   noncardiac chest
   nonpleuritic precordial
   parasternal chest
   pericardial
   pinching chest
   pleuritic
   pleuritic chest
   postprandial
   pounding
   precordial chest
   pressure
   pulsating
   radiating (to left arm, shoulder)
   referred cardiac
   reproducible
   rest
   retrosternal chest
   sharp
   squeezing
   squeezing chest
   stabbing
   sternal border

pain *(cont.)*
    substernal chest
    suffocating chest
    thoracic
    throbbing
    unrelenting
    unremitting
    viselike
    waning
    waxing and waning
pain abolished by breath-holding
pain accompanied by abdominal
    fullness
pain accompanied by nausea
pain accompanied by palpitations
pain accompanied by sensation of gas
pain accompanied by shortness of
    breath
pain accompanied by sweating
pain accompanied by weakness
pain aggravated by coughing
pain aggravated by deep breathing
pain aggravated by deep inspiration
pain continued unabated
pain control system (PCS),
    CADD-Prizm
pain following heavy meal
pain in chest
pain indistinguishable from angina
pain induced with methacholine
pain in sternal articulations
painless edema
pain "like being caught in a vise"
pain "like being crushed under a
    heavy load"
pain "like someone sitting on my
    chest"
pain on drinking cold liquid
pain on exposure to cold
pain on strong emotion
pain on swallowing
pain precipitated by emotional upset

pain precipitated by exertion
pain precipitated by strong emotion
pain radiating to back
pain radiating to epigastrium
pain radiating to jaw
pain radiating to left arm
pain radiating to neck
pain radiating to right arm
pain radiating to throat
pain rapidly extinguished by
    withdrawal of stimulus
pain relieved by antacids
pain relieved by belching
pain relieved by bowel movement
pain relieved by carotid massage
pain relieved by cimetidine
pain relieved by eating
pain relieved by food intake
pain relieved by leaning forward
pain relieved by passage of flatus
pain relieved by rest
pain reproduced by palpation
pain reproducible with moderate
    exercise
pain unaffected by position
pain unrelated to meals
pain unrelieved by nitroglycerin
pain when angry
pain when excited
P-A interval
paired beats
palate, high arched
pale thrombus
palliation
palliative operative procedure
palliative surgery
palliative therapy
pallid breath-holding spells
Pallister-Hall syndrome
pallor
    circumoral
    elevation

pallor of extremity
pallor of lower extremities
palmar pulses, palpable
Palmaz balloon-expandable iliac stent
Palmaz-Schatz coronary stent
Palmaz-Schatz stent (PSS)
Palmaz-Schatz stent prototype
Palmaz vascular stent
Palmeri QRS score
palpability
palpable A wave
palpable anterior motion
palpable aortic ejection sound
palpable apical impulse
palpable ejection click
palpable opening snap
palpable palmar pulses
palpable peripheral pulse
palpable popliteal pulse
palpable presystolic bulge
palpable pulmonic ejection sound
palpable S_3 or S_4
palpable systolic pulsation
palpable thrill
palpation
   fist
   precordial
palpation reproduces the pain
palpatory
palpitation, palpitations
   flip-flop
   flopping
   fluttering
palsy, cranial nerve
PAM (pulmonary artery mean)
   pressure
PAN (periarteritis nodosa)
pANCA (perinuclear antineutrophil
   cytoplasmic antibody)
panacinar emphysema
Pancoast syndrome
Pancoast tumor

Panacryl absorbable suture
Panafil enzymatic debriding agent
Panafil White ointment
panaortic
panarteritis nodosa
pancarditis
panchamber enlargement
pancreatitis, acute
pancuronium
panel, anergy
panel reactive antibodies (PRAs)
Paneth anuloplasty
paninspiratory crackles
panlobular emphysema
PanoGauze hydrogel-impregnated
   gauze
PanoPlex hydrogel dressing
pansinusitis
pansystolic mitral regurgitation
pansystolic murmur (PSM)
pantaloon embolus
pantyhose, support (see *stockings*)
panzerherz (dense pericardial
   calcification)
PaO$_2$ (arterial partial pressure of O$_2$)
   (mm Hg)
PAP (pulmonary alveolar proteinosis)
PAP (pulmonary artery pressure)
papaverine-soaked sponge
Papercuff disposable blood pressure
   cuff
papillary adenocarcinoma of the lung
papillary fibroelastoma
papillary muscle
   anterior
   posterior
   septal
papillary muscle rupture
papillary muscle dysfunction
papillary muscle infarction
papilledema
papillomas

papillomatosis
  laryngeal
  recurrent respiratory (RRP)
papillomavirus, human (HPV)
papillotome
  Apollo
  Apollo 3AC
Pappenheimer bodies
PA pulse amplitude
PAPVR (partial anomalous pulmonary
  venous return)
PA systolic pressure
para-arterial angiomatosis arteritis
paraaminosalicylic acid hypersensitivity
paracardiac mass
paracardiac-type total anomalous
  venous return
paracentesis of pericardium
parachute deformity of mitral valve
parachute mitral valve
parachute technique for distal
  anastomosis
paracicatricial emphysema
paracoccidioidomycosis
paracoronary right ventriculotomy
paracorporeal
paracostal sutures
paradoxic respiratory splitting
paradoxic splitting
paradoxical bronchospasm
paradoxical embolism
paradoxical embolus
paradoxically
paradoxical motion
paradoxical motion of the chest wall
paradoxical movement
paradoxical pulse
paradoxical septal motion
paraganglioma, cardiac
Paragon coronary stent
paragonimiasis

paragonimosis
Paragonimus westermani infection
Parahisian pacing electrode catheter
parainfluenza virus
paralysis of diaphragm
paralysis
  periodic
  phrenic nerve
paralytic chest
paramagnetic substances
paramagnetism
paramedian position
paramediastinal glands
parameter, parameters
  physiologic
  clinical
  ventricular function
parameters, respiratory
parameter study
paramyotonia congenita
paranasal sinuses
paraneoplastic process
paraneoplastic syndrome
parapharyngeal abscess
parapneumonic effusion
paraprosthetic leakage
paraprosthetic-enteric fistula
pararenal aortic aneurysm
pararenal aortic atherosclerosis
paraseptal emphysema
paraseptal position
parasite (pulmonary)
  Ascaris
  Echinococcus multilocularis
    (alveolaris)
  Entamoeba
  filaria
  hookworm
  liver fluke
  lung fluke
  Schistosoma haematobium
  Schistosoma japonicum

parasite *(cont.)*
  Schistosoma mansoni
  schistosomes
  Strongyloides
  tapeworms
  Toxocara
  Trichina
  Trichuris
parasitic circulation in angio-
  osteohypertrophic syndrome
parasitic infection, intestinal
parasitic infestation
parasitic pericarditis
paraspinal pleural stripe
parasternal bulge
parasternal chest pain
parasternal heave
parasternal incision
parasternal lift
parasternal long-axis view
parasternal lymph nodes
parasternal motion
  forceful
  sustained anterior
parasternal murmur
parasternal short-axis view
parasternal stainless steel wire
parasternal systolic lift
parasternal systolic murmur
parasternal view of heart
parasternal window
parasympathetic nervous system
parasystole
  atrial
  junctional
  ventricular
parathyroid hormone
parathyroidectomy
paratonia
paratracheal lymphadenopathy
paravalvular leak
paravertebral gutter

parchment heart syndrome
parchment right ventricle
Pardee T wave
parenchyma
  lung
  pulmonary
parenchymal hemorrhage
parenchymal infiltrates, pulmonary
parenchymal lung disease
parenchymal tumor mass
parent vein
parenteral bronchodilators
parenteral fluids
parenteral steroids
paresis
  hemidiaphragmatic
  vocal cord
paresthesia, paresthesias
  marching
  Nothnagel
  vasomotor
parietal band
parietal extension of infundibular
  septum
parietalis, pleura
parietal layer
parietal pericardium
parietal pleura
parietal pleurectomy
Parietaria judaica pollen allergen
parietoalveolar pneumonopathy
Park blade and balloon atrial
  septostomy
Park blade septostomy
Parkes Weber syndrome
Parks bidirectional Doppler flowmeter
Parodi anti-embolization device
  (PAEC)
parotitis
paroxysmal atrial fibrillation (PAF)
paroxysmal atrial tachycardia (PAT)
paroxysmal coughing

paroxysmal crisis, hypertensive
paroxysmal dyspnea
paroxysmal hyperpnea
paroxysmal hypertension
paroxysmal nocturnal dyspnea (PND)
paroxysmal nocturnal hemoglobinuria
    (PNH)
paroxysmal sneezing
paroxysmal supraventricular
    tachycardia (PSVT)
paroxysmal tachycardia
paroxysmal wheezing
paroxysmal wheezing dyspnea
paroxysms of cough
paroxysms of hypertension
parrot fever
pars membranacea
Parsonnet probe
partial anomalous pulmonary venous
    return (PAPVR)
partial collapse of lung
partial dislodgement
partial encircling endocardial
    ventriculotomy
partial exsanguination
partial graft preservation
partial left ventriculectomy (PLV)
partial lung collapse
partial occluding (or occlusion) clamp
partial-occlusion clamp
partial pericardial absence
partial pressure of arterial CO_2
    ($PaCO_2$)
partial pressure of arterial O_2 (PaO_2)
partial rebreather mask
partial reperfusion
partial thromboplastin time test
partial volume effect, artifact due to
particle debris
particle deposition
particle masks
particle radiotherapy

particle, ultrafine carbon
partition, atrial
parvovirus B19
parvus et tardus, pulsus
parvus pulse
PAS (pulmonary artery systolic)
    pressure
PAS-positive proteinaceous material
PASAR (permanent scanning anti-
    tachycardia) pacemaker
PASAR tachycardia reversion pace-
    maker
PASG (pneumatic antishock garment)
PAS/PAD (pulmonary artery systolic-
    pulmonary artery diastolic)
PASP/SASP (pulmonary to systemic
    arterial systolic pressure) ratio
Passage hemostasis valve (used in
    angiography and angioplasty)
Passager introducing sheath
passage of clots
passages, narrowing of bronchiolar
passer
    right-angle
    Schnidt (*not* Schmidt)
passive clot
passive filling
passive fixation lead
passive hyperemia
passive hyperimmune therapy (PHT)
passively congested lung tissue
passive pneumonia
passive smoking exposure
passive vascular congestion
passive venous distention
Passovoy defect
Passovoy mild hemorrhagic diathesis
PASTA (polarity-altered spectral selec-
    tive acquisition) imaging
paste, nitroglycerin
Pasys (single-chamber cardiac
    pacing system)

PAT (paroxysmal atrial tachycardia)
  with block
Patau syndrome (trisomy 13)
patch (see also *graft*)
  atriopulmonary
  autologous pericardial
  CardioFix Pericardium
  Carrel
  CV Peri-Guard
  Dacron Sauvage
  Dura-Guard
  felt
  Fluoropassiv thin-wall carotid
  Gore-Tex cardiovascular
  Gore-Tex soft tissue
  Graftpatch
  gusset-type
  kinking of
  large defibrillating
  MacCallum
  outflow cardiac
  pericardial
  Peri-Guard
  RapiSeal
  small defibrillating
  subcutaneous
  Supple Peri-Guard
  Teflon felt
  Teflon intracardiac
  Telectronics defibrillator
  transanular
  transdermal nitroglycerin
  Transvac transdermal
  Vascu-Guard
  vein
patch closure of septal defect
patch crinkling
patch electrode
  anterior anodal
  posterior cathodal
  subcutaneous

patch electrodes placed outside the
  pericardium
patch graft anuloplasty
patch graft aortoplasty
patch graft, Dacron onlay
patch graft of outflow tract
patching, transanular
patch lead, HV-1
patch lead placement, intrapericardial
patch placement, extrapericardial
patchplasty, profunda Dacron
patchy alveolar opacities
patchy atrophy of renal cortex
patchy consolidation
patchy infiltration, migratory
patchy inflammation of bronchioles
patchy migratory infiltrates
patchy zones of hemorrhagic exudate
patchy zones of purulent exudate
Patella's disease
patency
  arterial
  coronary artery
  coronary bypass graft
  ductus arteriosus
  graft
  vein
patency and valvular reflux of deep
  veins
patency of balloon-dilated vessel
patency of ductus arteriosus, persistent
patency of ductus venosus, persistent
patency of the radial artery-to-cephalic
  vein anastomosis
patency of vein graft
patency of vessel
patent artery
patent bifurcation
patent bronchus sign
patent ductus arteriosus (PDA)
patent ductus arteriosus closure

patent ductus arteriosus double
  umbrella closure
patent ductus arteriosus, silent
patent foramen ovale (PFO)
patent graft
patent trifurcation
patent, widely
Pathfinder catheter
pathogen (a quick-reference list of bac-
  teria, fungi, parasites, and viruses
  affecting the cardiovascular/thoracic
  system)
  Achromobacter
  Actinobacillus pleuropneumoniae
  Ancylostoma braziliense
  Ancylostoma duodenale
  Ascaris
  Ascaris lumbricoides
  Ascaris pulmonary parasite
  Ascaris suum
  Aspergillus niger
  Battey-avium complex infarction
  Chlamydia pneumoniae
  Clonorchis sinensis infection
  Corynebacterium pseudo-
    tuberculosis infection
  Dirofilaria immitis infection
  Echinococcus granulosus infection
  Eikenella infection
  Entamoeba pulmonary parasite
  Enterobacter aerogenes bronchitis
  Enterobacter agglomerans
  Enterobacter cloacae
  Enterobacteriaceae infection
  Escherichia coli
  filaria pulmonary parasite
  Francisella tularensis
  Friedländer bacillus
  Group A hemolytic streptococci
  Haemophilus infection
  Haemophilus influenzae
    (*H. influenzae*)

pathogen *(cont.)*
  Haemophilus influenzae bronchitis
  Haemophilus influenzae laryngitis
  Haemophilus influenzae pneumonia
  Helminthosporium
  Histoplasma myocarditis
  hookworm pulmonary parasite
  intraerythrocytic *Babesia*
  Kingella infection
  Klebsiella pneumoniae
  Klebsiella rhinoscleromatis
  Legionella pneumophila infection
  liver fluke pulmonary parasite
  lung fluke pulmonary parasite
  MAC (*Mycobacterium avium*
    complex)
  MAI *(Mycobacterium avium-*
    intracellulare)
  MOTT *(Mycobacterium* other than
    tuberculosis)
  MRSA (methicillin-resistant
    Staphylococcus aureus)
  Mycobacterium abscessus
  Mycobacterium alvei
  Mycobacterium avium complex
    (MAC)
  Mycobacterium avium-intracellu-
    lare (MAI) infection
  Mycobacterium fortuitum
  Mycobacterium gordonae
  Mycobacterium intracellulare
  Mycobacterium kansasii
  Mycobacterium simiae infection
  Mycobacterium tuberculosis
  Mycoplasma antibody titer
  Mycoplasma pneumoniae infection
  Necator americanus infection
  Neisseria infection
  Nocardia fungus
  Opisthorchis infestation
  Paragonimus westermani infection
  Peptostreptococcus

pathogen *(cont.)*
  Pneumocystic carinii pneumonia
    (PCP)
  Plasmodium falciparum infestation
  Pneumocystis carinii
  Pneumocystis jiroveci pneumonia
  Pseudomonas aeruginosa infection
  Pseudomonas bronchiectasis
  Pseudomonas cepacia
  Pseudomonas maltophilia
  Pseudomonas pneumonia
  rhinovirus
  Rickettsia burnetii infection
  Schistosoma haematobium
    pulmonary parasite
  Schistosoma japonicum pulmonary
    parasite
  Schistosoma mansoni pulmonary
    parasite
  schistosome (pulmonary parasite)
  Serratia marcescens
  Staphylococcus aureus infection
  Staphylococcus epidermidis
  Streptococcus haemolyticus
  Streptococcus mitis
  Streptococcus pneumoniae
  Streptococcus pyogenes
  Streptococcus sanguis
  Streptococcus viridans
  Strongyloides pulmonary parasite
  Strongyloides stercoralis infection
  tapeworm (pulmonary parasite)
  Thermoactinomyces sacchari
  Toxocara canis infestation
  Toxocara infection
  Toxocara pulmonary parasite
  Treponema pallidum infection
  Trichina pulmonary parasite
  Trichinella myocarditis
  Trichinella spiralis infection
  Trichosporon beigelii
  Trichuris pulmonary parasite

pathogen *(cont.)*
  Trypanosoma cruzi
  tubercle bacillus
  Veillonella
  viridans streptococcal
  Wuchereria bancrofti infection
  Yersinia infection
pathogenesis of bleeding syndrome
pathogenic coagulation process
pathognomonic symptoms
pathologic diagnosis
pathophysiologic changes in airways
  obstruction
pathophysiology
pathway
  ablation of accessory
  accessory (AP)
  accessory atrioventricular (AV)
  accessory conduction (ACP)
  alternative respiratory
  anomalous
  anomalous atrioventricular
    conduction
  antegrade
  antegrade fast
  anterior internodal
  atrio-His; atrio-Hisian; atriohisian
  atrioventricular (AV)
  AV (atrioventricular) nodal
  Bachmann
  bystander
  concealed accessory
  concealed atrioventricular
  dual AV nodal
  Embden-Meyerhof
  Embden-Meyerhof-Parnas
  fast
  flow
  free-wall accessory
  internodal
  left accessory
  multiple accessory

pathway *(cont.)*
    nodoventricular
    paranodal
    paraseptal accessory
    posterior septal
    preferential intranodal
    reentrant
    retrograde
    septal
    slow
    slow AV nodal
    Thorel
    Wenckebach
patient
    cardioverted
    rewarmed
patient-controlled analgesic (PCA)
    system
patient-directed beam-control
patient risk factors
Patrick-McGoon technique
pattern
    A fib (atrial fibrillation)
    bigeminal
    blood flow
    contractile
    DNA ploidy
    dP/dt upstroke
    early repolarization
    hemodynamic
    injury
    juvenile T-wave
    left ventricular contraction
    left ventricular strain
    M (on right atrial waveform)
    M-shaped mitral valve
    P pulmonale
    pseudoinfarct
    pulmonary flow
    pulmonary vascular
    QR
    respiratory

pattern *(cont.)*
    reticulogranular
    right ventricular strain
    RR' (RR prime)
    RSR' (RSR prime)
    S1Q3; S1Q3T3; S1S2S3
    speckled
    spectral
    strain
    tachypneic breathing
    trigeminal
    ventricular contraction
patulous
Paul-Bunnell test
Paul sign
pause, pauses
    asystolic
    compensatory
    full
    incomplete
    less-than-full
    noncompensatory
    postextrasystolic
    sinus
PAV (percutaneous aortic
    valvuloplasty)
PA Watch position-monitoring catheter
PAWP (pulmonary artery wedge
    pressure)
PBF (pulmonary blood flow)
PBLs (peripheral blood lymphocytes)
PBPC (peripheral blood progenitor
    cell)
PBPI (penile-brachial pressure index)
    to assess cardiac disease
PBVI (pulmonary blood volume index)
PBSC (peripheral blood stem cell)
    collections
PBV (percutaneous balloon valvulo-
    plasty)
PCA (patient-controlled analgesic)
    system

PCBS (percutaneous cardiopulmonary
bypass support)
PCD (programmable cardioverter-
defibrillator)
PCD ICD with biphasic shocks
PCD ICD active can model
(Medtronic)
PCD pulse generator
PCD tiered therapy
PCD Transvene implantable
cardioverter-defibrillator system
P cell
P congenitale
PCFP (postcatheterization false
aneurysm)
PCG (phonocardiogram,
phonocardiography)
PCICO (pressure-controlled intermit-
tent coronary occlusion)
PCL (paced cycle length)
PCNP (proliferating cell nuclear
protein)
pCO_2, PCO_2 (partial pressure of
carbon dioxide)
PCP (*Pneumocystis carinii* pneumonia)
prophylaxis
PCP (pulmonary capillary pressure)
PCPS (percutaneous cardiopulmonary
support)
PCr (phosphocreatine) analysis
PCR (polymerase chain reaction)
PCRA (percutaneous coronary
rotational atherectomy)
PCS (pain control system), CADD-
Prizm
PCS (proximal coronary sinus)
PCU (progressive care unit)
PCVD (pulmonary collagen vascular
disease)
PCWP (pulmonary capillary wedge
pressure)
PDA (patent ductus arteriosus)

PDA (peripheral directional
atherectomy)
PDA (posterior descending artery)
PDE isoenzyme inhibitor
PDF (probability density function)
PDP (postural drainage and
percussion)
PDS (polydioxanone suture)
PDS suture
PDS II Endoloop suture
PDS Vicryl suture
PDT guidewire
PDx pacing and diagnostic pacemaker
PE (pericardial effusion)
PE (pulmonary embolism)
PEA (pulseless electrical activity)
peacock sound
peak-and-trough drug levels
peak, carotid pulse
peak circumferential wall stress
peak dP/dt
peak early diastolic filling velocities
peaked P wave
peak exercise
peak expiratory flow (PEF)
peak expiratory flow rate (PEFR)
peak filling rate
peak flow
peak flow meter
peak flow variability
peak flow velocity
peak-inflation pressures
peak inspiratory pressure (PIP)
peak inspiratory pressure/positive
end-expiratory pressure
(PIP/PEEP) ventilation
peak late diastolic filling velocities
peak level of drug
peak of wave
peak regurgitant flow velocity
peak regurgitant wave pressure
peak systolic pressure

peak systolic velocity
peak tidal expiratory flow
peak-to-peak pressure gradient
peak velocity of blood flow on
    Doppler echocardiogram
Péan clamp
Péan forceps
PEAP (positive end-airway pressure)
pearls, Laënnec
Pearson chi-squared test (calculation
    used for artificial heart)
PEC (pulmonary ejection click)
$PECO_2$ (partial pressure of end-tidal
    $PECO_2$)
pectoral ectopia cordis
pectoral electrode
pectoral fremitus
pectoralis fascia
pectoralis major muscle
pectoralis major muscle flap
pectoralis major syndrome
pectoralis minor muscle
pectoriloquy
    aphonic
    whispered
    whispering
pectoris, angina (see *angina pectoris*)
pectus carinatum
pectus excavatum
pedal artery opacification
pedal edema
pedal pulses
    absent
    diminished
    intact
    palpable
pediatric biplane TEE (transesophageal
    echocardiography) probe
pediatric defibrillator paddles
pediatric laryngoscope
pedicle
    IMA (internal mammary artery)
    mammary

pedicle *(cont.)*
    musculofascial
    phrenic
    vascular
pedicled intercostal muscle flap
pedicle flap
Pedoff transducer (used in echo-
    cardiography)
pedunculated melanoma
pedunculated myxoma
pedunculated thrombus
peel-away guiding sheath
peel-away sheath
peeling back mechanism on electro-
    physiology study
PEEP (positive end-expiratory
    pressure)
PEF (peak expiratory flow)
PEFR (peak expiratory flow rate)
PEI (postexercise index)
PELA (peripheral excimer laser angio-
    plasty)
pelvic varices
Pemco prosthetic valve
Penaz methodology for monitoring
    blood pressure
pencil, electrocautery
pendelluft syndrome
penetrating aortic ulceration
penetrating atherosclerotic aortic ulcer
penetrating atherosclerotic ulceration
penetrating chest trauma
penetrating injury to aortic arch
penetrating injury to innominate artery
penetrating injury to superior vena
    cava
penetrating lung injury
penetrating trauma to heart
penetrating ulceration
penetrating wound of descending
    thoracic aorta
Penfield dissector
Penfield elevator

penicillin prophylaxis
penile-brachial pressure index (PBPI)
    to assess cardiac disease
Penn State total artificial heart (TAH)
Penn State ventricular assist device
    (VAD)
Pennington grasping forceps
Penrose drain
PentaCath 5-lumen thermodilution
    catheter
pentaerythritol tetranitrate (PETN)
pentalogy, Fallot
Pentax EB-1830 bronchoscope
Pentax FNL-10P2 nasopharyngoscope
Pentax FNL-13S nasopharyngoscope
Pentax FNL-15RP2 nasopharyngo-
    scope
penultimate
PEP (pre-ejection period)
PE Plus II balloon dilatation catheter
peptide, atrial natriuretic
Peptostreptococcus
perceived exertion scale, Borg
percent of predicted maximum heart
    rate
perceptual disturbances following open
    heart surgery
Perclose A-T (auto-tie) suture-
    mediated vessel closure device
Perclose closure device
Percor DL balloon catheter
Percor DL-II (dual-lumen) intra-aortic
    balloon catheter
Percor-Stat-DL catheter
PercuCut cut-biopsy needle
Percuflex APD all-purpose catheter
    with Fader Tip
percussion, auscultation and
percussion note
    drumlike
    dull
    flat

percussion *(cont.)*
    hyperresonant
    resonant
    tympanitic
percussion sound
percussion wave of carotid arterial
    pulse
PercuSurge GuardWire system
percutaneous abscess and fluid
    drainage (PAFD)
percutaneous aortic balloon valvulo-
    plasty (PABV)
percutaneous aspiration of pericardial
    cyst
percutaneous balloon aortic valvotomy
percutaneous balloon mitral valvulo-
    plasty
percutaneous balloon pulmonary
    valvotomy
percutaneous balloon valvuloplasty
    (PBV)
percutaneous cardiopulmonary bypass
    support (PCBS)
percutaneous cardiopulmonary
    support (PCPS), temporary
percutaneous closure device
percutaneous coil embolization
percutaneous coronary rotational
    atherectomy (PCRA)
percutaneous cutting needle
percutaneous dilational tracheostomy
    (PDT)
percutaneous endomyocardial biopsy
percutaneous groin puncture
percutaneous implantation of endovas-
    cular stent
percutaneous inferior vena cava (IVC)
    filter
percutaneous insertion
percutaneous insertion via femoral
    vein

percutaneous intra-aortic balloon counterpulsation
percutaneous intracoronary angioscopy
percutaneous lead introducer
percutaneously cannulated
percutaneously inserted
percutaneously introduced
percutaneous patent ductus arteriosus closure
percutaneous pericardial biopsy
percutaneous pericardioscopy
percutaneous puncture technique
percutaneous radiofrequency catheter ablation
percutaneous retrograde atherectomy
percutaneous revascularization
percutaneous technique
percutaneous thoracoscopy
percutaneous thrombolytic device (PTD)
percutaneous transatrial mitral commissurotomy
percutaneous transcatheter ductal closure (PTDC)
percutaneous transcatheter occlusion device
percutaneous transluminal angioplasty (PTA)
percutaneous transluminal carotid angioplasty
percutaneous transluminal coronary angioplasty (PTCA)
percutaneous transluminal coronary balloon angioplasty
percutaneous transluminal intra-arterial filtration system
percutaneous transluminal myocardial (or transmyocardial) revascularization (PTMR)
percutaneous transluminal septal myocardial ablation

percutaneous transmyocardial revascularization (PMR)
percutaneous transthoracic aspiration
percutaneous transtracheal aspiration
percutaneous transvenous mitral commissurotomy (PTMC)
percutaneous umbilical cord blood sampling (PUBS)
percutaneous umbrella closure of patent ductus arteriosus
PerDUCER pericardial access device
perennial fever
perennial rhinitis
Perez sign
perfluorocarbon blood substitute, oxygenated
perforated aortic cusp
perforating arteries
perforation
   cardiac
   transseptal
perforator
   first septal
   ligation of
   septal
   stripping of
perforator site reflux
perforator vessel
Performa angiographic catheter
performance (see *function*)
Performance irrigation device
Performr (RF-Performr) electrophysiology catheter (not Performer)
perfusate
perfuse
perfused
perfusion
   adequate coronary
   antegrade
   coronary
   diminished systemic

perfusion *(cont.)*
  extremity
  homogeneous
  hypothermic
  isolated heat
  luxury
  misery
  mosaic
  myocardial
  peripheral
  pulsatile
  regional (by mixed venous blood)
  retrograde cardiac
  retrograde cerebral (RCP)
  tissue
perfusion abnormality
perfusion and ventilation lung scan
perfusion catheter
perfusion defect
perfusionist, pump
perfusion lung scan
perfusion of myocardium
perfusion of underventilated lung
perfusion pressure
  diastolic
  transmyocardial
perfusion scintigraphy
perfusion time
perialveolar fibrosis
perianeurysmal retroperitoneal fibrosis
periaortic fibrosis
periaortic inflammation and fibrosis
periaortic neurectomy
periaortic nodes
periarterial sympathectomy
periarteritis, disseminated necrotizing
periarteritis nodosa (PAN)
peribronchial alveolar spaces
peribronchial connective tissue
peribronchial cuffing
peribronchial distribution
peribronchial fibrosis

peribronchial lymph nodes
peribronchiolar hemorrhage
pericardectomy (pericardiectomy)
pericardiaca, pleura
pericardiacophrenic vein
pericardial absence
  congenital
  partial
pericardial baffle
pericardial basket
pericardial biopsy, percutaneous
pericardial cavity
pericardial chyle with tamponade
pericardial closure
pericardial constriction, occult
pericardial cradle
pericardial cyst
pericardial diaphragmatic adhesions
pericardial disease
pericardial effusion
pericardial effusion with cardiac
  tamponade
pericardial flap
pericardial fluid
  evacuation of offending
  exudative
  transudative
pericardial fluid analysis
pericardial fluid aspiration
pericardial fold
pericardial fremitus
pericardial friction rub
pericardial hematoma
pericardial infusion
pericardial knock
pericardial lavage, continuous
pericardial pain
pericardial patch
pericardial reflection (on x-ray)
pericardial reserve volume
pericardial restraint
pericardial rub

pericardial sac
pericardial sinus (sinuses)
pericardial sling
pericardial space, free
pericardial stripping
pericardial tamponade
pericardial tap (tapping)
pericardial well
pericardial window operation
pericardiectomy (pericardectomy)
pericardiocentesis, diagnostic
pericardiocentesis needle
pericardiolysis
pericardioscopy, percutaneous
pericardiotomy syndrome
pericarditis
   actinomycotic
   acute
   acute benign
   acute fibrinous
   acute nonspecific
   acute rheumatic
   adhesive
   advanced tuberculous constrictive
   amebiasis
   amebic
   bacterial
   bread-and-butter
   calcific constrictive
   carcinomatous
   cholesterol
   chronic
   chronic constrictive
   chronic effusive
   constricting
   constrictive
   coxsackievirus
   drug-induced
   dry
   effusion-constrictive
   effusive-constricting
   enteroviral

pericarditis *(cont.)*
   epistenocardiac
   external
   fibrinous
   fibrous
   fungal
   gonococcal
   hemorrhagic
   idiopathic
   idiopathic benign
   infective
   inflammatory
   localized
   mediastinal
   meningococcal
   milk spot
   neoplastic
   nocardiosis
   noncalcific subacute constrictive
   nonpurulent
   obliterating
   obliterative
   occult constrictive
   parasitic
   Pick chronic constrictive
   pneumococcal
   pneumopyopericardium
   postcardiotomy
   postinfarction
   postirradiation
   postoperative
   postoperative constricting
   purulent
   pyopericardium
   radiation-induced
   restrictive
   rheumatic
   rheumatoid
   serofibrinous
   serous
   staphylococcal
   Sternberg

pericarditis *(cont.)*
    streptococcal
    subacute constrictive
    suppurative
    syphilitic
    traumatic
    tuberculous
    uremic
    viral
pericarditis calculosa
pericarditis, epistenocardiac
pericarditis-liver pseudocirrhosis
    syndrome
pericarditis-myocarditis syndrome
pericarditis obliterans
pericarditis sicca
pericarditis villosa
pericarditis with effusion
pericardium
    adherent
    autologous
    bread-and-butter
    calcified
    congenital absent
    congenitally absent
    diaphragmatic
    empyema
    fibrous
    inelastic
    inflamed
    nondistensible
    parietal
    pericardial
    serous
    shaggy
    soldier's patches of
    tenting of
    thickened
    visceral
pericardium calcareous deposits
pericardium exposed
pericardium fibrosum

pericardium opened in inverted T
    fashion
pericardium serosum
pericatheter thrombi
perichondritis
pericostal sutures
periendocarditis
    acute
    subacute
Periflow peripheral balloon catheter
perigraft hematoma
Peri-Guard patch
Peri-Strips
Peri-Strips Dry (bovine pericardium)
perihilar area
perihilar density
perihilar edema
perihilar edema haze
perihilar region
peri-infarction block
peri-infarction conduction defect
peri-infarction heart block
peri-infarctional defect
peri-infarctional ischemia
peri-infarction ischemia
perimedial dysplasia
perimembranous ventricular septal
    defect
Perimount Plus heart valve
Perimount RSR pericardial
    bioprosthesis
perimuscular plexus
perinatal respiratory distress syndrome
perinuclear antineutrophil cytoplasmic
    antibody (pANCA)
period
    absolute refractory (ARP)
    accessory pathway effective
        refractory
    antegrade refractory
    atrial effective refractory
    atrial refractory

period *(cont.)*
    diastolic filling
    effective refractory (ERP)
    ejection
    functional refractory (FRP)
    isoelectric
    isovolumetric
    isovolumic
    pacemaker amplifier refractory
    postventricular atrial refractory
      (PVARP)
    pre-ejection (PEP)
    presphygmic
    rapid filling (RFP)
    refractory
    relative refractory (RRP)
    retrograde refractory
    sphygmic
    symptom-free
    systolic ejection (SEP)
    ventricular effective refractory
      (VERP)
    ventricular refractory
    ventriculoatrial effective refractory
    vulnerable
    Wenckebach
periodic breathing
periodic chills
periodic dizziness
periodic edema
periodicity
    AV node Wenckebach
    circadian
periodic paralysis
period of isovolumic contraction
period of rapid ventricular filling
period of reduced ventricular filling
perioperative blood loss
perioperative complications
perioperative contamination of the
    mediastinal space
perioperative myocardial infarction

perioperative myocardial necrosis
perioperative plasmapheresis
perioperative stroke
perioral cyanosis
periorbital Doppler study
periorbital fullness
periosteal incision
periosteum
periostitis
peripancreatic arteries
peripartum cardiomyopathy
peripartum dilated cardiomyopathy
peripartum myocarditis
peripelvic collateral vessel
peripheral air-space disease
Peripheral AngioJet system
peripheral angiopathy
peripheral angioplasty
peripheral arterial cannula
peripheral blood flow
peripheral blood lymphocytes (PBLs)
peripheral blood progenitor cell
    (PBPC)
peripheral blood stem cell (PBSC)
    collections
peripheral cholesterol embolization
    syndrome
peripheral circulatory vasoconstriction
peripheral cutaneous vasoconstriction
peripheral cyanosis
peripheral directional atherectomy
    (PDA)
peripheral edema
peripheral embolus
peripheral excimer laser angioplasty
    (PELA)
peripheral infiltrates
peripheral intravenous infusion line
peripheral laser angioplasty (PLA)
peripherally inserted central catheter
    (PICC)
peripheral pulmonary stenosis

peripheral pulmonic stenosis
peripheral pulmonic systolic murmur
peripheral pulse (pulses)
peripheral pulse deficit
peripheral resistance
peripheral small airways study
peripheral vascular disease,
    arteriosclerotic
peripheral vascular resistance,
    decreased
peripheral vasodilators
peripheral vasodilatation
peripheral veins, absent
peripheral venous cannula
peripheral venous reservoirs
peripheral vessels
periphery of the lung
periphlebitis
    breast
    lateral thoracic vein
    sclerosing
    sclerosing breast
    thoracoepigastric vein
peripheral pulmonary artery stenosis
periprosthetic leak (leakage)
perirenal hematoma
peritoneal dialysis, continuous ambula-
    tory
peritoneovenous shunt
periumbilical area tenderness
perivalvular dehiscence
perivalvular disruption
perivalvular leak
perivascular canal
perivascular cell
perivascular distribution
perivascular edema
perivascular fibrosis
perivascular space of Virchow-Robin
perles
Perma-Flow coronary bypass graft
Perma-Hand braided silk suture

PermaMesh suture material
permanent disability
permanent idiopathic hypotension
permanent impairment
permanent lead introducer
permanent rate-responsive dual-
    chamber pacemaker
permanent rate-responsive pacemaker
permanent reciprocating atrioventricu-
    lar junctional tachycardia
Permathane Pacesetter lead pacemaker
PermCath double-lumen ventricular
    access catheter
permeability, increased capillary
permeability of capillaries
permeability-type pulmonary edema
pernicious anemia
pernicious myocarditis
peroneal area
peroneal artery
peroneal muscles
peroneal-tibial trunk
peroneal vein
peroneal vessel
perpetuation of atelectasis
persistent pulmonary hypertension of
    the newborn (PPHN)
Persantine Cardiolite stress test
Persantine stress test
Persantine thallium stress test
Persantine thallium scanning
Persantine thallium stress test
persistent bronchopleural fistula
persistent common atrioventricular
    canal
persistent fetal circulation
persistent marginal vein
persistent ostium primum
persistent ostium secundum
persistent patency of ductus arteriosus
persistent patency of ductus venosus
persistent splenomegaly

persistent truncus arteriosus
persistent upright T waves
personality type A
personality type B
perspiring
Perthes test for collateral circulation in
    varicose veins
pertussis
pertussoid eosinophilic pneumonia
pervenous catheter
PES (programmed electrical stimula-
    tion) interval
PET (positron emission tomography)
PET balloon, USCI
PET balloon with window and
    extended collection chamber
PET balloon Simpson atherectomy
    device
petechia (pl. petechiae)
petechial angioma
petechial hemorrhage
Petit sinus
PETN (pentaerythritol tetranitrate)
PET scan
pexelizumab
Peyrot thorax
PF-CVD (pulmonary fibrosis
    associated with collagen vascular
    disorders)
PFD (persistent fetal dispersion) of
    AV node
PFO (patent foramen ovale)
PFR (peak filling rate)
PF3 (platelet factor 3) syndrome
PFT (pulmonary function test)
PFTs (pulmonary function tests)
Pfuhl-Jaffé sign
PFWT (pain-free walking time) on
    treadmill
PG (pulse generator)
PGE_1 (prostaglandin E_1)

PHACE (posterior fossa brain malfor-
    mations, hemangiomas, arterial
    anomalies, coarctation of the aorta
    and cardiac defects, eye abnormali-
    ties) syndrome
pH interval
pH-stat strategy
phagocytized hemosiderin
phagocytosis
Phalen stress test
Phaneuf artery forceps
Phantom cardiac guidewire
pharmaceutical cardioversion
pharmacologic stress dual-isotope
    myocardial perfusion SPECT
pharmacologic stress echocardiography
pharmacologic stress technique
pharyngeal
pharyngitis
    acute
    catarrhal
    granular
    phlegmonous
    pneumococcal
    staphylococcal
    ulcerative
    viral
pharynx
phase (see also *period*)
    bradycardic agonal
    diastolic depolarization
    expiratory
    inspiration
    inspiratory
    plateau (in cardiac action
        potentials)
    prolonged expiratory
    prolonged inspiratory
    rapid early repolarization
    rapid filling
    rapid repolarization

phase *(cont.)*
 resting (of cardiac action potentials)
 upstroke (of cardiac action
  potentials)
phase angle
phase-shift velocity mapping
PHCA (profound hypothermic
 circulatory arrest)
P_2 heart sound (pulmonary valve
 closure)
phenomenon (pl. phenomena) (see
  also *sign, reaction*)
 aliasing
 anniversary
 Aschner
 Ashman
 Austin Flint
 booster
 Bowditch staircase
 coronary steal
 Cushing
 dip
 dip and plateau
 Doppler
 embolic
 Friedreich
 Gaertner (Gärtner)
 Gallavardin
 gap conduction
 Goldblatt
 Hering
 Kasabach-Merritt
 Katz-Wachtel
 Litten diaphragm
 no-reflow
 Raynaud
 R-on-T
 Schellong-Strisower
 staircase
 steal
 stone heart
 tactile precordial

phenomenon *(cont.)*
 treppe
 vasovagal
 Wenckebach
phenotype
 Cellano
 McLeod blood
phenylephrine
pheochromocytoma
 extra-adrenal
 intra-adrenal
 malignant
Philos DR pacemaker
Philos DR-T pulse generator
phlebectasia
 deep
 deep malformed
 diffuse
 superficial
phlebectomy
phlebitis
 adhesive
 anemic
 blue
 breast
 chest wall
 chlorotic
 migrating
 migratory
 obliterating
 obliterative
 plastic
 postvenography
 productive
 proliferative
 sclerosing breast
 septic
 superficial breast
 suppurative
phlebitis migrans
phlebodynia
phlebofibrosis

phlebogram, phlebography
  ascending
  ascending contrast
  direct puncture
  impedance
phleboid
phlebolith
phlebophlebostomy
phleboplasty
phleborheography
phleborrhagia
phleborrhaphy
phleborrhexis
phlebosclerosis
phlebosis
phlebostasis
phlebostenosis
phlebothrombosis
phlebotomy
  bloodless
  therapeutic
phlegm (see *sputum*)
phlegmasia
  cellulitic
  thrombotic
phlegmasia alba dolens puerperarum
phlegmasia cerulea dolens
phlegmonous pharyngitis
Phoenix single-chamber pacemaker
Phoenix total artificial heart
phonocardiogram (PCG)
phonocardiography, intracardiac
phonocardiographic
phonocatheter
phosphatase, histamine acid
phosphatidylglycerol levels
phosphatidylinositol
phosphocreatine (PCr)
phosphodiesterase inhibitors
phosphofructokinase
phosphoinositides
phospholamban

phospholipids
  autoantibodies to
  desaturated
phosphorus level, serum
phosphorylase kinase deficiency
phosphorylation
  mitochondrial
  oxidative
photoablation, laser
photoangioplasty
photocoagulation
  intraoperative laser (of ventricular
    tachycardia)
  laser
photodisruption
PhotoGenica V-Star pulsed-dye laser
photometer, HemoCue
Photon delivery system
Photon DR dual-chamber implantable
  cardioverter-defibrillator
photonic stimulator
photoplethysmography (PPG)
photoplethysmographic monitoring
photothermal sclerosis treatment of
  varicose veins
phrenic artery
phrenic nerve pacing
phrenic nerve paralysis
phrenic pedicle
PHT (passive hyperimmune therapy)
PHT (portal hypertension)
phthinoid chest
phthisis, aneurysmal
PHTN (pulmonary hypertension)
Phylax AV dual chamber implantable
  cardioverter-defibrillator (Biotronik)
Phymos 3D pacemaker
physical finding(s)
  cardinal
  salient
Physio anuloplasty ring (Carpentier-
  Edwards)

Physio-Control automatic and semi-automatic defibrillators (Medtronic)
Physio-Control bedside monitor
physiologic(al) anemia
physiologic fibrinolysis
physiologic pacing
physiologic regurgitation
physiologic shunt flow
physiologic solution
physiologic splitting of S_2
physiologic stress technique
physiologic third heart sound
Physio Partner support mechanism
Physios CTM 01 noninvasive cardiac transplant monitoring system
physiotherapy, vigorous chest
PI (pulmonic insufficiency)
PIB (peri-infarction block)
PIBC (percutaneous intra-aortic balloon counterpulsation)
PIC (plasmin inhibitor complex)
PICA (posterior inferior communicating artery)
Piccolo blood chemistry analyzer system
PICD (peri-infarction conduction defect)
Pick chronic constrictive pericarditis
Pick disease of heart
Pick syndrome
pickwickian syndrome
Pico-ST II low-profile balloon catheter
Picovir (pleconaril)
picture
   clinical
   hemodynamic
PIE (pulmonary infiltrates with eosinophilia)
PIE (pulmonary interstitial emphysema)
PIE (pulmonary infiltrate-eosinophilia) syndrome

Pierce-Donachy ventricular assist device (VAD)
pigeon breast
pigeon-breeder's lung
pigeon-breeder's pneumonitis
pigeon-breeder's syndrome
pigeon chest
pigeon-fancier's disease
pigeon-fancier's lung
piggy-back cardiac transplantation
pigmentation
pigmented macrophages
pigmenti, incontinentia
pigtail catheter
PIH (pregnancy-induced hypertension)
Pilling Weck Y-stent forceps
Pilling Wolvek sternal approximator
piloerection
Pilotip catheter guide
PIMS (programmable implantable medication system)
pinching chest pain
pincushion distortion, radiographic
pinked up (verb)
pinked up extremity
pink puffer
pink tetralogy of Fallot
Pinnacle pacemaker
Pins sign in pericarditis
PIP (peak inspiratory pressure)
pipestem arteries
PIP/PEEP (peak inspiratory pressure/positive end-expiratory pressure) ventilation
piriform (pyriform) sinus
pistol-shot femoral and radial pulse
pistol-shot sound in aortic regurgitation
pitch
Pitié-Salpetrière saphenous vein hook
pitting edema
Pittman IMA retractor system
Pixsys FlashPoint digitizer

PJC (premature junctional contraction)
PJT (paroxysmal junctional tachy-
    cardia)
PLA (peripheral laser angioplasty)
PLAATO (percutaneous left atrial
    appendage transcatheter occlusion)
    procedure
placebo effect
placement
    anular
    central venous line
    intracoronary stent
    intrapericardial patch lead
    poststent
    shunt
    subanular
placental souffle
placental transfusion syndrome
PLAC diagnostic test
PLA-I (platelet antigen)
planar exercise thallium-201
    scintigraphy
plane
    circular
    four-chamber
    frontal
    short-axis
    subadventitial
    subintimal cleavage
    transmedial
    transverse
    valve
    XY
    ZY
plane-type synovial joint
planimeter, -metry
planogram
plantar hyperplasia
plantar ischemia test for circulation
plantaris muscle
plaque, plaquing (noun)
    arterial
    arteriosclerotic

plaque *(cont.)*
    atheromatous
    atherosclerotic
    calcified
    concentric atherosclerotic
    coral reef
    disrupted
    eccentric
    eccentric atherosclerotic
    echogenic
    echolucent
    endocardial
    fatty
    fibrofatty yellow
    fibrotic
    fibrous
    fissured atheromatous
    flattening of
    Hollenhorst
    intimal
    intraluminal
    lipid-laden
    luminal
    noncompliant
    obstructive
    pleural
    pulverized
    residual
    sessile
    stenotic
    talc
    ulcerated
plaque cleaving
plaque compression
plaque constituents
plaque-containing artery
plaque cracker, LeVeen
plaque disintegration by laser pulses
plaque erosion
plaque fracture (or fracturing)
plaque redeposition
plaque regression
plaque remodeling

plaque rupture
plaque splitting
plaque tearing
plaque vaporization
plaquing
plaquing of arteries
Plasbumin
plasma
    fresh frozen
    platelet-rich
plasma aldosterone, circadian rhythm
plasma cell pneumonia, interstitial
plasma cells
plasma coagulation factors
plasma colloid osmotic pressure
plasma concentration
plasma expanders
plasma fibrinogen
plasma infusion, fresh frozen
plasma lactate, elevated
Plasmalyte A cardioplegic solution
plasmapheresis, perioperative
Plasma-Plex
plasma renin activity
    inappropriately elevated
    suppressed
Plasma-Saver
Plasmatein
Plasma TFE vascular graft
plasma thromboplastin component
    (PTC)
plasma viscosity
plasma volume expander (Hespan or
    hetastarch)
plasmin inhibitor complex (PIC)
plasminogen activator
    recombinant tissue-type
    tissue
    tissue-type
    urokinase-type
plasminogen activator inhibitor (PAI)
plasminogen deficiency

plasminogen streptokinase activator
    complex
Plasmodium falciparum infestation
plastic bronchitis
plastic clot
plastic phlebitis
plastic pleurisy
Plast-O-Fit thermoplastic bandage
    system
plasty, sliding
plate
    ground
    pusher
plateau
    elevated diastolic
    ventricular
plateau murmur
plateau phase in cardiac action
    potentials
plateau phenomenon, dip and
platelet
    blood
    HLA-type specific
    giant
platelet activating factor
platelet adhesiveness
platelet aggregation
platelet antiaggregant drugs
platelet count
platelet-derived growth factor
platelet factor 4
platelet-rich arterial plug
platelet-rich plasma
platelet-rich thrombus
platelet thrombosis or thrombus
platelet trapping
platelike atelectasis
platelike fibrous scar in lungs
platinum asthma
platysma layer
Plavix (clopidogrel bisulfate)
PLE (protein-losing enteropathy)

pledget, pledgets
   cotton
   oval
   Teflon felt
pledgeted double-armed sutures
pledgeted Ethibond suture
pledgeted everting mattress sutures
pledgeted mattress suture
pledgeted sutures
PlegiaGuard
Plegisol cardioplegic solution
pleomorphic mononuclear cells
Plesch test
plethora of findings
plethora, pulmonary
plethoric appearance
plethysmogram, plethysmography
   body box
   Doppler ultrasonic velocity detector
     segmental
   exercise strain gauge venous
   impedance (IPG)
   Medsonic
   strain-gauge
   venous
pleura (pl. pleurae)
   cervical
   congested
   costal
   diaphragmatic
   edematous
   inflamed
   mediastinal
   parietal
   pericardiac
   pulmonary
   roughened
   silicotic visceral
   visceral
   wrinkled
pleuracentesis
pleura costalis

pleuracotomy
pleura diaphragmatica
pleural adhesions, fibrous
pleural apical hematoma cap
pleural-based area of increased opacity
pleural biopsy
pleural biopsy needle
pleural cap, left
pleural carcinomatosis
pleural cavity
pleural crackle
pleural crepitation
pleural cupula (pl. cupulae)
pleural dissemination
pleural effusion
   chylous
   eosinophilic
   milky
pleural empyema
pleural exudate
pleural fibrosis, asbestos-induced
pleural fistula
pleural flap
pleural fluid, iridescent
pleural fremitus
pleural friction rub
pleuralgia
pleural implants, malignant
pleural margins
pleural mesothelium
pleural plaque
pleural poudrage
pleural pressure
pleural rales
pleural recesses
pleural reflection
pleural rub
   coarse
   creaking
   faint
   grating
   harsh

pleural *(cont.)*
  loud
  scratchy
  shuffling
  soft
pleural sac
pleural shock
pleural sleeve
pleural space
pleural studding
pleural tap
pleural thickening, diffuse
pleural trauma
pleura mediastinalis
pleura parietalis
pleura pericardiaca
pleura pulmonalis
pleura visceralis
pleurectomy, parietal
Pleur-evac suction tube
pleurisy
  acute
  acute fibrinous
  adhesive
  blocked
  cholesterol
  chronic
  chyliform
  chyloid
  chylous
  circumscribed
  costal
  diaphragmatic
  diffuse
  double
  dry
  encysted
  exudative
  fibrinopurulent
  fibrinous
  hemorrhagic
  ichorous

pleurisy *(cont.)*
  indurative
  interlobar
  interlobular
  mediastinal
  metapneumonic
  plastic
  pneumococcal
  primary
  proliferating
  pulmonary
  pulsating
  purulent
  sacculated
  secondary
  septic
  serofibrinous
  seropurulent
  serous
  single
  staphylococcal
  streptococcal
  suppurative
  typhoid
  visceral
  wet
pleurisy with effusion
pleuritic chest pain
pleuritic exudate
pleuritic pain
pleuritic rub
pleuritis
pleurodesis
pleurodesis via talc poudrage
pleurodynia
pleuropericardial incision
pleuropericarditis
pleuropneumonia-like organisms
  (PPLO)
pleuropulmonary adhesions
plexectomy
plexiform fibrosis

pneumonitis *(cont.)*
  congenital rubella
  cytomegalovirus
  early
  granulomatous
  hypersensitivity
  interstitial
  lipoid
  lymphocytic interstitial
  malarial
  manganese
  maple bark stripper's disease
  Mycoplasma (mycoplasmal)
  Pneumocystis
  pigeon breeder's
  radiation
  staphylococcal
  trimellitic anhydritic
  uremic
  ventilation
pneumonocirrhosis
pneumonopathy
  alveolar
  eosinophilic
  parietoalveolar
pneumonopexy
pneumonophthisis
pneumonorrhaphy
pneumonotomy
pneumopathy
pneumopericarditis
pneumopericardium, tension
pneumopleuritis
pneumopyopericardium pericarditis
pneumoscope
pneumotachograph
pneumothorax (pl. pneumothoraces)
  artificial
  blowing
  clicking
  closed
  congenital

pneumothorax *(cont.)*
  diagnostic
  extrapleural
  induced
  life-threatening
  open
  positive-pressure
  pressure
  simultaneous bilateral spontaneous
    (SBSP)
  spontaneous tension
  sucking
  tension
  therapeutic
  traumatic
  tuberculous
  uncomplicated
  valvular
Pneumovax
pneuPAC ventilator/resuscitator
PNH (paroxysmal nocturnal
    hemoglobinuria)
pO_2, (oxygen partial pressure or
    tension)
POBA (plain old balloon angioplasty)
pocket (see also *pouch*)
  air
  endocardial
  infraclavicular
  pacemaker
  pacemaker tissue
  rectus sheath
  regurgitant
  subcutaneous pacemaker
  subpectoral
Pockethaler
pockets of Zahn
poikilocyte
point
  A
  Arrhigi
  C

point *(cont.)*
  coaptation
  commissural
  D
  E
  Erb
  F
  J (junction)
  Mussey (de Mussey)
  null
  O
point of maximal intensity (PMI)
point of maximum impulse (PMI)
Poiseuille layer (or space)
poisoning, cyanide
poker back
Poland sequence syndrome
polar anemia
PolarCath catheter
Polaris-Dx steerable diagnostic
  catheter
Polaris 1.32 Nd:YAG laser
Polaris X steerable diagnostic catheter
polarity
polarity-altered spectral selective
  acquisition (PASTA) imaging
polarizing
Polar-Mate bipolar microcoagulator
polarographic oxygen method for
  determining cardiac output
Polar Vantage XL heart rate monitor
Polhemus-Schafer-Ivemark syndrome
pollen, mixed grass
pollinosis
pollutant, air
polyaneurysmatic
polyangiitis overlap syndrome
polyarteritis nodosa
polychondritis, relapsing
Poly GIA stapler
polycystic kidney disease

polycythemia
  compensatory
  primary
  secondary
  spurious
  true
polycythemia vera
polycythemic
polydactyly
Polydek suture
Polyderm foam wound dressing
polydioxanone suture (PDS)
PolyFlex lead pacemaker
PolyFlo catheter
polyfluorotetraethylene (PTFE) plastic
  graft material
polygenic hypercholesterolemia
PolyMemfoam wound dressing
polymer fume fever
polymerase chain reaction (PCR)
polymeric endoluminal paving stent
polymicrobial infection
polymorphic ventricular tachycardia
polymorphic VT/VF (ventricular
  tachycardia/ventricular fibrillation)
polymorphonuclear leukocytes
polymyositis
Polynesian bronchiectasis
polyolefin rubber diaphragm
polyp, cardiac
polypoid calcified irregular mass
Polyrox fractal active fixation lead
Polyskin II dressing
polysomnogram
polysomnography
Polysorb suture
polysplenia
polysplenia syndrome
Polystan perfusion cannula
Polystan venous return catheter
polytetrafluoroethylene (PTFE) fumes
polytetrafluoroethylene (PTFE) graft

polyunsaturated fats
polyurethane foam embolus
polyuria, nocturnal
polyvalvular dysplasia, congenital
PolyWic wound filling material
Pompe disease
Pompe glycogen storage disease,
  type II
Ponfick shadow
Pontiac fever
pontine intracerebral hemorrhage
pool, circulating fibrinogen
pooling of blood in extremities
pooling, venous
poor compliance
poor drainage of bronchial secretions
poorly controlled hypertension
poor outcome, portend a
poor prognosis
poor R-wave progression
poor short-term prognosis
popliteal artery aneurysmorrhaphy
popliteal artery entrapment syndrome
popliteal artery, infragenicular
popliteal artery occlusive disease
popliteal-blind peroneal graft
popliteal bypass
popliteal-distal bypass graft
popliteal fossa
popliteal in situ bypass
popliteal pulses, palpable
popliteal space
popliteal to distal in situ bypass
popliteal trifurcation
popliteal vein ligature
pop-off suture
Poppen-Blalock carotid clamp
poppet
  ball
  barium-impregnated
  disk

poppet *(cont.)*
  prosthetic heart valve
  prosthetic valve
popping sound
porcelain aorta
porcine heterograft
porcine valve prosthesis
porcine xenograft bioprosthesis
porcine xenograft, glutaraldehyde-
  preserved
pores of Kohn
porosity
porous electrode
porous tip electrode
porphyrins
port
  Aeon vascular access
  Angiotech cardiovascular
  A-port implant infusion
  BardPort implanted
  BodyFlex
  B-port implant infusion
  Ceredur vascular access
  injection
  noncoplanar multiple static
  Quinton vascular access
  RadPICC
  Rosenblatt implantable vascular
    access
  SEA (side entry access)
  side-arm pressure
  side entry access (SEA)
  SlimPort implantable vascular
    access
  Thora-Port
  Triumph-I vascular
  vent
  Vital-Port vascular access
  Xtent vascular access
portable chest x-ray
portable heart-lung machine
portable volume ventilator

Port-A-Cath
Port-A-Cath II low profile epidural
    system
portacaval anastomosis, end-to-side
portacaval shunt
port access CABG (PACAB)
Port-Access coronary artery bypass
    (PACAB) Port-Access minimally
    invasive
    cardiac surgery
portal hypertension (PHT)
portal, superolateral
Porta-Lung noninvasive extrathoracic
    ventilator (NEV)
portal vein thrombosis
portal venous clamp
portal venous-dominant phase (PVP)
    images (CT scan)
Porta Pulse 3 portable defibrillator
Portasonic nebulizer
portend, portends
portend a poor outcome
Porter syndrome
portion, conal
Portnoy ventricular cannula
portoportal anastomosis
portopulmonary bilharziasis
Porvidx noninvasive early lung cancer
    screening
port wine stain
Posadas disease
Posadas mycosis
Posadas-Wernicke coccidioidomycosis
Posadas-Wernicke disease
POSICAM medical imaging system
position
    anterior oblique
    catheter tip
    coaxial catheter tip
    45°
    Fowler
    infragenicular

position *(cont.)*
    infrapulmonary
    knee-chest
    lateral decubitus
    left anterior oblique (LAO)
    left lateral decubitus
    Nefertiti sniff
    noncoaxial catheter tip
    orthopnea
    orthopneic
    paramedian
    pulmonary capillary wedge
    right anterior oblique (RAO)
    right lateral decubitus
    semi-Fowler
    semilateral
    spiral
    squatting
    steep Trendelenburg
    suboptimal
    30°
    Trendelenburg
    wedge
position confirmed by fluoroscopy with
    aid of radiopaque marking on knot
position sensor, Hall-effect
positive deflection on EKG
positive end-airway pressure (PEAP)
positive end-expiratory pressure
    (PEEP)
positive inotropic effect
positive-pressure pneumothorax
positive-pressure ventilation (PPV)
positive skin test
positive tilt test
Positrol cardiac device
Positrol II catheter
positron emission tomography (PET)
positron emitters
Possis catheter
Possis epicardial pacing lead
postablation

postage-stamp-type skin graft
postangioplasty intracoronary radiation
   therapy (ICRT)
postangioplasty mural thrombosis
postangioplasty stenosis
post-arrest hypoxic encephalopathy
post balloon angioplasty restenosis
postcapillaries
postcapillary venules
postcardiac injury syndrome
postcardiotomy delirium
postcardiotomy intra-aortic balloon
   pumping
postcardiotomy lymphocytic
   splenomegaly
postcardiotomy pericarditis
postcardiotomy psychosis syndrome
postcardiotomy shock
postcardiotomy syndrome
postcatheterization
postcatheterization false aneurysm
   (PCFP)
postcatheterization injury
postcommissurotomy syndrome
postconversion electrocardiogram
postdeployment
postdevice anticoagulation
postductal type of coarctation
posterior anulus, redundant scallop of
posterior-aorta transposition of great
   arteries
posterior axillary line
posterior basal bronchi
posterior border of lung
posterior bronchi
posterior cathodal patch electrode
posterior coronary plexus (of heart)
posterior cusp
posterior descending artery (PDA),
   bifurcation of
posterior descending branch
posterior fascicular block

posterior fossa compression syndrome
posterior fossa hypertension
posterior free wall
posterior inferior communicating
   artery (PICA)
posterior intercostal artery
posterior intercostal branch
posterior interventricular groove
posterior interventricular sulcus
posterior interventricular vein
posterior lumbar vessel
posterior leaflet prolapse
posterior mediastinal lymph nodes
posterior mediastinum
posterior mitral valve leaflet
posterior papillary muscle
posterior parietal peritoneal incision
posterior patch aortoplasty (Nicks
   procedure)
posterior pericardial well
posterior pulmonary plexus
posterior rectus fascia exposed
posterior segment of lung
posterior semilunar valve
posterior table
posterior tibial pulse
posterior to the phrenic nerve
posterior ventricular branch
posterior wall myocardial infarction
posterior wall thickness
posterobasal wall myocardial infarction
posterolateral branch
posterolateral incision
posterolateral thoracotomy incision
posterolateral thoracotomy, left
posterolateral wall myocardial
   infarction
posteroseptal Kent bundle
postexercise tracing
postextrasystolic potentiation
postextubation stridor
posthemorrhagic anemia of newborn

postinfarction course
postinfarction failure
postinfarction unstable angina
postinfarction ventricular aneurysm
postinfarction ventricular septal defect
postinfectious bronchiectasis
postinflammatory pulmonary fibrosis
postirradiation pericarditis
postirradiation vascular insufficiency
postischemic recovery
postmalignant arrhythmia
postmastectomy lymphedema
   syndrome
post-MI (myocardial infarction)
   syndrome
postmortem clot
postmortem thrombus
postmyocardial infarction thrombolysis
postmyocardial infarction syndrome
postmyocardiotomy infarction
postmyocarditis dilated cardiomyopathy
postnasal catarrh
postnasal discharge
postnasal drainage
postnasal drip
postobstructive pneumonia
postoperative acute cholecystitis
postoperative bleeding
postoperative bronchopneumonia
postoperative cardiac function
postoperative choreiform movements
postoperative choreoathetosis
postoperative chylothorax
postoperative constricting pericarditis
postoperative mediastinal hemorrhage
postoperative oliguria
postoperative pericarditis
postoperative pneumomediastinum
postoperative pneumonia
postoperative pulmonary edema
postoperative renal failure

postoperative shock
postoperative transfusion
postpartum cardiomyopathy
postpartum myocardiopathy
postpartum thrombophlebitis
postperfusion lung syndrome
postperfusion pulmonary vasculitis
postperfusion syndrome
postpericardiotomy syndrome
postphlebitic incompetence
postphlebitic leg
postphlebitic neurosis
postphlebitic syndrome
postprandial angina
postprandial pain
postprandial syncope
postprimary tuberculosis
post-PTCA heparinization
post-PTCA residual stenosis
post-PVC sinus beat
postradiation fibrosis
postrepair
postshock escape interval
postshock PA
postshock pacing
postshock pacing period
postshock pause
postshock PW
postshock VVI pacing
poststenotic dilatation
poststent placement
poststreptococcal inflammatory
   process
postthrombolytic coronary reocclusion
postthrombotic syndrome
post-tourniquet occlusion angiography
posttransfusion purpura
posttransfusion syndrome
posttransplantation lymphoproliferative
   disorder (PTLD)
posttransplant coronary artery disease
posttussive inspiratory rhonchi

posttussive rales
posttussive rhonchi
posttussive syncope
postural drainage
postural drainage and percussion
  (PDP)
postural drainage with clapping and
  vibration
postural dyspnea
postural stimulation of aldosterone
postural stimulation test
postural syncope
posture, squatting
postvalvulotomy syndrome
postvenography phlebitis
postventricular atrial refractory period
  (PVARP)
Potain opening snap in mitral stenosis
Potain sign
potassium
  depressed serum
  ionic
potassium channel blocker
potassium channel openers
potassium chloride (KCl)
potassium chloride cardioplegia
potassium chloride repletion
potassium chloride solution
potassium concentration, 24-hour urine
potassium deficiency
potassium intoxication
potassium sparing
potassium-sparing diuretics
potassium-sparing effect
potassium wastage
potassium wasting
potassium-43 imaging agent (myocardial perfusion imaging)
potential
  action
  cardiac action
  membrane

potential *(cont.)*
  recruitment
  resting membrane
  tetrodotoxin
  ventricular late (VLP)
potentiation, postextrasystolic
Pottenger sign
Potts anastomosis
Potts anastomosis between descending
  aorta and left pulmonary artery
Potts aortic clamp
Potts aortic-pulmonary artery
  anastomosis
Potts bronchus forceps
Potts bulldog forceps
Potts clamp
Potts coarctation clamp
Potts-Cournand needle
Potts needle
Potts operation
Potts patent ductus clamp
Potts scissors
Potts shunt
Potts right-angled scissors
Potts-Satinsky clamp
Potts 60° angled scissors
Potts-Smith aortic occlusion clamp
Potts-Smith scissors
Potts-Smith side-to-side anastomosis
Potts-Smith tissue forceps
Potts-Smith vascular scissors
Potts thumb forceps
Potts vascular forceps
Potts vascular scissors
pouch
  blind
  Dacron
  pacemaker generator
poudrage
  intrapericardial
  pleural
  talc

pounding, heart
pounding in chest
pounding pain
Poupart ligament
povidone-iodine solution
Powerheart automatic external
    cardioverter-defibrillator
PowerPICC catheter
power-injector angiography
power pack, abdominal
P-P interval
PPA (plexogenic pulmonary
    arteriopathy)
PPAS (peripheral pulmonary artery
    stenosis)
PPD (purified protein derivative) skin
    test for tuberculosis
PPD skin test
PPH (primary pulmonary hyper-
    tension)
PPHN (persistent pulmonary hyperten-
    sion of the newborn)
PPLO (pleuropneumonia-like
    organisms)
PPM (posterior papillary muscle)
P pulmonale in leads II, III, aVF
P pulmonale syndrome
PPV (positive-pressure ventilation)
P-Q interval, short
P-QRS ratio
PRAs (panel reactive antibodies)
PRA (plasma renin activity) test
praecox, lymphedema
Pravigard PAC (buffered aspirin
    and pravastatin sodium)
PRBCs (packed red blood cells)
preablation
preacinar arterial wall thickness
preangioplasty stenosis
preaortic space, retropancreatic
precapillary pulmonary hypertension
precarious circulation

precarious condition
precatheterization
precautions, universal
precipitant
precipitated by exertion, angina
precipitating antibody
precipitating event
precipitating factor
precipitator
precipitously
precipitous rise in blood pressure
preclotted graft
preclotted Meadox woven double
    velour graft
preclotted patch graft
preclot the graft
preclotting of graft
preclude
Preclude pericardial membrane
precluding catheter passage, tortuosity
preconditioning ischemic stimuli
precordial chest pain
precordial clicking
precordial crunching
precordial discomfort
precordial honk
precordial impulse
precordial impulse amplitude
precordial impulse, bifid
precordial impulse contour
precordial impulse location
precordial knocking
precordial lead
precordial migraine
precordial motion
    heaving
    rocking
    trifid
precordial palpation
precordial thrill
precordial thump
precordial transition zone

precordium
    active
    anterior
    bulging
    lateral
Predator angioplasty balloon catheter
predicated on the assumption
predicted cardiac index
predilection
predispose
predisposed patient
predisposing factors
predominant flow loads
preductal coarctation of aorta
preeclampsia
pre-ejection interval
pre-ejection period (PEP)
pre-excitation (early ventricular
    depolarization)
pre-excitation atrioventricular
    conduction
pre-excitation syndrome
pre-excitation, ventricular
pre-exercise resting supine EKG
preexisting cardiopulmonary disease
preformed clot
preformed curves, catheter with
preformed guidewire
pregnancy-induced hypertension (PIH)
preformed peel-away guiding sheath
pregnancy-related hypertension
pregnancy, toxemia of
prehypertension
preinfarction angina
preinfarction syndrome
preload
    cardiac
    decreased ventricular
    left ventricular
    ventricular
preload reserve
Prelude vascular introducer sheath

premature atherosclerosis
premature atrial complex (PAC)
premature atrial contraction (PAC)
premature atrial depolarization
premature atrioventricular junctional
    complexes
premature battery depletion
premature closure of the ductus
    arteriosus
premature complex
    atrial
    junctional
premature contraction
    atrial
    atrioventricular junctional
    ventricular
premature depolarizations, atrial
premature heartbeat (extrasystole)
premature junctional contraction (PJC)
premature mid-diastolic closure of
    mitral valve
premature rewarming, retard
premature valve closure
premature ventricular beats
premature ventricular complex (PVC)
premature ventricular contraction
        (PVC)
    high-amplitude
    monomorphic
premature ventricular depolarizations
prematurity, apnea of
premedication
premonitory signs
premonitory symptoms
prenatal corticosteroid treatment
preoperative bronchoscopy
preoperative resting MUGA scan
prep
    Betadine
    Ioban
prepectorally
preperitoneal fat

preponderance
preponderant
prerenal azotemia
prescription (Rx)
presenile gangrene
preservation of native aortic valve
preserved left ventricular function
preserve the long thoracic nerve
pressor response, Cushing
pressors
pressor support
pressor therapy
pressure
   airway opening
   alveolar
   ambulant venous (AVP)
   ankle-arm
   AO or Ao (aorta)
   aortic
   aortic root
   arterial (ART or Art.)
   arterial peak systolic
   atmospheres of
   augmentation
   auto positive end-expiratory
   A wave (left or right atrial
     catheterization)
   back
   bilevel positive airway (BLPAP)
   blew off due to arterial
   blood (BP)
   brachial artery
   brachial artery cuff
   brachial artery end-diastolic
   brachial artery peak systolic
   C wave (right atrial catheterization)
   capillary
   cardiac filling
   central aortic
   central venous (CVP)
   cerebral perfusion
   chest

pressure *(cont.)*
   collapse of jugular venous
   continuous descending (CDP)
   continuous positive airway (CPAP)
   coronary artery perfusion (CPP)
   coronary wedge
   critical closing (CCP)
   cuff
   cuff blood
   diastolic blood (DBP)
   diastolic filling (DFP)
   diastolic perfusion
   diastolic pulmonary artery
   distal coronary perfusion
   Doppler blood
   elevated
   elevated jugular venous
   elevated pulmonary wedge
   end-diastolic
   end-expiratory
   end-inspiratory
   endocardial
   end-systolic (ESP)
   equalized diastolic
   extravascular
   femoral artery (FAP)
   filling
   high blood (HBP)
   high filling
   high interstitial
   high wedge
   increased pulmonary arterial
   intracardiac
   intrapericardial
   intrapleural
   intrapulmonary
   intrathoracic
   intrathoracic airway
   intraventricular
   intrinsic positive end-expiratory
   in vivo balloon
   jugular venous

pressure *(cont.)*
  LA (left atrium)
  left atrial (LAP)
  left atrial end-diastolic
  left subclavian central venous
    (LSCVP)
  left ventricular (LV)
  left ventricular cavity
  left ventricular end-diastolic
    (LVEDP)
  left ventricular filling
  left ventricular peak systolic
  left ventricular systolic (LVS)
  left-sided heart
  low wedge
  manual
  maximal respiratory
  maximum inflation
  mean
  mean airway (MAP)
  mean aortic
  mean arterial (MAP)
  mean atrial
  mean blood
  mean brachial artery
  mean circulatory filling
  mean left atrial
  mean pulmonary artery (MPAP)
  mean pulmonary artery wedge
  mean right atrial
  minimum blood
  PA (pulmonary artery) systolic
  PAD (pulmonary artery diastolic)
  PAS (pulmonary artery systolic)
  peak-inflation
  peak inspiratory (PIP)
  peak regurgitant wave
  peak systolic
  peak systolic aortic (PSAP)
  phasic
  plasma colloid osmotic
  pleural

pressure *(cont.)*
  positive end-expiratory (PEEP)
  pulmonary arterial wedge (PAWP)
  pulmonary artery (PAP)
  pulmonary artery diastolic (PAD)
  pulmonary artery end-diastolic
    (PAEDP)
  pulmonary artery mean (PAM)
  pulmonary artery peak systolic
  pulmonary artery/pulmonary
    capillary wedge
  pulmonary artery systolic (PAS)
  pulmonary artery wedge (PAWP)
  pulmonary capillary (PCP)
  pulmonary capillary wedge
    (PCWP)
  pulmonary venous capillary (PVC)
  pulmonary venous wedge
  pulmonary wedge
  pulse
  PV (pulmonary vein)
  PVC (pulmonary venous capillary)
  RA (right atrial)
  radial artery
  recoil
  regional cerebral perfusion (rCPP)
  right atrial (RAP)
  right heart
  right-sided heart
  right subclavian central venous
    (RSCVP)
  right ventricular (RVP)
  right ventricular diastolic (RVD)
  right ventricular end-diastolic
  right ventricular peak systolic
  right ventricular systolic (RVS)
  right ventricular volume
  RV (right ventricular)
  RVD (right ventricular diastolic)
  RVS (right ventricular systolic)
  segmental lower extremity Doppler
  stump

pressure *(cont.)*
  subatmospheric
  supersystemic pulmonary artery
  sustained maximal inspiratory
    (SMIP)
  SVC (superior vena cava)
  systemic
  systolic
  systolic blood (SBP)
  torr
  transcutaneous oxygen
  transmyocardial perfusion
  transpulmonary (P_{TP})
  turgor
  V wave (left or right atrial
    catheterization)
  venous
  wedge
  withdrawal
  X' (prime) wave (right atrial
    catheterization)
  Y wave
  zero diastolic blood
  Z point
pressure augmentation
pressure-controlled ventilator
pressure cuff
pressure difference, aortic-left
  ventricular
pressure equalization
pressure flow gradient
pressure gradient
  arteriovenous
  negligible
pressure gradient on pull-back
pressure injector
pressure-flow gradient
pressure in the chest
pressure-like sensation in chest
pressure loads, pure
pressure measurement
pressure oscillation

pressure overload
pressure pneumothorax
pressure pullback
pressure readings
pressure sensation
pressure support ventilation (PSV)
pressure transducer
pressure waveform
pressure waveform analysis
Pressurometer
presternal fascia
Presto cardiac device
presumptive diagnosis
presyncopal episode
presyncope
presystolic Austin Flint murmur
presystolic bulge, palpable
presystolic gallop rhythm
presystolic murmur (PSM)
presystolic pulsation
prethrombotic syndrome
pretibial edema
prevention of lung collapse
prevention of thrombus propagation
Price-Thomas bronchial forceps
Primaderm semipermeable foam
  dressing
Prima laser guidewire
Prima Plus stentless bioprosthesis
Prima pacemaker
Primapore absorptive wound dressing
primary aldosteronism
primary alveolar hypoventilation
primary amyloidosis
primary angiitis
primary angioplasty
primary atypical pneumonia
primary bronchi, right and left
primary chordal dysplasia
primary coccidioidomycosis
primary electrical disease

primary electrical ventricular tachycardia
primary endocardial fibroelastosis
primary hyperparathyroidism
primary hypertension
primary hypertrophic cardiomyopathy
primary hypotension
primary lung neoplasm
primary median sternotomy
primary myocardiopathy
primary pleurisy
primary prosthetic graft infection
primary pulmonary hypertension
primary thrombus
primary tuberculosis
primary varicose veins
Prime ECG (electrocardiographic)
mapping system
Primer compression dressing or wrap
primitive ventricle
Primopac diagnostic catheter
principal bronchus
principle
diamond anastomosis
Doppler
Fick
Frank-Starling
indicator fractionation
Prinivil (lisinopril)
P-R interval
prolongation of
short
shortening of
varying
Prinzmetal angina
Prinzmetal II syndrome
Prinzmetal variant angina
Prism-CL pacemaker
prism method for ventricular volume
proarrhythmia
proarrhythmic effect
proarrhythmic event

probe
AngeLase combined mapping-laser
blood flow
cardiac
Chandler V-pacing
cryosurgical
Doppler flow
echocardiographic
electromagnetic flow
Hagar
handheld exploring electrode
handheld mapping
Hemosonic hemodynamic monitor
and
nasopharyngeal temperature
nonimaging
nuclear
oligonucleotide
Parsonnet
pediatric biplane TEE
Robicsek vascular (RVP)
sapphire contact
Siemens-Elema AB pulse
transducer
Spectraprobe-Max
Teflon
temperature
transesophageal
Verbatim balloon
Xtent
Probe balloon-on-a-wire dilatation
system, USCI
Probe cardiac device
probe-patent anastomosis
probe-patent foramen ovale
probing catheter, USCI
Procardia XL (nifedipine)
procedural risk factors
procedure (see also *method,
operation, technique*)
adenosine echocardiography
advanced cardiac mapping

procedure *(cont.)*
    alcohol ablation to treat cardio-
        myopathy
    Alfieri mitral valve
    arterial switch
    Batista
    Bentall (for coronary ostial
        revascularization)
    Blalock-Hanlon
    Blalock-Taussig
    Brock
    Cabrol
    Cabrol I anastomosis
    Cabrol I tube graft
    Cabrol II modification of Bentall
    cardiokymography
    Cardiolite scan
    CardioTek (or Cardiotec) scan
    cardiotocography
    CAVH (continuous arteriovenous
        hemofiltration)
    Cox maze
    Damus-Norwood
    David
    debanding
    digital image fusion (DIF)
    domino
    Edwards-Kerr
    Eloesser
    endocardial resection (extended)
    endoluminal vascular repair
    endoscopic division of incompetent
        perforating veins
    extracardiac conduit Fontan
    femoral artery (or arterial)
        catheterization
    Fick
    flush aortogram
    Fontan conversion to an extra-
        cardiac conduit
    Fontan conversion to a lateral
        tunnel

procedure *(cont.)*
    Glenn shunt
    Heineke-Mikulicz
    high shear blood flow
    interventional
    intracoronary artery radiation
    intravenous fluorescein angiography
        (IVFA)
    IVOX artificial lung
    Judkins coronary arteriography
    Ko-Airan bleeding control method
    light reflection rheography
    magnetic resonance angioplasty
        (MRA)
    M-mode echocardiogram
    Mustard
    Nikaidoh
    percutaneous coil embolization
    percutaneous implantation of
        endovascular covered stent (for
        pseudoaneurysm repair)
    percutaneous intracoronary
        angioscopy
    percutaneous localization of
        pulmonary nodules using
        suture-ligated microcoils
    PLAATO (percutaneous left atrial
        appendage transcatheter
        occlusion)
    pulmonary artery banding
    Quaegebeur modification
    Rashkind balloon atrial septotomy
    Rastan-Konno
    sector scan echocardiography
    Senning
    Sones coronary arteriography
    sonographically guided human
        thrombin injection
    spatial vectorcardiography
    tattooing
    thrombin injection (into false
        aneurysm)

procedure *(cont.)*
  Todaro tendon resection
  transesophageal echocardiogram
  transfemoral endovascular stented
    graft
  transluminal stent-graft implanta-
    tion
  2-D echocardiography
  ultrasound-guided percutaneous
    thrombin injection
  ultrasound scan-guided compres-
    sion (to obliterate false
    aneurysm)
  ultrasound-guided tattooing
  vectorcardiography
procedure-related complications
process
  atherogenic
  jugular
  left ventricular posterior superior
  prominent xiphoid
  xiphoid
Pro-Clude transparent film wound
  dressing
proconvertin blood coagulation factor
ProCross Rely over-the-wire balloon
  catheter
ProCyte transparent adhesive film
  dressing
Prodec-DM drops
prodromal symptoms
prodrome (pl. prodromes)
productive cough
productive phlebitis
products
  fibrin
  fibrin split
profile
  automated physiologic
  biophysical (BPP)
  cardiac
  cardiac risk

profile *(cont.)*
  KDA
  respiratory
  serum lipid
Profile Plus dilatation catheter, USCI
Proflex 5 dilatation catheter
Pro-Flo XT catheter
Profore four-layer bandaging system
profound anxiety
profound cardiopulmonary deterioration
profound dyspnea
profound hypertension
profound hypothermia
profound hypothermic circulatory
  arrest (PHCA)
profoundly obtunded infant
profound peripheral eosinophilia
profound shock
profound volume depletion
profound weakness
profunda Dacron patchplasty
profunda femoris artery
profunda femoris pulse
profundaplasty
profunda popliteal collateral index
progeria syndrome
prognosis
  equivocal
  excellent
  favorable
  good
  grave
  grim
  guarded
  ominous
  poor
  poor short-term
  unfavorable
Programalith pacemaker
programmability of pacemaker rate

programmable cardioverter-
 defibrillator (PCD)
programmable implantable medication
 system (PIMS)
programmed electrical stimulation
 (PES)
programmed ventricular stimulation
 (PVS)
programmer wand
programming
 bidirectional pacemaker
 over-responsive
 phantom pacemaker
 unidirectional pacemaker
 unresponsive
progression
 inexorable
 poor R-wave (PRWP)
progressive angina
progressive anginal syndrome
progressive cardiomyopathic
 lentiginosis
progressive care unit (PCU)
progressive claudication
progressive coccidioidomycosis
progressive exercise intolerance
progressive hypercapnia
progressive interstitial pulmonary
 fibrosis
progressive intimal thickening
progressively severe fatigue
progressive malignant polyserositis
 with large effusions into pericardium, pleura, and peritoneum
progressive mitral regurgitation
progressive nodular pulmonary fibrosis
progressive parenchymal restriction
progressive pulmonary dystrophy
progressive respiratory distress
progressive shortness of breath
progressive systemic sclerosis
progressive weakness

prohibitive risk
projection (see also *position*, *view*)
 anterior
 fingerlike
 LAO (left anterior oblique)
 left lateral
 left posterior oblique
 RAO (right anterior oblique)
 right posterior oblique
 65° LAO
 steep left anterior oblique
 30° LAO
prolapse
 anterior leaflet
 holosystolic
 holosystolic mitral valve
 mitral
 mitral valve (MVP)
 mitral valve leaflet systolic
 posterior leaflet
 systolic
 tricuspid valve
prolapsed mitral valve leaflets
prolapsed tumor through mitral valve
 orifice
prolapsing scallop
prolapsing valve
Prolene suture
proliferating cell nuclear protein
 (PCNP)
proliferating pleurisy
proliferation
 alveoli
 collagen tissue
 connective tissue
 endothelial
 intimal
 myxomatous
 neointimal
proliferation of vascular smooth
 muscle cells (VSMC)
proliferative bronchiolitis

proliferative phlebitis
Prolith pacemaker
prolongation
    attenuated QT
    inspiratory
    QRS interval
    QT
    Q-T interval
    Q-T wave
    P-R
prolonged action
prolonged anticoagulation
prolonged aortic clamping
prolonged bed rest
prolonged clotting time
prolonged ejection time
prolonged expiration
prolonged expiration during quiet
    breathing
prolonged expiratory phase
prolonged in duration
prolonged inspiratory phase
prolonged interval
prolonged left ventricular impulse
prolonged P-R interval
prolonged pulmonary eosinophilia
prolonged Q-T interval, acquired
prolonged Q-T interval syndrome
prolonged rub
prolonged shock
prolonged standing
prominence
    hilar
    mediastinal
prominence of aorta
prominent central pulmonary artery
prominent fourth heart sound
prominent neck pulsations
prominent pulsus paradoxus
prominent S_3 (heart sound)
prominent septal lymphatics
prominent systolic venous impulses

prominent third heart sound
prominent U wave
prominent vascular pulsations
prominent ventricular diastolic gallop
prominent xiphoid process
promptly relieved by rest
Propac diagnostic catheter
propagated thrombus
propagation of thrombus
Propaq Encore vital signs monitor
Pro/Pel coating for catheters and
    guidewires
prophylactic antibiotics
prophylactic drug treatment
prophylactic effect
prophylactic implantation of
    pacemaker
prophylactic IVC filter
prophylactic measure
prophylactic pacing
prophylactic penicillin
prophylactic regimen
prophylaxis
    anticoagulant
    endocarditis
    low-dose heparin
    OKT3
    PCP (*Pneumocystis carinii*
        pneumonia)
    routine antimicrobial
    SBE (subacute bacterial
        endocarditis)
    topical antimicrobial
propranolol HCl
propria, lamina
prostacyclin therapy
prostaglandin infusion
prostaglandin synthesis inhibition
prostate carcinoma metastatic to heart
prosthesis (see also *valve*)
    Angelchik antireflux
    Angell-Shiley bioprosthetic valve

prosthesis *(cont.)*
  Angell-Shiley xenograft prosthetic
    valve
  Angiocor prosthetic valve
  aortic valve
  aortofemoral
  ATS Open Pivot bileaflet heart
    valve
  ball-and-cage valve
  ball-cage
  ball valve
  ball-valve type valve
  Baxter mechanical valve
  Beall disk valve
  Beall mitral valve
  Beall prosthetic valve
  Beall prosthetic mitral valve
  Beall-Surgitool ball-cage prosthetic
    valve
  Beall-Surgitool disk prosthetic
    valve
  Bianchi valve
  Biocor porcine stented aortic valve
  Biocor porcine stented mitral valve
  Biocor prosthetic valve
  Biocor stentless porcine aortic
    valve
  Bionit vascular
  bioprosthesis
  Bioprosthetic valve
  Bio-Vascular prosthetic valve
  Björk-Shiley convexo-concave disk
    prosthetic valve
  Björk-Shiley aortic valve
  Björk-Shiley convexo-concave
    60° valve
  Björk-Shiley floating disk
  Björk-Shiley mitral valve
  Björk-Shiley monostrut prosthetic
    valve
  Björk-Shiley monostrut 72° valve
  Björk-Shiley prosthetic aortic valve

prosthesis *(cont.)*
  Björk-Shiley prosthetic mitral valve
  Braunwald-Cutter ball prosthetic
    valve
  Braunwald-Cutter valve
  caged ball occluder prosthetic valve
  caged disk occluder prosthetic
    valve
  Capetown aortic prosthetic valve
  CarboMedics heart valve
  CarboMedics prosthetic heart valve
    (CPHV)
  Carpentier anuloplasty ring
  Carpentier-Edwards aortic valve
  Carpentier-Edwards bioprosthetic
    valve
  Carpentier-Edwards glutaraldehyde-
    preserved porcine xenograft
    bioprosthesis valve
  Carpentier-Edwards mitral anulo-
    plasty valve
  Carpentier-Edwards pericardial
    valve
  Carpentier-Edwards Perimount
    Plus pericardial bioprosthesis
  Carpentier-Edwards Perimount
    RSR pericardial bioprosthesis
  Carpentier-Edwards porcine
    prosthetic valve
  Carpentier-Edwards porcine
    SupraAnnular valve (SAV)
  Carpentier-Edwards valve
  Conform-X aortic heart valve
  convexo-concave (C-C) disk
    prosthetic valve
  Cooley-Cutter disk prosthetic valve
  Cooley Dacron
  Coratomic prosthetic valve
  CPHV OptiForm mitral valve
  Cross-Jones disk valve
  CryoLife-O'Brien porcine heart
    valve

prosthesis *(cont.)*

CryoLife-Ross porcine heart valve
CryoValve-SG valve
C-shaped silicone prosthesis
Cutter aortic valve
Cutter-Smeloff cardiac valve
DeBakey ball valve
DeBakey valve
DeBakey Vasculour
DeBakey-Surgitool prosthetic valve
Delrin frame of valve
De Vega
disk valve
double velour knitted Dacron
Duromedics aortic valve
Duromedics heart valve
Edmark mitral valve
Edwards-Duromedics bileaflet valve
Edwards-Duromedics prosthetic
 valve
Edwards Prima Plus stentless
 bioprosthesis
femorofemoral crossover
golf T-shaped polyvinyl
Gott shunt/butterfly heart valve
Guangzhou GD1 prosthetic valve
Hall Easy-Fit prosthetic heart valve
Hall-Kaster disk prosthetic valve
Hall-Kaster mitral valve
Hall-Kaster tilting-disk valve
Hall prosthetic heart valve
Hancock aortic valve
Hancock bioprosthetic valve
Hancock mitral prosthetic valve
Hancock M.O. II porcine
 bioprosthesis
Hancock pericardial prosthetic
 valve
Hancock porcine heart valve
Hancock porcine heterograft valve
Hancock porcine prosthetic heart
 valve

prosthesis *(cont.)*

Hancock prosthetic mitral valve
Hancock II porcine prosthetic valve
Hancock II tissue valve
Harken prosthetic valve
Hemex prosthetic valve
Hemobahn endovascular
Holter valve
Hufnagel prosthetic valve
Impra Carboflo vascular
intact Medtronic xenograft valve
Intact xenograft prosthetic valve
intraluminal sutureless
intravascular
Ionescu-Shiley aortic valve
Ionescu-Shiley bioprosthetic valve
Ionescu-Shiley bovine pericardial
 valve
Ionescu-Shiley heart valve
Ionescu-Shiley low-profile
 prosthetic valve
Ionescu-Shiley pericardial xenograft
 valve
Ionescu-Shiley standard pericardial
 prosthetic valve
Ionescu trileaflet valve
Ivalon
Jatene-Macchi prosthetic valve
Kaster mitral valve
Kay-Shiley disk valve
Kay-Shiley mitral valve
Kay-Suzuki disk prosthetic valve
Lillehei-Cruz-Kaster
Lillehei-Kaster disk prosthetic valve
Lillehei-Kaster mitral valve
Lillehei-Kaster pivoting-disk
 prosthetic valve
Lillehei-Kaster prosthetic mitral
 valve
Lillehei valve
Liotta-BioImplant LPB prosthetic
 valve

prosthesis *(cont.)*
   Lo-Por
   Lo-Por vascular graft
   low-profile prosthetic valve
   Magovern ball valve
   Magovern-Cromie
   Magovern-Cromie ball-cage
     prosthetic valve
   Meadox woven velour
   mechanical valve
   Medtronic-Hall heart valve
   Medtronic-Hall tilting-disk valve
   Medtronic prosthetic valve
   Medtronic-Hall heart valve
   Medtronic-Hall monocuspid tilting
     disk valve
   Microknit vascular graft
   Milliknit Dacron
   Milliknit vascular graft
   Mitroflow pericardial prosthetic
     valve
   Mitroflow Synergy PC stented
     pericardial bioprosthesis
   Mobius artificial heart valve
   Mobius vascular
   monostrut cardiac valve
   Mosaic porcine bioprosthesis
   Mosaic valve
   Neville tracheal and tracheo-
     bronchial
   Omnicarbon prosthetic heart valve
   Omniscience prosthetic heart valve
   Omniscience single leaflet cardiac
     valve
   Omniscience tilting-disk valve
   On-X aortic prosthetic heart valve
   OptiForm mitral valve
   outflow tract
   Passage hemostasis valve
   Pemco prosthetic valve
   Perimount Plus pericardial
     bioprosthesis

prosthesis *(cont.)*
   Perimount RSR pericardial
     bioprosthesis
   polyvinyl
   porcine heterograft
   prosthetic heart valve
   Puig Massana-Shiley anuloplasty
     valve
   Quattro mitral valve
   Rashkind double-disk occluder
   Ross pulmonary porcine valve
   Sauvage filamentous
   SLF vascular
   Smeloff-Cutter ball-cage prosthetic
     valve
   Smeloff-Cutter ball valve
   Sorin prosthetic valve
   Spitz-Holter valve
   Spotorno vascular
   Starr-Edwards
   Starr-Edwards aortic valve
   Starr-Edwards ball valve
   Starr-Edwards disk valve
   Starr-Edwards prosthetic aortic
     valve
   Starr-Edwards prosthetic mitral
     valve
   Starr-Edwards Silastic ball valve
   Stellite ring material of prosthetic
     valve
   stentless porcine aortic valve
   St. Jude bileaflet prosthetic valve
   St. Jude Medical aortic valve
   St. Jude Medical bileaflet tilting-
     disk aortic valve
   St. Jude Medical bileaflet valve
   St. Jude Medical Port-Access heart
     valve
   Sutter-Smeloff heart valve
   SynerGraft pulmonary heart valve
   SynerGraft tissue-engineered
     replacement heart valve

prosthesis *(cont.)*
   Surgitool prosthetic valve
   Tascon prosthetic valve
   Tekna mechanical heart valve
   tilting-disk aortic valve
   Top-Hat supra-anular aortic valve
   Toronto SPV aortic valve
   Toronto SPV bioprosthesis
   Ultracor prosthetic valve
   USCI Sauvage EXS side-limb
   Vascor porcine prosthetic valve
   Vasculour
   velour collar
   Wada-Cutter disk prosthetic valve
   Weavenit (and New Weavenit)
      Dacron prosthesis
   Wesolowski vascular
   Wessex prosthetic valve
   woven Teflon
   Xenomedica prosthetic valve
   Xenotech prosthetic valve
   XL-Endograft vascular
prosthesis dehiscence
prosthetic click
prosthetic heart valve (see *prosthesis*)
prosthetic heart valve poppet
prosthetic valve endocarditis (PVE)
prosthetic valve malfunction
prosthetic valve valvuloplasty
Prostigmin test
protamine, heparin reversed with
protamine sulfate, heparin neutralized
   with
protection
   cardiac
   myocardial
protective HDL cholesterol
Protect Point needle
protein
   anticoagulant protein S
   cardiac troponin T

protein *(cont.)*
   CHUK (conserved helix-loop-helix
      ubiquitous kinase)
   C-reactive
   dKa
   ESAT-6
   guanine-nucleotide-binding
   guanine nucleotide regulatory
   microsomal triglyceride transfer
      (MTP)
   NF-ATc (NFAT-3)
   Novel erythropoiesis stimulating
      (NESP)
   proliferating cell nuclear (PCNP)
   remnant-like particle (RLP)
      lipoprotein
   single-chain antigen-binding (SCA)
   thrombus precursor (TpP)
   SAA
   streptococcal M
   total
proteinaceous material
protein C deficiency
protein-losing enteropathy (PLE)
protein marker
   HLA-DR (histocompatibility
      antigen-DR)
   ICAM-1 (intercellular adhesions
      molecule-1)
proteinosis
   alveolar
   pulmonary alveolar
protein-rich material
protein S
protein troponin T
proteinuria
proteolytic attack
Proteus pneumonia
Proteus syndrome
prothrombin consumption test
prothrombin-proconvertin test

prothrombin time (PT)
pro time (PT, prothrombin time)
protocol
    ACT (activated clotting time)
    advanced cardiac life support
        (ACLS)
    Balke treadmill stress test
    Balke-Ware exercise stress testing
    Balke-Ware treadmill exercise
    Bruce exercise stress testing
    Bruce treadmill exercise stress
    cardiac rehabilitation
    CCU (cardiac care unit)
    CeQUAL
    chemoradiation
    chronotropic assessment exercise
        (CAEP)
    Cornell exercise stress testing
    Ellestad treadmill exercise
    exercise
    Kattus treadmill exercise
    LITE (low-intensity treadmill
        exercise)
    Mayo exercise treadmill
    McHenry treadmill exercise
    Mee
    modified Balke treadmill exercise
    modified Bruce treadmill exercise
    modified treadmill
    Naughton-Balke treadmill
    Naughton treadmill exercise
    pacing
    Reeves treadmill exercise
    rule-out MI (myocardial infarction)
        (ROMI)
    Sheffield exercise test
    Sheffield modification of Bruce
        treadmill
    Sheffield treadmill exercise
    slow USAFSAM treadmill exercise
    soft rule-out MI
    standard Bruce

protocol *(cont.)*
    standard Bruce treadmill exercise
    Stanford treadmill exercise
    TIMI II (thrombolysis in myocar-
        dial infarction)
    USAFSAM treadmill exercise
    ventilatory muscle training
    Weber exercise stress testing
protodiastolic gallop rhythm
protodiastolic reversal of blood flow
proton density
proton MRI
proton spectroscopy
prototype drug
prototypical holosystolic murmur
protozoal infestation
protozoal myocarditis
protozoa, tick-borne
protruding atheroma
protrusion, spoonlike (of leaflets)
protuberant abdomen
Proventil HFA (albuterol)
provocation (see *challenge*)
    aspirin inhalation
    HDM (house dust mites) bronchial
    methacholine bronchial
    oral aspirin
provocative
provocable ischemia
provoked by cold
provoked by dust
provoked by lying down
provoked by smoke
Prower factor X deficiency
proximal anastomosis
proximal and distal portion of vessel
proximal aortic endarterectomy
proximal circumflex artery
proximal clot
proximal coil
proximal coronary sinus (CS)
proximal hypertension

proximal popliteal artery
proximal segment
proximal thrombosis with distal
    embolization
Proximate flexible linear stapler
Proximate linear cutter surgical stapler
P-R prolongation
PR segment depression
PRS wave
Pruitt-Inahara balloon-tipped perfusion
    catheter
Pruitt-Inahara carotid shunt
prune-belly syndrome
prune juice sputum
pruned appearance of pulmonary
    vasculature
Prussian helmet sign
PRWP (poor R-wave progression)
PRx, PRx II ICD
PS (pulmonary sequestration)
PS (pulmonic stenosis)
PSA (pacing system analyzer)
PSAP (peak systolic aortic pressure)
pseudoaneurysm
    anastomotic
    aortic
    exploration of
    iatrogenic
    infected
    postcatheterization femoral (artery)
    ruptured
    superficial
pseudoaneurysm cavity
pseudoaneurysm of arteriovenous
    fistula
pseudoaneurysm resection
pseudoangina
pseudocapsule, tumor
pseudoclaudication syndrome
pseudocoarctation syndrome
pseudocolor B-mode display

pseudocyst of lung
pseudocyst, pulmonary
pseudofusion beat
pseudohemophilia, hereditary
pseudohypertrophy of calves
pseudohypoaldosteronism
pseudoinfarction
pseudolupus secondary to
    procainamide
pseudo-Meigs syndrome
pseudomembranous croup
pseudomitral leaflet
Pseudomonas aeruginosa infection
Pseudomonas bronchiectasis
Pseudomonas cepacia
Pseudomonas maltophilia
Pseudomonas pneumonia
pseudoperfusion beats, ventricular
pseudostratified columnar epithelium
pseudotruncus arteriosus
pseudotumor
pseudoxanthoma elasticum
pseudoxanthoma elasticum syndrome
P/S (pulmonic/systemic) flow ratio
PSG (peak systolic gradient)
psi, p.s.i. ("sigh") (pounds per square
    inch)
psittacosis
PSM (pansystolic murmur)
PSM (presystolic murmur)
P_2 sound, burying of
PSS (Palmaz-Schatz stent)
PST (paroxysmal supraventricular
    tachycardia)
PSV (pressure support ventilation)
PSVT (paroxysmal supraventricular
    tachycardia)
PSVT, slow-fast intranodal
psychogenic chest pain syndrome
psychogenic purpura
psychophysiologic hyperventilation

psychosis
   cardiac
   postcardiotomy
psyllium
P synchronous pacing
PT (prothrombin time), prolonged
PTA (percutaneous transluminal angio-
   plasty)
PTBD (percutaneous transluminal
   balloon dilatation)
PTC (plasma thromboplastin compo-
   nent)
PTCA (percutaneous transluminal
   coronary angioplasty)
PTCA catheter
PTCA catheterization
PTCA coronary angiogram
PTD (percutaneous thrombolytic
   device)
PTDC (percutaneous transcatheter
   ductal closure)
pterional incision
P terminal force abnormality
pterygoid chest
PTFE (polytetrafluoroethylene)
PTFE arterial graft material
PTFE graft
PTFE grafts seeded with smooth
   muscle cells
PTL (posterior tricuspid leaflet)
PTLD (posttransplantation lympho-
   proliferative disorder)
PTMC (percutaneous transvenous
   mitral commissurotomy)
PTMR (percutaneous transluminal
   myocardial (or transmyocardial)
   revascularization)
ptosis and miosis (Horner syndrome)
P_{TP} (transpulmonary pressure)
   (mm Hg)
PT/PTT (prothrombin time/partial
   thromboplastin time)

PTT (partial thromboplastin time)
PTT (pulmonary transit time)
public access defibrillation (PAD)
PUBS (percutaneous umbilical cord
   blood sampling)
PUCA (pulsatile catheter) pump
puerperium, hemodynamic changes
   during
puerperium myocardiopathy
puffer, pink
puff of smoke (moyamoya)
Puig-Massana anuloplasty
Puig-Massana-Shiley anuloplasty ring
Puig-Massana-Shiley anuloplasty valve
Pulec and Freedman classification of
   congenital aural atresia
pullback
   left heart
   pressure
pullback across the aortic valve
pullback arterial markings
pullback from ventricle
pullback pressure recording
pullback study
Pulmicort Turbuhaler (budesonide)
Pulmios inhaler
Pulmo-Aide nebulizer
pulmoaortic canal
pulmogram
pulmolithiasis
pulmonale, cor
pulmonales, vesiculae
pulmonalis
   pleura
   plexus
pulmonary abscess
pulmonary acid aspiration syndrome
pulmonary acini gigantism
pulmonary airway fibroblasts
pulmonary alveolar microlithiasis
pulmonary alveolar proteinosis (PAP)
pulmonary alveolus (pl. alveoli)

pulmonary and cardiac sclerosis
pulmonary angiitis
pulmonary angiitis-granulomatosis
  syndrome
pulmonary angiogram
  digital subtraction
  balloon occlusion
pulmonary angiography
pulmonary arterial circulation
pulmonary arterial hypertension
pulmonary arterial input impedance
pulmonary arterial markings
pulmonary arterial occlusion
pulmonary arterial pressure, increased
pulmonary arterial vent
pulmonary arterial wedge pressure
pulmonary arteries, intra-acinar
pulmonary arteriolar vasoconstriction
pulmonary arteriosclerosis
pulmonary arteriovenous aneurysm
pulmonary arteriovenous fistula
pulmonary arteritis
pulmonary artery
  aberrant left
  anomalous
  dilated
pulmonary artery agenesis
pulmonary artery apoplexy
pulmonary artery banding procedure
pulmonary artery bifidity
pulmonary artery catheter-associated
  endocarditis
pulmonary artery catheter, balloon-
  tipped flow-directed
pulmonary artery catheter-related
  bacteremia
pulmonary artery catheter-related
  candidemia
pulmonary artery compression
  ascending aorta aneurysm
pulmonary artery debanding
pulmonary artery end-diastolic
  pressure (PAEDP)

pulmonary artery engorgement
pulmonary artery flotation
pulmonary artery hypertension
pulmonary artery hypoplasia
pulmonary artery incisura
pulmonary artery mycotic aneurysm
pulmonary artery obstruction-Manson
  schistosomiasis
pulmonary artery oxygen saturation
pulmonary artery plication
pulmonary artery pressure (PAP)
pulmonary artery stenosis, peripheral
pulmonary artery wedge pressure
  (PAWP)
pulmonary aspiration of gastric
  contents
pulmonary atresia
pulmonary auscultation
pulmonary autograft procedure
pulmonary AV O_2 difference
pulmonary banding
pulmonary barotrauma
pulmonary bed
pulmonary blood flow
pulmonary blood flow redistribution
pulmonary capillary endothelial cells
pulmonary capillary endothelium
pulmonary capillary hemangiomatosis
pulmonary capillary pressure (PCP)
pulmonary capillary wedge position
pulmonary capillary wedge pressure
  (PCWP)
pulmonary capillary wedge tracing
pulmonary carcinomatosis
pulmonary cartilage
pulmonary cavitation
pulmonary cavity
pulmonary circulation
pulmonary cirrhosis
pulmonary compliance, reduced
pulmonary compression by pleural
  fluid or gas

pulmonary function tests (PFTs)
  determination of all lung volumes
  diffusing capacity
  flow-volume loop
  maximum inspiratory and
    expiratory pressures
  MVV (maximal voluntary
    ventilation)
  spirometry
pulmonary function testing device
pulmonary gangrene
pulmonary gas exchange
pulmonary hemorrhage
pulmonary hilus
pulmonary histiocytosis
pulmonary hypertension
  familial
  hypoxic
  secondary
pulmonary hypoperfusion
pulmonary hypoperfusion unmasked
  by ductus arteriosus closure
pulmonary idiopathic hemosiderosis
pulmonary incompetence
pulmonary infarct (see *infarct*)
pulmonary infarction (see *infarction*)
pulmonary infiltrate (see *infiltrate*)
pulmonary infiltrates, sulfasalazine-
  induced
pulmonary infiltrates with eosinophilia
  (PIE)
pulmonary infiltration eosinophilia
pulmonary insufficiency
pulmonary interstitial emphysema
  (PIE)
pulmonary interstitial idiopathic
  fibrosis
pulmonary Kaposi sarcoma
pulmonary ligament
pulmonary metastasectomy
pulmonary microcirculation
pulmonary microvasculature

pulmonary nodule percutaneous
  localization using suture-ligated
  microcoils
pulmonary nodule, solitary
pulmonary obliterative arteriolitis
pulmonary orifice
pulmonary origin of the coronary
  artery, anomalous
pulmonary osteoarthropathy
pulmonary outflow obstruction
pulmonary outflow tract
pulmonary overdistention
pulmonary overexpansion
pulmonary parasites
pulmonary parenchyma
pulmonary parenchymal changes
pulmonary parenchymal disease
pulmonary parenchymal infiltrates
pulmonary parenchymal injury
pulmonary parenchymal window
pulmonary plethora (pulmonary
  vascular engorgement)
pulmonary pleura
pulmonary pleurisy
pulmonary plexus
pulmonary pseudocysts
pulmonary rales
pulmonary rhonchi
pulmonary scars
pulmonary schistosomiasis
pulmonary secretions, amber-colored
pulmonary sequelae
pulmonary sequestration (PS)
pulmonary sling syndrome
pulmonary sounds in Warthin sign
pulmonary stenosis
pulmonary stenosis-ostium secundum
  defect syndrome
pulmonary stenosis-patent foramen
  ovale syndrome
pulmonary strongyloidiasis
pulmonary sulcus tumor

pulmonary suppuration
pulmonary surfactant
pulmonary/systemic flow ratio
pulmonary TB (tuberculosis)
pulmonary thromboembolism (PTE)
pulmonary thromboendarterectomy
pulmonary thrombosis
pulmonary tissue
pulmonary toilet, aggressive
pulmonary toxicity
pulmonary tractotomy
pulmonary trunk
pulmonary trunk idiopathic dilatation
pulmonary trunk murmur
pulmonary tuberculosis (TB)
pulmonary valve
pulmonary valve anulus
pulmonary valve atresia
pulmonary valve atresia-intact
    ventricular septum syndrome
pulmonary valve closure
pulmonary valve deformity
pulmonary valve dysplasia
pulmonary valve insufficiency
pulmonary valve stenosis
pulmonary valve stenosis dilatation
pulmonary valvular stenosis
pulmonary vascular bed
pulmonary vascular bed impedance
pulmonary vascular disease
pulmonary vascular disease, Heath-
    Edwards classification of
pulmonary vascular markings
pulmonary vascular obstruction
pulmonary vascular pattern
pulmonary vascular redistribution
pulmonary vascular reserve
pulmonary vascular resistance (PVR)
    increased
    Wood units of
pulmonary vascular resistance index
    (PVRI)

pulmonary vasculature
pulmonary vasoconstriction, hypoxic
pulmonary vasoreactivity
pulmonary vein apoplexy
pulmonary vein atresia
pulmonary vein, congenital stenosis of
pulmonary vein fibrosis
pulmonary vein stenosis
pulmonary vein to left atrium baffle
pulmonary vein wedge angiography
pulmonary veno-occlusive disease
pulmonary venous anomalous drainage
    to hepatic vein
pulmonary venous anomalous drainage
    mitral stenosis syndrome
pulmonary venous anomalous drainage
    to right atrium
pulmonary venous congestion
pulmonary venous connection
    partial anomalous
    total anomalous
pulmonary venous drainage
pulmonary venous hypertension
pulmonary venous obstruction
pulmonary venous return
pulmonary venous system
pulmonary venous wedge pressure
pulmonary venous-systemic air emboli
pulmonary ventilation
pulmonary vesicles
pulmonary vessels
pulmonary wedge angiography
pulmonary wedge pressure (PWP)
pulmonary wedge elevated
pulmonary wedge resection
pulmonic atresia
pulmonic atresia with intact ventricular
    septum
pulmonic component, markedly accen-
    tuated
pulmonic component of murmur
pulmonic ejection sound, palpable

pulmonic regurgitation
pulmonic stenosis, peripheral
pulmonic stenosis-ventricular septal
   defect
pulmonic stenosis with intact
   ventricular septum
pulmonic systolic murmur
pulmonic valve
pulmonic valve dysplasia
pulmonic valve stenosis
pulmonis (also pulmonum), alveoli
Pulmosonic nebulizer
PulmoSphere
Pulsar Max II pacemaker system
Pulsar NI pacemaker
pulsatile abdominal mass
pulsatile assist device (PAD)
pulsatile catheter (PUCA) pump
pulsatile cutaneous vascular anomaly
pulsatile flow, dampened
pulsatile lavage system
pulsatile mass
pulsatile perfusion
pulsatile tinnitus
pulsatile ventricular assist device
pulsatility index (PI)
pulsating empyema
pulsating hematoma
pulsating hepatomegaly
pulsating pain
pulsating pleurisy
pulsating vein
pulsation
   capillary
   carotid arterial
   cervical vein
   discrete
   expansile
   hepatic vein
   jugular venous
   large vein
   left ventricular

pulsation *(cont.)*
   lower sternal
   mean venous
   palpable systolic
   precordial
   presystolic
   prominent neck
   prominent vascular
   suprasternal
   transient ectopic
   transmitted carotid artery
   venous (3 cm above the sternal
      angle)
pulsation balloon
Pulsavac III wound debridement
   system
pulse, pulses (see also *beat, impulse*)
   abdominal
   abrupt
   absence of
   absent
   allorhythmic
   alternating
   anacrotic
   anadicrotic
   anatricrotic
   "a" peak of jugular venous
   apex
   apical
   arterial
   atrial liver
   atrial venous
   atriovenous
   biferious
   bifid arterial
   bigeminal
   bilaterally symmetric
   bisferiens
   bisferious
   bounding arterial
   bounding peripheral
   bounding water-hammer

pulse *(cont.)*
  brachial
  brisk bifid arterial
  cannon ball
  capillary
  cardiac
  cardiac apex
  carotid
  carotid arterial (CAR)
  catadicrotic
  catatricrotic
  centripetal venous
  chaotic
  character of
  collapsing
  Corrigan
  coupled
  C point of cardiac apex
  c wave of jugular venous
  dampened obstructive
  delayed femoral
  diastolic collapse of venous
  dicrotic
  dicrotic arterial
  diminished pedal
  diminution of
  distal
  Doppler
  dorsalis pedis
  dorsal pedal
  dropped-beat
  easily palpable
  elastic
  entirely chaotic
  entoptic
  equal
  external carotid
  femoral
  filiform
  formicant
  frequent
  full

pulse *(cont.)*
  full and equal
  h peak of jugular venous
  hard
  high-tension
  incisura of
  infrequent
  intermittent
  irregular
  irregular but patterned
  irregularly irregular
  jerky
  jugular
  jugular venous
  Kussmaul paradoxical
  labile
  low-tension
  lower extremity
  Monneret
  monocrotic
  movable
  nonpalpable
  palpable palmar
  palpable peripheral
  palpable popliteal
  paradoxic
  paradoxical
  parvus
  pedal
  peripheral
  pistol-shot femoral
  pistol-shot radial
  plateau-type
  polycrotic
  popliteal
  posterior tibial
  pressure
  profunda femoris
  prominent systolic venous
  quadrigeminal
  quick
  Quincke

pulse *(cont.)*
  Quincke capillary
  radial
  rapid
  reduced
  regular
  regularly irregular
  resting
  retrosternal
  RF
  Riegel
  running
  sharp
  short
  slow
  small water-hammer
  soft
  spike-and-dome
  strong
  symmetric
  synchronous carotid arterial
  tardus
  tense
  thready
  tidal wave
  tremulous
  tricrotic
  trigeminal
  trip-hammer
  trough of venous
  ulnar
  undulating
  unequal
  unilateral loss of
  vagus
  venous
  vermicular
  vibrating
  v peak of jugular venous
  water-hammer
  weak peripheral
  wide

pulse *(cont.)*
  wiry
  x depression of jugular venous
  x descent of jugular venous
  y descent of jugular venous
pulse amplitude
pulse character
pulse count increment
pulse deficit
pulse Doppler interrogation
pulsed Doppler transesophageal
  echocardiography
pulsed Doppler ultrasound
pulsed infrared laser
pulsed laser ablation
pulsed lavage
PulseDose technology
pulsed ultrasound
pulse duration
pulsed volume recorder (PVR) testing
pulsed-wave Doppler recording
pulse generator of pacemaker (see
  generator)
pulse generator pocket erosion
pulse inversion harmonic imaging
pulseless bradycardia
pulseless disease
pulseless electrical activity (PEA)
pulselessness
pulseless syndrome
pulse oximeter
pulse oximetry devices
pulse pressure
Pulse Pro heart rate monitor
Pulse Spray infusion catheter
  (AngioDynamics)
pulse rate, baseline standing
pulse reappearance time
pulses altered by changes in position
PulseSpray
pulse voltage
pulse volume recording (PVR)

pulse wave
pulse width
pulsus alternans
pulsus bigeminus
pulsus bisferiens (or biferiens)
  (biferious pulse)
pulsus celer
pulsus paradoxus, prominent
pulsus parvus
pulsus parvus et tardus
pulsus tardus
pulverization
pulverized plaque particulate matter
Pulvules
pump
  angle port
  AutoCat
  AutoCAT automatic intra-aortic
    balloon
  balloon
  Bard cardiopulmonary support
  Bard TransAct intra-aortic balloon
  Bio-Medicus
  Bio-Pump centrifugal blood
  blood
  BVS (biventricular support) system
  CADD (computerized ambulatory
    drug delivery)
  calcium
  Cancion
  cardiac balloon
  Carmeda Bio-Pump centrifugal
    blood
  Chronofusor infusion
  Cobe/Stockert dual head
  CoolFlow infusion (used in electro-
    physiology procedures)
  Cormed
  Curlin 2000 Plus portable infusion
  Datascope System 90 balloon
  ECG asynchronous
  ECG synchronous

pump *(cont.)*
  Emerson
  Hemopump
  Impella intracardiac
  intra-aortic balloon (IABP)
  ion
  KAAT II Plus intra-aortic balloon
  Kangaroo
  LVAS (left ventricular assist
    system) implantable
  Master Flow Pumpette
  McKinley EpM infusion
  Medtronic Hemopump
  Mobius open heart
  muscular venous
  Novacor
  Orqis
  priming of the
  PUCA (pulsatile catheter)
  pulmonary artery balloon (PABP)
  push-pull
  Reitan catheter
  Sarns centrifugal
  Sarns Delphin centrifugal
  Sarns 7400 pulsatile
  Sarns S10K II
  Sorin dual head
  St. Jude Medical Lifestream
    centrifugal
  sodium
  stroke volume
  sump
  TandemHeart
  Thoratec
  Travenol
  Travenol infusion
  volumetric infusion
pump failure, Cedars-Sinai classifica-
  tion of
pumping capacity of heart
pumping of the ventricles

pumping, postcardiotomy intra-aortic balloon
pump lung syndrome
pump oxygenator
pump perfusionist
pump reserve
pump standby
pump support
pump technician
punch
    aortic
    circular
    Hancock aortic
    Karp aortic
    Medtronic aortic
    Sweet sternal
punch aortotomy
puncture
    arterial
    blind percutaneous (of subclavian vein)
    groin
    iatrogenic
    percutaneous
    transseptal
    venous
    ventricular
pupillary constriction
pupils, Argyll Robertson
PuraPly wound dressing
pure pressure loads
pure red cell aplasia
Puri-Clens wound cleanser
purified 38-kDa protein antigen
Puritan-Bennett ventilator
Purkinje arborization
Purkinje cells
Purkinje cell tumor
Purkinje fibers
Purkinje network
Purkinje system
Purmann method

purple toes syndrome
purpura
    Henoch-Schönlein
    immune thrombocytopenic
    posttransfusion
    Schönlein-Henoch
    thrombocytopenic
    thrombotic thrombocytopenic
pursed-lip breathing
pursestring effect
purse-stringing effect
purse-string suture
purulent bronchitis
purulent drainage
purulent endocarditis
purulent exudate in pleural cavity
purulent fluid
purulent material
purulent pericardial exudate
purulent pericarditis
purulent pleurisy
purulent sputum
push-pull pump syndrome
pus in pleural cavity
putrid empyema
putrid odor
putrid sputum
Puzzle stent
PV (pulmonic valve)
PVARP (postventricular atrial refractory period)
PVB (premature ventricular beat)
PVC (premature ventricular contraction)
    bigeminal
    early-cycle
    monomorphic
    multifocal
    multiform
    paired
    unifocal
PVC (pulmonary venous congestion)

PVCs in a bigeminal pattern
PVD (peripheral vascular disease)
PVE (prosthetic valve endocarditis)
P vector
PVER (paced ventricular evoked
    response)
PvO_2 (venous oxygen tension)
PVOD (pulmonary veno-occlusive
    disease)
PVR (peripheral vascular resistance)
PVR (pulmonary vascular resistance)
PVR (pulse volume recorder)
PVRI (pulmonary vascular resistance
    index)
PVS (programmed ventricular
    stimulation
PW (posterior wall)
PW (pulse width)
P wave
    bifid
    biphasic
    broadened
    depressed
    diphasic
    flattened
    inverted
    low-amplitude
    nonconducted
    notched

P wave *(cont.)*
    peaked
    pointed
    retrograde
    tall
    terminal negativity of
    upright
    widened
P-wave amplitude
PWT (posterior wall thickness)
pyelography, excretory intravenous
pyknic
pyogenic bacteria
pyopericardium pericarditis
pyopneumothorax
pyothorax
PYP (pyrophosphate) myocardial scan
pyramidal hemorrhagic zone
pyramidal-shaped structure
pyramid method for ventricular
    volume
pyridine sulfonylurea class of drugs
pyridoxylated stroma-free hemoglobin
    (SFHb)
pyriform (piriform) sinus
pyrogen reaction
pyroglycolic acid sutures
pyrophosphate (PYP) myocardial scan
pyrosis (heartburn)

Q, q

Q (cardiac output)
Q (perfusion)
QCA (quantitative coronary
    arteriography)
Q-cath catheterization recording
    system
Qdose inhaler
QEEG (quantitative electro-
    encephalography)
Q fever endocarditis
Q-H interval of jugular venous pulse
QO_2 (oxygen consumption)
QOL (quality of life) index
Q Port
QR pattern
QRS complex (see also *complex*)
    fusion
    narrow
    normal
    normal voltage
    preexcited
    slurring of
    wide
QRS complex duration
QRS duration
QRS interval
QRS alternans

QRS changes
QRS complex
QRS interval
QRS loop, counterclockwise superiorly
    oriented frontal
QRS score
QRS-ST junction
QRS synchronized shock
QRS-T changes
QRS-T angle, wide
QRS-T complex
QRS-T interval
QRS vector
QRS vertical axis
QS complex
QS deflection
Qsma (superior mesenteric artery
    blood flow)
Q-Stress treadmill
QS wave
QS_2 (total electromechanical systole
    on phonocardiogram)
QS_1, QS_2 interval
QT dispersion
QT interval, absolute
Q-T_c interval (corrected QT interval)
QT prolongation

Q-T interval prolongation
Q-T interval sensing pacemaker
Q-T prolongation
Q-T syndrome, long
Quad-Lumen drain
quadrangular resection
quadrangulation of Frouin
QuadraPulse radiofrequency catheter
quadrigeminy
quadrilateral space syndrome
quadripolar catheter
Quadripolar cutting forceps
quadripolar electrode catheter
quadripolar steerable electrode
    catheter
quadruple rhythm
Q-U interval
Quaegebeur modification of Carpentier
    repair
Quain fatty degeneration of the heart
Quain fatty heart
quality of A_2, tambour
quality of breath sounds
quality of life (QOL) index
Quanticor catheter
QuantiFERON-TB
quantification
quantify
quantitation of ischemic muscle
quantitative analysis
quantitative coronary arteriography
quantitative electroencephalography
    (QEEG)
Quantum Maverick coronary balloon
    dilatation catheter
Quantum PTCA catheter
Quantum pacemaker
quasitransmural endocardial incision
Quattro mitral valve
Quénu-Muret sign
QuickDraw venous cannula
QuickFlash radial artery catheter

Quick method
Quick one-stage prothrombin time test
QuickSeal arterial closure system
QuickSilver hydrophilic-coated
    guidewire
Quick-Tap paracentesis system
Quick test
quickWIT (wire insertion tool)
quiescent heart, electromechanically
Quik-Prep, Quinton
Quincke angioedema disease
Quincke capillary pulsations
Quincke disease
Quincke edema
Quincke pulse
Quincke sign
quinidine
quinolone antibiotics
quinolones
quinsy
Quinton catheter
Quinton computerized exercise EKG
    system
Quinton electrode
Quinton PermCath
Quinton Quik-Prep
Quinton-Scribner shunt
Quinton vascular access port
quotient
    respiratory (RQ)
    RQ (respiratory)
QVAR (beclomethasone dipropionate)
Q wave
    large
    left precordial
    nondiagnostic
    pathologic
    septal
Q-wave infarctions
Q wave in the right precordial leads
Qwikstart catheter

R, r

RA (rotational atherectomy)
Raaf Cath (vascular catheter)
RAAPI (resting ankle-arm pressure
    index)
RACAT (rapid acquisition computed
    axial tomography)
racemaker (runaway artificial
    pacemaker)
rachitic rosary
racing of heart
RAD (reactive airways disease)
RAD (reversible airways disease)
RAD (right axis deviation)
radial artery catheter
radial artery graft
radial artery line
radial artery pressure
radial artery to cephalic vein
    anastomosis
radial artery to cephalic vein fistula
radial pulse
radial vascular thermal injury
radiate ligament
radiating chest pain
radiating to axilla
radiating to the clavicle

radiation fibrosis
radiation-induced cardiomyopathy
radiation-induced pericarditis
radiation nephritis
radiation pericardial disease
radiation pneumonitis
radiation toxicity syndrome
radical, hydroxyl
radicular arteries
radicularis anterior magna, arteria
radicularis magna
radiculitis, cervical
radio frequency (rf) field
radioactive aerosol
radioactive fibrinogen scan
radioactive labeling
radioactive string markers
radioactive xenon gas inhalation
radioactivity in lungs
radiocontrast-induced nephropathy
radioenzymatic technique
Radiofocus Glidewire
radiofrequency ablation (RFA)
    transaortic
    transseptal
radiofrequency ablation therapy

radiofrequency catheter ablation
(RFCA, RCA)
radiofrequency energy
radiofrequency energy in percutaneous
myocardial revascularization
(RF-PMR)
radiofrequency modification,
transcatheter
radiofrequency percutaneous myocardial revascularization (RF-PMR)
radiofrequency thermal ablation
radiographic control
radiographic pincushion distortion
radioimmunoassay (RIA)
radioisotope (see *imaging agent*)
radioisotope lung scan
radioisotope stent
radiolabeled fibrinogen
radiolucent foci
radionuclear venography
radionuclide angiocardiography,
equilibrium
radionuclide angiogram (RNA)
radionuclide cineangiography
radionuclide gated blood pool scanning
radionuclide ventriculography, bicycle
exercise
radiopaque FEP sheath with stepped
tissue dilator
radiopaque wire of counteroccluder
buttonhole
radiotherapy, particle
radiotracer
RadiStop radial compression system
Radius coronary stent delivery
catheter
RadPICC catheter
RadPICC port
RAE (right atrial enlargement)
Raeder-Arbitz syndrome
ragpicker's disease
RAI (radioimmunoassay)

railroad track sign
Rainbow ABC aerosol dispenser
rake retractor
R-albuterol
rale, rales (see also *rhonchi*)
amphoric
atelectatic
basilar
bibasilar
border
bronchial
bubbling
cavernous
cellophane
clicking
coarse
collapse
consonating
crackling
crepitant
diffuse
diffuse inspiratory crepitant
dry
expiratory
extrathoracic
fine
fine crepitant
guttural
gurgling
hollow
inspiratory
laryngeal
marginal
metallic
mucous
musical
moist
pleural
post-tussive
pulmonary
sibilant
sonorous

rale *(cont.)*
  sticky
  subcrepitant
  tinkling
  tracheal
  Velcro
  vesicular
  wet
  whistling
rale indux (crepitant rale)
rale redux (subcrepitant sound)
rales clear with coughing
rales clear with deep breathing
rales, rhonchi, or wheezes
rales, wheezes, rhonchi, or rubs
Raman spectroscopy
Ramirez shunt
rami subendocardiales
ramp atrial pacing
ramp decrement
ramping
ramp overdrive pacing
ramp pacing
RAMP Reader
ramp technique of atrial pacing
ramus branch
ramus intermedius artery branch
ramus medialis branch
ramus medianus
Randall stone forceps for thromboendarterectomy
Rand microballoon
R- and S-wave pattern over precordium,
  reversal of
Ranexa (ranolazine)
Raney clamp
Ranger PTCA catheter
range, therapeutic (of drug)
RAO (right anterior oblique)
RAO position (or view) for cardiac
  catheterization
RA (right atrium) oxygen saturation

RAP (remote access perfusion)
  cannula raphe
RAP (right atrial pressure)
rapid atrial pacing
rapid breathing
rapid deceleration injury
rapid early repolarization phase
Rapide suture
Rapid Exchange (RX) coronary stent
  delivery system
rapid-exchange PTCA balloon angioplasty catheter
Rapid Exchange vein graft stent
  delivery system
rapid filling phase
rapid filling wave
rapid fluid expansion
Rapidgraft arterial vessel substitute
rapid heartbeat
rapid inspiratory flow rates
rapid oscillatory motion
rapid pulse
rapid repolarization phase
rapid respirations
rapid respiratory rate
rapid sequence intravenous pyelogram
  (IVP)
rapid shallow breathing
rapid thoracic compression technique
Rapid-Trak balloon
Rapid-Trak catheter
Rapid-Trak guidewire
Rapid-Trak stent
Rapid-Trak stent delivery system
rapid ventricular rate
rapid ventricular response
RapiSeal patch
RA (right atrial) pressure
Raptor PTCA balloon
RaptorRail PTCA dilatation catheter
RaptorRail stent
RAS (rotational atherectomy system)

Rashkind atrial septostomy
Rashkind balloon atrial septostomy
Rashkind balloon atrial septotomy
Rashkind blade septostomy
Rashkind cardiac device
Rashkind double-disk occluder
Rashkind double umbrella device
Rashkind-Miller atrial septostomy
Rashkind occluder
Rashkind septostomy balloon catheter
Rasmussen mycotic aneurysm
RASON (respirable or radiolabeled
    antisense oligonucleotides)
Rasor blood pumping system (RBPS)
rasp (raspatory)
    Alexander-Farabeuf rib
    Doyen rib
    Haight
rasping bruit
rasping cough
rasping sound
raspy
RAST (radioallergosorbent) test
Rastan-Konno procedure
Rastelli atrioventricular canal defect
    (type A, B, or C)
Rastelli operation for correction of
    large ventricular septal defects
Rastelli operation for transposition of
    the great arteries
rate
    aldosterone secretion
    atrial (AR)
    auricular
    basic
    circulation
    complication
    echo intensity disappearance
    erythrocyte sedimentation (ESR)
    exercise-induced heart
    glomerular filtration
    heart (HR)

rate *(cont.)*
    intrinsic heart
    KVO (keep vein open)
    left ventricular filling
    magnet
    maximal heart
    maximum predicted heart (MPHR)
    mean circumferential fiber
        shortening (MCFSR)
    pacemaker adaptive
    peak exercise heart
    peak expiratory flow (PEFR)
    peak filling (PFR)
    percent of predicted
    predetermined heart
    predicted maximum heart
    pulse
    rapid respiratory
    rapid ventricular
    reduced glomerular filtration
    respiratory (RR)
    resting heart
    sed (sedimentation)
    sinus
    slew (SR)
    slowing of heart
    standby
    stroke ejection
    systolic ejection (SER)
    target heart
    time-to-peak filling (TPFR)
    variable response
    ventricular
    washout
    Westergren sedimentation
rate-adaptive pacemaker
rate and incline of treadmill
rate and rhythm of heartbeat
rate and rhythm, regular (RRR)
rated capacity of cardiac pump
rate hysteresis
rate limit

rate-modulated pacemaker
rate-modulated pacing
rate-responsive pacemaker, permanent
rate-sensing lead
RATG (rabbit antithymocyte globulin)
rating of perceived exertion (RPE)
ratio
  a/A
  AH/HA or AH-HA
  AO/AC or AO-AC (aortic valve
    opening to aortic valve closing)
  aortic root
  BR (breathing reserve)
  breathing reserve (BR)
  cardiothoracic (CTR)
  CK/AST or CK-AST
  conduction (number of P waves to
    number of QRS)
  E/A or E-A or E to A
  ESP-ESV
  ESWI-ESVI (end-systolic wall
    stress index to end-systolic
    volume)
  FEV_1–FVC; FEV_1 to FVC
  ID/OD (internal diameter-outside
    diameter)
  I–E (inspiration to expiration)
  I–E (inspiratory to expiratory)
  INR (international normalized)
  inverse inspiratory–expiratory time
  LA-AR (left atrium-aortic root
    or left atrium to aortic root)
  left atrial to aortic (root) (LA-Ao)
  left to right ventricular pressure
  left ventricular systolic time
    interval
  maximum diameter to minimum
    diameter
  mean total cholesterol to HDL
  orifice-anulus or orifice to
    anulus
  PASP–SASP (pulmonary to sys-
    temic arterial systolic pressure)

ratio (cont.)
  P-QRS
  P-S flow (pulmonic-systemic)
  pulmonary–systemic blood flow
  pulmonary to systemic flow
  R/S amplitude
  R/S wave
  risk–benefit
  RVP–LVP (right ventricular to left
    ventricular systolic pressure)
  RV6/RV5 or RV6-RV5 voltage
  RV/TLC or RV-TLC
  septal to free wall
  T–D (thickness to diameter of
    ventricle)
  VLDL-TG to HDL-C
rattle, death
rattling bruit
rattling cough
rattling sound
Rauchfuss triangle
Raulerson spring-wire introduction
  syringe
Raulerson syringe
rauwolfia derivative
R_{AW} (airway resistance)
raw irritated throat
rawness in chest
Raynaud disease
Raynaud gangrene
Raynaud phenomenon
Raynaud syndrome
Ray-Tec x-ray detectable sponge
Razi cannula introducer
RBBB (right bundle branch block)
RBC (red blood cell) count
RBC indices
  MCH (mean corpuscular
    hemoglobin)
  MCHC (mean corpuscular
    hemoglobin concentration)
  MCV (mean corpuscular volume)

RBC, technetium-99m-labeled
RBPS (Rasor blood pumping system)
RCA (right coronary artery)
RCA (rotational coronary
  atherectomy)
rCBV (regional cerebral blood
  volume)
RCP (retrograde cerebral perfusion)
rCPP (regional cerebral perfusion
  pressure)
RCM (restricted cardiomyopathy)
RDS (respiratory distress syndrome)
RDW (red cell diameter width)
RDX coronary radiation catheter
  delivery system
reabsorbable suture
reaccumulation
reactance
reaction (see also *effect, phenomenon,*
    test)
  allergen-induced bronchial
  allergic
  allograft
  anaphylactic
  anaphylactoid
  atopic
  cell-mediated
  cytotoxic
  delayed
  Eisenmenger
  foreign body
  granulomatous
  homograft
  hypersensitivity
  immune-complex-mediated
  inflammatory
  inflammatory granulomatous
  Jaffé rate
  Koch
  Liebermann-Burchard
  pneumococcus capsule swelling
  pyrogen

reaction *(cont.)*
  tuberculin
  vagal
reaction recovery time
reactive airways disease (RAD)
reactive airways dysfunction syndrome
reactive arterioles
reactive disease of smooth muscle
reactive hyperemia
reactivity, bronchial
Reader paratrigeminal syndrome
Real coronary artery scissors
real-time chirp Z transformer
real-time Color Flow Doppler imaging
  of blood flow
real-time 4-D ultrasound
real-time images
real-time 2-D Doppler flow-imaging
real-time ultrasonography
ream out (verb)
reapproximated
Rebar microcatheters
rebound, heparin
rebreather, partial
rebreathing mask
recalcitrant
recanalization
  argon laser
  laser
  percutaneous transluminal coronary
  peripheral laser (PLR)
recanalization
recanalization of total coronary
  occlusion
recanalization technique
recanalized artery
recanalized ductus
recanalizing
receptor
  adrenergic
  airway epithelial irritant
  alpha

receptor *(cont.)*
   alpha-adrenergic
   alpha$_1$-adrenergic
   beta
   beta-adrenergic
   beta$_1$-adrenergic
   beta$_2$-adrenergic
   decreased beta-adrenergic
   juxtacapillary
   LDL
   small airways stretch
recessed balloon septostomy catheter
recession of eyeball
recession, rib
recipient
   double lung transplant (DLT)
   SLT (single-lung transplant)
recipient heart
reciprocal changes
reciprocal depression of ST segments
reciprocating atrioventricular
   tachycardia
reciprocating conduction
reciprocating permanent atrioventricular junctional tachycardia
reciprocating rhythm
reciprocating tachycardia
recirculation
recoarctation of the aorta
recognizable structural disease,
   absence of
recognizable trigger
recoil
   arterial
   catheter
   elastic
recoil pressure
recombinant hemoglobin (rHbl.l)
recombinant immunoblot assay (RIBA)
recombinant tissue plasminogen
   activator (rt-PA)
reconditioning, left ventricular

reconstitution of blood flow in artery
reconstitution via the profunda (deep
   femoral artery)
reconstitution via collaterals
reconstruction
   anular
   aortic
   aortic anular
   Dor
   gated 3-D
   patch graft
   respiration gated 3-D
   three-dimensional
   transanular patch
reconstruction of aorta
recontouring of esophagus
recording
   color Doppler
   continuous-wave Doppler
   pullback pressure
   pulsed-wave Doppler
   simultaneous
recording electrode
recovery of donor organs for transplantation
recovery period of myocardium
recovery time
   corrected sinus node
   sinus node
recovery, uneventful
recrudescence
recrudescent toxoplasmosis
recruitment
recruitment potential
rectilinear biphasic waveform for
   external defibrillation
rectilinear coordinates
rectus muscle split longitudinally
rectus sheath incised
rectus sheath pocket
recumbency
recumbent

recurrence
  distant
  locoregional
  systemic
recurrent bronchiectasis
recurrent cardiac arrest
recurrent ductus
recurrent episodes
recurrent intractable ventricular tachycardia
recurrent laryngeal nerve
recurrent, not-so-sudden cardiac death
recurrent pulmonary embolism
recurrent respiratory infections (RRI)
recurrent respiratory papillomatosis
  (RRP)
recurring ectopic beats
red-cedar asthma
red cell aplasia
red cell diameter width (RDW)
red clot
reddish brown sputum
redeposition of atherosclerotic plaque
red hepatization of lung
Redifocus guidewire
RediFurl TaperSeal IAB catheter
RediGuard flexible IAB catheter
  redirection of inferior vena cava
redistributed thallium scan
redistribution
  flow
  pulmonary blood flow
  pulmonary vascular
redistribution myocardial image
redistribution of pulmonary vascular
  blood flow
red-streaked sputum
red tissues
reduced alveolar ventilation
reduced breath sounds
reduced cardiac output
reduced circulation

reduced compliance of chamber
reduced diffusing capacity
reduced exercise tolerance
reduced glomerular filtration rate
reduced peripheral pulses
reduced plasma volume
reduced pulmonary compliance
reduced sewing ring (RSR) reduced
  stroke volume
reduced signal intensity in the center
  of the blood vessels on MR
  angiograms
reduced systemic cardiac output
reductase inhibitors
reduction, afterload
reduction in thoracic volume
reduction of blood viscosity
redundant aortic leaflets
redundant carotid artery
redundant chordae tendineae
redundant mitral valve leaflets
redundant scallop of posterior anulus
Reed anuloplasty technique
Reed ventriculorrhaphy
re-endothelialization
reentrant circuit
reentrant loop
reentrant rhythm
reentrant supraventricular tachycardia
reentrant tachycardia
reentry
  anisotropic
  atrial
  atrioventricular (AV) nodal
  Bachmann bundle
  bundle branch (BBR)
  functional
  intra-atrial
  SA nodal
  sinus nodal
reentry circuit
Reeves treadmill exercise protocol

reexsanguination
reexpansion of lung
reexpansion pulmonary edema
referred pain
REFI (regional ejection fraction
    image)
refill, capillary
reflectant
reflection
    epicardial
    pericardial (on x-ray)
reflectivity, high
reflex (see also *phenomenon*, *sign*)
    abdominocardiac
    Abrams heart
    Aschner
    atriopressor
    Bainbridge
    baroreceptor
    Bezold-Jarisch
    bregmocardiac
    carotid sinus
    Churchill-Cope
    conditioned
    coronary
    Cushing
    deep tendon (DTR)
    diving
    Erben
    heart
    hepatojugular
    Hering-Breuer
    hyperactive carotid sinus
    inverted oculocardiac
    Livierato
    Lovén
    McDowall oculovagal
    oculocardiac
    psychocardiac
    pulmonocoronary
    vagal
    vascular
    vasopressor

reflex *(cont.)*
    ventilatory
    viscerocardiac
reflex cough
Reflex steerable guidewire from
    Cordis
reflex syncope
Reflotron bedside theophylline test
reflux
    abdominojugular
    acid
    greater saphenous vein
    hepatojugular
    perforator site
    superficial vein
reflux esophagitis
refractoriness, ventricular
refractory angina
refractory asthma
refractory atrial fibrillation
refractory congestive heart failure
refractory heart failure
refractory hypertension
refractory hypoxemia
refractory lactic acidosis
refractory period of myocardium
        (see also *period*)
    effective
    functional
    relative
refractory to medical therapy
refractory to treatment
refractory ventricular fibrillation
refractory ventricular tachycardia
Refsum disease
Reg. (regurgitation)
Regency SR+ single-chamber, rate-
    responsive pulse generator
regeneration, tissue-guided
regimen
    antirejection
    desensitizing
    exercise

regimen *(cont.)*
  prophylactic
  stepped-care antihypertensive
region
  aortic anular
  dark
  perihilar
  watershed
regional compliance
regional cerebral blood volume
    (rCBV)
regional cerebral perfusion pressure
    (rCPP)
regional ejection fraction image
    (REFI)
regional left ventricular function
regional myocardial uptake of thallium
regional perfusion by mixed venous
    blood
regional venous hypertension
regional ventricular function
regional wall motion abnormality,
    left ventricular
regional wall motion assessment
Regional Organ Procurement Agency
    (ROPA)
regression
  multiple logistic
  plaque
  spontaneous
  univariate logistic
regular irregularity
regular rate and rhythm
regular rate and rhythm without gallop
    or rub
regular sinus rhythm (RSR)
regulation
  defective volume
  volume
regurgitant CV waves
regurgitant flow
regurgitant jet

regurgitant lesion
regurgitant mitral valve murmur
regurgitant murmur
regurgitant orifice
regurgitant orifice area (ROA)
regurgitant pandiastolic flow
regurgitant pocket
regurgitant stream
regurgitant velocity
regurgitant volume
regurgitation (Reg.)
  aortic (AR)
  aortic valve
  congenital
  congenital aortic
  congenital mitral (CMR)
  Dexter-Grossman classification of
    mitral
  Grossman scale for
  ischemically mediated mitral
  massive aortic
  mitral valve
  pansystolic mitral
  paravalvular
  physiologic
  pulmonary
  pulmonic (PR)
  pulmonic valve
  silent
  transient tricuspid (of infancy)
  tricuspid (TR)
  tricuspid orifice
  tricuspid valve
  trivial mitral
  valvular (VR)
regurgitation of sour fluid
rehabilitation, cardiac
rehabilitation exercises
Rehbein rib spreader
Rehfuss tube
rehydrated

Reichek method of calculating end-
    systolic wall stress
Reilly bodies
reimplantation, coronary ostial
reimplantation technique
reinfarction
reinforced second sound
Reinhoff clamp
Reinhoff-Finochietto rib spreader
reintimalization
Reitan catheter pump
Reiter disease
rejection
    borderline severe
    cardiac transplant (allograft)
    chronic
    chronic humoral
    delayed xenograft (DXR)
    focal moderate
    hyperacute
    low moderate
    resolved
    resolving
    severe acute
rejection crisis
relapse
relapsing polychondritis
relation
    end-diastolic pressure-volume
    end-systolic pressure-volume
    force-frequency
    force-length
    force-velocity
    Frank-Starling (of the heart)
relationship
    anecdotal
    Frank-Starling
relative hypoxia
relative refractory period (RRP)
relative shunt flow
relaxation
    isovolumic (IVR)
    period of isovolumic

relaxation time (in MRI scan)
    T1
    T2
relaxing factor, endothelium-derived
Relay pacemaker
release, Valsalva
Relia-Flow device
relieved by antacids
relieved by rest, angina
remission
    clinical
    spontaneous
remnant
    ductal
    heart
remnant-like particle (RLP) lipo-
    protein
remodeling of thrombus
remodeling, ventricular
Remodulin (treprostinil sodium)
remote access perfusion (RAP)
    cannula
remote history
removable Herbst appliance
renal arteriography
renal artery aneurysm
renal artery occlusion
renal atrophy
renal cholesterol embolization
    syndrome
renal cocktail
renal cortex, patchy atrophy of
renal duplex scan
renal dyspnea
renal failure
    chronic
    postoperative
renal function impairment
renal hemangiopericytoma
renal hypertension
renal parenchymal disease
renal sclerosis

renal shutdown
renal thromboendarterectomy,
    transaortic
renal vasculitis
renal vein renin, differential
renal vein thrombosis (RVT)
Rendu-Osler-Weber disease or syn-
    drome (also *Weber-Osler-Rendu*)
renin
    circulating
    differential renal vein
    plasma
renin activity, suppressed plasma
renin-angiotensin system
renin-dependent hypertension
renin levels, serum
renin-secreting tumor
renin suppression
renovascular disease
renovascular hypertension
Rentrop infusion catheter
reocclusion, postthrombolytic coronary
repair (see also *operation*)
    aortic valve (AV)
    Barbero-Marcial
    Brom
    conotruncal
    endograft
    Fontan
    hemitruncus
    infrarenal aortic
    intraventricular tunnel
    Takeuchi
    Trusler
    tunnel
repeated bouts of coughing
repeated sneezing
Repel bioresorbable barrier film
reperfuse
reperfusion
    controlled aortic root
    coronary

reperfusion *(cont.)*
    normokalemic
    partial
reperfusion edema after lung trans-
    plantation
reperfusion in acute myocardial
    infarction
reperfusion injury of postischemic
    lungs
reperfusion therapy
repetition time (TR)
repetitive maximal inspiratory
    maneuvers against closed shutter
repetitive monomorphic ventricular
    tachycardia
repetitive sneezing
replacement
    aortic root
    aortic valve (AVR)
    ascending aneurysm
    mitral valve (MVR)
    orthotopic total heart
repletion, potassium chloride
RepliCare hydrocolloid dressing
    material
Repliderm collagen-based dressing
repolarization
    atrial
    early
    early rapid
    final rapid
    transient
    ventricular
repolarization phase, rapid early
reproducible pain
Request devices (used in heart
    catheterization)
rerouting, intraventricular
rescue defibrillation
rescue PTCA
rescue shock
rescue, surgical

resectability
resection (see also *operation*)
  anatomic pulmonary
  aneurysm
  bronchial sleeve
  en bloc vein
  endocardial
  endocardial-to-epicardial
  infundibular
  lung
  lung tumor
  pseudoaneurysm
  quadrangular
  selective subendocardial
  stapled pulmonary
  subaortic
  thoracoscopic wedge
  Todaro tendon
  transhiatal
  transmural
  video-assisted thoracoscopic wedge
  wedge (of lung)
  wedge-shaped sleeve aneurysm
reserve
  cardiac
  contractile
  coronary flow (CFR)
  diastolic
  left ventricular systolic functional
  myocardial perfusion (MPR)
  preload
  pulmonary vascular
  pump
  regional contractile
  stenotic flow (SFR)
  suboptimal cardiac
  systolic
  ventricular
reserve force
reserve mechanism, heart rate
reservoir
  cardiotomy
  peripheral venous

residua
residual deficit, significant
residual gradient
residual plaque
residual pulmonary dysfunction
residual thermal collagen damage
  (RTCD)
residual volume (RV)
residual volume/total lung capacity
  (RV/TLC)
resilient artery
reinfection tuberculosis
resistance
  acquired multidrug
  airway (R_{AW})
  arteriolar
  calculated
  coronary vascular
  decreased peripheral vascular
  decreased systemic
  expiratory
  fixed pulmonary valvular
  increased airways
  increased cerebral vascular
  increased outflow
  increased peripheral
  increased pulmonary vascular
  index of runoff
  lead
  multidrug
  multiple drug
  nasal airway
  peripheral
  peripheral vascular (PVR)
  pulmonary
  pulmonary arteriolar
  pulmonary vascular (PVR)
  systemic
  systemic vascular (SVR)
  total peripheral (TPR)
  total pulmonary (TPR)
  vascular
  vascular systemic

resistance *(cont.)*
  viscous
  Wood units index of
resistive breathing through fixed
  orifice
resistivity
resolution stage
Resolve drainage catheter
resolved (or resolving) rejection
resonance
  bandbox
  cough
  cracked-pot
  skodaic
  tympanic
  vesicular
  vesiculotympanic
  vocal
  whispering
  wooden
resonant frequency
resonant percussion note
resorption, fluid
resorption of dependent edema fluid
RESPeRATE apparatus
RespiGam
Respihaler
respiration
  abdominal
  absent
  accelerated
  accessory muscles of
  amphoric
  artificial
  asthmoid
  Austin Flint
  Biot
  Bouchut
  bronchial
  bronchocavernous
  bronchovesicular
  cavernous

respiration *(cont.)*
  cerebral
  Cheyne-Stokes
  cogwheel
  collateral
  controlled diaphragmatic
  Corrigan
  costal
  deep
  diaphragmatic
  divided
  electrophrenic (EPR)
  forced
  gasping
  granular
  grunting
  harsh
  Holger Nielsen artificial
  indefinite
  inhibited
  interrupted
  jerky
  Kussmaul
  Kussmaul-Kien
  labored
  meningitic
  metamorphosing
  mouth-to-mouth
  nervous
  paradoxical
  periodic
  puerile
  rapid
  rude
  Schafer artificial
  Seitz metamorphosing
  shallow
  Silvester artificial
  slow
  splinting
  stertorous
  supplementary

respiration *(cont.)*
  suppressed
  thoracic
  transitional
  tubular
  unlabored
  vesiculocavernous
  vicarious
  wavy
  wheezing
  whistling
respiration gated three-dimensional
  reconstruction
respirations per minute
respirator (see also *ventilator*)
  BABYbird
  BABYbird II
  Bear
  Better Breathing HEPA-tech half-
    mask
  Bird
  cabinet
  cuirass
  Engström
  Servo
  tank
  volume
respiratory acidosis
respiratory airway asymmetry
respiratory alkalosis
respiratory allergies
respiratory or radiolabeled antisense
  oligonucleotides (RASON)
respiratory apparatus
respiratory arrest
respiratory assist, mechanical
respiratory bronchiole
respiratory bronchiolitis-associated
  interstitial lung disease
respiratory burst activity
respiratory chain
respiratory chain complex I deficiency

respiratory chain enzymatic complex
respiratory complications
respiratory compromise
respiratory decompensation
respiratory-dependent pacemaker
respiratory depression and apnea from
  drug overdose
respiratory distress at rest
respiratory distress syndrome (RDS)
  of newborn
respiratory distress with grunting
respiratory droplets
respiratory effort
respiratory embarrassment
respiratory epithelium
respiratory excursions full and equal
respiratory failure, hypoxemic
respiratory flora, moderate growth of
  normal
respiratory frequency
respiratory gate
respiratory gating
respiratory infection, self-limiting
respiratory insufficiency
respiratory irritants
respiratory isolation
respiratory modulation of vascular
  impedance
respiratory muscle weakness
respiratory noise
respiratory ordered phase encoding
  (ROPE)
respiratory parameters
respiratory pattern
respiratory physical therapy
respiratory profile
respiratory quotient (RQ)
respiratory rate (RR)
respiratory sinus arrhythmia (RSA)
respiratory spasm
respiratory status, compromised
respiratory stertor

respiratory stridor
respiratory syncytial virus (RSV)
respiratory syncytial virus pneumonia
respiratory syncytial virus bronchiolitis
respiratory therapy
respiratory tract obstruction,
    mechanical
respiratory tract specimen
respiratory triggering
Respirgard II nebulizer
respirologist
Respironics CPAP (continuous positive
    airway pressure) machine
Respironics nasal mask
Respitrace machine
response
    abnormal ejection fraction
    baroreceptor-mediated
    blunted chronotropic
    cardioinhibitory
    controlled ventricular
    Cushing
    Cushing pressor
    early asthmatic
    humoral
    hypotensive
    late asthmatic
    rapid ventricular
    slow ventricular
    torque
    tyramine
    vagal
    vasoactive
    vasoconstrictor
    vasodepressor
    vasodilatory
    ventricular
    visuomotor
    Wenckebach upper rate
    whole body inflammatory
Response electrophysiology catheter

response rate, variable
responsiveness, airway
Res-Q AICD (automatic implantable
    cardioverter-defibrillator)
Res-Q Micron implantable
    cardioverter-defibrillator
rest
    angina at
    breathlessness at
    ectopic (of thyroid tissue)
    embryonic cell (in the septum)
rest angina
rest dyspnea
Restcue CC dynamic air therapy
restenosis or re-stenosis, in-stent (ISR)
re-stenosis after angioplasty
re-sternotomy, resternotomy
rest force
rest images
resting electrocardiogram
resting end-systolic wall stress
resting heart
resting heart rate
resting imaging
resting MUGA scan, preoperative
resting phase of cardiac action
    potentials
resting pulse
resting-redistribution thallium-201
    scintigraphy
resting regional myocardial hypo-
    perfusion
rest LV function
rest pain
rest-related angina
rest RV function
rest thallium-201 myocardial imaging
Reston foam wound dressing
restoration of sinus rhythm
Restore alginate wound dressing
restricted fluid intake

restriction
  dietary sodium
  exercise
  fluid
restrictive airway disease
restrictive bulboventricular foramen
restrictive cardiac syndrome
restrictive cardiomyopathy
restrictive defect
restrictive hemodynamic syndrome
restrictive hemodynamics
restrictive lung disease
restrictive myocardial disease
restrictive-obstructive lung disease,
  mixed
restrictive pattern
restrictive pericarditis
restrictive ventilatory defect
restrictive ventilatory pattern
results
  hemodynamic
  suboptimal
resuscitate, resuscitated
resuscitation
  cardiac
  cardiopulmonary (CPR)
  closed chest cardiopulmonary
  fluid
  mouth-to-mouth
resuscitative devices
resuscitative thoracotomy
resuscitator (see *ventilator* or
  respirator)
resuspension of aortic valve
resuture
retained secretions
retard premature rewarming
retention
  carbon dioxide (CO_2)
  fluid
  salt

retention *(cont.)*
  sodium
  water
reticularis, livedo
reticulation
reticulocyte count
reticuloendothelial system
reticulogranular appearance
reticulogranular pattern
reticulonodular infiltrates
reticulum
  endoplasmic
  sarcoplasmic
retinal angioid streaks
retinal exudate
retinopathy, hypertensive
retracted leaflets
retraction
  chest-wall
  clot
  costal
  inspiratory
  intercostal
  late systolic
  midsystolic
  mild subcostal
  postrheumatic cusp
  sternocleidomastoid
  sternum
  substernal
  suprasternal
  systolic
retraction on inspiration, chest
retractions and grunting
retraction wave
retractor
  Allison lung
  Ankeney sternal
  Army-Navy
  atrial
  Axius Vacuum surgical
  Beckman

retractor *(cont.)*
  Bookwalter
  Burford
  Chaux
  Collins
  Cooley atrial
  Crawford aortic
  Cushing vein
  Davidson scapular
  Deaver
  DeBakey-Cooley
  EndoRetract
  eXpose
  Favaloro sternal
  Finochietto
  Garrett
  Gelpi
  Green
  Haight-Finochietto rib
  handheld
  Harrington
  Hartzler rib
  Himmelstein sternal
  IMA (inferior mesenteric artery)
  Joe's hoe
  Kelly
  Kirklin atrial
  leaflet
  lung
  malleable
  malleable ribbon
  Miller-Senn
  Ochsner
  Octopus
  Omni
  Omni-Tract adjustable wishbone
  ophthalmic
  Pittman IMA
  rake
  Richardson
  Rosenkranz pediatric
  Sachs vein

retractor *(cont.)*
  SaphLITE
  SaphLITE II
  Sauerbruch
  self-retaining table-mounted
  Semb lung
  Senn
  small rake
  Spacekeeper
  Space-OR flexible internal
  sternal
  U.S. Army
  vein
  Volkmann
  Weitlaner
Retract-O-Tape surgical vessel loops
retraining, left ventricular
retrieval device, Innovante
retrocardiac infiltrate
retrocardiac space
retroesophageal right subclavian artery
retroesophageal subclavian artery
retrofascial
retrograde aortogram
retrograde arterial catheterization
retrograde atherectomy
retrograde atrial activation mapping
retrograde blood flow across valve
retrograde blood velocity
retrograde cerebral perfusion (RCP)
retrograde conduction
retrograde coronary sinus infusion
retrograde fashion
  advanced in a
  catheter advanced in a
retrograde femoral arterial approach
retrograde filling of vessels
retrograde infusion of cardioplegic
  solution
retrograde injection
retrogradely (backward)

retrograde percutaneous femoral artery
   approach for cardiac catheterization
retrograde perfusion
retrograde refractory period
retrograde ventriculoatrial conduction
retropancreatic preaortic space
retroperfusion
   coronary sinus
   synchronized
retroperitoneal aneurysmectomy
retroperitoneal approach
retroperitoneal bleeding
retroperitoneal fibrosis, perianeurysmal
retroperitoneal hematoma
retroperitoneal space
retroperitoneal tunnel
retroperitoneal tunneling
retropharyngeal abscess
retrosternal chest pain
retrosternal pain
Retrox fractal active fixation lead
return
   anomalous
   anomalous pulmonary venous
   central arterial
   infracardiac type total anomalous
      venous
   paracardiac type total anomalous
      venous
   pulmonary venous
   supracardiac type total anomalous
      venous
   systemic venous
   total anomalous pulmonary venous
   total anomalous venous
   venous
return of sinus rhythm
return to baseline
REV procedure (intraventricular repair
   of anomalies of ventriculoarterial
   connection)

revascularization (see also *operation*)
   Bentall operation for coronary
      ostial
   Cabrol II coronary ostial
   cardiac hybrid
   coronary
   coronary ostial
   direct myocardial (DMR)
   heart
   infrainguinal
   intraoperative transmyocardial
      (ITMR)
   myocardial
   off-pump beating heart
   percutaneous
   percutaneous transluminal myocar-
      dial (or transmyocardial)
      (PTMR)
   percutaneous transmyocardial
      (PMR)
   radiofrequency percutaneous
      myocardial (RF-PMR)
   RF-PMR (radiofrequency energy
      in percutaneous myocardial
      revascularization)
   surgical
   target lesion (TLR)
   transmyocardial (TMR)
   VCAB (ventriculocoronary artery
      bypass)
   VCAB (ventricle-to-coronary artery
      bypass)
   Vineberg cardiac
revascularized
Reveal insertable loop recorder
   implantable heart monitor
Reveal Plus insertable loop recorder
Reveal XVI PET/CT imaging system
Revelation microcatheters
reversal of ventricular tachycardia
reversal, shunt

reverse Berman angiographic balloon
  catheter
reversed arm leads
reversed coarctation
reversed differential cyanosis
reverse distribution
reversed greater saphenous vein
reversed splitting
reversed 3 sign
reversed with protamine, heparin was
reverse immunoassay
reversible airways disease (RAD)
reversible atrial pacing
reversible defect
reversible ischemia
reversible obstructive airway disease
  (ROAD)
reversible ventricular fibrillation
reversible ventricular tachycardia (VT)
rewarm
rewarmed patient
rewarming, retard premature
Reynolds number
Reynolds vascular clamp
RF (radiofrequency)
RFA (radiofrequency ablation)
RFCA (radiofrequency catheter
  ablation)
RF-generated thermal balloon catheter
RFP (rapid filling period)
RF-Performr electrophysiology
  catheter (not Performer)
RF-PMR (radiofrequency energy in
  percutaneous myocardial revascu-
  larization)
RF-PMR (radiofrequency percutaneous
  myocardial revascularization)
RF (rapid filling) pulses
RFW (rapid filling wave)
RF wave of cardiac apex pulse
RF (rheumatic fever)
rhabdomyoblast

rhabdomyoma of heart
rhabdomyosarcoma, cardiac
rhabdomyosarcoma of the heart
rHb1.1 (recombinant hemoglobin)
RHC (respirations have ceased)
RHD (rheumatic heart disease)
rheography, light reflection
Rheolog device to measure blood
  viscosity
rhEPO or rHuEPO (recombinant
  human erythropoietin)
rheumatic adherent pericardium
rheumatic aortic insufficiency
rheumatic aortic stenosis
rheumatic aortitis
rheumatic carditis
rheumatic chorea
rheumatic endocarditis
rheumatic fever (RF)
rheumatic heart disease (RHD)
rheumatic lesion
rheumatic myocarditis
rheumatic nodule
rheumatic pericarditis
rheumatic pneumonia
rheumatic valvular deformity
rheumatic valvulitis
rheumatism, articular
  acute
  subacute
  desert
rheumatoid-arthritis-associated
  interstitial lung disease
rheumatoid arthritis (RA) factor
rheumatoid arthritis-pneumoconiosis
rheumatoid lung disease
rheumatoid lung silicosis
rheumatoid nodule
rheumatoid pericarditis
rheumatoid pneumoconiosis
rhinovirus
rhizomelic chondrodysplasia punctata
  (RCP)

Rh-null syndrome
rhomboideus muscle
rhomboid major muscle
rhonchi (pl. of rhonchus) (see also
      rale)
   coarse
   coarse sibilant expiratory
   high-pitched
   humming
   low-pitched
   musical
   post-tussive inspiratory
   pulmonary
   scattered
   sibilant
   sonorous
   whistling
rhonchi on forced exhalation
rhonchus (pl. rhonchi)
rHuEPO or rhEPO (recombinant
   human erythropoietin)
rhythm
   accelerated atrioventricular (AV)
      junctional
   accelerated idioventricular (AIVR)
   atrial escape
   atrial gallop
   atrioventricular junctional escape
   atrioventricular nodal
   AV (atrioventricular)
   AV junctional
   AV nodal (idionodal)
   AVNR (atrioventricular nodal)
   baseline
   bigeminal
   cardiac
   coronary nodal
   coronary sinus (CSR)
   coupled
   dual
   ectopic
   embryocardia

rhythm *(cont.)*
   escape
   fibrillation
   gallop
   idiojunctional rhythm
   idioventricular (IVR)
   irregularly irregular heart
   junctional
   junctional escape
   mu
   nodal
   nodal escape
   normal sinus (NSR)
   paced
   pacemaker
   parasystolic
   pendulum
   predominant
   presystolic gallop
   protodiastolic gallop
   pulseless idioventricular
   quadruple
   reciprocal
   reciprocating
   reentrant
   regular
   regular sinus (RSR)
   regularly irregular heart
   sinoatrial
   sinus
   sinusoidal irregular
   slow escape
   supraventricular
   systolic
   tic-tac
   transitional
   triple
   ventricular
   wide complex
Rhythm Catheter, The
rhythm disturbance
rhythmical

rhythmic auscultatory cadence
rhythmicity
rhythm runs, benign idioventricular
rhythm strip
RIA (radioimmunoassay)
rib, ribs
 hypoplastic horizontal
 retracted
RIBA (recombinant immunoblot assay)
rib approximator, Bailey
Ribberts thrombosis
rib guillotine
rib notching
rib recession
rib-resecting incision
rib spaces, narrowed
rib spreader
RIC fluid exchange resuscitation
 catheter
Richardson retractor
richly cellular exudate
Rickettsia burnetii infection
rickettsial myocarditis
rickettsial pneumonia
ridge
 broad maxillary
 fibromuscular
 septal
 supra-aortic
 supracoronary
riding embolus
Ridley syndrome
Riegel pulse
Riesman myocardosis
right and retrograde left heart
 catheterization
right-angle chest tube
right-angle clamp
right-angled telescopic lens
right ankle indices
right anterior oblique (RAO) position
right anterior oblique projection

right aortic arch with mirror image
 branching
right atrial appendage
right atrial chamber
right atrial enlargement
right atrial extension of uterine
 leiomyosarcoma
right atrial patch positioned over the
 right atrioventricular sulcus
right atrial pressure (RAP)
right atrial sarcoma
right atrioventricular valve
right atrium
right axis deviation
right border of heart
right bundle branch block (RBBB)
right bundle branch block with left
 anterior (or posterior) hemiblock
right bundle branch heart block
 (RBBB)
right carotid endarterectomy
Right Clip
right coronary artery, dominant
right coronary cusp
right coronary plexus (of heart)
right femoral artery
right fibrous trigone
right first intercostal space
right free-wall pathway
right-handedness, ventricular
right heart catheter
right heart failure
right heart pressure
right internal jugular artery
right internal jugular (IJ) vein
right internal mammary anastomosis
right Judkins catheter
right lateral decubitus position
right-left disorientation
right main stem bronchus
right middle lobectomy
right middle lobe lingula

right middle lobe subsegments
right middle lobe syndrome
right minithoracotomy
right second intercostal space
right semilunar valve
right-sided empyema
right-sided heart failure
right-sided pneumonia
right subclavian artery, retro-
    esophageal
right to left shunt of blood
right-to-left shunt with pulmonic
    stenosis
right upper lobe
right upper sternal border
right ventricle
    augmented filling of
    double-outlet
    parchment
    Taussig-Bing double-outlet
right ventricle adherent to posterior
    table of sternum
right ventricle outflow tract
right ventricle-pulmonary artery
    conduit
right ventricle to aorta baffle
right ventricle-to-ear time
right ventricle to pulmonary artery
    conduit
right ventricular assist device (RVAD)
right ventricular bypass tract
right ventricular cardiomyopathy,
    arrhythmogenic
right ventricular chamber
right ventricular coil
right ventricular conduction defect
right ventricular dysplasia, arrhythmo-
    genic
right ventricular ejection fraction
    (RVEF)
right ventricular end-diastolic volume
    (RVEDV)

right ventricular endocardial sensing
    lead
right ventricular endomyocardial
    biopsy
right ventricular end-systolic volume
    (RVESV)
right ventricular failure
right ventricular hypertrophy (RVH)
right ventricular hypoplasia
right ventricular impulse, hyper-
    dynamic
right ventricular inflow view
right ventricular infundibulectomy
right ventricular infundibulum
right ventricular lift
right ventricular myocardial aplasia
right ventricular obstruction, intraven-
    tricular
right ventricular outflow obstruction
right ventricular outflow tract
right ventricular overload
right ventricular patch positioned over
    the atrioventricular sulcus
right ventricular pressure (RVP)
right ventricular preponderance
right ventricular stroke work (RVSW)
right ventricular stroke work index
    (RVSWI)
right ventricular systolic time interval
right vocal cord
rigor, frank
Riley-Day syndrome
rimlike calcium distribution
RIND (reversible intermittent or
    ischemic neurologic deficit)
Rindfleisch, fold of
ring
    anuloplasty
    aortic subvalvular
    atrioventricular
    biofragmentable anastomotic
        (BAR)

ring *(cont.)*
  Carpentier
  Carpentier-Edwards (CE)
  Carpentier-Edwards Physio
    anuloplasty
  congenital (of aortic arch)
  Crawford suture
  double-flanged valve sewing
  Duran anuloplasty
  Medtronic anuloplasty
  mitral
  mitral valve
  Physio anuloplasty (Carpentier-
    Edwards)
  prosthetic valve sewing
  prosthetic valve suture
  Puig Massana-Shiley anuloplasty
  Sculptor flexible anuloplasty
  sewing
  St. Jude anuloplasty
  supra-anular suture
  supravalvar
  tricuspid valve
  universal valve prosthesis sewing
  valve
  vascular
ring dissector
ring of Vieussens
ring shadows with air-fluid levels
ripple, triple
rise, trajectory of creatinine (cr)
risk
  formidable
  prohibitive
  surgical
risk/benefit ratio
risk factors
  cardiac risk
  incremental
  patient
  procedural
risk index, Detsky modified cardiac

Riva-Rocci manometer
Rivas vascular catheter
Rivero-Carvallo maneuver
Rivero-Carvallo sign
Rivetti-Levinson intraluminal shunt
Riviere sign
Riza-Ribe needle
R-lactate enzymatic monotest
RLP (remnant-like particle) lipopro-
  tein
R-Med Plug
RMVT (repetitive monomorphic
  ventricular tachycardia)
RNA (radionuclide angiogram), gated
RNS terminal
RNV (radionuclide ventriculogram)
ROA (regurgitant orifice area)
ROAD (reversible obstructive airway
  disease)
roaring in ears
Roadrunner guidewire
Robert Jones bulky soft dressing with
  Hemovac drainage
Robertson sign
Robicsek closure of median
  sternotomy
Robicsek vascular probe (RVP)
Robinson catheter
robot, da Vinci
Robotrac passive retraction system
robust
Rochester-Mixter artery forceps
rocking precordial motion
Rocky Mountain spotted fever
Rodriguez-Alvarez catheter
Rodriguez catheter
roentgenkymography
roentgenogram, chest
roentgenographic control
roentgenographic silhouette
Roger bruit
Roger disease

Roger murmur
Roger syndrome
Roger ventricular septal defect
Rokitansky disease
R/O (rule out)
Rolleston rule for systolic blood
pressure
Romaña sign
Romano-Ward syndrome
Romberg-Wood syndrome
Romhilt-Estes score for left ventricular
hypertrophy
ROMI (rule out myocardial infarc-
tion); romied (slang past tense for
MI ruled out)
R1 Rapid Exchange balloon catheter
rongeur
Bethune
Cushing
Giertz
Kerrison
Sauerbruch
Semb
thoracic
R on T (R wave on T wave)
R on T phenomenon on EKG
R on T ventricular premature
contraction
roof, Dacron
roof of coronary sinus
room air
room air arterial blood gases
Roos test to detect thoracic outlet
syndrome
root
aortic
dilated aortic
root of lung
ROPA (Regional Organ Procurement
Agency)
ROPE (respiratory ordered phase
encoding)

ropelike cord (in thrombophlebitis)
ropy sputum
Roques syndrome
rose fever
Rosenbach syndrome
Rosenblatt implantable vascular access
port
Rosen-Castleman-Liebow syndrome
Rosen guidewire
Rosenkranz pediatric retractor system
Rosenthal syndrome
Ross aortic valve replacement
procedure
Ross pulmonary porcine valve
Ross switch procedure
Rostan asthma
Rostan syndrome
Rotablator atherectomy device
Rotacaps
ROTACS guidewire
RotaLink Plus rotational atherectomy
device
RotaLink rotational atherectomy
device
rotary cutter
rotating bur
rotating tourniquets for pulmonary
edema
rotation
counterclockwise
neck
rotation therapy, continuous lateral
rotational atherectomy (RA)
rotational atherectomy system (RAS)
rotational coronary atherectory (RCA)
rotavirus
RotaWire Floppy Gold guidewire
Rotch sign in pericardial effusion
Rotex II biopsy needle
Rothschild sign in tuberculosis
Roth spots
roticulating endograsper

Roticulator stapler
Roticulator, suture
Rotoresect device
Roubin-Gianturco flexible coil stent
roughened pleurae
roughened state of pericardium
roughening of lining of artery
rough murmur
rough zone
Rougnon de Magny syndrome
Rougnon-Heberden angina pectoris
round atelectasis
rounded border of lung
roundworm infestation
routine antimicrobial prophylaxis
roving handheld bipolar electrode
Royal Flush angiographic flush
    catheter
Royer-Wilson syndrome
Rozanski precordial lead placement
    system
RPA (right pulmonary artery)
RPE (rating of perceived exertion)
R-P interval
RPM (real-time position management)
    tracking system
rpm (rotations per minute)
R-Port Premier implantable vascular
    access system
RPV (right pulmonary vein)
RQ (respiratory quotient)
RR (respiratory rate)
RR cycle
RR interval
RR' (RR prime) pattern
RRI (recurrent respiratory infections)
RRP (rate-responsive pacing)
RRP (relative refractory period)
RRR (regular rate and rhythm)
RSA (respiratory sinus arrhythmia)
rS deflection
RS complex (also rS complex)

RSCVP (right subclavian central
    venous pressure)
RS4 pacemaker
Rsma (superior mesenteric artery
    resistance)
RSR (reduced sewing ring)
RSR (regular sinus rhythm)
R/S ratio; wave ratio
RSR' triphasic pattern (on EKG)
RS-T segments
RSV (regurgitant stroke volume)
RSV (respiratory syncytial virus)
    bronchiolitis
RSV pneumonia
RTCD (residual thermal collagen
    damage)
R-to-R scanning
rt-PA (recombinant tissue plasminogen
    activator) thrombolysis
RTCD (residual thermal collagen
    damage)
RT segment, elevated
RTV total artificial heart
R-2 defibrillator pads
rub
    coarse friction
    creaking friction
    faint friction
    friction
    grating friction
    harsh friction
    loud friction
    pericardial
    pericardial friction
    pleural
    pleural friction
    pleuritic
    prolonged
    scratchy friction
    shuffling friction
    soft friction
    three-component friction

rubber band, Vesseloops
rubber, vulcanizing silicone
rubbery mass
rubbery sputum
rubbing sound
rubedo
rubella, maternal
rubeola
Rubinstein-Taybi syndrome
rubor, dependent
ruborous
ruddy cyanosis
rudimentary outlet chamber
rudimentary ventricular chamber
Ruel forceps
rufous
Ruiz-Cohen round expander
rule
    Simpson
    Trusler
rule of bigeminy
rule out (R/O)
rule out myocardial infarction (ROMI)
rumble
    Austin Flint
    booming
    crescendo
    diastolic
    mid-diastolic (or middiastolic)
    protodiastolic
rumbling murmur
Rumel catheter
Rumel myocardial clamp
Rumel thoracic forceps
Rumel tourniquet device
Rummo syndrome
Rundles-Falls syndrome
runaway pacemaker
running continuous absorbable suture
runoff
    absent
    aortic

runoff *(cont.)*
    arterial
    digital
    distal
    inadequate
    single-vessel
    suboptimal
    three-vessel
    two-vessel
    vessel
runoff arteriogram
runoff resistance, index of
runoff vessel
runoff views, aortofemoral arteri-
    ography with
runs of arrhythmia
runs of atrial fibrillation
runs of PVCs (premature ventricular
    contractions)
runs of tachycardia
runs of ventricular tachycardia,
    spontaneously occurring
runs of VPCs (ventricular premature
    contractions)
runting syndrome
rupture
    abdominal aortic aneurysm
    arterial
    cardiac
    chordae tendineae
    chordal
    contained aneurysmal
    interventricular septal
    myocardial
ruptured aneurysm
ruptured aortic cusp
ruptured capillaries
ruptured chordae
ruptured chordae tendineae
ruptured emphysematous bleb
ruptured pseudoaneurysm
ruptured thoracic duct

rupture of arch
  papillary muscle
  plaque
  ventricular free wall
  ventricular septal
  vessel
rupture of blebs on surface of lungs
rupture of bullae on surface of lungs
rupture of emphysematous bleb
rupture of emphysematous bulla in
  apex of lung
rupture of heart muscle
rupture of lung
rupture of membranes (ROM)
rupture of myocardium
rupture with bleeding
Russell-Silver syndrome
Russian tissue forceps
rusty sputum
RV (residual volume)
RV (respiratory volume)
RVA (right ventricular apical) electrogram
RVAD (right ventricular assist device),
  Thoratec
RVBF (reversed vertebral blood flow)
RVCD (right ventricular conduction
  defect)
RVD (right ventricular diastolic)
  pressure
RVD (right ventricular dimension)
RVE (right ventricular enlargement)
RVEDP (right ventricular end-
  diastolic pressure)
RVEDV (right ventricular end-
  diastolic volume)
RVEF (right ventricular ejection
  fraction)
RVESV (right ventricular end-systolic
  volume)

RVFW (right ventricular free wall)
RVH (right ventricular hypertrophy)
RVID (right ventricular internal
  diameter)
RVM (right ventricular mass)
R voltage
RVOT (right ventricular outflow tract)
RVP (right ventricular pressure)
RVP (Robicsek vascular probe)
RVP–LVP (right ventricular to left
  ventricular systolic pressure) ratio
RV (right ventricle) pressure
RVS (right ventricular systolic)
  pressure
RV strain
RVSTI (right ventricular systolic time
  interval)
RVSW (right ventricular stroke work)
RVSWI (right ventricular stroke work
  index)
RVT (renal vein thrombosis)
RV/TLC or RV-TLC (residual vol-
  ume/total lung capacity)
RV/TLC or RV-TLC (respiratory vol-
  ume to total lung capacity) ratio
R' (R prime) wave
R wave (on EKG)
  low-amplitude
  tall right precordial
  upright
R-wave amplitude
r wave of jugular venous pulse
R wave progression, poor (on EKG)
R wave upstroke, slurred (on EKG)
Rx5000 cardiac pacing system
RX stent delivery system
Rx (prescription) therapy
Rythmol (propafenone)

S, s

S_1 (first heart sound)
S_1 amplitude
S_1Q3 pattern
S_1Q3T3 pattern
S_1-S_2 interval (heart sounds)
S_1-S_3 interval (heart sounds)
S_1-S_2-S_3 pattern (heart sounds)
S_2 (second heart sound)
    audible expiratory splitting of
    fixed splitting of
    paradoxical splitting of
    physiologically split
S_3 (third heart sound)
    audible
    palpable
    prominent
S_3 gallop
S_4 (fourth heart sound)
S_4 abolished by breath holding
S_4 abolished by sitting up
S_4 abolished by standing up
S_4, exaggerated
S_4 palpable
SA (sinoatrial)
SAA protein
SAB (sinoatrial block)
SAB (stereotactic aspiration biopsy)

Sabathie sign
Sable balloon catheter
Sabreloc spatula needle
sac
    air
    alveolar
    aneurysmal
    false
    heart
    pericardial
    pleural
    terminal air
    wrapped aneurysmal
saccular aneurysm
saccular appearance, lobulated
saccular bronchiectasis
saccular mass
sacculated pleurisy
Sachs vein retractor
Sack-Barabas syndrome
saclike spaces
sacrospinalis muscle
SACT (sinoatrial conduction time)
saddle embolism or embolus
saddle leather friction rub
Sade modification of Norwood
    procedure

503

SaECG (signal-averaged electrocardiogram)
Saf-Clens chronic wound cleanser
SAF-Gel hydrogel dressing
SAFT (Synthetic Aperture Focusing
Technique) in intravascular ultrasound imaging
sagging ST segment
sagittal image
sagittal plane loop
sagittal tomogram
Sahli method of measuring hemoglobin calorimetrically
saint (see *St. Jude, St. Thomas*)
Salbutamol Nebuamp (salbutamol
sulfate)
salicylate ingestion
salient history
salient physical findings
saline
    cold
    half normal (0.45% NaCl)
    heparinized
    iced
    normal (0.9% NaCl)
    topical cold
    warm
saline flush
saline irrigation
saline lavage
saline loading
saline solution
Salkowski test
salmonellosis
saloon door approach in MIDCAB
(minimally invasive direct coronary
artery bypass) procedures
salt edema
salt intake, excessive
salt-restricted diet
salt restriction
salt retention
salvage of limb

salvage of myocardium
salvage therapy
salvo of echoes
salvo of premature ventricular
complexes
salvo of ventricular tachycardia
Salzman test
SAM (systolic anterior motion) on
2-D echocardiogram
sampling, adrenal vein
sampling error
Samuels forceps
Samuels hemoclip
Samuels Micro-Scler catheter
SAN (sinoatrial node)
Sanchez-Cascos cardioauditory
syndrome
sandbag
Sanders sign in constrictive pericarditis
Sandrock test for thrombosis
sandwich patch closure, anterior
Sanfilippo syndrome
sanguineous exudate
sanguineous pleural exudate
San Joaquin Valley coccidioidomycosis
San Joaquin Valley disease
San Joaquin Valley fever
SA (sinoatrial)
SA nodal reentry tachycardia
SA node (also called *sinus*)
Sansom rhythmical murmur
Sansom sign in pericardial effusion
SaO$_2$ (arterial oxygen saturation)
saphenectomy site
saphenofemoral junction
saphenous varices
saphenous vein, veins
    arm and lesser (ALSVs)
    greater
    lesser
    nonreversed
    reversed
    small

saphenous vein bypass graft
saphenous vein bypass graft disease
saphenous vein graft (SVG)
saphenous vein incompetence
SAPHFinder surgical balloon
    dissector
SaphLITE/SaphLITE II retractor
    system
SAPHtrak balloon dissector
sapphire contact probe
saralasin infusion
sarcoid, Boeck
sarcoidosis
sarcoma
    cardiac
    cherry-red endobronchial lesions of
        Kaposi's
    endobronchial Kaposi
    intrathoracic Kaposi
    Kaposi epicardial
    myocardial infiltration by Kaposi
    pulmonary Kaposi
    right atrial
sarcomere, A bands of
sarcoplasmic reticulum
Sarns ABLD system
Sarns aortic arch cannula
Sarns centrifugal pump
Sarns Delphin 9000 centrifugal pump
Sarns electric saw
Sarns 5000 Console heart-lung
    machine
Sarns H.E.L.P. unit
Sarns 9000 heart-lung machine
Sarns occluder 5000 system
Sarns occluder 7000 system
Sarns S10K II blood pump
Sarns 7000 MDX heart-lung machine
Sarns 7400 pulsatile pump module
Sarns 7800 centrifugal pump system
Sarns two-stage cannula
Sarns ventricular assist device

Sarns wire-reinforced catheter
Sarot artery forceps
Sarot bronchus clamp
SARS (severe acute respiratory
    syndrome)
SAS (supravalvular aortic stenosis)
Satinsky aortic clamp
Satinsky scissors
Satinsky vascular clamp
Satinsky vena cava clamp
satisfactory threshold
saturated fats
saturation
    aortic oxygen
    arterial oxygen (SaO$_2$)
    decreased arterial hemoglobin
    low oxygen
    mixed venous
    oxygen (O$_2$)
    oxyhemoglobin
    PA (pulmonary artery) oxygen
    RA (right atrium) oxygen
Sauerbruch retractor
Sauerbruch rib shears
Sauerbruch rongeur
sausaging of a vein
Sauvage arterial graft
Sauvage filamentous prosthesis
Sauvage filamentous velour Dacron
    arterial graft material
SAVVI synchronous pacemaker with a
    single lead
saw
    Gigli
    Hall sternal
    mechanical
    oscillating sternotomy
    Sarns electric
    sternotomy
    Stryker
sawtooth configuration
SB (sinus bradycardia)

SBE (subacute bacterial endocarditis)
SBE prophylaxis
SBF (systemic blood flow)
SBP (systolic blood pressure)
SBSP (simultaneous bilateral sponta-
neous pneumothorax)
SC (systolic click)
SCAD (spontaneous coronary artery
dissection)
SCA-EX catheter with rotating blades
SCA-EX ShortCutter catheter with
rotating blades
scalar EKG
scale (see also *classification, criteria,
index, score*)
Borg (perceived exertion)
Abbreviated Injury
Exercise Self-efficacy Scale
Health Failure Self-Care Behavior
Scale, revised
scalene node biopsy
scalenus anterior muscle
scalenus anticus muscle hypertrophy
scalenus anticus syndrome
scalenus minimus
scalloped commissure
scalloped luminal configuration
scalloping
scallop of posterior anulus, redundant
scallop, prolapsing
scalp edema
scalp electrode
scalpel
Hemo-Cath
UltraCision ultrasonic knife
ultrasonic
scalp pH
scan
attenuation
biphasic helical CT scan
Captopril-stimulated renal
cardiac

scan *(cont.)*
Cardiolite (^{99m}Tc sestamibi)
Cardiotec or CardioTec (^{99m}Tc
teboroxime)
cine CT (computed tomography)
cine view in MUGA (cinematograph in multiple gated
acquisition)
computerized tomography (CT)
coronary artery scan (CAS) by
Ultrafast CT
dipyridamole thallium-201
duplex
dynamic helical
gallium
gated equilibrium blood pool
high-resolution computed
tomography
hot spot
^{125}I (I 125) fibrinogen
^{131}I-iodocholesterol
^{131}I meta-iodobenzylguanide
(^{131}I-MIBG)
isotope-labeled fibrinogen
MUGA (multiple gated acquisition)
blood pool radionuclide
myocardial perfusion
perfusion and ventilation lung
perfusion lung
PET
^{31}P nuclear magnetic resonance
PYP (pyrophosphate technetium)
myocardial
radioactive fibrinogen
radionuclide gated blood pool
redistributed thallium
renal duplex
rest thallium-201
resting MUGA
R to R
scintillation
serial duplex

scan *(cont.)*
   SPECT thallium
   stress thallium
   ^{99m}Tc glucoheptonate
   ^{99m}Tc pyrophosphate myocardial
   thallium
   ultrafast CT
   ventilation lung
   ventilation-perfusion lung
   xenon 133 scan (^{133}Xe)
scan decrement
scanner
   ATL duplex
   ATL real-time Neurosector
   Evolution XP ultrafast CT
   Lumiscan 150
   Signa I.S.T. MRI
   Somatom Plus-S CT
   spiral XCT (x-ray computed
      tomography)
   Vision 1.5-T Siemens MRI
Scanning-Beam Digital X-ray (SBDX)
   system
scan pacing
scanty findings
scanty mucoid sputum
scapula
   inferior tip of
   wing-like protrusion of
   winged
scar
   arrhythmogenic
   dense
   infarcted
   myocardial
   nonviable
   pulmonary
   scarred
   well-demarcated
   zipper
scar formation on myocardium
scarification of pleura

Scarpa method
Scarpa triangle
scarred fibrotic media
scarring
   apical
   endocardial
   interstitial
   selective
scarring of valve
scar tissue
scattered rhonchi
scattering of sound waves
SCD (sudden cardiac death)
Schafer artificial respirations
Schatz-Palmaz tubular mesh stent
Schede operation for leg varicose
   veins
Schede resection of thorax for chronic
   empyema
Schede thoracoplasty
schedule, dose-escalation
Scheie syndrome
Schellong-Strisower phenomenon
Schepelmann sign in dry pleurisy
Schick sign of tuberculosis
Schick stridor heard on expiration
Schiff test
Schistosoma haematobium
Schistosoma infection
Schistosoma japonicum
Schistosoma mansoni
schistosomiasis
   cardiopulmonary
   Manson
   pulmonary
schistosomiasis japonica syndrome
Schlichter test
Schmincke-Bernheim syndrome
Schneider catheter
Schneider PTCA instruments
Schneider-Shiley catheter
Schneider Wallstent

Schneider wire
Schnidt clamp
Schnidt passer
Scholten endomyocardial biopsy
  forceps
Scholten endomyocardial bioptome
Schonander film changer
Schonander technique
Schönenberg syndrome
Schönlein disease
Schönlein purpura
Schoonmaker femoral catheter
Schoonmaker multipurpose catheter
Schroeder syndrome
Schrötter syndrome
Schuco nebulizer
Schultze acroparesthesia
Schultze test
Schwarten balloon dilatation catheter
Schwarten LP guidewire
Schwartz clamp
Schwartz test for patency of deep
  saphenous veins
sciatic artery, persistent
SciMed Express balloon
SciMed Express Monorail balloon
SciMed membrane oxygenator
SciMed NC Ranger PTCA catheter
SciMed Radius coronary stent
SciMed SSC Skinny catheter
scimitar deformity
scimitar-shaped flap
scimitar-shaped shadow
scimitar sign on chest radiograph
scimitar syndrome
scimitar vein
Scinticore multicrystal scintillation
  camera
scintigram, scintigraphy
  AMA-Fab (antimyosin monoclonal
    antibody with Fab fragment)
  dipyridamole thallium-201
  dual intracoronary

scintigram *(cont.)*
  exercise stress-redistribution
  exercise thallium
  gated blood pool
  indium-111 (^{111}In)
  infarct-avid hot-spot
  ^{131}I-19-iodocholesterol
  labeled FFA (free fatty acid)
  metaiodobenzylguanidine (MIBG)
  microsphere perfusion
  myocardial
  myocardial cold-spot perfusion
  myocardial perfusion
  NEFA (non-esterified fatty acid)
  perfusion
  planar thallium
  pulmonary
  pyrophosphate
  resting-redistribution thallium-201
  SPECT thallium
  ^{99m}Tc-PYP (pyrophosphate)
  thallium perfusion
  thallium-201 myocardial
scintillation camera
scintillation, migrainous-like
scintillation scan
scintirenography
scintiscan (scintigraphy)
scintiscanning of lungs
scissors
  bandage
  Beall circumflex artery
  Church
  coronary artery
  Crafoord thoracic
  curved
  DeBakey endarterectomy
  DeBakey valve
  DeMartel vascular
  Diethrich coronary
  Diethrich valve
  dissecting
  Duffield

scissors *(cont.)*
    Evershears II bipolar curved
    Finochietto thoracic
    Haimovici arteriotomy
    Harrington-Mayo thoracic
    hook
    Howell coronary
    iris
    Kantrowitz vascular
    Karmody venous
    Lincoln
    Lincoln-Metzenbaum
    Litwak mitral valve
    Lloyd-Davies
    Mayo curved
    Mayo straight
    Metzenbaum curved
    Metzenbaum straight
    microvascular
    Mills arteriotomy
    Nelson
    Potts right-angled
    Potts 60° angled
    Potts-Smith vascular
    Real coronary artery
    right-angle
    Satinsky
    Smith
    Snowden-Pencer
    Spencer
    Stille-Mayo
    straight
    Strully
    thoracic
    valve
    Westcott
    Willauer thoracic
    Wilmer
SCL (sinus cycle length)
Sclavo PPD solution (tuberculin
    purified protein derivative)
Sclavo Test-PPD (tuberculin purified
    protein derivative)

SCLC (small-cell lung cancer)
scleroderma
sclerosing breast periphlebitis
sclerosing breast phlebitis
sclerosing mediastinitis
sclerosis
    arterial
    arteriocapillary
    arteriolar
    calcified
    coronary
    endocardial
    medial calcific
    Mönckeberg
    photothermal
    progressive systemic
    pulmonary and cardiac
    renal
    segmental vein
    subendocardial
    tuberous
    valvular
    vascular
    venous
sclerosis of aorta
sclerotherapy
sclerotic coronary arteries
sclerotic degeneration
SCLS (systemic capillary leak
    syndrome)
SCOOP 1 transtracheal oxygen
    catheter
SCOOP 2 catheter with distal and
    side openings
scooping, nonspecific (on EKG)
scope, Jako anterior commissure
score (see also *classification, criteria,*
    index, scale)
    Agatston
    Baylor bleeding
    CASS
    Cooperman event probability
    coronary artery scoring

score *(cont.)*
 defibrillatory efficacy
 Detsky modified cardiac risk index
 Dripps-American Surgical
  Association
 Duke treadmill exercise
 Estes EKG
 Gensini coronary artery disease
 Goldman
 Goldman cardiac risk index
 mean wall motion
 QRS
 Romhilt-Estes left ventricular
  hypertrophy
 Selvester QRS
 TAPSE (tricuspid anular plane
  systolic excursion)
 wall motion
Scoring Balloon catheter
scotoma
scout films
scratch
 Means-Lermans
 systolic
scratchy friction rub
scratchy murmur
scratchy throat
screen, collagen vascular
screw, atrial
screw-in lead
screw-in lead pacemaker
screw-in straight atrial lead
screw-on epimyocardial lead
screw-on lead
scrub typhus
Sculptor flexible anuloplasty ring
SCV-CPR (simultaneous compression-
 ventilation CPR)
SD (standard deviation)
SDAP (single donor apheresis
 platelets)
SDB (sleep-disordered breathing)

SDBP (systemic diastolic blood
 pressure)
SD Plasma
SDPS (protamine solution)
SE (standard error)
Sea-Clens wound cleanser
seagull bruit
seagull murmur
seal and suction
sealant
 CoSeal resorbable synthetic
  fibrin
 FloSeal matrix hemostatic
 FocalSeal
 FocalSeal-L
 FocalSeal-S
seal, underwater
Sea-Clens wound cleanser
SEA (side entry access) port
SeaSorb alginate wound dressing
seated, valve is
seating of valve
Sebastiani syndrome
Sechrist Air/O$_2$ blender
secondary atrioventricular heart block
secondary bacterial infection
secondary cardiomyopathy
secondary cartilaginous joint
secondary chordal dysplasia
secondary coccidioidomycosis
secondary endocardial fibroelastosis
secondary erythrocytosis
secondary extravasation of intravascular contents
secondary hypertension
secondary lymphedema
secondary median sternotomy
secondary myocardiopathy
secondary pacemaker
secondary pleurisy
secondary venous insufficiency
second branch of artery

second component
second-degree atrioventricular block
second diagonal branch
second-hand smoke
second heart sound, loud pulmonic
    component
second heart sound, single
second intercostal space
second left interspace
second order chordae
second pulmonic sound, accentuated
second sound followed by opening
    snap
second sound, reinforced
secretion
    ACTH
    ADH (antidiuretic hormone)
    amber-colored pulmonary
    bronchial
    liquification of
    mucopurulent
    nonpurulent pulmonary
    retained
    thickened
secretion-filled medium-sized bronchi
sector echocardiography
secundum and sinus venosus defects
secundum atrial septal defect (ASD)
sed (sedimentation) rate
sedentary lifestyle
sedimentation rate, Wintrobe
Sedlackova syndrome
Seecor pacemaker
seeding
    cell
    graft
seesaw (to-and-fro) murmur
segment
    accessory
    akinetic
    amplitude and slope of ST
    angulated

segment *(cont.)*
    anterior
    anterior basal
    anterobasal
    anterolateral
    apex
    apical
    arterial
    bronchopulmonary
    coarcted
    contiguous
    depressed PR
    depressed ST
    diaphragmatic
    distal
    elevated RT
    elevated ST
    endarterectomized
    expansile aortic
    hypokinetic
    infarcted lung
    inferior
    inferior basal
    inferoapical
    inferoposterior
    nonfilling venous
    noninfarcted
    ostial
    posterior
    posterobasal
    posterolateral
    P-R
    proximal
    RS-T
    septal wall
    septum
    ST
    ST-T
    superior
    Ta
    TQ
    upsloping ST
    venous

segmental agenesis
segmental atelectasis
segmental bowel infarction
segmental bronchi
   cardiac
   lateral
   lateral basal
   medial
   medial basal
   posterior
   posterior basal
   superior
segmental bronchus
segmental ischemia
segmental lesion
segmental limb pressure
segmental lower extremity Doppler
   pressures
segmental orifice
segmental perfusion abnormality
segmental plethysmography
segmental pneumonia
segmental resection
segmental vein sclerosis
segmental wall motion
   akinetic
   dyskinetic
   hyperkinetic
   hypokinetic
segmental wall motion abnormality
segmentectomy of lung
segs (segmented neutrophils)
Segura Lock hub
Sehrt clamp
Sehrt compressor
SEI (subendocardial infarction)
Seitz bronchial inspiration
Seitzinger tripolar cutting forceps
Seitz sign
seizure
SELCA (smooth excimer laser
   coronary angioplasty)

Seldinger needle
Seldinger percutaneous technique
Seldinger technique, modified
Selection AFm (atrial fibrillation)
   monitor
selective arteriogram
selective cannulization
selective coronary arteriography
selective coronary cineangiography
selective dopamine agonists
selective scarring of posterobasal
   portion of left ventricle
selective vascular ligation
selective visualization
Select Performance balloon dilatation
   catheter
self-aspirating cut-biopsy needle
self-breath-holding
self-expandable stent
self-expanding stent
self-inhibition, pacemaker
self-limited
self-limiting respiratory
   infection
self-positioning balloon
self-retaining retractor
self-retaining table-mounted retractor
   system
Selman vessel forceps
Selverstone cardiotomy hook
Selverstone carotid clamp
Selvester QRS score
SEM (systolic ejection murmur)
Semb forceps
Semb lung retractor
Semb rongeur
semicircularis, linea
semiclosed endarterectomy
semi-Fowler position
semilateral position
semilunar (aortic and pulmonary)
   valves

semilunar aortic valve regurgitation
semilunar pulmonic valve regurgitation
semilunar valve cusp
senescent aortic stenosis
Sengstaken-Blakemore tube
senile arteriosclerosis
senile emphysema
senile myocarditis
senile nevus
Senning atrial baffle repair
Senning intra-atrial baffle
Senning operation for transposition
Senn retractor
sensation
    flip-flop
    fluttering
    globus
    pressurelike
    squeezing
    suffocating
sensing
    afterpotential
    integrated bipolar
    intrinsic
    P
    pacemaker
    R-wave
sensing error
sensing sensitivity
sensing specificity
sensing spike
sensing threshold
sensing wire
sensitivity
    airway
    baroreflex
    pacemaker
    sensing
Sensi-Touch anesthesia delivery
    system
Sensi-Touch anesthesia needle
Sensolog pacemaker

sensor
    Hall-effect position
    minute ventilation
    muscle activity
    respiration
    temperature
    vibration
sensorium
Sensor Kelvin pacemaker
Sensor-Medics metabolic cart
Sensormedics 3100A ventilator
Sensor PTFE-nitinol guidewire with
    hydrophilic tip
sensory impairment
Sentinel implantable cardioverter-
    defibrillator
sentinel nodes
SEP (systolic ejection period)
separation
    aortic cusp
    leaflet
Seprafilm tissue barrier
SEPS (subfascial endoscopic
    perforating vein surgery)
SEPS (subfascial endoscopic
    perforator surgery)
sepsis
    catheter-related (CRS)
    gram-negative
    overwhelming
septa
    alveolar
    thickened alveolar
septal accessory pathway
septal amplitude
septal arcade
septal band
septal cardiac defect
septal collateral
septal cusp of right atrioventricular
    valve

septal defect
    atrial
    atrioventricular
    interventricular
septal dip
septal hypertrophy, asymmetric
septal hypokinesis
septal hypoperfusion on thallium scan
septal infarction
septal leaflet
septal necrosis
septal papillary muscle
septal pathway
septal perforation
septal perforator branch
septal perforators
septal ridge
septal separation
septal thickness
septal wall thickness
septation
septectomy
    atrial
    Blalock-Hanlon atrial
    Blalock-Hanlon partial atrial
septic bronchitis
septic emboli
septic embolization
septic embolus
septic endocarditis
septic lung syndrome
septic myocarditis
septic pelvic thrombophlebitis with
    emboli
septic phlebitis
septic pleurisy
septic pulmonary emboli
septic pulmonary infarction
septic shock
septic thrombosis
septic tonsillitis

septicemia
septomarginal trabecula
    (pl. trabeculae)
septostomy
    balloon
    balloon and blade
    balloon atrial
    blade
    blade and balloon atrial
    blade atrial
    Mullins transseptal blade and
        balloon atrial
    Park blade and balloon atrial
    Rashkind balloon
    Rashkind balloon atrial
    Rashkind blade
    Rashkind-Miller atrial
    transcatheter knife blade atrial
septotomy, balloon atrial
septum (pl. septa)
    anteroapical trabecular
    asymmetric hypertrophy of
    atrial
    atrioventricular
    bronchial
    bulbar
    canal
    conal
    conus
    dyskinetic
    infundibular
    intact ventricular
    interatrial (IAS)
    interventricular (IVS)
    membranous
    muscular atrioventricular
    sinus
    thickened
    ventricular
septum primum
septum secundum

sequela (pl. sequelae)
  clinical
  pulmonary
  significant
sequence
  A-B-C (airway, breathing, circulation) (in cardiopulmonary resuscitation)
  C-A-B (circulation, airway, breathing) (in cardiopulmonary resuscitation)
  conventional pulse
  echo-planar
  gradient-echo imaging
  gradient-echo pulse
  Klippel-Feil
  single breath-hold
  spin-echo imaging
sequential balloon inflation
sequential bypass graft
Sequential Compression Device, Kendall
sequential CT images
sequential dilatations
sequential graft
sequential in situ bypass
sequential monophasic shocks
sequential obstruction
sequential pacing
sequestered lobe of lung
Sequestra 1000 blood processing system
sequestration, third space
Sequicor pacemaker
Sequoia ultrasound system
sequoiosis asthma
SER (systolic ejection rate)
Serevent (salmeterol xinafoate)
serial cardiac isoenzymes
serial changes
serial CPK and LDH isoenzymes
serial cut film technique

serial duplex scan
serial EKG tracings
serial electrophysiologic testing (SET)
serial lesions
serial samples of blood
serial tracings
serine proteinase inhibitor
seriography
Seroche syndrome
serofibrinous pleurisy
seroma, graft
seropositive
seropositivity
seropurulent pleurisy
serosanguineous fluid
serosum, pericardium
serotonin
serous exudate
serous exudation
serous pericarditis
serous pericardium
serous pleurisy
serrated catheter
Serratia marcescens
serratus anterior muscle
serum (pl. sera)
serum aspergillus precipitins
serum cardiac enzymes
serum cryptococcal antigen
serum electrophoresis
serum fibrinogen
serum iron
serum lactate level, elevated
serum lipid level
serum lipid profile
serum magnesium
serum myoglobin (Mb) concentration
serum phosphorus level
serum potassium concentration
serum prothrombin conversion accelerator (SPCA)
serum renin levels

serum titer
Servelle-Martorell syndrome
Servomotor
Servo respirator
sessile plaque
sestamibi Tc-99m SPECT with
  dipyridamole stress test
sestamibi technetium-99m stress test
SET (serial electrophysiologic testing)
SET three-lumen thrombectomy
  catheter
7E3 monoclonal antiplatelet antibody
17-hydroxylase deficiency
seventh intercostal space
7-3 rule
7-valent vaccine
severe acute rejection
severe acute respiratory syndrome
  (SARS)
severe acidosis
severe cardiopulmonary failure
severe exertion
severe infarction
severe oxygen debt
severe respiratory distress
sewing capsule
sewing ring
sew-on lead
Sex After MI Knowledge Test
SF wave of cardiac apex pulse
SFA (subclavian flap aortoplasty)
SFA (superficial femoral artery)
SFHb (stroma-free hemoglobin,
  pyridoxylated)
SFR (stenotic flow reserve)
SGOT (serum glutamic-oxaloacetic
  transaminase)
SGPT (serum glutamic-pyruvic
  transaminase)
shadow
  bat's wing (on x-ray)
  butterfly (on x-ray)

shadow *(cont.)*
  cardiac
  discoid
  fusiform
  hilar
  large thymus (obscuring cardiac
    silhouette)
  linear
  Ponfick
  toothpaste
  tramlines
  tumorlike
  widened heart
shadowing, acoustic
Shadow over-the-wire balloon catheter
shag, aortic
shagging of cardiac borders
shaggy aorta syndrome
shake test
shaking chills
shaking sound
Shaldon catheter
shallow breathing
shallow respirations
shapeable guidewire
Shapiro sign
sharp and blunt dissection
sharp border of lung
sharp carina
sharp dissection
sharp pain
sharp pulse
sharp, stabbing pain
sharp waves
shaver catheter
Shaver-Ridell syndrome
Shaver syndrome
shears
  Bethune rib
  Gluck rib
  LaparoSonic coagulating shears
    for autograft harvesting

shears *(cont.)*
    Sauerbruch rib
    Shoemaker rib
    Stille-Giertz rib
sheath
    Ancure EZ Path catheter
    angioplasty
    arterial
    catheter
    check-valve
    Cook transseptal
    Cordis
    femoral artery
    French
    GlideCath
    Guidant
    guiding
    Hemaquet
    InnerVasc
    Innovante
    introducer
    Mullins
    Mullins transseptal
    Passager introducing
    peel-away
    preformed peel-away guiding
    Prelude vascular introducer
    radiopaque FEP
    rectus
    Shuttle flexor (used as guiding
      catheter)
    side arm
    Silastic
    Spectranetics (SLS)
    tearaway
    transseptal
    USCI angioplasty guiding
    vascular
    venous
    X-Sept
sheath and side-arm
sheath-dilator, Mullins transseptal

sheathed insertion technique
sheathless, flexible, pre-wrapped
    double-lumen IAB catheter
sheathless insertion technique
sheath with side-arm adapter
sheepskin boot
Sheffield exercise test protocol
Sheffield modification of Bruce
    treadmill protocol
Sheffield treadmill exercise protocol
shell, ejection
shepherd's hook or crook deformity
Sherpa guiding catheter
Shibley sign
shift
    mediastinal
    ST segment
    superior frontal axis
shift to the left (white blood cells)
shift to the right (white blood cells)
shifting pacemaker syndrome
Shiley guiding catheter
Shiley-Ionescu catheter
Shiley 795 A (Dideco) autotransfusion
    system
Shiley tracheotomy tube
Shimazaki area-length method
Shinobi Plus guidewire from Cordis
Shinobi steerable guidewire from
    Cordis
Shirley wound drain
shivering
SHJR4s (side-hole Judkins right,
    curve 4 French, short)
shock
    advanced cardiogenic
    bacteremic
    biphasic
    biphasic electrical
    cardiogenic
    circulatory
    committed defibrillation

shock *(cont.)*
  DC electrical
  diastolic
  defibrillation
  distributive
  40 joule rescue
  hemorrhagic
  hypovolemic
  initial
  joule
  noncardiogenic
  obstructive
  pleural
  pneumonia-induced septic
  postcardiotomy
  postoperative
  profound
  prolonged
  QRS synchronized
  rescue
  septic
  sequential monophasic
  simultaneous
  spurious
  toxic
  vasogenic
  viremic
shock blocks
shocking electrode
shocking lead
shock lung
shock lung syndrome
shocky appearance
Shoemaker rib shears
Shone anomaly
Shone syndrome
short-acting bronchodilators
short-axis parasternal view
short-axis plane
short-axis plane on echocardiography
short-axis slice
short-axis view

shortening
  fractional myocardial
  mean rate of circumferential
  median percent
shortening fraction
shorthand vertical mattress stitch
shortness of breath (SOB)
  intermittent
  severe
shortness of breath at rest
shortness of breath with low-level
  exercise
short P-Q interval
short P-R interval
short pulse
short Q-T phenomenon
short rib-polydactyly syndrome
Short syndrome
short-term anticoagulation
shortwindedness *or* short-windedness
shots, guiding
shoulder-hand syndrome
shoulder of the heart
shower of echoes
Shprintzen velocardiofacial syndrome
shrinkage, graft
shudder, carotid
shudder of carotid arterial pulse
shuffling friction rub
shunt
  Allen-Brown vascular access
  Anastaflo intravascular
  aorta to pulmonary artery
  aorticopulmonary
  aortopulmonary
  apicoaortic
  arteriovenous (A-V)
  ascending aorta to pulmonary
    artery
  Axius Vacuum
  bidirectional
  Blalock

shunt *(cont.)*
  Blalock-Taussig
  Buselmeier
  cardiac
  cardiovascular
  Cordis-Hakim
  coronary anastomotic
  Davidson
  Denver PAK (percutaneous access
    kit)
  Denver pleuroperitoneal
  descending aorta-pulmonary artery
  descending thoracic aorta to
    pulmonary artery
  dialysis
  extracardiac
  extracardiac right-to-left
  Flo-Thru Intraluminal
  Glenn
  Gore-Tex
  Gott
  Holter
  intracardiac
  intracardiac right-to-left
  intracardial
  intrapericardial aorticopulmonary
  intrapulmonary
  ISCI
  Javid
  Javid endarterectomy
  left-to-right
  modified Blalock-Taussig
  net
  peritoneovenous
  portacaval
  portasystemic vascular
  Potts
  Pruitt-Inahara carotid
  Quinton-Scribner
  Ramirez
  reversed (right-to-left)
  right-to-left (reversed)

shunt *(cont.)*
  Rivetti-Levinson intraluminal
  subclavian artery to pulmonary
    artery
  subclavian-pulmonary
  Sundt
  supracardiac
  Thomas
  Thomas vascular access
  transjugular intrahepatic porto-
    systemic (TIPS or TIPSS)
  vena cava to pulmonary artery
  venoarterial
  ventriculoatrial
  ventriculoperitoneal
  ventriculopleural
  Vitagraft arteriovenous
  Wakabayashi
  Warren splenorenal
  Waterston
  Waterston-Cooley
shunted blood
shunt flow
  anatomic
  physiologic
  relative
shunting
  aortopulmonary
  atrial right-to-left
  central aortopulmonary
  intracardiac
  intrapulmonary
  venoarterial
shunting of blood
  left-to-right
  marked
  right-to-left
shunt passer
shunt placement
shunt reversal
Shur-Clens wound cleanser
shutdown, renal

Shuttle flexor sheath (used as guiding
    catheter)
shuttle technique, bronchoscopic
Shy-McGee-Drager syndrome
SI (sinus irregularity)
SI (stroke index)
sibilant rales
sibilant rhonchi
sicca
    laryngitis
    pericarditis
sickle cell anemia
sickle cell–thalassemia disease
sickle cell trait
sickle chest syndrome
sicklemia
sickling test
sickness
    acute mountain
    altitude
    decompression
    hypobarism-acute mountain
    mountain
sick sinus node
sick sinus syndrome (SSS)
    extrinsic
    intrinsic
SICOR (computer-assisted cardiac
    catheter recording system)
side-arm adapter, sheath with
side-arm pressure port
side arm sheath
side-biting clamp
side branch occlusion
side-by-side transposition of great
    arteries
side-cutting spatulated needle
side entry access (SEA) port
side-hole catheter
siderosis, welder's
siderotica, pneumoconiosis
side-to-side anastomosis

sidewinder catheter
side-wire pacing lead
SIDS (sudden infant death syndrome)
Siemens-Albis bicycle ergometer
Siemens electrode
Siemens-Elema AB pulse transducer
    probe
Siemens-Elema pacemaker
Siemens-Pacesetter pacemaker
Siemens PTCA/open heart table
Siemens Servo 300 ventilator
Siemens Servo 900C ventilator
SieScape ultrasound imaging
sieve, vena caval
Siewert syndrome
sighing
sighing breathing
sighing dyspnea
sigmoid omentum
sign
    Abrahams
    ace of spades (on angiogram)
    air crescent (on chest x-ray)
    amputation
    angel wing
    antler (on x-ray)
    aortic arch aneurysm
    aortic nipple
    apical cap
    applesauce
    Auenbrugger
    Baccelli (of pleural effusion)
    bagpipe
    Bamberger
    Bard
    Becker
    Bethea
    Biermer
    Biot
    Bird
    Bouillaud
    Bozzolo

sign *(cont.)*
  Branham
  Branham arteriovenous fistula
  Braunwald
  Broadbent
  Broadbent inverted
  Brockenbrough
  Brockenbrough-Braunwald
  Cardarelli
  cardinal
  cardiorespiratory
  carotid string
  Carvallo
  Castellino
  Cegka
  Claybrook
  clenched fist
  Corrigan
  cortical
  coughing
  crescent
  Cruveilhier
  cuff
  D'Amato
  de la Camp
  Delbet
  Delmege
  de Musset (aortic aneurysm)
  d'Espine
  Dorendorf
  Drummond
  Duroziez
  E (on x-ray)
  Ebstein
  Ellis
  Ewart
  Federici
  figure 3
  finger tip
  Fischer
  Fleischner
  focal neurologic

sign *(cont.)*
  Frank
  Franz
  Friedreich
  Fürbringer
  Gerhardt
  Glasgow
  gloved finger
  gooseneck (on x-ray)
  Grancher
  Greene
  Grocco
  Grossman
  Gunn crossing
  Hall
  Hamman
  Hamman pneumopericardium
  Heim-Kreysig
  Hill
  Homans
  Hoover
  Hope
  Huchard
  Jaccoud
  Jackson
  jugular
  Jürgensen
  Karplus
  Katz-Wachtel
  Kellock
  knuckle
  Korányi
  Korányi-Grocco
  Kussmaul
  Kussmaul venous
  Laënnec
  Lancisi
  Landolfi
  Levine
  liver-jugular
  Livierato
  Mahler

sign *(cont.)*
  Mannkopf
  McGinn-White
  Meltzer
  Moschcowitz (of arterial occlusive
    disease)
  Müller (Mueller) aortic
    regurgitation
  Musset (de Musset)
  Nicoladoni-Branham
  Oliver-Cardarelli
  ominous
  Osler
  pad
  patent bronchus
  Paul
  Perez
  Pfuhl
  Pfuhl-Jaffé
  Pins
  plumb-line
  Potain
  Pott
  Pottenger
  premonitory
  Prevel
  Prussian helmet
  Quénu-Muret
  Quincke
  rabbit ear
  railroad track
  reversed 3 (on x-ray)
  Rivero-Carvallo
  Riviere
  Robertson
  Rotch
  Rothschild
  Sabathie
  Sanders
  Sansom
  Schepelmann
  Schick

sign *(cont.)*
  scimitar
  Seitz
  Shapiro
  Shibley
  Skoda
  Smith
  spinal
  square-root
  Sterles
  Sternberg
  3
  trapezius ridge
  Traube aortic regurgitation
  vein
  vital
  Weill
  Westermark
  Williams
  Williamson
  wind sock (echocardiogram)
  Wintrich
SignaDress hydrocolloid dressing
  material
Signa I.S.T. MRI scanner
signal (see also *signaling*)
  Doppler
  magnetic resonance
  mosaic-jet
signal-averaged electrocardiogram
  (SaECG)
signal blooming
signal dephasing
signal intensity
signaling, myocardial adrenergic
signal magnification
signal void
signature, echo
signif (significant)(ly)
significant axis deviation
significant, clinically
significant residual deficit

significant sequelae
Sigvaris compression stockings
SIHC (surgically implanted hemo-
  dialysis catheter)
Silastic bead embolization
Silastic catheter
Silastic electrode casing
Silastic H.P. tissue expander
Silastic loop
Silastic sheath
Silastic tape
Silastic tubing
Silastic vessel loop
"sil-ee-um" (psyllium)
silent infarction
silent ischemia
silent mitral stenosis
silent myocardial infarction
silent patent ductus arteriosus
silent regurgitation
silhouette
    cardiac (large thymus shadow
      obscuring)
    enlarged cardiac
    luminal
    roentgenographic
    widened cardiac
silhouette image
silhouette technique
silicone dioxide inhalation
silicone rubber, vulcanizing
Silicore catheter
silicosis
    complicated
    conglomerate
    infective
    non-nodular
    rheumatoid lung
    simple
    simple nodular
silicotic fibrosis of lung
silicotic lung

silicotic mediastinitis
silicotic nodule with central necrosis
silicotic visceral pleura
silicotuberculosis
silk sutures
Silk guidewire
silo-filler's disease
silo-filler's lung
silver clip
silver finisher's lung
silver-iontophoretic catheter
Silverlon wound packing strips
Silverman II syndrome
silver polisher's lung
Silver-Russell syndrome
SilverSpeed guidewire
Silver syndrome
silver wire effect
silver wiring
Silvester artificial respirations
SIMA (single internal mammary
  artery) reconstruction
Simmons-type sidewinder catheter
Simon foci
Simon nitinol percutaneous IVC filter
simple acroparesthesia
simple arteriovenous anastomosis
simple arteriovenular (arteriolovenular)
  anastomosis
simple pulmonary eosinophilia
simple silicosis
simplex, xanthoma tuberosum
Simplus catheter
Simplus PE/t dilatation catheter
Simpson atherectomy
Simpson atherectomy catheter
Simpson atherectomy device, PET
  balloon
Simpson Coronary AtheroCath (SCA)
  system
Simpson method to calculate LV
  volume and LVEF

Simpson peripheral AtheroCath
Simpson-Robert catheter
Simpson rule method for ventricular volume
Simpson rule volume method
Simpson Ultra-Low Profile II balloon catheter
simultaneous aneurysmectomy
simultaneous balloon inflation
simultaneous bilateral spontaneous pneumothorax (SBSP)
simultaneous individual stapling (SIS)
simultaneous pacing and coronary blood flow measurement
simultaneous pacing and coronary sinus lactate sampling
simultaneous recording
simultaneous shocks
simultaneous waveforms, truncated exponential
SIMV (synchronized intermittent mandatory ventilation)
SIMV-PC ventilator
sine-wave pattern on electrocardiogram
Singh-Vaughan-Williams classification of arrhythmias
single atrium
single atrium syndrome
single-bore cannula
single breath-hold sequence on CT scan
single-cannula atrial cannulation
single-chain antigen-binding (SCA) protein
single-chamber pacing
single-channel ECG
single donor apheresis platelets (SDAP)
single extrastimuli
single-lung transplantation
single-outlet heart
single pleurisy

single-punch fenestration
single second heart sound
single-slice long-axis tomograms
Singleton-Merten syndrome
single ventricle
single ventricle syndrome
single ventricle with pulmonic stenosis
single-vessel disease
single-vessel runoff
Singley forceps
Singulair (montelukast sodium)
singultus
sinistrocardia
Sin Nombre virus (SNV)
sinoatrial (SA)
sinoatrial block
sinoatrial branch
sinoatrial bundle in heart
sinoatrial conduction time (SACT)
sinoatrial exit block
sinoatrial heart block
sinoatrial node (SA or S-A node)
   Flack
   Koch
sinoatrial node artery
sinoatrial node dysfunction
sinoatrial node infarction
sinoatrial rhythm
sinoauricular heart block
sinoauricular node
sinobronchitis
sinopulmonary infection
sinotubular junction
sinus
   accessory
   aortic
   aortic valve
   carotid
   coronary (CS)
   coronary (of Valsalva)
   distal coronary (DCS)
   left coronary

sinus *(cont.)*
   middle coronary (MCS)
   noncoronary
   oblique
   pericardial
   Petit
   proximal coronary (PCS)
   pulmonary
   subeustachian
   transverse
   Valsalva
   venous
sinus arrest
sinus aneurysm, aortic
sinus arrhythmia
sinus beat, post-PVC
sinus bradycardia
sinus cycle length (SCL)
sinus exit block
sinus impulse
sinus-initiated QRS complex
sinus irregularity (SI)
sinusitis-bronchiectasis syndrome
sinus mechanism
sinus nodal reentry
sinus node automaticity
sinus node depression
sinus node dysfunction
sinus node recovery time, corrected
sinus node reentry
sinus of Morgagni
sinus of pulmonary trunk
sinus of Valsalva
sinus of venae cavae
sinusoidal irregular rhythm
sinusoids
sinus pause
sinus retroperfusion, coronary
sinus rhythm, normal
sinus rhythm return
sinus segment
sinus septum

sinus slowing
sinus tachycardia
sinus venarum cavarum
sinus venosus defect
sinus venosus syndrome
sinus venous defect
SiPAP
Sirius catheter
Sirius stent
sirolimus
SIS (simultaneous individual stapling)
   lobectomy
site
   arrhythmogenic
   de-airing
   saphenectomy
SiteGuard MVP transparent adhesive
   film dressing
Site-Rite and Site-Rite II ultrasound
   system
site of maximal intensity
sitting-up view
situs
   atrial
   D-loop ventricular
   L-loop ventricular situs
situs ambiguus of atria
situs atrialis solitus
situs concordance
situs inversus totalis
situs solitus
   atrial
   visceral
situs viscerum inversus
SIVD (subcortical ischemic vascular
   dementia)
sivelestat
sixth intercostal space
60° left anterior oblique projection
sizer, prosthetic valve
sizing, balloon
Sjögren syndrome

SK (streptokinase)
skeletal breathing
skeletal emphysema
skin blanching with pressure
skin prick test, DPT-positive
skin, taut
skin testing
skin wheal (*not* weal)
skin wheal diameter
Skinny dilatation catheter
Skinny over-the-wire balloon catheter
SkinTegrity hydrogel dressing
skipped beat
skipping a heartbeat
skodaic bruit
skodaic resonance
skodaic tympany
Skoda sign
sl (slight)(ly)
Slalom balloon dilatation catheter
slate-gray cyanosis
slave balloon
slaved programmed electrical
    stimulation
slaved PS
SLE (systemic lupus erythematosus)
sleep apnea, obstructive
sleep-disordered breathing (SDB)
sleep dysfunction
sleeve pneumonectomy
slew rate (SR)
SLF stent
SLF vascular prosthesis
slice
    apical short-axis
    basal short-axis
    horizontal long-axis
    mid-ventricular short-axis
    short-axis
    tomographic
    vertical long-axis
slice format

sliding plasty
Slim-Cath catheter
SlimPort implantable vascular access
    port
sling
    pericardial
    pulmonary artery
    vascular
sling ring complex
Slinky catheter
Slinky catheter PTCA (percutaneous
    transluminal coronary angioplasty)
slip-in connection
slipping rib syndrome
slip-tip connector
slitlike costomediastinal recess
slitlike lumen
slitlike opening
slitlike orifice
slit-shaped vessel lumen
sliver of aneurysmal wall
SLMD (symptomatic left main
    disease)
slope
    closing (on echo)
    D to E (of mitral valve)
    decreased E to F (E-F)
    disappearance
    E to F (of mitral valve)
    flat diastolic
    flattened E to F
    opening (on echo)
    ST/HR (ST segment/heart rate)
slope of valve opening
sloping, downward
slot blot analysis
sloughing of skin from necrosis
slow-channel blocking drugs
slow-fast atrioventricular node reentry
    tachycardia
slow-fast tachycardia
slow filling wave

slow-flow lesions
slow-flow malformation
slow-flow vascular anomaly
slowing of electrical conduction
slowing of heart rate
slow inspiration, inhalation by
slow-pathway conduction
slow-pathway modification
slow-reacting substance of anaphylaxis
    (SRS-A)
SLP (systolic pressure determination)
SLS (Spectranetics laser sheath) laser
SLT (single-lung transplant) recipient
sludging of blood
sluggishly flowing blood
slush
    ice
    topical cooling with ice
Sly syndrome
SM (systolic murmur)
SMA (Sequential Multiple Analyzer)
        chemistry panel (SMA-6,
        SMA-12, SMA-17, SMA-20)
    albumin
    alkaline phosphatase
    ALT (alanine aminotransferase)
        (formerly SGPT)
    AST (aspartate aminotransferase)
        (formerly SGOT)
    BUN (blood urea nitrogen)
    calcium
    cholesterol
    creatinine
    glucose
    LDH (lactic dehydrogenase)
    phosphorus
    SGOT (now AST)
    SGPT (now ALT)
    sodium
    total protein
    triglyceride
    uric acid

SMA (superior mesenteric artery)
small airway dysfunction
small airways stretch receptors
small airways study, peripheral
small aorta syndrome
small cardiac vein
small-cell carcinoma of the lung
small-cell lung cancer (SCLC)
small-cuff syndrome
small defibrillating patch
small feminine aorta
small-lunged emphysema
Small Particle Aerosol Generator
    nebulizer
small patch lead
small rake retractor
small saphenous vein
small-vessel stenting
small water-hammer pulse
SMAP (systemic mean arterial
    pressure)
smart defibrillator
SmartFlow device
smart foam dressing
Smart-Inflate diagnostic ultrasonog-
    raphy
Smart-Inflate heart monitor
SmartKard digital Holter system
SmartMist asthma management system
SmartNeedle
SmartScore
smear, fungal
Smec balloon catheter
Smeloff-Cutter ball-cage prosthetic
    valve
Smeloff prosthetic valve
smile (or smiling) incision
SMIP (sustained maximal inspiratory
    pressure)
Smith-Lemli-Opitz syndrome
Smith-Magenis syndrome
Smith murmur

Smith scissors
Smith sign
Smithwick hook
smoke inhalation
smokelike echoes
smoker respiratory syndrome
smoker's cough
smoking, pack-years of cigarette
smooth excimer laser coronary angio-
    plasty (SELCA)
smooth glistening membrane
smooth muscle, reactive disease
SMPV (superior mesenteric-portal
    vein)
SMT (septomarginal trabecula)
SMV (superior mesenteric vein)
Sn-mesoporphyrin (SnMP)
Sn-protoporphyrin
snake graft
snap
    high-pitched opening
    mitral opening
    opening (OS)
    palpable opening
    valvular
snare, caval
sneezing
    frequent
    paroxysmal
    repeated
    repetitive
    staccato
Snider match test for pulmonary
    ventilation
sniffles
sniff test
snorer, nonapneic
snowman deformity
Snowden-Pencer forceps
Snowden-Pencer scissors
snowman appearance of heart
    (on x-ray)

snowman heart
snowplow effect
snowplow occlusion
SNRT (sinus node recovery time)
snuff taker's pituitary disease
snugged down, suture
snugly
SNV (Sin Nombre virus)
SO_2 (oxygen saturation)
soaked in thrombin, coil
soaker catheter
soap bubble appearance of exudate
SOB (shortness of breath)
SOD (superoxide dismutase), recombi-
    nant human
sodium
    decreased exchangeable
    erythrocyte
    metrizoate
sodium channel blocker
sodium concentration, 24-hour urine
sodium content of foods
sodium-induced asthma
sodium nitroprusside
sodium pertechnetate Tc 99m
sodium retention
sodium-restricted diet
Sofsorb absorptive dressing
Soft-Cell catheter
SoftCloth absorptive dressing
soft friction rub
SOF-T guidewire
Softgut surgical chromic suture
soft heart sounds
Softip diagnostic catheter
soft murmur (low grade)
Soft N Dry Merocel sponge
soft pulse
Softouch guiding catheter
Soft-Vu Omni flush catheter
Sof-Wick drain sponge
Sof-Wick dressings

soft x-ray
Solcotrans drainage/reinfusion system
soldier's heart syndrome
soldier's patches of pericardium
soldier's spot
soleal vein
soleal vein thrombosis
soleus muscle
solid edema of lung
solid pulmonary nodule (SPN)
solitary lung nodule
solitary mass
solitary pulmonary nodule
solitus
   atrial situs
   situs
   visceral situs
Solo catheter with Pro/Pel coating
Solomon syndrome
SoloSite nonsterile hydrogel dressing
SoloSite wound gel
solution (see also *cardioplegic solu-
   tions*; *medications*)
   albumin
   antibiotic
   bacitracin-kanamycin
   balanced salt
   bibiotic
   Buckberg
   carbonated saline
   cardioplegic
   Celsior organ preservation
   cold blood hyperkalemic
      cardioplegic
   cold cardioplegic
   cold lactated Ringer
   cold potassium
   cold topical saline
   cooling
   colloid
   crystalloid cardioplegic
   dextran and saline

solution *(cont.)*
   dextran, saline, papaverine, and
      heparin
   E2F Decoy
   fixative
   Gey
   hand-agitated
   Hank balanced salt
   hemostatic
   heparinized saline
   HK-Cardiosol organ preservation
   hyperkalemic crystalloid
      cardioplegic
   hyperosmotic
   ice slush
   ice-cold physiologic
   intracellular-like, calcium-bearing
      crystalloid (ICS)
   leukocyte-depleted terminal blood
      cardioplegic
   Lugol fixative
   Melrose
   Monsel's hemostatic
   Myers
   normal saline (NS)
   papaverine
   physiologic
   potassium chloride
   povidone-iodine
   priming
   saline
   Sclavo PPD solution (tuberculin
      purified protein derivative)
   uncrystallized cardioplegic
   University of Wisconsin (for donor
      heart preservation)
somatic symptoms
somatic tremor
somatomedin C
Somatom Plus-S CT Scanner
Somatom Volume Zoom computed
   tomography system

somatostatin
somatotropin-releasing hormone
somnolence
Sonazoid ultrasound contrast agent
Sondergaard cleft (interatrial groove)
Sones arteriography technique
Sones brachial cutdown technique
Sones cardiac catheter
Sones cardiac catheterization
Sones Cardio-Marker catheter
Sones cineangiography technique
Sones coronary arteriography
Sones coronary cineangiography
Sones guidewire
Sones Hi-Flow catheter
Sones selective coronary arteriography
sonicated albumin microbubbles
sonicated contrast medium
Sonifer sonicating system
SonoCT (real-time spatial compound
    imaging)
sonogram
sonographically guided human
    thrombin injection
sonography
    Acuson computed
    duplex pulsed-Doppler sonography
    sonolucent area or zone
SonoHeart handheld digital echocar-
    diography system
sonorous rales
sonorous rhonchi
Sonos 500 2.5 MHz ultrasonographic
    transducer
sonotherapy, intravascular
Soprano cryoablation system
SorbaView composite wound dressing
Sorin dual head pump module
Sorin heart-lung machine
Sorin pacemaker
Sorin prosthetic valve
soroche

SOS guidewire
Soto USCI balloon
souffle
    cardiac
    continuous mammary
    funic
    funicular
    mammary (sound on auscultation)
    systolic mammary
sound (see also *bruit, fremitus,*
    murmur, rale)
    abnormal heart
    absent breath
    adventitious breath
    adventitious heart
    adventitious lung
    A_2 (aortic closure) heart
    amphoric breath
    aortic ejection
    aortic second
    atrial
    atrial gallop
    auscultatory
    bandbox
    Beatty-Bright friction
    bell
    bellows
    booming diastolic rumble
    bottle
    brass
    breath
    bronchial breath
    bronchovesicular breath
    cannon
    cat mewing
    cavernous breath
    clapping
    clear ringing musical note
    cogwheel breath
    coin
    cracked-pot sound
    crackling

sound *(cont.)*
  diastolic
  discrete
  distant breath
  distant heart
  dull wooden nonmusical note
  eddy
  ejection (E)
  faint breath
  filing
  first heart (S_1)
  fixed splitting of second heart
  flapping
  flapping rustle
  fourth heart (S_4)
  friction
  gallop
  heart
  hippocratic
  humming top
  inspiratory-expiratory breath
  Korotkoff
  Lermans-Means systolic grating
  light crackling
  M_1 (mitral valve closure) heart
  mammary souffle
  metallic
  muffled breath
  muffled heart
  new leather
  P_2 (pulmonic closure) heart
  pacemaker heart
  paradoxical splitting of second
  heart
  paradoxically split S_2
  parchment
  parchment rubbing
  peacock
  percussion
  pericardial friction
  physiologic heart
  physiologic splitting of second heart

sound *(cont.)*
  physiologic third heart
  pistol-shot
  pistol-shot femoral
  pleuritic
  popping
  prominent third
  prosthetic valve
  pulmonary component of second
    heart
  pulmonic ejection
  rasping
  rattling
  reduced
  reduced breath
  ringing
  rippling
  rubbing
  rustle of silk
  rustling
  S_1 (first heart sound)
  S_2 (second heart sound)
  S_3 (third heart sound)
  S_4 (fourth heart sound)
  sail
  sawing
  second heart (S_2)
  second pulmonic
  shaking
  single second heart
  snapping
  souffle (heart puffing sound)
  splashing
  split
  split apical first
  succussion
  summation (SS)
  suppressed
  systolic ejection
  systolic grating
  T_1 (tricuspid valve closure) heart
  tambour (drum)

sound *(cont.)*
    third heart (S$_3$)
    tick-tack
    to-and-fro
    transitory
    tubular breath
    tumor plop heart
    tympanitic
    ubiquitous
    valvular ejection
    ventricular filling (third heart
      sound)
    ventricular gallop
    vesicular breath
    water-wheel
    weak heart
    white
    widely split second heart
    wood
sound reflector
source, defibrillator power
Southern blot analysis or test
Southern blot hybridization
Southwestern blot test
S/P (status post)
space
    anatomical dead
    antecubital
    anterior mediastinal
    apical air (on x-ray)
    Burns
    dead
    echo-free
    epicardial
    fifth intercostal
    first intercostal
    fourth intercostal
    free pericardial
    His perivascular
    Holzknecht
    intercellular
    intercostal

space *(cont.)*
    interpleural
    interscalene
    interstitial
    intravascular
    left fifth intercostal
    left intercostal (LICS)
    peribronchial alveolar
    pericardial
    pleural
    Poiseuille
    popliteal
    posterior septal
    retrocardiac
    retropancreatic preaortic
    right first intercostal
    right second intercostal
    second intercostal
    seventh intercostal
    sixth intercostal
    third intercostal
Spacekeeper retractor
Spacemaker balloon dissector
space-occupying lesions
Space-OR flexible internal retractor
spade-shaped valvulotome
Spanish toxic oil syndrome
sparkling appearance of myocardium
spasm
    bronchial
    catheter-induced
    catheter-induced coronary artery
    coronary
    coronary artery (CAS)
    diffuse arteriolar
    inspiratory
    postbypass
    respiratory
    vascular
    venous
spasm of bronchial smooth muscles
spasmodic croup

spasmodic rhinorrhea
spastic contractions
spastic heart
spatial vectorcardiography
spatula, spatulated, spatulating
SPCA (serum prothrombin conversion
    accelerator)
specificity, sensing
specimen collecting device
specimen, respiratory tract
speckle, blood
speckled pattern
SPECT (single photon emission
    computed tomography)
SPECT thallium scan
SPECT thallium scintigram
SPECT thallium test
SPECT tomography
Spectracef (cefditoren pivoxil)
Spectraflex pacemaker
spectral Doppler
spectral analysis
spectral pattern
Spectranetics excimer laser for
    coronary angioplasty
Spectranetics laser sheath (SLS)
Spectraprobe-Max probe
Spectrax programmable Medtronic
    pacemaker
Spectrax SXT pacemaker
spectrofluorometry
spectroscopy
    fluorescence
    magnetic resonance
    proton
SpectRx test to measure LDL and
    HDL cholesterol levels
specular echo
Speedy balloon catheter
spell
    anginal
    cyanotic hypoxic

spell (cont.)
    fainting
    hypercyanotic
    hypoxemic
    hypoxic
    pallid breath-holding
    sneezing
    syncopal
    tetrad
    violent sneezing
Spencer stitch curved scissors
Spens syndrome
SpermaTex preshaped mesh
sphenoidal sinusitis
spherical lesion
spherical mass
spherocytosis, hereditary
sphincter incontinence
sphingolipidosis
Sphygmocorde
sphygmography
sphygmomanometer, cuff
SPIDER (steady-state projection
    imaging with dynamic echo-train
    readout)
spider angioma (pl. angiomata)
spider cells
spider nevus (pl. nevi)
spider x-ray view
spike
    atrial
    H and H' (H prime)
    sensing
    wave
spike-and-dome configuration
spike-dome configuration
spike-Q interval
spiking fever
spin density
spin-echo imaging sequence
spin-echo sequence
spinal needle

spinal sign in pleurisy
spindle, aortic
spindle-shaped arterial
spindly limbs
Spinhaler turbo-inhaler
spinocerebellar ataxia
spiral dissection
spiral position
spiraling dissection
spirals, Curschmann
spiral XCT (x-ray computed tomography) scanner
spiral x-ray computed tomography (SXCT)
Spira-Valve implantable device
Spirexx stent and stent delivery system
Spiriva (tiotropium)
spirochetal infection
spirochetal myocarditis
spirometer
    incentive
    MultiFEV
    SpiroScan
    Tissot
spirometry
    FEV_1 (forced expiratory volume in 1 second)
    full-volume loop
    FVC (forced vital capacity)
    incentive
    MMEF (mean maximal expiratory flow)
spirometry after bronchodilator
spirometry before bronchodilator
spironolactone
SpiroScan spirometer
spitting up blood
Spitz-Holter valve
splanchnic vasculature
splanchnic vessels
splashing bruit

splash, succussion
splenic flexure syndrome
splenic follicular arteriolitis
splenic hilar vasculitis
splenomegaly
    Opitz thrombophlebitic
    persistent
    postcardiotomy lymphocytic
splenorenal anastomosis
splenorenal arterial bypass graft
splenosis, thoracic
splint, pneumatic
splinter hemorrhage
splinting of the chest
splinting on deep breathing
splinting respirations
splint-type tear
split apical first sound
split sheath catheter
splitting
    audible
    fixed
    narrow expiratory
    narrow inspiratory
    paradoxic
    paradoxic respiratory
    physiologic
    plaque
    reversed
    widened respiratory
splitting of S_1 or S_2 heart sounds
splitting of first heart sound, wide
splitting of second heart sound, wide
SPN (solid pulmonary nodule)
sponge
    Collastat collagen hemostatic
    4 x 4
    laparotomy
    papaverine-soaked
    Ray-Tec
    stick
    Surgifoam absorbable gelatin

sponge and needle counts
sponge dissector
spongiosa of mitral valve
spontaneous breathing
spontaneous cardioversion
spontaneous closure of defect
spontaneous coronary artery dissection
  (SCAD)
spontaneous echo contrast
spontaneous infantile ductal aneurysm
spontaneous pneumothorax
spontaneous regression
spontaneous remission
spontaneous subsidence
spontaneous tension pneumothorax
spontaneous thrombosis
spontaneous transient vasoconstriction
spoon forceps
spoonlike protrusion of leaflets
sporadic hypertriglyceridemia
spores, fungal hyphae and
spot
  Brushfield
  cold
  hot
  milk
  Roth
  soldier's
  Tardieu
spot-film fluorography
Spotorno coronary stent
Spotorno prosthesis
Spotorno suture
Spotorno valve
Spotorno vascular prosthesis
Spotorno vascular stent
spray-as-you-go anesthesia technique
spray, lidocaine
spreader
  Bailey rib
  Burford rib
  Burford-Finochietto rib

spreader *(cont.)*
  Davis rib
  DeBakey rib
  Favaloro-Morse rib
  Finochietto rib
  Haight rib
  Harken rib
  Lemmon sternal
  Lilienthal rib
  Medicon
  Miltex rib
  Morse sternal
  Nelson rib
  Rehbein rib
  Reinhoff-Finochietto rib
  Tuffier rib
  Weinberg rib
  Wilson rib
Spring catheter with Pro/Pel coating
spring-loaded vascular stent
springwater cyst
spring-wire guide
spring-wire introduction syringe
Sprinter balloon catheter
Sprinter stent
Sprinter stent delivery system
Sprint Quattro Secure lead by
  Medtronic
spur, calcific
spurious findings
spurious polycythemia
spurious shocks
sputum (pl. sputa)
  abundant
  albuminoid
  blood-flecked
  blood-streaked
  blood-tinged
  bloody
  brick-red in color
  brown
  chunky

sputum *(cont.)*
 clear
 clear viscous
 copious
 dark
 fetid
 foul-tasting
 frothy at the top (of layered)
 gelatinous
 gelatinous mottled
 globular
 grayish
 green
 green-yellow
 greenish and turbid in the middle
  (of layered)
 greenish-yellow
 icteric
 moss-agate
 mucoid
 mucopurulent
 nonfetid
 nummular
 opalescent
 pink
 pinkish
 prune juice
 purulent
 putrid
 red-streaked
 reddish brown
 ropy
 rubbery
 rusty
 scant, scanty
 tenacious
 thick
 thick with pus at the bottom (of
  layered)
 viscid
 viscous
 watery

sputum *(cont.)*
 white
 whitish
 yellow
 yellowish-green
sputum aeruginosum
Spyglass angiography catheter
SpyroDerm dressing
S-QRS interval
SQS-20 subcuticular skin stapler
Squirt wound irrigation system
SR guidewire
stabilization device, acrobat heart
Stabilizer Plus steerable guidewire
Stabilizer steerable guidewire
Stabilizer XS steerable guidewire
Staccato drug delivery device
STAE (subsegmental transcatheter
 arterial embolization)
stage, Brunnstróm
staged closure
stagnation, blood flow
stain, Wright's stain
standard error
Staphylococcus epidermidis
staple
 En Garde
 Glycoprene surgical
 Lactoprene surgical
 Max-Prene surgical
 Osteoprene surgical
staple-line reinforcement buttress
stapled pulmonary resection
stapler
 anastomosis
 Endo-GIA suture
 Poly GIA
 Proximate flexible linear
 Proximate linear cutter surgical
 Roticulator
 SQS-20 subcuticular skin
static apnea

statin drugs
StatLock hemodialysis catheter
StatLock Universal Plus anchor of
    catheter
Stat Profile pHOx blood gas critical
    care analyzer
STAT-Site M Hgb test system
status asthmaticus
stay sutures
ST depression
steady-state projection imaging with
    dynamic echo-train readout (SPI-
    DER)
ST elevation
steal, carotid
steal phenomenon
steal syndrome
steam autoclaved
Steell murmur
steep left anterior oblique view
steep Trendelenburg position
steerable catheter
steerable electrode catheter
steerable guidewire system
steering, electronic independent beam
Steerocath-A ablation catheter
Steerocath catheter
Steerocath-Dx octapolar and valve
    mapping catheter
Steerocath-T ablation catheter
Steidele complex
Steidele syndrome
Steinert disease
stellar nevus
stellate ganglion block
stellectomy
Stellite ring material of prosthetic
    valve
stem
    AF (axillofemoral)
    axillofemoral (AF)
    left main (bronchus)

stem *(cont.)*
    main (carina)
    right main (bronchus)
stem bronchus
STE MI (ST-segment elevation in
    myocardial infarction)
stenocardia
stenosing ring of left atrium
stenosis (pl. stenoses)
    acquired mitral
    American Heart Association
        classification of
    aortic (AS)
    aortic valvular
    aortoiliac
    atypical aortic valve
    Austin Flint murmur of relative
        mitral
    bicuspid valvular aortic
    branch pulmonary
    bronchial
    buttonhole mitral
    calcific aortic
    calcific bicuspid valvular
    calcific mitral
    calcific senile aortic valvular
    calcific valvular
    carotid artery
    common pulmonary vein
    congenital aortic
    congenital aortic valvular
    congenital mitral valve
    congenital pulmonary
    congenital subaortic
    congenital subvalvular aortic
    congenital supravalvular aortic
    congenital tricuspid
    congenital valvular aortic
    coronary artery
    coronary luminal
    coronary ostial
    critical

stenosis *(cont.)*
   critical coronary
   critical valvular
   cross-sectional area
   culprit
   diffuse
   discrete
   discrete subaortic
   discrete subvalvular aortic (DSAS)
   dynamic subaortic
   eccentric
   external iliac
   femoropopliteal atheromatous
   fibromuscular subaortic
   fishmouth mitral
   fixed-orifice aortic
   flow-limiting
   focal
   focal eccentric
   granulation
   hemodynamically significant
   high-grade
   hypercalcemia supravalvular aortic
   hypertrophic infundibular
      subpulmonic
   hypertrophic subaortic
   idiopathic hypertrophic subaortic
      (IHSS)
   infrainguinal bypass
   infrarenal
   infundibular
   infundibular pulmonary
   infundibular pulmonic
   infundibular subpulmonic
   innominate artery
   interrenal
   linear
   luminal
   membranous
   membranous subvalvular aortic
   mitral (MS)
   mitral valve

stenosis *(cont.)*
   multifocal short
   muscular subaortic
   napkin-ring
   noncalcified
   noncalcified coronary
   noncritical
   nonrheumatic aortic
   nonrheumatic valvular aortic
   ostial
   peripheral arterial
   peripheral pulmonary
   peripheral pulmonary artery
      (PPAS)
   peripheral pulmonic
   post-PTCA
   postangioplasty
   preangioplasty
   pulmonary
   pulmonary artery
   pulmonary artery branch
   pulmonary valve
   pulmonary valvular
   pulmonary vein
   pulmonic (PS)
   pulmonic (with intact ventricular
      septum)
   relative mitral
   renal artery
   rheumatic aortic
   rheumatic aortic valvular
   rheumatic mitral
   rheumatic tricuspid
   segmental
   senescent aortic
   severe
   silent mitral
   subaortic
   subclavian artery
   subinfundibular pulmonary
   subpulmonary
   subpulmonic

stenosis *(cont.)*
    subpulmonic infundibular
    subtle mitral
    subvalvar aortic
    subvalvular aortic
    subvalvular congenital aortic
    supra-aortic
    supraclavicular aortic
    suprarenal
    supravalvar aortic
    supravalvular
    supravalvular aortic (SAS, SVAS)
    supravalvular pulmonic
    tapering
    tight
    tricuspid (TS)
    tricuspid valve
    true mitral
    tubular
    tunnel subaortic
    tunnel subvalvular aortic
    unicusp aortic
    valvar aortic
    valvular aortic
    valvular pulmonic
stenosis area
stenosis diameter
stenosis length
stenosis of coronary orifices
stenosis of saphenous vein
stenosis of unicuspid aortic valve
stenosis with a spastic component
stenotic but patent tricuspid valve
stenotic coronary artery
stenotic isthmus
stenotic lesion
stenotic valve
stent (see also *stent-graft*; *stenting*)
    Acculink self-expanding
    ACS Multi-Link coronary
    ACS OTW (over-the-wire) HP
      (high pressure) coronary

stent *(cont.)*
    ACS RX Multi-Link
    activated balloon expandable
      intravascular
    Ancure
    AngioStent balloon-expandable
    Angiotech
    balloon-expandable
    balloon-expandable, fixed tubular
      mesh stainless steel
    balloon-expandable flexible coil
    balloon-expandable intravascular
    balloon-expandable stainless steel
      (BE-SS)
    Bard XT coronary
    biodegradable
    BiodivYsio phosphorylcholine-
      coated coronary
    Biostent
    Bridge Assurant biliary
    BX Agile
    Bx Sonic balloon expandable
    BX Velocity Rx with Hepacoat
      balloon-expandable
    Bx Velocity sirolimus-coated
      coronary
    CardioCoil coronary
    Cardiovasc
    CBAS vascular
    Cerebrence
    coil vascular
    Constant
    Contour closed end
    Contour (with HydroPlus coating)
    Contour VL Percuflex
    Cordis coronary
    Cordis tantalum
    Cragg Endopro System 1
    CrossFlex LC coronary
    Cypher sirolimus-eluting
    Dacron
    DISA S-Flex coronary

stent *(cont.)*
 DoubleStrut
 Driver
 drug-eluting (DES)
 Dumon tracheobronchial
 EES (expandable esophageal stent)
 Elastalloy Ultraflex Strecker nitinol
 Endeavor
 endoluminal
 endovascular
 expandable coronary
 Express
 Express II coronary
 Fluency
 Fluency XX
 Fulcrum
 GenStent biologic therapy
 GFX coronary
 Gianturco
 Gianturco-Roubin flexible coil
 Guidant Multi-Link Tetra coronary
 Harrell Y
 heat-expandable
 helical coil
 Hepamed-coated Wiktor
 interdigitating coil
 Innovante
 InStent CarotidCoil
 InStent self-expanding and balloon
  expandable
 In-Time
 IntraCoil self-expanding nitinol
 intracoronary
 IntraStent DoubleStrut LD
 intravascular
 INX stainless steel
 IRIS coronary
 Jocath
 Jography
 Joguide
 Litespeed
 Luminexx biliary

stent *(cont.)*
 Mardis firm (with HydroPlus
  coating)
 Magic Wallstent
 Medivent vascular
 Medtronic AVE BeStent with
  Discrete Technology over-the-
  wire coronary
 Memotherm nitinol self-expanding
 metal
 Micro-Driver
 MicroStent II over-the-wire PTCA
 MINI Crown
 Mobius vascular
 Multilink Duet noncoated coronary
 Multilink Penta coronary
 Multilink Tetra coronary
 Navius
 NexStent carotid
 NIR
 NIR ON
 NIR Prince (or NIR pRINce)
 NIR with SOX over-the-wire
  coronary
 NIRflex coronary
 NIRoyal
 Niroyal Elite Monorail coronary
 nitinol thermal memory
 Omnir
 OmniStent
 Outcomes by Design
 Palmaz balloon-expandable
 Palmaz balloon-expandable iliac
 Palmaz vascular
 Palmaz-Schatz (PSS)
 Palmaz-Schatz coronary
 Paragon coronary
 percutaneous implantation of
  endovascular
 polymeric endoluminal paving
 Puzzle
 radioisotope

stent *(cont.)*
Radius coronary
Rapid Exchange (RX) coronary
Rapid Exchange (RX) vein graft
Rapid-Trak
RaptorRail
Roubin-Gianturco flexible coil
RX
Schatz-Palmaz tubular mesh
self-expandable
self-expanding
Sirius
SLF
Spirexx
Spotorno coronary
Spotorno vascular
spring-loaded
spring-loaded vascular
Sprinter
S660 small vessel
S670 coronary
S7 coronary
S7 with Discrete Technology
over-the-wire coronary
S7 with Discrete Technology
Rapid Exchange coronary
stainless steel mesh
Strecker balloon-expandable
Strecker tantalum
Stretch VL Flexima
Symbiant
Symbiot
Symphony
thermal memory
Thunder high scaffolding over-the-
wire vein graft
tracheal
Transiel vascular
T–Y tracheobronchial
Ultraflex self-expanding
Wallstent spring-loaded
VascuCoil peripheral vascular

stent *(cont.)*
Versafit
Wiktor
Wiktor balloon expandable
coronary
Wiktor GX coronary
wire-mesh self-expandable
XT radiopaque coronary
Xtent
Y
ZETA coronary
Zipper
zig-zag
stent asymmetry
stent delivery system, constant
stent deployment
stent embolization
stent expansion
stent fracture
stent-graft (also stent-grafting)
AneuRx stent-graft system
Aorfix
endovascular
Hemobahn nitinol
Jocath
Jography
Joguide
Talent LPS endoluminal
Tiason
Zenith AAA endovascular
stenting (see *stent*)
bailout
intracoronary
multivessel
small-vessel
stentless porcine aortic valve
stentless valve
Stentloc device for holding and release
stents during surgery
stent migration
stent-mounted allograft valves
stent-mounted heterograft valve

stent placement, intracoronary
stent recanalization
stent thrombosis
stent-vessel wall contact
stepdown unit
stepped-care antihypertensive regimen
stepped tissue dilator
stepup (or step-up)
Steri-Cath suction catheter
Steri-Drape
sterilely prepped and draped
Steri-Strips
Sterles sign
sternal angle
sternal angle of Louis
sternal articulations, pain in
sternal border
   left
   lower left
   mid-left
sternal cartilage
sternal edge
sternal joint
sternal lift
sternal marrow
sternal pleural reflection
sternal reflection
sternal splitting
sternal wire suture
Sternberg myocardial insufficiency
Sternberg pericarditis
Sternberg sign in pleurisy
Sterneedle tuberculin test
sternoclavicular angle
sternoclavicular joint
sternoclavicular junction
sternocleidomastoid muscle
sternocleidomastoid retraction
sternocostal joint
sternocostal surface of heart
sternohyoid muscle
sternopericardial ligament

sternothyroid muscle
sternotomy
   median
   midline
   primary median
   secondary median
   transverse
sternotomy incision
sternum
   anterior bowing of
   burning sensation over
   nonunion of operated
sternum retraction
sternutation
steroid dependent
steroid-eluting active fixation lead
steroidogenesis, adrenal
steroids
   adrenal
   parenteral
stertorous breathing
stertor, respiratory
Stertzer brachial guiding catheter
Stertzer-Myler extension wire
stethoscope
   bell of
   diaphragm of
   E-Scope electronic
   nuclear
Stevens-Johnson syndrome
Stewart-Hamilton technique for cardiac
   output
ST/HR slope (ST segment/heart rate)
STI (systolic time interval)
stick (venipuncture or arterial
   puncture)
stick tie
sticky exudate
sticky rales
Stifcore aspiration needle
stiff guidewire
stiff heart syndrome

stiffness
   aortic
   lung
   myocardial
   ventricular
stiff noncompliant lungs
stigmata of stroke
Still early systolic murmur
Stille-Crawford clamp
Stille-Giertz rib shears
Stille-Mayo scissors
still-heart surgery
Still murmur
Stimucath continuous nerve block
   catheter
stimulant, alpha-adrenoceptor
stimulation
   atrial single and double extra-
   inotropic
   programmed electrical (PES)
   programmed ventricular (PVS)
   slaved programmed electrical
   transvenous electrode (of atrium)
   ventricular single and double extrastimulation threshold of pacemaker
stimulator
   Bloom DTU 201 external
   Bloom programmable
   high-voltage pulsed galvanic
   InSync multisite cardiac
stimuli (pl. of stimulus)
   afterpotential
   ischemic
   noxious
   paired
   preconditioning ischemic
   premature
Stinger and Stinger S ablation
   catheters
Stinger SL catheter
S-T interval
stippling of lung fields

stitch (see *suture*)
St. Jude anuloplasty ring
St. Jude Aries 700 intra-aortic balloon
   pump
St. Jude bileaflet prosthetic valve
St. Jude composite valved conduit
St. Jude 4F Supreme catheter
St. Jude Medical bileaflet valve
St. Jude Medical composite graft
St. Jude Medical Lifestream
   centrifugal pump
St. Jude Medical Port-Access heart
   valve system
St. Jude valve prosthesis
Stockert/Shiley venous occluder
stockinette (stockinet)
stockings (also *support hose*)
   antiembolism
   compression
   elastic
   Jobst
   Jobst-Stride support
   Jobst-Stridette support
   pneumatic
   Sigvaris compression
   Stride support
   TED (thromboembolic disease)
   thigh-high compression
   Vairox high compression vascular
   Venes II medical
   Zimmer antiembolism support
Stokes-Adams attack
Stokes-Adams disease
Stokes-Adams syndrome
stoma
   coronary artery
   tracheostomy
stomach, thoracic
stone heart phenomenon
stone heart syndrome
Stoney method
Stoney technique

stony mass
stooped posture
stopcock
   Marquis
   three-way
stoppage of heart
stored energy
stored ventricular electrogram
Stormer balloon catheter
Stormer over-the-wire balloon dilatation catheter
Storq steerable guidewire
Storz bronchoscope
Storz infant bronchoscope
Storz needle cannula
straddling atrioventricular valves
straddling embolus
straddling of tricuspid valve
straight AP pelvic injection
straight-back syndrome
straight biopsy cup forceps
straight chest tube
straight flush percutaneous catheter
straight Hasson grasper
strain
   left ventricular (LV)
   right ventricular (RV)
   Valsalva
strain gauge, mercury-in-Silastic
straining heart muscle
strain pattern on EKG
strandy pulmonic infiltrate
strap cells
strap muscle
Stratasorb composite wound dressing
strategy
   alpha-stat
   pH-stat
stratified clot
stratified squamous epithelium
Stratus cardiac troponin I test
Strauss method

straw-colored fluid
straw, fungus-laden
streaking, coarse
streaks
   atherosclerotic fatty
   retinal angioid
stream, regurgitant
Strecker balloon-expandable stent
Strecker tantalum stent
strep throat
streptococcal carditis
streptococcal empyema
streptococcal M proteins
streptococcal pericarditis
streptococcal pleurisy
streptococcal sore throat
streptococcus (pl. streptococci)
   alpha
   anhemolytic
   beta
   gamma
   group A, B, C (etc.)
   hemolytic
   indifferent
   nonhemolytic
   viridans
Streptococcus (S.)
Streptococcus hemolyticus
Streptococcus mitis
Streptococcus pneumoniae
Streptococcus pyogenes
Streptococcus sanguis
Streptococcus scarlatinae
Streptococcus viridans
streptokinase (SK)
streptokinase resistance test
streptokinase thrombolysis
stress
   high-fluid shear
   mechanical
   occupational
   pharmacologic
   shear

stress erythrocytosis
stress images
stress imaging
stress management
stress perfusion and rest function by
    sestamibi-gated SPECT
stress perfusion scintigraphy
stress test
    dipyridamole thallium
    isometric exercise
    Persantine thallium
    submaximal
stress testing of cardiac response
stress thallium scan
stress thallium-201 myocardial
    imaging
stress ulcer
stress-induced
stress-injected sestamibi-gated SPECT
    with echocardiography
stretch, abnormal airways
STRETCH cardiac device
stretched lung
Stretch VL Flexima stent
stricture, anastomotic
Stride support stockings
stridor
    mild to moderate
    postextubation
    respiratory
stridulous breathing
striking asymmetry
stringlike bands of fibrous tissue
string-of-beads appearance
string sign
strip
    bovine pericardium
    cardiac monitor
    EKG monitor
    felt
    rhythm
    transtelephonic rhythm

stripe, paraspinal pleural
stripper
    Alexander rib
    Babcock vein
    Dunlop thrombus
    Emerson vein
    endarterectomy
    external vein
    internal vein
    Matson rib
    Mayo vein
    Meyer vein
    Nabatoff vein
    olive-tipped
    Trace vein
    vein
    Webb vein
stripper cable
stripper with bullet end
stripping
    pericardial
    varicose vein
stripping of multiple communicators
stripping of perforators and communi-
    cators
stroke
    cardiogenic embolic
    embolic
    thromboembolic (TE)
stroke distance, Doppler-derived
stroke ejection rate
stroke force
stroke index (SI)
stroke power
stroke syndrome
stroke volume (SV)
    adequate
    augmented
    back
    cardiac
    decreased
    reduced

stroke volume index (SVI)
stroke volume pump
stroke work
stroma
stroma-free hemoglobin solution
Strongyloides stercoralis infection
strongyloidiasis, pulmonary
structural weakness of bronchial wall
    supports
structure, pyramidal-shaped
structures
    central hilar
    superior mediastinal
Strully scissors
strut
    tricuspid valve
    valve
    valve outflow
strut chordae
Stryker saw
ST segment abnormality
ST segment alteration
ST (segment) and T wave abnor-
    malities (same as ST-T wave)
ST-segment changes
ST segment coved
ST segment depressed
ST-segment depression
    downsloping
    exercise-induced
    horizontal
    reciprocal
    slight
    upsloping
ST-segment displacement
ST-segment distortion
ST-segment elevated
ST-segment elevation
    marked
    slight
ST-segment isoelectric
ST-segment monitoring

ST-segment sagging
ST-segment shift
ST-segment upsloping
ST-segment vector forces
ST-T abnormalities
ST-T wave
ST-T wave changes
Stuart blood coagulation factor
Stuart-Prower blood coagulation factor
Stuart-Prower factor X deficiency
studding, pleural
study (see also *procedure, test, trial*)
    APRICOT (aspirin versus Coumadin
        in prevention of reocclusion and
        recurrent ischemia after success-
        ful thrombolysis)
    Bogalusa Heart
    cardiac wall motion
    cardiovascular radioisotope scan
        and function
    carotid duplex
    Coronary Artery Surgery (CASS)
    Doppler flow
    electrocardiogram microbubble
    electromagnetic blood flow
    electrophysiologic (EP)
    enzyme
    Familial Atherosclerosis Treatment
        (FATS)
    first-pass
    follow-up duplex
    Framingham
    gated blood pool
    gated blood (pool) cardiac wall
        motion
    GISSI (Italian Group for the Study
        of Survival in Myocardial
        Infarction)
    International (of Infarct Survival)
        (ISIS)
    MILIS (Multicenter Investigation
        for the Limitation of Infarct
        Size)

study *(cont.)*
  Oslo
  parameter
  periorbital Doppler
  PIOPED (Prospective Investigation
    of Pulmonary Embolism
    Diagnosis)
  pull-back
  spiral x-ray computed tomography
    (SXCT)
  STILE (Surgery versus Thrombo-
    lysis for Ischemia of the Lower
    Extremity)
  stress perfusion scintigraphy
  TIMI-IIA (Thrombolysis in
    Myocardial Infarction)
  TIMI-IIB (Thrombolysis in
    Myocardial Infarction)
  TOPS (Treatment of Post-
    Thrombolytic Stenoses)
  virology
  wall motion
stump, bronchial
stump ligature in vascular surgery
stump of a resected bronchus
stump pressure
stump-related neovascularity
stunning, myocardial
stuporous
Sturge-Weber syndrome
ST vector
stylet
  blunt
  straight
  transseptal
Stylus cardiovascular suture
Stypven time test for deficiency
  of factor X
sub (subendocardial)
subacute allergic pneumonia
subacute bacterial endocarditis (SBE)
subacute bronchopneumonia

subacute cardiac tamponade
subacute constrictive pericarditis
subacute interstitial myocarditis
subacute mountain sickness
subacute stent thrombosis (SAT)
subadventitial plane
subadventitial tissue
subanular mattress sutures
subanular placement of sutures
subanular region
subaortic curtain
subaortic glands
subaortic muscle
subaortic resection
subaortic stenosis, discrete
subarachnoid hemorrhage, diffuse
subatmospheric pressure
subcapsular hematoma
subcarinal area
subcarinally
subclavia, ansa
subclavian approach for cardiac
  catheterization
subclavian artery
subclavian artery stenosis
subclavian flap aortoplasty (SFA)
subclavian junction
subclavian loop
subclavian peel-away sheath
subclavian-pulmonary shunt
subclavian steal syndrome (SSS)
subclavian turndown technique
subclavian vein, blind percutaneous
  puncture of
subclavian vein catheterization
subclavicular approach
subclavicular area
subcommissural suture anuloplasty of
  neoaortic valve
subcoronary aortic valve implantation
subcortical intracerebral hemorrhage
subcortical ischemic vascular dementia
  (SIVD)

subcostal approach
subcostal artery
subcostal branch
subcostal nerve
subcostal retractions, mild
subcostal window
subcrepitant rales
subcutaneous array electrode
subcutaneous emphysema
subcutaneous hemangioma
subcutaneous patch
subcutaneous patch electrode
subcutaneous pocket
subcutaneous sutures
subcutaneous tissue
subcutaneous tunnel
subcutaneous veins
subcuticular closure
subcuticular layer
subcuticular skin closure
subcuticular suture
subdermal suture
subendocardial fibroelastosis
subendocardial infarct
subendocardial infarction (SEI)
subendocardial injury
subendocardial ischemia
subendocardial myocardial infarction
subendocardial necrosis
subendocardial resection
subendocardial sclerosis
subendocardium
subendothelial hyalinization
suberosis
    cork worker's
    maple-bark worker's
subeustachian sinus
subfascial endoscopic perforating vein
    surgery (SEPS)
subfascial endoscopic perforator
    surgery (SEPS)
subfascially

subglottic area
subglottic edema
subinfundibular pulmonary stenosis
subintimal cleavage plane
subintimal dissection
subisthmic coarctation, atypical
subjective symptoms
sublingual nitroglycerin
sublingual varices
submassive pulmonary embolism
submaximal exercise
submaximal exercise test
submaximal stress test
submersion syndrome
Sub-Microinfusion catheter
submucosal arterial malformation
submucous resection
submuscular patch lead
suboptimal cardiac reserve
suboptimal position
suboptimal results
suboptimal runoff
suboptimal visualization
suboptimally visualized
subpectoral implantation of pulse
    generator
subpectoral pocket
subperiosteal resection
subphrenic abscess
subpleural blanketing technique
subpleural bleb
subpleural curvilinear lines
subpulmonary conus underdevelop-
    ment
subpulmonary ventricular septal defect
subpulmonic fluid
subpulmonic infundibular stenosis
subpulmonic obstruction
subpulmonic outflow
Subramanian clamp
subrectus placement
subsegment of lung

subsegmental bronchus
subsegmental perfusion abnormality
subsegmental transcatheter arterial
     embolization (STAE)
subsegments, right middle lobe
subsidence, spontaneous
substances, paramagnetic
substernal angle
substernal burning discomfort
substernal chest pain
substernal discomfort
substernal pain
substernal retractions
substitute, oxygenated perfluorocarbon
     blood
subtherapeutic theophylline level
subtle mitral stenosis
subtotal graft excision
subtotal lesion
subtraction, digital
Subtraction Ictal SPECT Co-registered
     to MRI (SISCOM) imaging system
subtraction films, manual
subvalvular aneurysm
subvalvular aortic obstruction
subvalvular aortic stenosis
subvalvular congenital aortic stenosis
subvalvular obstruction
subxiphoid approach
subxiphoid echocardiography view
subxiphoid implantation
subxiphoid incision
subxiphoid view
successful conversion
succussion sound
succussion splash
sucking pneumothorax
Sucquet-Hoyer anastomosis
Sucquet-Hoyer canal
suction
     Frazier
     nasotracheal
     underwater seal and

suction bottle
suction line, aortic vent
suction tip
     Andrews
     Yankauer
suction-type electrode
sudden blockage of coronary artery
sudden cardiac death (SCD)
sudden death, adult
sudden infant death syndrome (SIDS)
suffocating chest pain
suffocating sensation
suffocating thoracic dystrophy
Sugita right angle aneurysm clamp
Sugiura vascular surgery procedure for
     esophageal varices
suitable candidate
sulcus (pl. sulci)
     atrioventricular
     posterior interventricular
     pulmonary
sulcus terminalis
sulfasalazine-induced pulmonary
     infiltrates
sulfonamides
sulfonylureas
sulfur colloid, technetium bound to
SULP II catheter
Sumida cardioangioscope
summation beat
summation gallop (S_3 and S_4)
summation sound (SS)
summer asthma
summit, ventricular septal
sump catheter
sump drain
sump pump
Sundt-Kees clip for aneurysms
Sundt shunt
Super Arrow-Flex central venous
     catheter
superdominant left anterior descending
     artery

superficial angioma
superficial breast phlebitis
superficial cardiac dullness
superficial cardiac plexus
superficial crepitation
superficial femoral artery
superficial femoral artery occlusion
superficial femoral vein
superficial posterior compartment
superficial pseudoaneurysm chamber
superficial vein
superficial vein reflux
superimposed bronchial infection
superimposed mycoplasma pneumonia
superimposed pulmonary infection
superior border of heart
superior border of rib
superior bronchus
superior caval defect
superior caval obstruction
superior costotransverse ligament
superior epigastric artery
superior genicular artery
superior intercostal artery
superior intercostal vein
superior lobe of lung
superior margin of inferior rib
superior marginal defect
superior mediastinal structures
superior mediastinum
superior mesenteric artery (SMA)
superior mesenteric artery blood flow
(Qsma)
superior mesenteric artery resistance
(Rsma)
superior mesenteric artery syndrome
superior mesenteric-portal vein
(SMPV)
superior mesenteric vein (SMV)
superior phrenic branch
superior pulmonary vein
superior segment

superior thoracic aperture
superior thyroid artery
superior vena cava lead
superior vena cava obstruction
superior vena cava, penetrating injury
to
superior vena cava (SVC) syndrome
Super-9 guiding cardiac device
supernormal conduction
supernormal excitation
superoinferior heart
superolaterally
superolateral portal
superoxide dismutase (SOD), recombinant human
superselective embolization
SuperStat hemostatic agent
superstiff wire
SuperStitch
SuperTorque diagnostic catheter
SuperTorque Plus diagnostic catheter
super stress test
supersystemic pulmonary artery
pressure
supervene
supine bicycle exercise treadmill
supine hypotensive syndrome
supine hypotensive syndrome of
pregnancy
supplemental oxygen
Supple Peri-Guard patch
supply
accessory blood
collateral
support
hemodynamic
inotropic
mechanical circulatory
mechanical ventilatory
pump
temporary percutaneous cardiopulmonary
ventilatory

support hose (see *stockings*)
supportive therapy
suppressed breath sounds
suppressed cough reflex
suppressed plasma renin activity
suppression
    overdrive
    renin
suppression of arrhythmia
suppression of breath sounds
suppurative lung disease
suppurative pericarditis
suppurative phlebitis
suppurative pleurisy
suppurative pulmonary infection
supra-anular constriction
supra-anular suture ring
supra-aortic ridge
supra-aortic Takayasu arteritis
supra-aortic stenosis
supra-aortic trunk
supracardiac shunt
supracardiac type total anomalous
    venous return
supraceliac aorta
supraceliac aorta-femoral artery
    bypass graft
supraceliac aorta-visceral artery bypass
    graft
supraceliac aortic bypass graft
supraceliac aortofemoral bypass graft
supraclavicular aortic stenosis,
    uncomplicated
supraclavicular lymph nodes
supraclavicular murmur
supraclavicular nerve
supraclavicular node
supraclavicular systolic murmur
supraclavicular triangle
supraclinoid internal carotid artery
supracoronary ridge
supracristal defect

supracristal septal defect
supracristal ventricular defect
supracristal ventricular septal defect
supradiaphragmatic aorta
supraglottic edema
supra-Hisian (or suprahisian) block
supramanubrial systolic thrill
supramesocolic
suprapleural membrane
suprarenal aneurysm, mycotic
suprarenal stenosis
suprasternal bulging
suprasternal notch
suprasternal notch incision
suprasternal notch thrill
suprasternal notch view on echocar-
    diogram
suprasternal retraction on inspiration
suprasternal window
supravalvar aortic stenosis
supravalvar aortic stenosis syndrome
supravalvar ring
supravalvular aortic stenosis (SAS,
    SVAS)
    Brom repair of
    congenital
supravalvular aortic stenosis syndrome
supravalvular aortogram
supravalvular mitral stenosis
supravalvular pulmonic stenosis
supraventricular arrhythmia (SVA)
supraventricular crest (SVC)
supraventricular ectopic levels
supraventricular ectopic pacemaker
supraventricular rhythm
supraventricular tachyarrhythmia
    (SVT)
supraventricular tachycardia (SVT),
    inducible sustained orthodromic
supraventricular tachydysrhythmias
supraventricularis, crista
Supreme electrophysiology catheter

SureCuff for catheter fixation
SurePress compression dressing or
    wrap
Suresite transparent adhesive film
    dressing
surface active extract of saline lavage
    of bovine lungs surface coils
surface cooling initiated by circulating
    water
surface, endothelial
surface-induced deep hypothermia
surface phagocytosis
surface tension of lungs
surfactant (see also *medications*)
    bovine lavage extract
    Curosurf (poractant alfa)
    Exosurf (colfosceril palmitate)
    heterologous
    homologous
    human amniotic fluid derived
    lung
    natural
    pulmonary
    Survanta
    synthetic
surfactant activity
surfactant deficiency
surfactant depletion
Surfit ("sure-fit") adhesive
surgery (see *operation*)
    beating-heart
    invasive
    lung volume reduction
    minimally invasive (MIS)
    palliative
    still-heart
    video-assisted thoracic (VATS)
surgical cardiac tamponade
surgical emphysema
surgical extirpation
surgical field
surgical intensive care unit

surgical intervention
surgically curable hypertension
surgically implanted hemodialysis
    catheter (SIHC)
surgically induced complete heart
    block
Surgical Nu-Knit hemostatic material
surgical rescue
surgical revascularization
surgical stumps of bronchi
surgical venous interruption
surgical wedge resection
Surgicel gauze
Surgidac braided polyester suture
    material
Surgidine
Surgifoam absorbable gelatin sponge
Surgilase 150 laser
Surgilase CO_2 laser
Surgilene suture
Surgilon suture
Surg-I-Loop
Surgi-Prep (Betadine, povidone-iodine)
Surgitool 200 prosthetic valve
Survanta pulmonary surfactant for
    neonates
surveillance
susceptible, susceptibility
suspended heart syndrome
sustained anterior parasternal motion
sustained apical impulse
sustained hypertension
sustained left ventricular heave
sustained maximal inspiratory pressure
    (SMIP)
sustained or nonsustained reciprocating
    tachycardia
SutraSilk nonabsorbable silk suture
Sutter-Smeloff heart valve prosthesis
suture (also *stitch*)
    absorbable
    alternating blue and white mattress

suture *(cont.)*
  anchoring
  angle
  atraumatic
  Auto Suture
  basting
  Biosyn suture
  black
  blue and white mattress
  blue and white Tycron
  Bondek absorbable
  braided
  braided silk
  bridle
  buried
  buttressed mattress
  Caprosyn
  cardiovascular silk
  catgut
  chromic
  chromic catgut
  circular
  circumferential
  CloseSure
  coated
  collagen
  collagen absorbable
  continuous
  cotton
  Dacron
  Dacron-bolstered
  Dagrofil
  deep
  Deklene
  Dermalene
  Dermalon
  Dexon
  Dexon II
  Dexon Plus
  DG (Davis & Geck) Softgut
  double-armed
  doubly ligated

suture *(cont.)*
  dural tenting
  end-to-side
  En Garde
  EPTFE (expanded polytetrafluoro-
    ethylene) vascular
  Ethibond
  Ethicon
  Ethiflex
  Ethilon
  everting
  everting mattress
  figure-of-8
  Flexon steel
  Frater
  Glycoprene
  Gregory stay
  gut
  guy
  heavy silk
  heavy wire
  horizontal
  horizontal mattress
  imbricating
  intermittent
  interrupted
  interrupted pledgeted
  intracuticular
  inverted
  inverting
  Jocath
  Jography
  Joguide
  Lactoprene
  Lembert
  locked
  locking
  loop
  Magnetic Controlled Suturing
    (MCS)
  mattress
  mattress-type

suture *(cont.)*
  Maxon
  Mersilene
  Mersilene braided nonabsorbable
  Mersilk braided silk
  Monocryl suture (polyglecaprone
    25)
  monofilament absorbable
  monofilament nylon
  monofilament polypropylene
  nonabsorbable
  noneverting
  Novofil
  Nurolon
  nylon
  nylon paracostal
  over-and-over
  over-and-over whip
  Panacryl absorbable
  paracostal
  patch-reinforced mattress
  PDS (polydioxanone suture) II
  Perma-Hand braided silk Endoloop
  PDS Vicryl
  pericostal
  Perma-Hand
  plain
  plastic
  pledgeted
  pledgeted double-armed
  pledgeted Ethibond
  pledgeted mattress
  Polydek
  polydioxanone (PDS)
  polypropylene
  Polysorb
  pop-off
  Potts tie
  preplaced
  Prolene
  pursestring or purse-string
  pyroglycolic acid

suture *(cont.)*
  Rapide
  reabsorbable
  retention
  running
  running continuous absorbable
  seromuscular-to-edge
  shorthand vertical mattress stitch
  silk
  simple
  single-armed
  skin staples
  Softgut surgical chromic
  Spotorno
  stainless steel wire
  staples
  stay
  Steri-Strips
  sternal wire
  stitch
  subanular mattress
  subcutaneous
  subcuticular
  subdermal
  SuperStitch
  Surgidac braided polyester
  Surgilene
  Surgilon
  SutraSilk nonabsorbable silk
  Sutureloop
  swaged-on
  synthetic
  Synthofil
  tack-up
  Teflon
  Teflon-pledgeted
  Teflon-pledgeted mattress
  tenting
  Tevdek
  Tevdek pledgeted
  Thiersch
  through-and-through

suture *(cont.)*
    through-and-through continuous
    through-the-wall mattress
    Ti-Cron
    tie-over stent
    traction
    transfixion
    transfixation
    transfixing Vicryl
    Trumbull
    T12
    Tycron
    U double-barrel
    umbilical tape
    undyed
    undyed braided polyglycolic acid
    vertical
    Vicryl
    whipstitch
    white
    white silk
    wing
    wire
suture anchor (see *anchor*)
suture beads (on cannula ports)
suture bites
suture guide, McGuire
sutureless electrode lead
sutureless myocardial electrode
suture-ligated
suture-ligated embolization microcoils
suture ligation
suture ligature
Sutureloop
suture passer, Carter-Thomason
suture Roticulator
Suture Strip Plus
Suture Trimmer accessory to The
    Closer
Suture/VesiBand organizer
SV (stroke volume)
SVA (supraventricular arrhythmia)

SVAS (supravalvular aortic stenosis)
SVC (superior vena cava) syndrome
SVC (supraventricular crest)
SVG (saphenous vein graft)
SVI (stroke volume index)
SvO_2 (venous oxygen saturation)
SVPC (supraventricular premature
    contraction)
SVR (systemic vascular resistance)
SVRI (systemic vascular resistance
    index)
SVT (supraventricular tachyarrhythmia)
SVT (supraventricular tachycardia)
swaged-on suture
swallowed electrode
swallow syncope
swallowing, difficulty
Swan aortic clamp
Swan-Ganz balloon-flotation catheter
Swan-Ganz flow-directed catheter
Swan-Ganz guidewire TD catheter
Swan-Ganz pacing TD catheter
Swan-Ganz pulmonary artery catheter
Swan-Ganz radial artery pressure
    monitoring line
Swan-Ganz technique for cardiac
    catheterization
Swan-Ganz thermodilution catheter
swan-neck catheter
Swartz SL Series Fast-Cath introducer
S wave
    deep
    slurred
    systolic
    wide
sweats, drenching
Sweet sternal punch
swelling, ankle
swelling resolves overnight
SWI (stroke work index)
Swing DR1 DDDR pacemaker
swing test

swirling smokelike echoes
swiss roll technique
Swiss cheese appearance
Swiss cheese ventricular septal defect
swollen throat
swollen tissues
sword-fighting (of thoracoscopic ports)
Swyer-James syndrome
Swyer-James unilateral hyperlucency
   of lung
SXCT (spiral x-ray computed tomog-
   raphy)
Sydenham chorea
Sydenham cough
Symbiant catheter
Symbiant distal protection device
Symbiant guidewire
Symbiant stent
Symbiant stent delivery system
Symbion cardiac device
Symbion/CardioWest 100-mL total
   artificial heart (TAH)
Symbion J-7 70-mL ventricle total
   artificial heart (TAH)
Symbion Jarvik-7 artificial heart
Symbion pneumatic assist device
Symbios pacemaker
Symbiot stent
symmetric pulmonary congestion
symmetrical chest or thorax
symmetrical mediastinal adenopathy
symmetrical phased array
sympathetic chain
sympathectomy
   cardiac
   high thoracic left
   lumbar
   periarterial
   regional cardiac
sympathetic trunk
sympathicotonic orthostatic
   hypotension

sympathomimetic activity
sympathomimetic amines, cardiac
sympathomimetic drug
Symphony stent
symphysis pubis
symptomatic digitalis-induced
   bradyarrhythmia
symptomatology
symptom complex
symptom-free period
symptom-limited exercise test
symptom reproduced with exertion
symptoms
   brachiocrural
   Buerger
   Burghart
   cardinal
   characteristic
   cognitive
   concomitant
   constitutional
   equivocal
   faciobrachial
   factitious
   florid (fully developed)
   nostril
   objective
   Oehler
   pathognomonic
   premonitory
   prodromal
   somatic
   subjective
   Tar
   transitory
   vegetative
symptom triad, classical
synchronicity
synchronized DC cardioversion
synchronized intermittent mandatory
   ventilation (SIMV)
synchronous carotid arterial pulse

synchronous mode of pacemaker
synchrony
    atrioventricular (AV)
    bilateral
    loss of AV (atrioventricular)
    out of
    ventricular
Synchrony system
syncopal attack
syncopal spell
syncope
    Adams-Stokes
    afferent nerve stimulation
    arrhythmia-induced
    cardiac
    cardiogenic
    cardioinhibitory carotid sinus
    carotid sinus
    cerebral carotid sinus
    cerebrovascular
    cough
    defecation
    deglutition
    diver's
    drug-induced
    effort
    exertional
    glossopharyngeal
    glossopharyngeal-vagal
    malignant vasovagal
    micturition
    near
    neurally mediated
    neurocardiogenic
    neuroregulatory
    ocular cardiac reflex
    orthostatic
    positional
    postprandial
    post-tussive
    postural
    pressor-postpressor

syncope *(cont.)*
    reflex
    swallow
    temporal lobe
    tussive
    vagal
    vagal carotid sinus
    vagovagal
    vasodepressor
    vasodepressor carotid sinus
    vasovagal
    vertiginous
    X
syncope anginosa
syncytial virus, respiratory
syncytium
    circular
    horseshoe-shaped
syndactyly
syndrome
    AAIR pacemaker
    Aase
    absent pulmonary valve
    acid-pulmonary-aspiration
    acute aortic regurgitation
    acute chest
    acute coronary
    acute febrile mucocutaneous lymph
        node
    acute radiation
    acute respiratory distress (ARDS)
    Adams-Stokes
    adult respiratory distress (ARDS)
    Afzelius
    Alagille
    ALCAPA (anomalous origin of left
        coronary artery from the
        pulmonary artery)
    Aldrich
    Alexander
    allergic alveolitis
    Alport

syndrome *(cont.)*
   alveolar capillary block
   Angelman
   angina
   angina decubitus
   angina with normal coronaries
   anginal
   anomalous first thoracic rib
   anterior chest wall
   anticholinergic
   antiphospholipid (APS)
   antiphospholipid-antibody
   anxiety
   aorta coarctation
   aortic arch
   aortic arch calcification-osteo-
      porosis-tooth-buds hypoplasia
   aortic arch hypoplasia
   aortic bifurcation
   Apert
   apical systolic click-murmur
   Archer
   Arneth
   Arnold-Chiari
   arrhythmogenic right ventricular
      dysplasia
   arteriohepatic dysplasia
   arthropathy-camptodactyly
   atherosclerotic occlusive
   athletic heart
   atypical chest pain
   autoerythrocyte sensitization
   Ayerza
   Babinski
   bagasse worker
   Balint
   Barlow
   Bartter
   basilar artery
   Becker
   beer and cobalt
   beer drinker

syndrome *(cont.)*
   Behçet
   Bernard-Soulier
   Bernheim
   Bernheim-Schmincke
   Beuren
   bird fancier's
   Blackfan-Diamond
   Bland-Garland-White
   blue finger
   blue of Gregoire (Gregoire's blue
      leg)
   blue toe (trash foot)
   blue velvet
   Bouillaud
   Bouveret-Hoffmann
   Bradbury-Eggleston
   bradycardia-tachycardia
   brady-tachy (slang for
      bradytachycardia)
   bradytachycardia
   bradytachydysrhythmia
   Brett
   Brock
   Brock middle lobe
   bronchial cartilage absence-
      bronchiectasis-bronchomalacia
   bronchial carcinoma myasthenia
   bronchial cast
   bronchiectasis-megaesophagus-
      osteopathy
   bronchiolitis obliterans (BOS)
   Brugada
   bubbly lung
   buckled innominate artery
   Buckley
   Budd-Chiari
   Burke
   caffeine heart
   caisson
   capillary leak
   capillary leakage

syndrome *(cont.)*
    Caplan
    carcinoid
    cardiac neurosis
    cardiac radiation
    cardiac-limb
    cardioauditory
    cardiocutaneous
    cardiofacial
    cardioinhibitory carotid sinus
    cardiopathia nigra
    cardiovascular-arm
    cardiovocal
    carnitine deficiency
    carotid sinus (CSS)
    Carpenter
    cast
    CATCH 22 (cardiac defects,
        abnormal facial features, thymic
        hypoplasia, cleft palate, and
        hypocalcemia)
    cat eye
    Cayler
    Ceelen-Gellerstedt
    celiac artery compression
    celiac axis
    cerebrocardiac
    cervical aorta
    Chandra-Khetarpal
    Charcot-Weiss-Baker
    CHARGE (colobomas, choanal
        atresia, mental and growth
        deficiency, genital and ear
        anomalies)
    Chiari-Budd
    cholesterol pericarditis
    chronic hyperventilation
    Churg-Strauss
    circulatory hyperkinetic
    Clarke-Hadfield
    Clerc-Levy-Cristeco (CLC)
    click

syndrome *(cont.)*
    click-murmur
    CLC (Clerc-Levy-Cristeco)
    cobbler chest
    Cockayne
    Coffin-Siris
    Colinet-Caplan
    congenital central hypoventilation
    congenital rubella
    concealed Wolff-Parkinson-White
    Conn
    Conradi-Hünermann
    Corvisart
    cork worker
    Cornelia de Lange
    coronary artery steal
    coronary steal
    coronary-subclavian steal
    Corrigan
    costal margin
    costochondral junction
    costoclavicular
    costosternal
    cotton-mill fever
    CREST (calcinosis cutis,
        Raynaud phenomenon,
        esophageal dysmotility,
        sclerodactyly, telangiectasia)
    cri du chat (short-arm deletion-5)
    croup
    Cruveilhier-Baumgarten
    cryptophthalmos
    Currarino-Silverman
    Cushing
    cutis laxa
    Cyriax
    Da Costa
    Davies
    Davies-Colley
    dead arm (DAS)
    declamping shock
    defibrinating

syndrome *(cont.)*

DeGimard
de Lange
De Martini-Balestra
Demons-Meigs
Determann
Diamond-Blackfan
DiGeorge
Dilantin
diphasic postcardiotomy
disseminated intravascular
    coagulation
Doehle-Heller
double outlet–left ventricle (DOLV)
double outlet–right ventricle
    (DORV)
Down
Dressler
Dusard
dysbarism
Dysshwannian
Eaton-Lambert
Edwards
effort
Ehlers-Danlos
Eisenmenger
elfin facies
Elliotson
Ellis-van Creveld
Elsner
eosinophil lung
eosinophilia-myalgia
eosinophilia-pulmonary tuberculosis
Erdheim I
erythrocyte autosensitization
external carotid steal
factor III platelet deficiency
Fahr-Volhard
Fallot
Fanconi-Hegglin
fat embolism (FES)
Fechtner

syndrome *(cont.)*

Feldaker
FG
fibrinogen-fibrin conversion
Fiedler
Fissinger-Rendu
flapping valve
floppy valve
florid Marfan
Fluckiger
Foix-Alajouanine
folded lung
Forney
Forrester
Friedel Pick
Frimodt-Moller
fulminant acute eosinophilic
    pneumonia-like
extrinsic sick sinus
funnel chest
G
Gailliard
Gaisböck
Gallavardin
gastrocardiac
giving up-given up
GLH (Green Lane Hospital)
Goldenhar
Goodpasture
Gorlin
Gouley
Gowers
Graham-Burford-Mayer
Gsell-Erdheim
Guillain-Barré
Hale
Hamman
Hamman-Rich
hand-heart
Hantavirus pulmonary
Harbitz
Harkavy

syndrome *(cont.)*
Harris
Hayem-Widal
heart and hand
heart-hand
heart-hand II
Heberden
Hegglin
HELLP (hemolysis, elevated liver
    enzymes, and low platelets)
hemangioma-thrombocytopenia
hemopleuropneumonia
heterotaxy
Hippel-Lindau
Hislop-Reid
holiday heart
hollow chest
Holmes
Holt-Oram
homocystinuria
Horner
Hughes-Stovin
Hunter
Hurler
Hurler-Scheie
Hutchinson-Gilford progeria
Hutinel-Pick
hyperdynamic heart
hypereosinophilic
hyperimmunoglobulinemia E
hyperkinetic heart
hyperlucent lung
hypersensitive carotid sinus
hypersensitive xiphoid
hypertelorism-hypospadias
hyperviscosity
hypogenetic lung
hypoplastic aorta
hypoplastic left-heart (HLHS)
hypoplastic left ventricle
hypoplastic right-heart
hypotonic

syndrome *(cont.)*
idiopathic hypereosinophilic
idiopathic long QT interval
idiopathic respiratory distress
    (IRDS)
iliocaval compression
immotile cilia
inappropriate antidiuretic hormone
    (SIADH)
incomplete Kartagener
incontinentia pigmenti
infantile
inferior vena cava
inframammary
intercoronary steal
intermediate coronary
intrinsic sick sinus
Irukandji
ischemic heart
ischemic heart disease
Ivemark
Janus
Jarcho-Levin
Jervell and Lange-Nielsen
Jeune
Jeune-Tommasi
Kabuki make-up
Kaposi-Besnier-Libman-Sacks
Kartagener
Kasabach-Merritt
Kast
Katayama
Kaufman-McKusick
Kawasaki
Kearns-Sayre
Kearns-Shy
Kemp-Elliot-Gorlin
King
Klauder
Klein-Waardenburg
Klippel-Feil
Klippel-Trénaunay

syndrome *(cont.)*
  Klippel-Trénaunay-Weber
  Kostmann
  Kousseff
  Kugelberg-Welander
  Kurtz-Sprague-White
  Kussmaul
  Labbé
  LAMB (lentigines, atrial myxoma,
    blue nevi)
  Lambert-Eaton
  Larsen
  Laslett-Short
  Laubry-Pezzi
  Laubry-Soulle
  Laurence-Moon-Biedl
  Laurence-Moon-Biedl-Bardet
  lazy leukocyte
  Leigh
  Leitner
  Lenègre
  Lenz
  LEOPARD
  Leriche
  lethal multiple pterygium
  Lev
  Lewis
  LGL (Lown-Ganong-Levine) variant
  Lian-Siguier-Welti venous
    thrombosis
  Libman-Sacks endocarditis
  Liddle
  locked lung
  Löffler (Loeffler) endomyocardial
  Loehr-Kindberg
  long QT (LQTS)
  long QTc interval
  low cardiac output
  low-flow
  Lown-Ganong-Levine (LGL)
  low-output
  low-renin essential hypertension

syndrome *(cont.)*
  low salt
  lupus-like
  Lutembacher
  Macleod
  Maffucci
  mal de Meleda
  Malin
  Manson schistosomiasis-pulmonary
    artery obstruction
  manubriosternal
  maple-bark worker
  Marable
  Marchiafava-Micheli
  Marfan
  marfanoid hypermobility
  Marie-Bamberger
  Maroteaux-Lamy
  Martorell
  Martorell-Fabre
  MAS (Morgagni-Adams-Stokes)
  Master
  mastocytosis
  maternal hypotension
  maternal rubella
  Maugeri
  McArdle
  McKusick-Kaufman
  MCLS
  Meadows
  Meigs
  Meigs-Cass
  Mendelson
  Ménière
  midaortic
  middle aortic
  middle lobe
  midsystolic click–late systolic
    murmur
  milk leg
  Miller
  Miller-Dieker

syndrome *(cont.)*
    Millikan-Siekert
    Minot–von Willebrand
    mitral click
    mitral click-murmur
    mitral regurgitation–chordal
       elongation
    mitral valve prolapse
    Mönckeberg
    Mohr
    Monday fever
    Mondor
    Monge
    Morgagni-Adams-Stokes (MAS)
    Morquio
    Morquio I
    Moschcowitz
    Mounier-Kuhn
    Moynahan
    MSA (multiple system atrophy)
    mucocutaneous lymph node
    mulibrey nanism
    multiple system atrophy (MSA)
    myxoma with facial freckling
    nail-patella
    NAME (nevi, atrial myxoma,
       myxoid neurofibroma,
       ephelides)
    nervous heart
    nonhypertension
    Noonan
    nutrition heart
    Opitz-Frias
    organic dust
    organic dust toxic
    Ormond
    Ortner
    Osler-Libman-Sacks
    osteogenesis imperfecta
    ovarian hyperstimulation
    pacemaker
    pacemaker twiddler's

syndrome *(cont.)*
    Page
    Paget-Schrötter (Schroetter)
    Paget-von Schrötter
    Pallister-Hall
    Pancoast
    paraneoplastic
    parchment heart
    Parkes Weber
    Patau (trisomy 13)
    pectoralis major
    pendelluft
    pericardiotomy
    pericarditis-liver pseudocirrhosis
    perinatal respiratory distress
    peripheral cholesterol embolization
    PF-III (platelet factor III)
    Pick
    pickwickian
    PIE (pulmonary infiltrate-
       eosinophilia)
    pigeon breeder's
    placental transfusion
    P mitrale
    Poland sequence
    Polhemus-Schafer-Ivemark
    polyangiitis overlap
    polysplenia
    popliteal artery entrapment
    Porter
    post-cardiac injury
    postcardiotomy
    postcardiotomy psychosis
    postcoarctation
    postcommissurotomy
    posterior fossa compression
    post-MI
    postmyocardial infarction
    postperfusion
    postperfusion lung
    postpericardiotomy
    postphlebitic

syndrome *(cont.)*
    postthrombotic
    postvalvulotomy
    P pulmonale
    preexcitation
    preinfarction
    prethrombotic
    primary mitral valve prolapse
    Prinzmetal II
    progeria
    progressive anginal
    prolonged QT interval
    Proteus
    pseudoclaudication
    pseudocoarctation
    pseudo-Meigs
    pseudoxanthoma elasticum
    psychogenic chest pain
    pulmonary acid aspiration
    pulmonary dysmaturity
    pulmonary sling
    pulmonary stenosis-ostium
        secundum defect
    pulmonary stenosis-patent foramen
        ovale
    pulmonary valve atresia-intact
        ventricular septum
    pulmonary venous anomalous
        drainage-mitral stenosis
    pulseless
    pump lung
    purple toes
    push-pull pump
    QT
    quadrilateral space
    radiation toxicity
    Raeder-Arbitz
    Raynaud
    reactive airways dysfunction
    renal cholesterol embolization
    Rendu-Osler-Weber
    respiratory distress (of newborn)

syndrome *(cont.)*
    restrictive cardiac
    restrictive hemodynamic
    Rh-null
    Ridley
    right middle lobe
    Riley-Day
    Roger
    Romano-Ward
    Romberg-Wood
    Roques
    Rosen-Castleman-Liebow
    Rosenbach
    Rosenthal
    Rostan
    Rougnon de Magny
    Royer-Wilson
    Rubinstein-Taybi
    Rummo
    Rundles-Falls
    runting
    Russell-Silver
    Sack-Barabas
    Sanchez-Cascos cardioauditory
    Sanfilippo
    scalenus anticus
    Scheie
    schistosomiasis japonica
    Schmincke-Bernheim
    Schönenberg
    Schroeder
    Schrötter (Schroetter)
    scimitar
    Sedlackova
    septic lung
    Seroche
    Servelle-Martorell
    severe acute respiratory syndrome
        (SARS)
    shaggy aorta
    Shaver
    Shaver-Ridell

syndrome *(cont.)*
    shifting pacemaker
    shock lung
    Shone
    short rib-polydactyly
    Short
    shoulder-hand
    Shprintzen
    Shy-Drager
    Shy-McGee-Drager
    sick sinus (SSS)
    Siewert
    Silver
    Silverman II
    Silver-Russell
    single atrium
    single ventricle
    Singleton-Merten
    sinus venosus
    sinusitis-bronchiectasis
    Sjögren
    slipping rib
    Sly
    small aorta
    small-cuff
    Smith-Lemli-Opitz
    smoker respiratory
    soldier's heart
    Solomon
    Spanish toxic oil
    Spens
    splenic flexure
    Srb (no vowel)
    Steidele
    Stevens-Johnson
    stiff heart
    Stokes-Adams
    stone heart
    straight back
    stroke
    subclavian steal (SSS)
    submersion

syndrome *(cont.)*
    sudden infant death (SIDS)
    superficial vena cava
    superior mesenteric artery
    superior vena cava (SVC)
    supine hypotensive (of pregnancy)
    supravalvar aortic stenosis
    supravalvular aortic stenosis
    surdocardiac
    suspended heart
    SVC (superior vena cava)
    Swan-Ganz
    Swyer-James
    syphilitic aorta
    systemic capillary leak (SCLS)
    systemic inflammatory response
    systolic click-late systolic murmur
    systolic click–murmur
    tachycardia-bradycardia
      (slang, tachy-brady)
    taffy candy
    Takayasu
    TAR (thrombocytopenia-absent
      radius)
    Taussig-Bing
    Taussig-Snellen-Alberts
    Terry
    thoracic outlet
    thoracic outlet compression
    thrombocytopenia-absent radius
      (TAR)
    thromboembolic
    Tietze
    tight-collar
    Townes
    Townes-Brocks
    toxic oil
    toxic shock
    transfusion
    transplant lung
    trash foot
    Treacher Collins

syndrome *(cont.)*
    trisomy 13(D)
    trisomy 13-15
    trisomy 18(E)
    trisomy 21 (Down)
    trisomy 11q
    trisomy 22
    22q11.2 deletion (22q11DS)
    twin transfusion
    twin-twin transfusion
    tropical eosinophilia
    Trousseau
    tuberous sclerosis
    turkish sabre
    Turner
    Turpin
    twiddler's
    Uhl
    Ullrich-Noonan
    unroofed coronary sinus
    upper-limb cardiovascular
    Upshaw-Schulman
    uremic cardiac
    vagal syncope
    vanishing lung
    Vaquez-Osler
    vascular
    vascular ring
    vasovagal
    VATER (vertebral anomalies, anal
        atresia, tracheoesophageal
        fistula, radial and renal
        anomalies)
    velocardiofacial (VCF)
    vena cava
    venous phlebitis-gangrene
    vertebral artery
    vertebral basilar artery
    visceral cholesterol embolization
    von Willebrand
    Von Rokitansky
    von-Hippel-Lindau

syndrome *(cont.)*
    VSD (ventricular septal defect) and
        absent pulmonary valve
    Waardenburg
    WAGR (Wilms tumor, aniridia,
        genitourinary involvement, and
        retardation)
    wandering pacemaker
    Ward-Romano
    Waterhouse-Friderichsen
    Weber-Osler-Rendu
    Wegener
    Weingarten
    Weisenburg
    Weiss-Baker
    Werner
    wet lung
    white lung
    Willebrand (von Willebrand)
    Williams
    Williams elfin facies
    Williams-Beuren
    Williams-Campbell
    Wilson-Mikity
    Winiwarter-Manteuffel-Buerger
    Wiskott-Aldrich
    Woakes
    Wolff-Parkinson-White (WPW)
    Wolf-Hirschhorn
    WPW (Wolff-Parkinson-White)
    X
    xiphoid process
    XO (Turner)
    XXXY and XXXXX
    Young
    Zeek
    Ziegler
syndrome of inappropriate antidiuretic
    hormone (SIADH)
syndrome X
SynerG detachable coil system
SynerGraft pulmonary heart valve

SynerGraft tissue-engineered replacement heart valve
Synergyst DDD pacemaker
synostosis
synovial sarcoma of the heart
synpneumonic empyema
Syntel latex-free embolectomy catheter
Synthaderm dressing
Synthaderm synthetic (polyurethane) occlusive wound dressing
synthetic absorbable film
Synthetic Aperture Focusing Technique (SAFT) in intravascular ultrasound imaging
synthetic patch angioplasty
synthetic surfactant
Synthofil suture
syphilis, cardiovascular
syphilitic aneurysm
syphilitic aorta syndrome
syphilitic aortic regurgitation
syphilitic aortitis
syphilitic myocarditis
syphilitic pericarditis
syringe
   Arrow Raulerson
   CoverTip safety
   IntelliSystem 25 disposable inflation
   Medallion
   MM coronary
   Osciflator balloon inflation
   Raulerson
   Raulerson spring-wire introduction
   spring-wire introduction
   Vaclok
Syringe Avitene delivery system for a collagen hemostat
system
   Access MV beating-heart bypass
   AccuNet embolic protection
   Achieve off-pump

system *(cont.)*
   Acolysis ultrasound intravascular thrombolysis
   Advantx LC+ cardiovascular imaging
   Aerocel pulmonary delivery
   air-driven implantable left ventricular assist (LVAS)
   Aloka color Doppler blood flow imaging
   Altaire open MR imaging
   Ancure minimally invasive endovascular
   AneuRx stent-graft
   AngioJet Rheolytic thrombectomy
   AngioJet XMI Rheolytic thrombectomy
   AnnuloFlo anuloplasty ring
   aortic connector
   Argyle Turkel safety thoracentesis
   arrhythmia mapping
   Atricure bipolar radiofrequency
   BacT/Alert automated blood culture
   BacTec (BACTEC) automated blood culture
   Bard CPS
   Bard percutaneous cardiopulmonary support (CPS)
   Belos VR-T ICD home monitoring
   Biojector 2000 jet injection system for drug delivery
   BioZ system digital noninvasive cardiac function monitoring
   Bridge Assurant biliary stent delivery
   Cardiofreezer cryosurgical
   cardiohemic
   CardioSEAL septal occlusion
   CASE computerized exercise EKG
   Cath-Finder tracking
   CathScanner ultrasound imaging

system *(cont.)*
 Cenflex central monitoring
 CGR biplane angiographic
 Checkmate intravascular
  brachytherapy
 Chemo-Port per venam catheter
 circumflex
 circumflex coronary
 closure
 COBE Spectra Apheresis
 codominant
 collateral
 CollectFirst
 conducting
 conduction
 conductive (conduction)
 Constant stent delivery
 continuous-wave laser
 Continuum MR-compatible
  infusion
 Cook Micropuncture catheter
 Cordis Checkmate
 COROSKOP C cardiac imaging
 Cosgrove-Edwards anuloplasty
 CPS (cardiopulmonary support)
 Crit-Line III blood monitoring
 CryoCor cardiac cryoablation
 Desilets introducer
 Digitron digital subtraction imaging
 dominant left coronary artery
 dominant right coronary
 Driver stent delivery
 dual-coronary
 Echovar Doppler
 Eclipse TMR holmium laser
 800 Series Blood Gas and Critical
  Analyte
 Ekos drug delivery
 Embol-X arterial cannula and filter
 Enabler circulatory support
 Encompass cardiac network
 Endeavor stent delivery

system *(cont.)*
 EndoSaph vein harvest
 engorged collecting
 ENTec Coblator plasma surgery
 EPT-1000 cardiac ablation
 Equinox occlusion balloon
 Evolve Cardiac Continuum
 Express2 coronary stent
 extracranial carotid
 E-Z Tac soft-tissue reattachment
 F.A.S.T. (First Access for Shock
  and Trauma) 1
 FastPack blood analyzer
 FiberScan laser
 Flowtron DVT pump
 Frank lead
 Frank XYZ orthogonal lead
 Frostline linear cryoablation
 GenESA
 GuardWire angioplasty
 Guidant Multi-Link Tetra coronary
  stent
 greater saphenous
 Haemonetics Cell-Saver
 HDI 1000 ultrasound
 heart assist
 HeartMate II air-driven implant-
  able left ventricular assist
  (LVAS)
 HeartMate vented electric LVAS
  (left ventricular assist system)
 Heartport Port-Access
 HeartSaver VAD (ventricular assist
  system)
 Heartstring proximal seal
 Helios diagnostic imaging
 Hemasure r/LS red blood cell
  filtration
 hexaxial reference
 HomMed Monitoring
 Horizon AutoAdjust CPAP

system *(cont.)*
HP (Hewlett-Packard) SONOS
5500 ultrasound imaging
His-Purkinje (HPS)
His-Purkinje conduction
Hombach lead placement
IDIS (intraoperative digital
subtraction) angiography
Infant Flow nasal CPAP
Integrity AFx AutoCapture pacing
Intuitive surgical telemanipulation
Isocam SPECT imaging
Itrel 3 spinal cord stimulation
Innovator Holter
kallikrein-kinin
lesser saphenous
Leukotrap RC (red cell) storage
Liposorber LA-15
Litespeed endovascular grafting
Luminexx biliary stent delivery
MAP digital inflation
Mason-Likar 12-lead ECG
MEDDARS cardiac catheterization
analysis
Medtronic AVE BeStent with
Discrete Technology over-the-
wire coronary stent delivery
Medtronic Interactive Tachycardia
Terminating
Medtronic Octopus tissue
stabilizing
Metrix atrial defibrillation
Micro-Driver stent delivery
microvascular anastomotic coupler
microwave cardiac ablation
Mirage nasal ventilation mask
Myotherm XP cardioplegia
delivery
Nellcor Symphony blood pressure
monitoring
Neotrend blood gas monitoring
Niroyal Elite Monorail coronary
stent

system *(cont.)*
NIR premounted stent delivery
NIR with SOX over-the-wire
coronary stent
Novacor left ventricular assist
(LVAS)
Oasis thrombectomy
Octopus 3 tissue stabilizing
OnLineABG monitoring
orthogonal lead
Pacefinder pacemaker lead
placement
pacemaker tester
Pasys
PCA (patient-controlled analgesic)
PCD Transvene implantable
cardioverter-defibrillator
PercuSurge GuardWire
percutaneous transluminal intra-
arterial filtration
Peripheral AngioJet
Photon delivery
Physios CTM 01 noninvasive
cardiac transplant monitoring
Piccolo blood chemistry analyzer
Port-A-Cath II low profile epidural
Prime ECG (electrocardiographic)
mapping
Probe balloon-on-a-wire dilatation
Profore four-layer bandaging
pulmonary venous
pulsatile lavage
Pulsar Max II pacemaker
Pulsavac III wound debridement
PulseSpray
Purkinje
Q-cath catheterization recording
QuickSeal arterial closure
Quick-Tap paracentesis
Quinton computerized exercise
EKG
RadiStop radial compression

system *(cont.)*
  Rapid Exchange (RX) coronary
    stent delivery
  Rapid Exchange (RX) vein graft
    stent delivery
  Rapid-Trak stent delivery
  Rasor blood pumping (RBPS)
  RDX coronary radiation catheter
    delivery
  reticuloendothelial
  Robotrac passive retraction
  Rosenkranz pediatric retractor
  Rozanski lead placement
  RPM (real-time position manage-
    ment) tracking
  R-Port Premier implantable
    vascular access
  Rx5000 cardiac pacing
  RX stent delivery
  saphenous
  Sarns ABLD
  Sarns occluder 5000
  Sarns occluder 7000
  Scanning-Beam Digital X-ray
    (SBDX)
  Sensi-Touch anesthesia delivery
  Sequestra 1000 blood processing
  Sequoia ultrasound
  SICOR computer-assisted cardiac
    catheterization recording
  SieScape ultrasound imaging
  single-chamber cardiac pacing
    (Pasys)
  Site-Rite and Site-Rite II ultra-
    sound
  SmartKard digital Holter
  SmartMist asthma management
  Solcotrans drainage/reinfusion
  SOMATOM Volume Zoom
    computed tomography
  SonoHeart handheld digital
    echocardiography

system *(cont.)*
  Soprano cryoablation
  Spirexx stent delivery
  Sprinter stent delivery
  Squirt wound irrigation
  STAT-Site M Hgb test
  steerable guidewire
  Symbiant stent delivery
  Synchrony
  SynerG detachable coil
  S7 coronary stent with Zipper
    delivery
  T (sarcolemma)
  TAG (tissue anchor guide)
  Talent LPS endoluminal stent-graft
  Techstar percutaneous vascular
    surgery
  Techstar XL percutaneous vascular
    surgery
  Thora-Klex chest drainage
  Tomcat Guidance (for guidewires)
  transesophageal pacing
  transluminal lysing
  TriActiv saphenous vein graft
    disease treatment
  Triage cardiac
  triaxial reference
  TriVex transilluminated powered
    phlebectomy
  TRON 3 VACI cardiac imaging
  Tru-Close wound drainage
  Trufill n-BCA liquid embolic
  ultrasonic nebulization
  underwater chest drainage
  USCI Probe balloon-on-a-wire
    dilatation
  VasoView balloon dissection
  VasoView Uniport endoscopic
    saphenous vein harvesting
  Vaxcel implantable vascular access
  VenaFlow compression
  Venodyne compression

system *(cont.)*
   vertebral artery
   Virtuoso portable three-dimensional
     imaging
   V_1-like ambulatory lead
   V_5-like ambulatory lead
   Voluson ultrasound
   Viagraph computerized exercise
     EKG
   Wallstent endoprosthesis with
     Unistep catheter delivery
   water-seal drainage
   X-PRESS vascular closure
   Xillix LIFE-Lung
   Zenith AAA endovascular graft
   Zipper delivery
systema cardiovasculare
systema conducens cordis
systema respiratorium
systemic and topical hypothermia
systemic anticoagulation with heparin
systemic arterial circulation
systemic arterial oxygen desaturation
systemic arterial vasoconstriction
systemic AV O_2 difference
systemic blood
systemic capillary leak syndrome
   (SCLS)
systemic carnitine deficiency
systemic circulation
systemic diastolic blood pressure
   (SDBP)
systemic disorders affecting heart
   function
systemic heparin anticoagulation
systemic heparinization
systemic hypertension
systemic hypoperfusion
systemic inflammatory response
   syndrome
systemic lupus erythematosus
systemic mean arterial pressure
   (SMAP)

systemic metastases
systemic necrotizing vasculitis
systemic oxygen saturation measured
   after balloon-occluding each
   collateral
systemic perfusion, diminished
systemic pressure
systemic-pulmonary artery shunt
systemic resistance, vascular
systemic sclerosis
   fibrosing alveolitis associated with
   progressive
systemic sepsis
systemic to pulmonary artery anastomosis
systemic vascular resistance (SVR)
systemic vascular resistance index
   (SVRI)
systemic vasculitis
systemic venous hypertension
systemic venous return
systole
   aborted
   atrial
   cardiac
   coupled premature
   electromechanical
   end of
   extra
   premature atrial
   premature junctional
   premature ventricular
   total
   ventricular
   ventricular ectopic
systolic anterior motion (SAM) of
   mitral valve
systolic anterior motion (SAM) on
   2-D echocardiogram
systolic blood pressure (SBP)
systolic bulge, late
systolic click (SC)

systolic click–murmur syndrome
systolic diameter (of LV)
systolic-diastolic blood pressure
systolic-diastolic window
systolic ejection click
systolic ejection murmur (SEM)
systolic ejection period (SEP)
systolic ejection sound
systolic fractional shortening
systolic gradient
systolic grating sound
systolic heart failure
systolic hypertension
systolic impulse
systolic mammary souffle
systolic murmur (SM), graded from
   1 to 6

systolic pressure
systolic pressure determination (SLP)
systolic pressure-time index
systolic prolapse of mitral valve leaflet
systolic reserve
systolic retraction
systolic retraction of apex
systolic S waves
systolic scratch
systolic thrill
systolic time interval (STI)
systolic trough
systolic upstroke time
systolic velocity-time integral
systolic whoop
Szabo-Berci needle drivers

T, t

TAAA (thoracoabdominal aortic
   aneurysm) surgery
tabagism (nicotinism)
tab, fibrous
table
   anterior
   posterior
table of the sternum
TAC atherectomy catheter
TACE (transcatheter arterial
   chemoembolization)
tachyarrhythmia
   atrial
   digitalis-induced
   drug refractory atrial
   drug-resistant
   ectopic
   lethal
   malignant ventricular
   paroxysmal
   paroxysmal ventricular
   supraventricular
   sustained ventricular
   ventricular
Tachyarrhythmia Detection Software
tachybrady

tachycardia
   accelerated idioventricular
   acceleration of
   accessory pathway reentrant
      paroxysmal supraventricular
   antidromic
   antidromic AV reciprocating
   antidromic AV reentrant
   antidromic circus-movement
   antidromic reciprocating
   atrial
   atrial automatic
   atrial ectopic automatic
   atrial paroxysmal (APT)
   atrial reentrant
   atrial reentrant paroxysmal
      supraventricular
   atrioventricular nodal
   atrial reentry
   atrioventricular junctional
   atrioventricular nodal (AVNT)
   atrioventricular nodal reentrant
      (AVNRT)
   atrioventricular node re-entry
   atrioventricular reciprocating
      (AVRT)

tachycardia *(cont.)*
   atypical AV nodal re-entry
   automatic atrial
   automatic ectopic (AET)
   AV (atrioventricular)
   AV nodal re-entrant
   AV nodal re-entrant paroxysmal
     supraventricular
   AV nodal re-entry (reentry)
   AV reciprocating
   benign ventricular
   bidirectional ventricular
   bundle branch block (BBB)
   bundle branch reentrant ventricular
   chaotic atrial
   circus movement (CMT)
   concealed accessory pathway (AP)
   concealed bypass-type
   congenital ventricular
   double
   drug-refractory
   ectopic atrial
   ectopic supraventricular
   endless-loop
   exercise-aggravated ventricular
   exercise-induced ventricular
   fast-slow AV nodal reentrant
   focal ventricular
   hemodynamically unstable
     ventricular
   hypokalemia-induced ventricular
   idiopathic ventricular
   idioventricular
   incessant
   incessant ectopic atrial
   incessant focal atrial
   incisional macroreentrant atrial
   inducible
   intra-atrial reentrant
   intractable ventricular
   junctional
   macro-reentrant

tachycardia *(cont.)*
   malignant ventricular
   monomorphic
   monomorphic ventricular
   multifocal atrial (MAT or MFAT)
   multiform
   narrow-complex
   nodal reentrant
   nodoventricular
   nonparoxysmal atrioventricular
     junctional
   nonparoxysmal automatic atrial
   nonparoxysmal AV junctional
   nonparoxysmal AV nodal
   nonparoxysmal reciprocating
     junctional (NPRJT)
   nonsustained monomorphic
     ventricular
   nonsustained polymorphic
     ventricular
   nonsustained ventricular (NSVT)
   NPJT (nonparoxysmal AV
     junctional)
   orthodromic
   orthodromic AV reentrant
   orthodromic reciprocating (ORT)
   orthodromic supraventricular
   orthostatic
   pacemaker-mediated
   parasystolic ventricular
   paroxysmal
   paroxysmal atrial (PAT)
   paroxysmal junctional (PJT)
   paroxysmal sinus
   paroxysmal supraventricular
     (PSVT)
   permanent reciprocating
     atrioventricular junctional
   pleomorphic
   polymorphic ventricular
   primary electrical ventricular
   rapid nonsustained ventricular

tachycardia *(cont.)*
  reciprocating
  reciprocating atrioventricular
  reciprocating permanent
    atrioventricular junctional
  reentrant
  reentrant supraventricular
  reflex
  refractory
  repetitive monomorphic ventricular
    (RMVT)
  repetitive paroxysmal ventricular
  resting
  runs of
  SA (sinoatrial) nodal reentry
  salvos of ventricular
  self-terminating
  sinoatrial (SA) reentrant
  sinus
  sinus reentrant
  slow retrograde
  slow-fast
  slow-fast atrioventricular node
    reentry
  slow-fast AV nodal reentrant
  supraventricular (SVT)
  sustained ventricular
  torsades de pointes ventricular
  transvenous cryoablation of
    supraventricular
  ventricular (VT)
  wide QRS
  wide-complex
  Wolff-Parkinson-White reentrant
  WPW (Wolff-Parkinson-White)
tachycardia-bradycardia syndrome
tachycardiac
tachycardic
tachydysrhythmia
Tachylog pacemaker
tachypnea, transient
tachypneic breathing pattern

tacked
tack up (verb)
tack-up sutures
tacrolimus
Tactilaze angioplasty laser catheter
tactile fremitus
tactile precordial phenomena
TAD guidewire
TAE (transcatheter arterial embolization)
taffy candy syndrome
TA-55 stapling device
Tagarno 3SD cine projector for
  angiography
tagged blood cells
tagging cine magnetic resonance
tagging, myocardial
TAG (tissue anchor guide) system
TAH (total artificial heart),
  electromechanical
tailored to fit
Takayasu aortitis
Takayasu arteritis, supra-aortic
Takayasu pulseless disease
Takayasu syndrome
Take-apart scissors and forceps
takedown of adhesions
takedown of Fontan operation
takedown of laryngostomy
takedown of Mustard baffle
takeoff
  aortic
  artery
  high (of left coronary artery)
takeoff of acute marginal branch
takeoff of left anterior descending
  coronary artery
takeoff of vessel
Takeuchi repair
taking down of adhesions
talc
talc plaque

talc pneumoconiosis
talc poudrage
talc slurry
talcum powder
Talent LPS endoluminal stent-graft
  system
Talent pacemaker
tall right precordial R waves
tambourlike
tambour quality of A_2
tambour sound
tamponade
  cardiac
  chronic
  florid cardiac
  full-blown cardiac
  heart
  low-pressure cardiac
  medical cardiac
  pericardial
  pericardial chyle with
  subacute cardiac
  surgical cardiac
TandemHeart
tandem lesion
Tandem cardiac device
tangential constriction
tangential incision
tangentially
tangential orientation
Tango catheter
tank respirator
tank-type body ventilator
TA-90 stapler
tanned red cells (TRC) test
tantalum bronchogram
tantalum, knitted
tap (tapping), pericardial
TAP (transesophageal atrial pacing)
tape
  braided
  Cath-Secure

tape *(cont.)*
  compression
  Dacron
  Elastikon elastic tape
  silastic
  umbilical
  vascular
  white cotton umbilical
tapering, abrupt
tapering doses
tapering occlusion
tapering off
tapering stenosis
tape ligature
TAPSE (tricuspid anular plane
  systolic excursion) score
TAPVC (total anomalous pulmonary
  venous connection)
TAPVR (total anomalous pulmonary
  venous return)
Tar symptoms
TAR (thrombocytopenia-absent radius)
  syndrome
Tardieu spot
tardive cyanosis
tardus et parvus, pulsus
tardus, pulsus
target heart rate
target lesion
target lesion revascularization (TLR)
TARP (total atrial refractory period)
T artifact
Tascon prosthetic valve
Ta segment (electrocardiography)
TASH (transcoronary ablation of
  septal hypertrophy)
TAT (thrombin-antithrombin III
  complex)
TA-30 autosuture
TA-30 4.5 mm staples
TAT inhibitor
tattooing procedure

taurine deficiency
Taussig-Bing anomaly
Taussig-Bing congenital anomaly of
    heart
Taussig-Bing congenital malformation
Taussig-Bing double-outlet right
    ventricle
Taussig-Bing syndrome
Taussig-Snellen-Alberts syndrome
taut pericardial effusion
taut skin
TAV (transcutaneous aortovelography)
Tawara atrioventricular node
TB (tuberculin) skin test
TB (tuberculosis)
TBB (transbronchial biopsy)
TBNA (transbronchial needle aspira-
    tion)
TBT (transcervical balloon tuboplasty)
TCBF (total cerebral blood flow)
TCCS (transcranial color-coded sonog-
    raphy)
T cells
TCL (tachycardia cycle length)
Tc 99m or ^{99m}Tc (technetium)
TCP (total cavopulmonary connection)
TDD (thoracic duct drainage)
TDI (toluene diisocyanate)
T'd incision
TDI sensitivity
T/D or T-D (thickness to diameter of
    ventricle) ratio
TD2 torque device
TE (echo delay time)
TE (thromboembolic) stroke
team, donor
tear
    eccentric
    intimal
    linear
    splint-type
tearaway sheath

tear in ascending aorta
tear in descending aorta
tearing, plaque
teased off
tea-taster's cough
TEB (thoracic electrical bioimped-
    ance)
teboroxime cardiac scan for
    myocardial infarction
TEC (transluminal extraction catheter)
TECAB (totally endoscopic coronary
    artery bypass)
tecadenoson
TEC atherectomy device
technetium (see *imaging agent*)
technetium bound to DTPA
technetium bound to serum albumin
technetium bound to sulfur colloid
technetium 99m-labeled fibrinogen
technetium 99m venogram
technetium pyrophosphate scanning
Techni-Care surgical scrub
technician, pump
technique (see also *method,*
    operation, procedure)
    acquisition
    adjunctive
    Amplatz
    antegrade transseptal approach
        in valvuloplasty
    anterior sandwich patch closure
    aseptic
    Bentall
    Bentall inclusion
    Blalock-Hanlon
    bolus-chase
    bronchoscopic shuttle
    button
    Carpentier
    Carrel
    clamp-and-sew
    clavicotomy

technique *(cont.)*
  claviculectomy
  claviculotomy
  cough CPR
  Damus-Kaye-Stansel (DKS)
  De Vega
  Dor
  dos Santos
  Dotter
  Dotter-Judkins
  double-umbrella
  double-wire atherectomy
  draw-back stent deployment
  dye dilution
  ECG signal-averaging
  ECG-gated multislice MRI
  elephant-trunk
  equilibrium radionuclide
    angiocardiography
  esophageal balloon
  eversion
  extracorporeal carbon dioxide
  extrastimulus
  fat-suppressed breath-hold
  first-pass
  flow mapping
  fluoroscopic road-mapping
  free-flap anastomotic reconstruction
  Frouin
  gated
  graft seeding
  Gruentzig angioplasty
  Gruentzig PTCA
  hybrid open-endoluminal
  inclusion
  indicator-dilution
  intravascular MRI
  J loop (on catheterization)
  Jerome Kay
  Judkins cardiac catheterization
  Judkins femoral catheterization
  Kawashima

technique *(cont.)*
  kissing atherectomy
  kissing balloon
  lasing
  Lecompte
  Linton open subfascial division
  Lown
  Mee
  modified Seldinger
  Mullins blade
  multiphasic multislice MRI
  multiple chord, center line
    echocardiogram
  multislice multiphase spin-echo
    imaging
  multislice spin-echo
  Nikaidoh
  noninvasive
  Nambudripad's Allergy Elimina-
    tion (NAET)
  noninvasive
  no-touch (in vascular anastomosis)
  open subfascial division technique
    in treatment of varicose veins
  parachute (for distal anastomosis)
  Patrick-McGoon
  PCICO (pressure-controlled inter-
    mittent coronary occlusion)
  percutaneous
  percutaneous Judkins
  percutaneous puncture
  percutaneous transfemoral
  pharmacologic stress
  physiologic stress
  Potts
  pressure half-time
  radioenzymatic
  rapid thoracic compression
  Rashkind
  recanalization
  Reed anuloplasty
  reimplantation

technique *(cont.)*
   sandwich
   Schonander
   Seldinger
   Seldinger percutaneous
   serial cut film
   sheathed insertion
   sheathless insertion
   silhouette
   Sones arteriography
   Sones brachial cutdown
   Sones cardiac catheterization
   Sones cineangiography
   Sones coronary arteriography
   Stewart-Hamilton cardiac output
   Stoney
   subclavian turndown
   subpleural blanketing
   swiss roll
   test and ablate
   T-graft configuration
   thermal dilution
   thermodilution (for measuring
     cardiac output)
   Trusler aortic valve
   two-layer latex and Marlex closure
   two-stick or three-stick
   upgated
   Waldhausen and Nahrwold
   Waldhausen subclavian flap
   Waterston-Cooley
   whiplash technique for reposition-
     ing a catheter with a trocar
     under fluoroscopy
   wraparound
   xenon computed tomography
     (XeCT)
Techstar percutaneous closure device
Techstar percutaneous vascular surgery
   system
Techstar XL percutaneous vascular
   surgery system

Tecothane catheter
TED, T.E.D. (thromboembolic
   disease)
TED, T.E.D. antiembolism stockings
TED, T.E.D. thigh-high stockings
tedious dissection
TEE (transesophageal echocardi-
   ography) imaging
teeth-chattering chills
Teflon Bardic plug
Teflon catheter
Teflon felt bolster
Teflon felt pledget
Teflon-fluon fumes
Teflon graft or patch
Teflon intracardiac patch
Teflon pledget
Teflon-pledgeted mattress suture
Teflon suture
Tegaderm dressing
Tegagel hydrogel dressing and sheet
Tegagen HG alginate wound dressing
Tegagen HI alginate wound dressing
Tegapore contact-layer wound dressing
Tegasorb hydrocolloid wafer dressing
Teichholz ejection fraction in
   echocardiogram
Teichholz equation for left ventricular
   volume
Tekna mechanical heart valve
Tektronix oscilloscope
telangiectasia
   cutaneous
   hereditary hemorrhagic
   Osler hereditary hemorrhagic
telangiectasias in the bathing suit area
telangiectasis, bilateral juxtafoveal
   (BJT)
telangiectatic angioma
telangiectatic lesions
Telangitron
Telectronics defibrillator patches

Telectronics endocardial defibrillation
(DF) lead system
Telectronics endocardial defibrillation/
rate-sensing/pacing lead
Telectronics endocardial pacing lead
Telectronics Guardian ATP II ICD
Telectronics pacemaker electrode
Telectronics pacing lead
Telectronics PASAR antitachycardia
pulse generator
telemetric mitral valve repair
telemetry
telephone monitoring of EKG
telephone transmission of EKG
Teletrast absorbable surgical gauze
Telfa dressing
Telfa pad
temperature
core
esophageal
normothermic
temperature probe, nasopharyngeal
temperature-sensing pacemaker
temporal arteritis
temporal artery
temporal lobe syncope
temporary atrial pacing wire
temporary cardiac pacing
temporary pacing catheter
temporary percutaneous cardiopulmonary support
temporary tracheostomy
tenacious bronchial exudate
tenacious mucoid plugs
tenacious mucus
tenacious secretions
tenacious sputum
tenderness
calf muscle
chest wall
periumbilical area

tendineae
chordae
ruptured chordae
tendinosum, xanthoma
tendinous hiatus
tendon
left ventricular false
Todaro
Tendril DX implantable pacing lead
Tendril SDX pacing lead
tennis racquet cells
Tennis Racquet angiography catheter
tense pulse
Tensilon (edrophonium chloride) test
tension
alveolar wall
decreased inspired oxygen
epicardial
ventricular wall
tension pneumatocele
tension pneumopericardium
tension pneumothorax
tensionless anastomosis
tension-time index (TTI)
tensor apparatus
tent
croup
mist
tentative diagnosis
tented up
tenting of pericardium
tent-shaped T waves
teratogenicity
teratoma
cardiac
malignant (of the heart)
terazosin HCl
terminal air sacs
terminal air space
terminal aortic thrombosis
terminal bronchioles

terminal crest of right atrium
terminal edema
terminal inversion
terminalis
   crista
   sulcus
terminal negativity of P wave
terminal, RNS
Terry syndrome (oxygen toxicity to
   retina)
tertiary spread of tumor
Terumo sheath
tesla
test (see also *assay, analysis, testing*)
   Abigram vascular diagnostic
   acid-fast
   ACM (automated cardiac flow
      measurement) technology
   Actalyke activated clotting time
      (ACT)
   adenosine stress
   Adson
   Albumin Cobalt Binding
   alkaline phosphatase antialkaline
      phosphatase (APAAP) antibody
   Allen
   Allen circulator
   alternans noninvasive cardiac
      diagnostic
   Amplicor *Mycobacterium*
      tuberculosis
   Amplified *Mycobacterium*
      tuberculosis direct (MTD)
   ANA (antinuclear antibody)
   Anderson-Keys total serum
      cholesterol
   antihyaluronidase
   Anti-MPO (p-ANCA) ELISA
      autoimmune
   APACHE CV risk predictor
   antistreptolysin-O titer
   antistreptozyme (ASTZ)

test *(cont.)*
   Apt
   APTT clotting
   ASO titer
   ASTZ (antistreptozyme)
   atrial pacing
   atrial pacing stress
   BacTec (BACTEC) culture
   baseline pulmonary function
   Bernstein acid infusion
   bicycle ergometer
   bicycle ergometer exercise
   bicycle exercise
   blood culture
   breath excretion
   Brodie-Trendelenburg (for varicose
      veins)
   bronchial provocation
   bronchoprovocation
   capillary fragility
   capillary resistance
   carbon monoxide diffusion capacity
   cardiokymographic (CKG)
   carotid sinus
   CAST (Cardiac Arrhythmic
      Suppression Trial)
   Cholestech LDX system with the
      TC (total cholesterol) and
      glucose panel
   Cholesterol Manager home
      cholesterol management kit
   Cholesterol 1,2,3 noninvasive
      testing device
   CholesTrak
   Clauss modified method of plasma
      fibrinogen measurement
   coccidioidin
   coin
   cold agglutinins
   cold pressor (Hines and Brown)
   cold pressor exercise
   collagen vascular screen

test *(cont.)*
   collateral circulation
   computerized texture analysis
      of lung nodules and lung
      parenchyma
   contraction stress (CST)
   Coombs
   costoclavicular
   ^{11}C palmitate uptake
   ^{11}C propranolol uptake
   Crampton
   creatine phosphokinase (CPK)
   C3a serum level
   cuff
   culture and sensitivity
   cytological
   Dehio
   dehydrocholate
   diaphragmatic stimulation
   dipyridamole echocardiography
   dipyridamole handgrip
   dipyridamole infusion
   dipyridamole thallium stress
   direct Coombs
   dobutamine exercise stress
   dobutamine stress
   Donath-Landsteiner
   DPT-positive skin prick
   drip
   drop (for pneumoperitoneum)
   Duke
   dynamic exercise
   800 Series Blood Gas and Critical
      Analyte System
   elastic fibers stain
   electrophysiologic
   EliSpot
   equivocal exercise
   ergonovine provocative
   erythrocyte sedimentation rate
      (ESR)
   euglobulin lysis

test *(cont.)*
   exercise
   exercise stress
   exercise thallium-201 stress
   exercise tolerance (ETT)
   fibrinogen determination
   functional intact fibrinogen (FiF)
   Fisher exact
   flat-hand
   fungal
   Gibbon and Landis
   Goethlin
   graded exercise tolerance
   graded treadmill
   handgrip exercise
   handgrip stress
   hanging drop (for pneumo-
      peritoneum)
   HDM (house dust mites) bronchial
      provocation
   head-up tilt
   Heart Failure Knowledge
   Heartscan heart attack prediction
   Helisal rapid blood
   HemaStrip-HIV 1/2 whole blood
   Henle-Coenen
   heparin neutralized thrombin time
      (HNTT)
   Hess capillary
   high-dose thrombin time (HiTT)
   high shear blood flow
   Hines and Brown
   Howell
   hydrogen
   hyperabduction
   hyperemia
   hyperventilation
   ^{123}I heptadecanoic acid uptake
   immunohistochemistry
   indirect Coombs
   inhalation bronchial challenge
   injection (for pneumoperitoneum)

test *(cont.)*
    intermediate tuberculin
    isometric exercise
    isometric exercise stress
    isometric stress
    Kleihauer-Betke
    Kobert
    Korotkoff
    Kveim
    lactate dehydrogenase (LDH)
    Landis-Gibbon
    Levine
    Lewis and Pickering
    Liebermann-Burchard
    lipid
    low-range heparin management
      (LHMT)
    lung diffusion
    Mantoux
    Master two-step (2-step) exercise
    Matas
    match
    maximal exercise
    meniscus of saline (for pneumo-
      peritoneum)
    methacholine bronchial provocation
    mirror
    Mono-Vacc
    Moschcowitz
    MTD (*Mycobacterium tuberculosis*
      direct)
    multiple-puncture tuberculin
    multiple sleep latency (MSLT)
    MycoAKT latex bead agglutination
    Nambudripad's Allergy Elimi-
      nation Technique (NAET)
    New Leaf cardiopulmonary
      performance
    Newman-Keuls
    N-geneous HDL cholesterol
    niacin
    noninvasive

test *(cont.)*
    nonstress (NST)
    Northern blot
    Oliver-Rosalki method of testing
      serum CPK
    one-stage clotting
    one-stage prothrombin time
    pacemaker threshold
    Pachon
    PaO_2
    partial thromboplastin time
    passive tilt
    Paul-Bunnell
    Pearson chi-squared (calculation
      used for artificial heart)
    Persantine Cardiolite stress
    Perthes
    Phalen stress
    PLAC diagnostic
    plantar ischemic
    plasma renin activity (PRA)
    Plesch
    polymerase chain reaction (PCR)
    polysomnogram
    Porvidx noninvasive early lung
      cancer screening
    PPD (purified protein derivative)
      skin (for tuberculosis)
    positive skin
    positive tilt
    postmyocardial infarction exercise
    postural stimulation of aldosterone
    PPD (purified protein derivative)
    primed lymphocyte (PLT)
    Prostigmin (neostigmin)
    prothrombin
    prothrombin consumption
    prothrombin-proconvertin
    provocative
    PT/PTT
    pulmonary function (PFT)
    Quick

test *(cont.)*

  Quick one-stage prothrombin time
  Reflotron bedside theophylline
  R-lactate enzymatic monotest
  Roos (to detect thoracic outlet
    syndrome)
  Salkowski
  Salzman
  Sandrock
  scalene
  Schiff
  Schlichter
  Schultze
  Sclavo PPD
  Sclavo test-PPD (tuberculin
    purified protein derivative)
  sestamibi Tc-99m SPECT with
    dipyridamole stress
  Sex After MI Knowledge
  sickle cell
  sickling
  skin-prick
  SmartScore
  Snider match
  sniff
  Southern blot hybridization
  Southwestern blot
  SpectRx
  SPECT thallium
  Sterneedle tuberculin
  spirometric
  STAT-Site M Hgb
  Stratus cardiac troponin I
  streptokinase resistance
  stress
  Stypven time
  submaximal treadmill exercise
  super stress
  swing
  symptom-limited maximal exercise
  TB (tuberculin)
  teichoic acid antibody

test *(cont.)*

  thallium stress
  thallium-201 exercise
  t-HIAA
  tilt
  Tine test PPD (tuberculin purified
    protein derivative)
  tine tuberculin
  tolazoline
  tourniquet
  treadmill (TMT)
  treadmill exercise (TET)
  treadmill stress (TMST)
  Trendelenburg
  Triage BNP (B-type natriuretic
    peptide)
  Tris-buffer infusion
  tuberculin (TB)
  Tuberculin Mono-Vacc
  Tuberculin Tine test, Old
  Tubersol
  Tuffier
  two-step exercise
  Valsalva
  VAP cholesterol
  ventilation
  VEX (vasodilator plus exercise)
    treadmill
  voltammetry
  von Recklinghausen
  Waaler-Rose
  Western blot
  Williamson
  Zwenger
test and ablate technique
test battery
testing (see also *test*)
  extrastimulus (EST)
  mycobacteria susceptibility
  nuclear gated blood pool
  serial electrophysiologic (SET)
  stress
  upright tilt-

test-occluded, vessel was
Test of Incremental Respiratory
    Endurance (TIRE) software
test of vasomotor function
test result
    false negative
    false positive
tet (slang for tetralogy of Fallot)
TET (treadmill exercise test)
tethered ventricular assist device
tetrad spells
tetrahedron chest
tetralogy of Fallot (TOF)
    atypical
    pink
tetralogy of Fallot plus atrial septal
    defect
tetrapolar esophageal catheter
tetrodotoxin effect
tetrodotoxin potential
tet (tetralogy of Fallot) spell
Tevdek suture
Texas catheter
TGA (transposition of great arteries)
T-graft configuration technique
thalassemia
    alpha
    beta
thalassemia major
thalassemia minor
thalassemia–sickle cell disease
thallium clearance
thallium defect
thallium imaging
thallium injection
thallium myocardial perfusion imaging
thallium perfusion study
thallium, regional myocardial uptake
    of
thallium scintigraphy
thallium SPECT (thallium-201 single-
    photon emission computed tomo-
    graphic) imaging

thallium stress test
thallium treadmill
thallium-201 myocardial imaging
thallium-201 myocardial scintigraphy
thallium uptake
thallium washout
thatched roof worker's lung
thebesian circulation
thebesian foramen
thebesian valve
thebesian vein
Theden method
T-helper lymphocyte alveolitis
theophylline (sustained-release form)
theophylline toxicity
theorem
    Bayes (exercise stress testing)
    Bernoulli
Thera-Boot compression dressing or
    wrap
therapeutic anticoagulation
therapeutic blood level of drug
therapeutic bronchoscopy
therapeutic embolization
therapeutic intervention
therapeutic modality
therapeutic phlebotomy
therapeutic pneumothorax
therapeutic range (of drug)
therapeutic thoracentesis
therapeutic trial
therapy
    ablation
    abort
    Acapella chest physical
    adjunctive
    adjuvant
    aerosol
    alcohol ablation
    antagonist
    anthelminthic
    antianginal

therapy *(cont.)*
   antibacterial
   antibiotic
   anticoagulant
   antihypertensive
   antimicrobial
   antitachycardiac pacing
   antiviral
   aspirin
   beta-adrenergic blocker
   BioBypass PVD (peripheral
      vascular disease) angiogen
      (gene-based)
   bronchodilator
   cardiac rehabilitation
   cardiac resynchronization (CRT)
   cardiac shock wave (CSWT)
   circulator boot
   coronary radiation (CRT)
   cardiotherapy
   chemical ablation (for arrhythmia)
   chest PT (physical therapy)
   chronotropic
   concomitant antiarrhythmic
   continuous lateral rotation
   continuous nebulization (CNT)
   cortisone in congenital vascular
      defect
   corticosteroid in hemangioma
   dietary
   diuretic
   drug
   efficacy of drug
   empiric
   empirical
   empiric bronchodilator
   endolaser venous (ELVT)
   exercise
   fibrinolytic
   GenStent biologic
   heparin anticoagulation
   home ambulatory inotropic

therapy *(cont.)*
   immunosuppressive
   immunotherapy
   inotropic
   intracoronary thrombolytic
   intravascular red light (IRLT)
   intravascular sonotherapy
   K (vitamin) antagonist
   lipid-lowering
   local thrombolytic
   multidrug
   nebulization
   neoadjuvant
   nonballoon (stents, atherectomy,
      and excimer laser angioplasty)
   palliative
   passive hyperimmune (PHT)
   PCD tiered
   physiotherapy
   pressor
   prostacyclin
   quinidine
   radiofrequency ablation
   refractory to medical
   reperfusion
   respiratory
   respiratory physical
   Restcue CC dynamic air therapy
   Rx (prescription)
   salvage
   sclerotherapy
   step-care hypertensive
   supportive
   thrombolytic
   tiered
   tiered tachyarrhythmia
   transcatheter sclerotherapy
   transfusion
   transplacental drug
   triple-drug
   updraft
   vaso-occlusive angiotherapy (VAT)

therapy *(cont.)*
    ventricular fibrillation
    ventricular resynchronization
    ventricular tachycardia
    vitamin K antagonist
    weight loss
therapy zones
Theriflash drug delivery device
thermal compression
thermal dilution technique
thermal memory stent
Thermedics cardiac device
thermistor catheter
thermistor electrode
thermistor plethysmography
Thermoactinomyces sacchari
Thermocardiosystems left ventricular
    assist device
thermodilution balloon catheter
thermodilution cardiac output
thermodilution catheter
thermodilution ejection fraction
thermodilution method for determining
    cardiac output
thermodilution method of cardiac
    output measurement
thermodilution Swan-Ganz catheter
thermography, blood vessel
thermophilic actinomycete
ThermoRod implants for thermal
    ablation of tissue
Thermos pacemaker
TherOx 0.014 infusion guidewire
THI needle
thiamine deficiency
thiazide diuretics
thick border of lung
thick echo
thickened adventitia
thickened alveolar septa
thickened degenerated intima, friable
thickened mitral valve

thickened pericardium
thickened secretions
thickened valvular leaflets
thickening
    balloon-injured carotid intimal
    diffuse pleural
    focal intimal
    intimal
    mottled
    pleural
thickening of arterial intima, diffuse
thickening of interstitial structures,
    coarse
thickening of valve
thickening of valve leaflets
thickening of ventricular wall
thick mucus secretions
thickness
    interventricular septal (IVST)
    intima-media (IMT)
    IVS wall
    posterior LV wall
    posterior wall (PWT)
    septal
    septal wall
    ventricular free wall
    wall
thickness of sputum
thick sputum
thick-walled ventricle
thick yellowish-green discharge
Thiersch suture
thigh claudication
thigh-high antiembolic stockings
thigh-high TEDs (thromboembolic
    disease) (hose or stockings)
thin border of lung
thin fibrous cap
ThinLine EZ bipolar cardiac pacing
    lead
THINSite dressing
THINSite with Biofilm dressing

thin-walled atrium
thiocyanate blood level
thiocyanate toxicity
thionamides
third-degree atrioventricular (AV)
  block
third-generation device (first-, second-
  fourth-, etc.)
third heart sound, physiologic
third intercostal space
third left interspace
third order chordae
third space sequestration
30° position
30° right anterior oblique
  projection
38-kDa (38-kilodalton)
38-kDa antibodies
38-kDa protein antigen, purified
Thomas-Allis forceps
Thomas vascular access shunt
Thompson carotid artery clamp
Thomsen disease
thoracentesis
  diagnostic
  therapeutic
thoracentesis fluid
thoracentesis needle
thoracic aneurysm
thoracic aorta
thoracic aorta aneurysm
thoracic aorta, descending
thoracic aorta-femoral artery bypass
  graft
thoracic aortic dissection
thoracic aortography
thoracic arch aortogram
thoracic asymmetry
thoracic cage configuration
thoracic catheter
thoracic cavity
thoracic deformity

thoracic duct
thoracic duct drainage (TDD)
thoracic duct injury
thoracic empyema
thoracic fistula
thoracic gas volumes
thoracic great vessel
thoracic great vessel injury
thoracic inlet
thoracic inlet syndrome
thoracic kyphosis, loss of
thoracicoabdominal fistulectomy
thoracicoabdominal incision
thoracicogastric fistulectomy
thoracicointestinal fistulectomy
thoracic outlet compression syndrome
thoracic outlet syndrome
thoracic outlet, widened
thoracic pain
thoracic rongeur
thoracic scissors
thoracic spine (T spine)
thoracic splenosis
thoracic stomach
thoracic trauma, blunt
thoracic vertebrae (T1-T12)
thoracic wall, abdominal
thoracoabdominal aneurysm
thoracoabdominal aorta
thoracoabdominal aortic aneurysmectomy
thoracoabdominal aortic aneurysm
  (TAAA) surgery
thoracoabdominal approach
thoracoabdominal asymmetry
thoracoabdominal incision
thoracoabdominal nerves
thoracoabdominal wall
thoracodorsal vein
thoracoepigastric vein
thoracoepigastric vein periphlebitis
thoracofemoral conversion

thoracolaparotomy
thoracophrenolaparotomy
thoracoplasty
Thoracoport (laparoscopy port)
thoracoscope (see *endoscope*)
"thorascopic" (misspelling of thoracoscopic)
thoracoscopic apical pleurectomy
thoracoscopic implantation
thoracoscopic lung biopsy
thoracoscopic resection, video-assisted
thoracoscopic repair of diaphragmatic defect
thoracoscopic talc pleurodesis
thoracoscopic wedge resection, video-assisted
thoracoscopy
   transpleural
   video-assisted (VAT)
thoracoscopy cannula
thoracoscopy of lung, video-assisted
thoracoscopy trocar
thoracostomy (see *thoracotomy*)
thoracotomy (pl. thoracotomies)
   anterolateral
   anterolateral muscle-sparing lateral
   bilateral anterior
   bilateral staged
   closed tube
   left lateral
   left posterolateral
   limited
   posterolateral
   resuscitative
   transverse anterior
Thora-Klex chest drainage system
Thoralon biomaterial in coronary artery bypass graft
Thor angioplasty dilatation catheter
Thora-Port
Thoratec BVAD, BiVAD (biventricular assist device)

Thoratec cardiac device
Thoratec RVAD (right ventricular assist device)
Thoratec VAD (ventricular assist device)
thorax (see also *chest*)
   asymmetrical
   barrel-shaped
   cylindrical
   Peyrot
   squared off
   symmetrical
Thorel bundle of muscle fibers in heart
Thorel pathway
thready pulse
threatened vessel closure post-PTCA
three-antigen recombinant immunoblot assay
three-block claudication
three-component friction rub
3-D (three-dimensional)
3-D CE (three-dimensional contrast-enhanced) magnetic resonance angiography technique
3-D echocardiography (3DE)
3-DE (three-dimensional echocardiography)
3-D FT magnetic resonance angiography (3-dimensional Fourier transform)
3-D gadolinium-enhanced MR angiography
3-D IVUS (three-dimensional intravascular ultrasound)
3-D reconstruction
3-D time of flight magnetic resonance angiographic sequences (3DTOF MR angiographic sequences)
3-D transesophageal echocardiography
three-pillow orthopnea
3-prong (or three-prong) rake blade

3 sign
three-step test
3:2 block ("three to two")
three-turn electrode
three-vessel coronaropathy
three-vessel coronary disease
three-vessel runoff
three-way catheter
three-way stopcock connector
three-way valve (of catheter)
thresher's lung
threshing fever
threshold
    anaerobic
    capture
    defibrillation (DFT)
    high pacing
    implant
    lead
    myocardial
    pacemaker
    pacemaker stimulation
    pacing
    pain
    satisfactory
    sensing
    sensitivity
    stimulation
threshold current
threshold for arrhythmia
threshold load training
threshold of activation
threshold rate of excretion
thrill
    aneurysmal
    aortic
    apical
    arterial
    basal precordial
    crescendo-systolic
    dense
    diastolic

thrill *(cont.)*
    diastolic apical
    excellent
    faint
    palpable
    parasternal systolic
    precordial
    presystolic
    purring
    supramanubrial systolic
    suprasternal notch
    systolic
    vibratory
throat
    inflamed
    irritated
    raw
    scratchy
    strep
    swollen
throbbing pain
thrombectomy
thrombi (pl. of thrombus)
thrombin
    coil soaked in
    topical
thrombin-antithrombin III complex
    (TAT)
thrombin injection (into false
    aneurysm)
Thrombinar
thrombin inhibitor
thrombin-soaked Gelfoam
thrombin time
thromboangiitis obliterans, Winiwarter-
    Buerger
thromboarteriectomy
thromboatherosclerotic process
thrombocytopenia
    heparin-induced
    Werlhof autoimmune
thrombocytopenia-absent radius (TAR)
    syndrome

thrombocytopenic purpura
  primary
  secondary
thrombocytosis, essential
thromboembolectomy
thromboembolic disease (TED)
thromboembolic syndrome
thromboembolism
  aortic
  catheter-induced
  deep venous
  pulmonary
  venous
thromboembolization
thromboendarterectomized
thromboendarterectomy
  aortoiliofemoral
  carotid
  femoral
  pulmonary
  transaortic renal
thrombogenesis
thrombogenic
thrombogenicity
thromboglobulin plasma level
thrombolysis
  anistreplase
  catheter-directed
  Eminase
  intracoronary
  intravenous coronary
  post myocardial infarction
  rt-PA (recombinant tissue
    plasminogen activator)
  streptokinase
  t-PA (tissue plasminogen activator)
  urokinase
thrombolytic agent or drug
thrombolytic enzymes
thrombolytic therapy
thrombolytic treatment of coronary
  thrombosis

thrombo-obliterative process
thrombopathia
thrombophlebitis
  anterior chest wall
  breast
  femoral
  iliofemoral
  migratory
  Mondor
  postpartum
thrombophlebitis cerulea dolens
thromboplastic material into the
  circulation
thromboplastin
thromboresistance
thrombosed graft
thrombosis (see also *thrombus*)
  abdominal aorta
  acute aortic
  agonal
  aortic
  aortoiliac
  arterial
  atrial
  atrophic
  axillary vein traumatic
  capsular
  cardiac
  cavernous sinus
  central splanchnic venous (CSVT)
  cerebral
  coronary arterial
  coronary artery
  creeping
  deep venous (DVT)
  de novo
  digital vessel
  dilatation
  effort
  femoropopliteal
  hepatic vein
  iliofemoral vein

thrombosis *(cont.)*
  infective
  intracardiac
  intravascular
  intraventricular
  left atrial
  left ventricular
  Lian-Siguier-Welti venous
  limb-threatening
  luminal
  marantic
  marasmic
  mesenteric arterial
  mesenteric venous
  migrating
  mural
  necrotizing
  nonpyogenic
  plate
  platelet
  portal vein
  postangioplasty mural
  postoperative
  propagating
  proximal
  puerperal
  pulmonary
  pulmonary artery
  renal vein
  Ribberts
  septic
  soleal vein
  spontaneous
  stent
  subacute stent (SAT)
  superficial venous
  terminal aortic
  traumatic
  venous
thrombosis in pulmonary vessels
thrombosis in situ of pulmonary
  arteries

thrombosis of aortic aneurysm,
  induced
ThromboSol
thrombotic gangrene
thrombotic microangiopathy
thrombotic occlusion
thrombotic pulmonary arteriopathy
  (TPA)
thrombotic thrombocytopenic purpura
thromboxanes (TxA1 and TxB2)
thrombus (pl. thrombi) (see also
    thrombosis)
  adherent
  agonal
  agony
  anular
  antemortem
  apical
  ball
  ball valve
  blood plate
  blood platelet
  calcified
  calf vein
  coral
  currant jelly
  fibrin
  fibrin-rich
  hyaline
  infective
  intra-arterial
  intracardiac
  intracavitary
  intravascular
  laminated
  laminated intraluminal
  laser desiccation of
  lateral
  luminal
  marantic
  marasmic
  migratory

thrombus *(cont.)*
  mixed
  mobile
  mural
  nonocclusive luminal
  obstructive
  occluding
  occlusive
  occlusive arterial
  organized
  organizing
  pale
  parietal
  pedunculated
  pericatheter
  plate
  platelet
  platelet-rich
  postmortem
  primary
  propagated, propagating
  propagation of
  red
  remodeling of
  saddle
  stratified
  traumatic
  white
thrombus formation
thrombus inhibitor
thrombus nidus
thrombus precursor protein (TpP)
thrombus propagation, prevention of
through-and-through injury
through-and-through sutures
through-the-scope balloon dilator
through-the-wall mattress sutures
Thruflex PTCA balloon catheter
thrust
  apical
  brief anterior
  cardiac

thrust *(cont.)*
  double systolic outward
  left ventricular
  presystolic outward
thrusting ventricles
thumping of heart in chest
thump, precordial
thumpversion (striking patient's chest)
Thunder high scaffolding over-the-wire
  vein graft stent
thymoma of the heart
thymus gland
  blood supply of
  lymph vessels of
  veins of
thyrocardiac disease
thyroid artery
thyroid cartilage
thyroid hormone deficiency
thyroid hormone excess
thyroid studies
thyrotoxic heart disease
thyrotoxicosis, neonatal
thyrotoxicotic cardiomyopathy
TIA (transient ischemic attack)
Tiason catheter
Tiason stent-graft
Tiason vascular graft
tibial artery disease
tibial in situ bypass
tibial outflow tracts, blind
tibial-peroneal trunk
tibial vessel Doppler waveforms
tibioperoneal occlusive disease
tick-borne protozoa
tick-tack sound
Ti-Cron suture (also Tycron)
tidal breathing
tidal expiratory flow, peak
tidal flow, midexpiratory
tidal inspiratory flow-volume
tidal volume (TV)

tidal volume, decreased
tidal volume of 10 mL/kg
tidal wave of carotid arterial pulse
tie
  free
  plastic
  tracheotomy
tie gun
Tielle absorptive dressing
tie-over stent suture
tiered tachyarrhythmia therapy
tiered therapy for ventricular fibrillation, defibrillation, and bradycardia
  pacing
tiered-therapy ICD
tiered-therapy programmable cardioverter-defibrillator (PCD)
Tietze syndrome
tigering
tight asthmatic
tight-collar syndrome
tightener, wire
tight lesion
tightness in the chest
tightness of chest
tilt table protocol
tilt test
  head-up
  positive
timbre métallique
time, times
  acceleration
  activated partial thromboplastin
    (APTT)
  aortic ischemic
  arm-to-tongue
  atrial activation
  atrioventricular
  bleeding
  cardiopulmonary bypass
  carotid ejection
  circulation

time *(cont.)*
  conduction
  contralateral washout
  corrected sinus node recovery
    (CSNRT)
  cross-clamp
  deceleration
  diastolic perfusion
  donor heart-lung
  donor organ ischemic
  Duke bleeding
  echo delay
  ejection (ET)
  high-dose thrombin (HiTT)
  insensitive
  inspiratory and expiratory (Ti, Te)
  ischemic
  isovolumic contraction
  isovolumic relaxation (IVRT)
  Ivy bleeding
  left ventricular ejection (LVET)
  maximum inflation
  maximum walking (MWT)
  mean pulmonary transit (MTT)
  myocardial contrast appearance
    (MCAT)
  pain-free walking (PFWT) (on
    treadmill)
  partial thromboplastin (PTT)
  perfusion
  prothrombin (PT)
  pulmonary transit (PTT)
  pulse reappearance
  pump
  reaction recovery
  relaxation
  right ventricle-to-ear
  sinoatrial conduction (SACT)
  sinus node recovery (SNRT)
  systolic upstroke
  T1 relaxation (in MRI)
  T2 relaxation (in MRI)

time *(cont.)*
 total cross-clamp
 total ischemic
 two-stage prothrombin
 venous filling (VFT)
 venous return (VRT)
 ventricular activation (VAT)
 ventricular isovolumic relaxation
 washout
time activity curve of contrast agent
timed imaging
Timeless Performance vena cava filter
time of heartbeat
time-out, ventriculoatrial
time-to-peak contrast (TPC)
time-to-peak filling rate (TPFR)
TIMI (thrombolysis in myocardial
 infarction) classification
TIMI grading system for patency
TIMI II, IIA, IIB protocol
timothy grass
Tine Test PPD (tuberculin purified
 protein derivative)
tine tuberculin test
tined atrial J pacing/defibrillation lead
tined J lead
tined lead
tined lead pacemaker
Tine Test PPD (tuberculin purified
 protein derivative)
tinkling rales
tinnitus, pulsatile
tip
 Andrews suction
 catheter
 directable (of bronchoscope)
 Frazier suction
 leaflet
 mitral valve leaflet
 Neon (for a catheter)
 tonsil suction
 valve
 Yankauer suction

TIPS or TIPSS (transjugular intrahepatic portosystemic shunt)
TIRE (Test of Incremental Respiratory
 Endurance) software
Tissot spirometer
Tissucol biologic adhesive
Tissucol fibrin-collagen material for
 hemostasis
tissue
 apical
 cone of apical
 cryopreserved homograft
 devitalized
 gangrenous
 granulation
 hematopoietic
 indurated
 subadventitial
 subcutaneous
 tuberculosis granulation
tissue acidosis
tissue active
tissue adhesive, Glycoprene
tissue borne
tissue breakdown
tissue contrast
tissue cutting
tissue expander
 PMT AccuSpan
 Silastic H.P.
 T-Span
tissue factor pathway inhibitor
Tissue-Guided Regeneration
tissue inflow valve
tissue-interface barrier, Vitacuff
TissueLink Monopolar Floating Ball
 for hemostasis tissue migration,
 mesenchymal
tissue outflow valve
tissue perfusion
tissue plasminogen activator (t-PA)
tissue thromboplastin
tissue veil

tissue viability
Ti, Te (inspiratory and expiratory times)
Titanium VasPort implantable vascular access device
Titan Mega PTCA dilatation catheter
Titan PTCA dilatation catheter
titer
    antistreptolysin-O (ASO)
    cold agglutinin
    Mycoplasma antibody
    serum
titrated dose or dosing
titration of dosage
Titrator
TKO (to keep open), intravenous
TKO-type I.V. (to keep open [the vein])
^{201}Tl (thallium-201)
^{201}Tl stress imaging
Tl (thallium) myocardial imaging
TLC (total lung capacity)
TLC (total lymphocyte count)
TLC (triple-lumen catheter)
T loop (vectorcardiography)
TLR (target lesion revascularization)
TLV (total lung volume)
T (thymus-dependent) lymphocytes
TMR (transmyocardial revascularization)
TNB (transthoracic needle biopsy)
TMST (treadmill stress test)
TMT (treadmill test)
TNB (Tru-Cut needle biopsy)
TNKase (tenecteplase)
to-and-fro murmur
Todaro tendon resection
Todaro, triangle of
Todd units for ASO titer
toe ulceration
toenails, thickened

toes, purple
TOF (tetralogy of Fallot)
toilet (toilette)
    aggressive pulmonary
    pulmonary
    tracheal
    tracheostomy
tolazoline test
tolerance, exercise
Tomcat Fighter guidewire
Tomcat Guidance System (for guidewires)
Tomcat guidewire
Tom Jones closure
tomogram
tomograph (x-ray)
    single-slice long-axis
    stacked
tomographic slices
tomography
    biplanar cardiac blood pool
    computerized axial (CAT)
    dynamic single photon emission
    exercise thallium-201
    GE single-photon emission computerized
    myocardial perfusion
    positron emission (PET)
    rapid acquisition computed axial (RACAT)
    seven-pinhole
    single photon emission computed (SPECT)
    slant-hole
    SPECT (single photon emission computed)
tomoscintigraphy
T_1 heart sound (tricuspid valve closure)
T1 relaxation time (in MRI)
T1-weighted image

tone
   hyperactive sympathetic
   postural
tongue
   chicken heart
   geographic
tongue of vein material
toothed Adson tissue forceps
toothpaste shadows
Topaz II SSIR pacemaker
Top-Hat supra-anular aortic valve
topical antimicrobial prophylaxis
topical cold saline
topical cooling of heart with saline
topical cooling with ice slush
topical drugs
topical ice
topical lavage
topical lidocaine spray
topical myocardial hypothermia
topically cooled
top normal limits in size
topographic
topographical
topography
   arterial
   ventricular
   vessel
Toprol XL (metoprolol succinate)
TORCH titer
Torcon catheter
Torcon NB selective angiographic
   catheter
Toronto SPV aortic valve
Toronto SPV bioprosthesis
torqueability
torque, constant clockwise (of
   electrode tip)
torque-directed nonballoon catheter
torque response
torque tube catheter
torr pressure

torsades de pointes ventricular tachycardia
torsemide
tortuosity and elongation
tortuosity of blood vessel
tortuosity of superficial veins
tortuosity of veins
tortuosity precluding catheter passage
tortuous aorta
tortuous arterial curves
tortuous emptying
tortuous veins
tortuous vessel
torus aorticus
Toshiba echocardiograph machine
total absence of pericardium
total alternans
total anomalous pulmonary venous
   connection
total anomalous pulmonary venous
   drainage
total anomalous pulmonary venous
   return
total anomalous venous return
total artificial heart (TAH) (see *artifi-*
   cial heart and *heart*)
total atrial refractory period (TARP)
total body heparinization
total body water
total cavopulmonary artery conversion
   and arrhythmia surgery
total cavopulmonary connection (TCP)
total heart replacement, orthotopic
Total-Lo
total lung capacity (TLC)
total lung volume (TLV)
totally endoscopic coronary artery
   bypass (TECAB)
total parenteral nutrition (TPN)
total peripheral resistance (TPR)
total valvectomy
totalis, situs inversus

tour de force
tourniquet
   caval
   Esmarch
   Medi-Quet surgical
   rotating (for pulmonary edema)
   Rumel myocardial
   vena caval
tourniquet inflated to 300 mm Hg
tourniquet test for collateral circulation
Townes-Brocks syndrome
Townes syndrome
toxemia of pregnancy
toxic appearance
toxic fumes
toxic gas inhalation
toxic insult
toxicity
   cyanide
   cyclosporine
   digitalis
   dose-limiting
   oxygen
   pulmonary
   theophylline
   thiocyanate
toxic myocarditis
toxic oil syndrome
toxic pneumonia
toxic shock
toxic shock syndrome
toxic vapor inhalation
Toxocara canis infection
toxoplasmosis, recrudescent
toxoplasmotic myocarditis
TP segment on EKG
t-PA (tissue plasminogen activator)
t-PA thrombolysis
TPA (thrombotic pulmonary
   arteriopathy)
TPC (time to peak contrast)
   (myocardial)

TPEG (transluminally placed endovas-
   cular grafts)
TPFR (time to peak filling rate)
T-piece oxygen
TPM (turning-point morphology)
TPN (total parenteral nutrition)
TpP (thrombus precursor protein)
TPR (temperature, pulse, and
   respiration)
TPR (total peripheral resistance)
TPR (total pulmonary resistance)
TQ segment
TR (repetition time)
TR (tricuspid regurgitation)
trabecula (pl. trabeculae)
trabecula septomarginalis
trabeculae carneae cordis
trabeculated atrium
trabeculation, endocardial
trace edema
trace Hematest positive
Trace vein stripper
tracer (see *radioisotope*)
tracer activity
tracer dose
trachea
tracheal anastomosis
tracheal aspiration through artificial
   airway
tracheal aspiration through natural
   airway
tracheal bifurcation
tracheal bronchial lavage
tracheal caliber
tracheal cartilage
tracheal deviation
tracheal displacement, anterior
tracheal hook
tracheal injury, concomitant
tracheal rales

tracheal ring
  first
  second
  third
tracheal stenosis
tracheal toilet
tracheal tug
tracheitis
  acute
  catarrhal
tracheobronchial fistula
tracheobronchial lavage
tracheobronchial lymph nodes
tracheobronchial secretions
tracheobronchial tract
tracheobronchial tree
tracheobronchial tuberculosis
tracheobronchitis
tracheobronchomalacia, acquired
tracheobronchomegaly
tracheoesophageal fistula (TEF)
tracheoesophageal fistulectomy
tracheomalacia
tracheostomy
  mediastinal
  temporary
tracheostomy collar
tracheostomy stoma
tracheostomy toilet
tracheostomy tube
tracheotomizing
tracheotomy
tracheotomy ties
Tracheotwist tracheostomy tube
Trachi-Naze artificial nose
Trachi-Naze laryngectomy filter
tracing
  electrocardiographic
  flat
  monitor lead
  postexercise
  pulmonary capillary wedge

track valve
trackability
Tracker catheter
Tracker-18 Soft Stream catheter
tracking limit
tracking over the guidewire
tracking, P
tracking T
Tracleer (bosentan)
tract, tracts
  aberrant AV bypass
  atrio-His
  atrio-Hisian (atriohisian) bypass
  atriofascicular
  atriofascicular bypass
  atrionodal bypass
  blind tibial outflow
  Brechenmacher
  bypass
  fasciculoventricular bypass
  free-wall
  inflow
  internodal
  James atrionodal bypass
  James intranodal
  left ventricular inflow
  left ventricular outflow (LVOT)
  nodoventricular bypass
  outflow
  pulmonary conduit outflow
  pulmonary outflow
  respiratory
  right ventricular bypass
  right ventricular inflow
  right ventricular outflow (RVOT)
  tracheobronchial
  ventricular flow
  ventricular outflow
traction suture
tractotomy, pulmonary

training
   threshold load
   ventilatory muscle
trajectory, missile
trajectory of creatinine (Cr) rise
tramlines shadow
transabdominal left lateral retroperitoneal maneuver
TransAct intra-aortic balloon pump
transaminase, glutamic oxaloacetic
transanular patching
transaortic approach
transaortic endarterectomy
transaortic extraction endarterectomy
transaortic gradient
transaortic radiofrequency ablation
transaortic renal thromboendarterectomy
transapical endocardial ablation
transarterial pacemaker insertion
transatrial approach
transatrial surgical approach
transaxial images
transbronchial biopsy (TBB)
transbronchial lung biopsy
transbronchial needle aspiration
   (TBNA)
transcarotid balloon valvuloplasty
transcatheter ablation
transcatheter anterograde valvotomy
transcatheter arterial chemoembolization (TACE)
transcatheter arterial embolization
   (TAE)
transcatheter embolization
transcatheter fenestration
transcatheter His bundle ablation
transcatheter intervention
transcatheter knife blade atrial
   septostomy
transcatheter occlusion of ASD with
   button device

transcatheter patent ductus arteriosus
   closure
transcatheter radiofrequency ablation
transcatheter radiofrequency modification
transcatheter sclerotherapy
transcervical balloon tuboplasty (TBT)
transcoronary ablation of septal hypertrophy (TASH)
transcranial color-coded sonography
   (TCCS)
transcranial Doppler sonography
transcranial Doppler ultrasonography
transcrural
transcutaneous drive lines
transcutaneous extraction catheter
   atherectomy
transcutaneous femoral artery
   puncture
transdermal nitroglycerin
transdiaphragmatic approach
transdiaphragmatic implantation
transducer
   arterial line
   Bentley
   Diasonics
   epicardial Doppler flow
   Gould Statham pressure
   Hewlett-Packard
   high-fidelity pressure
   Meritrans disposable blood
      pressure
   Metricath catheter and
   Millar catheter-tip
   M-mode
   Pedoff
   pressure
   Siemens-Elema AB pulse
   Sonos 500 2.5 MHz ultra-
      sonographic
   Statham strain-gauge
   strain-gauge

transducer *(cont.)*
　TruWave pressure
　Ultramark 8
transducer-tipped catheter
Transeal transparent adhesive film
　dressing
transect, transected
transection
　beveled
　traumatic aortic
transection of aorta
transesophageal Doppler color flow
　imaging
transesophageal echocardiography
　(TEE)
transesophageal echocardiography,
　biplane
transesophageal imaging
transesophageal pacing
transesophageal echocardiographic
　probe
transesophageal transducer
transfemoral arteriogram
transfemoral endovascular stented
　graft procedure
transfemoral Fogarty embolectomy
transfemoral liver biopsy
transfer, free-tissue
transfixation suture
transfixion suture
transfixing Vicryl suture
transfusion, transfusions
　autogenous blood
　autologous blood
　homologous blood
　intraoperative autologous (IOAT)
　massive blood
　multiple blood
　twin-to-twin
transfusional hemosiderosis
transfusion syndrome
transfusion therapy

transgress (verb)
transhiatal esophagectomy
transhiatal resection for esophageal
　carcinoma
Transiel vascular stent
transient apnea
transient cerebral ischemia
transient decrease of consciousness
transient ECG changes
transient ectopic pulsation
transient infiltrate
transient infiltrations of lungs
transient ischemic attack (TIA)
　crescendo
　ipsilateral hemispheric carotid
　limb-shaking
transient ischemic carotid insufficiency
transient left ventricular dilatation
transient loss of consciousness
transient monocular blindness
transient perfusion defect
transient repolarization changes
transient tachypnea of the newborn
　(TTN)
transient tricuspid regurgitation of
　infancy
transient ventricular tachycardia (VT)
TransiGel hydrogel-impregnated gauze
transition zone
transitional cells
transitional rhythm
transitory symptoms
transitory weakness
transjugular intrahepatic portosystemic
　shunt (TIPS or TIPSS)
translingual nitroglycerin
translocation of coronary arteries
translucent depression in interatrial
　septum
translumbar aortography
transluminal angioplasty, percutaneous
transluminal balloon angioplasty

transluminal coronary artery angioplasty complex
transluminal endovascular graft placement
transluminal extraction catheter (TEC)
transluminal intra-arterial filtration system, percutaneous
transluminally placed endovascular
grafts (TPEG)
transluminally placed stented graft
transluminal lysing system
transluminal stent-graft implantation
transmedial plane
transmediastinal pacemaker electrode
insertion
transmitral flow
transmitral gradient
transmitted carotid artery pulsations
transmucosal nitroglycerin
transmural atrial ablation
transmural cryoablation
transmural infarct
transmural linear lesions on the
beating heart
transmural myocardial infarction
transmural steal
transmyocardial perfusion pressure
transmyocardial revascularization
(TMR)
transnasal approach
transnasally
transoral approach
transorally
Transorbent multilayer dressing
transpectoral approach
transperitoneal approach
transplacental drug therapy
transplant, transplantation
allogeneic
cardiac
double-lung
heart

transplant *(cont.)*
heart and lung
heart-lung
heterotopic
heterotopic heart
kidney
living related (LRT)
Lower-Shumway cardiac
lung
orthotopic heart
piggy-back cardiac
single-lung
syngenesioplastic
valved venous
transplant lung syndrome
transpleural thoracoscopy
transport, mucociliary
transport of cholesterol by lipoproteins
transposed aorta
transposition
atrial
carotid-subclavian
congenitally corrected
corrected great arteries
great arteries
great vessels
Jatene
Mustard procedure for
partial (of great vessels)
Senning procedure for
ventricular
transposition of great arteries (TGA)
complete
corrected (CTGA)
anterior-aorta
posterior-aorta
side-by-side
transposition of great vessels
transposition of pulmonary veins
transpulmonary echo ultrasound
reflectors
transpulmonary pressure (P_{TP})

transpulmonary pressure gradient
transpulmonic gradient
Trans-Scan
transseptal angiocardiography
transseptal antegrade approach in
  valvuloplasty
transseptal approach
transseptal cardiac catheterization
transseptal extended atriotomy
transseptal left heart catheterization
transseptal perforation
transseptal puncture
transseptal radiofrequency ablation
transstenotic pressure gradient
transtelephonic ICD interrogation
transtelephonic monitoring
transthoracic approach
transthoracic echocardiography (TTE)
transthoracic imaging
transthoracic needle aspiration biopsy
transthoracic needle aspiration,
  ultrasound-guided
transthoracic needle biopsy (TNB)
transthoracic pacemaker electrode
  insertion
transthoracic 3DE
transtracheal aspiration
transtricuspid approach
transudates
transudation of fluid
transudative pericardial fluid
Transvac transdermal patch
transvalvar gradient
transvalvular gradient
Transvene electrode
Transvene lead system
transvenous approach
transvenous cryoablation of supraventricular tachycardia
transvenous defibrillation
transvenous electrode
transvenous electrode stimulation of
  atrium

transvenous endomyocardial biopsy
transvenous implantation
transvenous insertion of vena caval
  filter
transvenous lead defibrillator
transvenous pacemaker insertion
transvenous pacing
transvenous ventricular demand
  pacemaker
transventricular aortic valvotomy,
  closed
transventricular approach
transventricular dilator
transverse anterior thoracotomy
transverse anterior thoracotomy
  incision
transverse aortic arch hypoplasia
transverse aortotomy
transverse arch
transverse arteriotomy
transverse diameter
transverse heart
transverse incision
transverse pericardial sinus
transverse plane
transverse sternotomy
transverse submammary incision
transverse venotomy
transversus thoracic muscle
transxiphoid approach for pacemaker
  lead
trap
  embolus
  Lukens
trapdoor flap method (for ALCAPA)
trapdoor incision
trapdoor-type aortotomy
trapezius muscle
Trapper catheter exchange device
trapping, air
trash foot (blue toe syndrome)
trash foot (embolization of small
  vessels in feet)

Traube murmur
Traube aortic regurgitation sign
trauma
    blunt chest
    blunt thoracic
    penetrating cervicomediastinal
        venous
traumatic aortic injuries in children
traumatic aortic transection
traumatic emphysema
traumatic pericarditis
traumatic pneumothorax
traumatic tap
traumatic thrombus
traumatic tricuspid incompetence
trauma to heart
    nonpenetrating
    penetrating
Travenol pump
Treacher Collins–Franceschetti
    syndrome
Treacher Collins syndrome
treadmill
    Astrand
    Borg exertion scale on
    Ellestad
    exercise
    motorized
    Q-Stress
treadmill exercise stress test
treadmill exercise test (TET)
treadmill inclination, incremental
    increases in
treadmill slope
treadmill speed, incremental increases
    in
treadmill stress test (TMST, TST)
treadmill testing
treatment (see also *therapy*)
    adjunctive
    conjunctive
    empiric

treatment *(cont.)*
    IPPB
    nebulizer
    noninvasive
    prenatal corticosteroid
    updraft
Tredex powered bicycle
tree
    arterial
    bronchial
    coronary
    coronary artery
    iliocaval
    tracheal-bronchial
    tracheobronchial
tree-in-winter appearance (on x-ray)
trefoil balloon catheter
Treitz ligament
Trellis infusion catheter and system
Trendelenburg excision of varicose
    veins
Trendelenburg position
Trendelenburg test for valve
    competency
Trendelenburg test for varicose veins
trendscriber
trendscription
Treponema pallidum infection
treppe ("staircase") phenomenon of
    Bowditch
TriActiv system to treat saphenous
    vein graft disease
triad
    acute compression
    adrenomedullary
    Beck
    classical (of symptoms)
    Cushing
    Grancher
    Kartagener
    Osler
triad asthma

Triage BNP (B-type natriuretic peptide) test
Triage cardiac system
trial (see also *study*)
   BARI
   BASIS (Basel Antiarrhythmic Study of Infarct Survival)
   CABG-Patch (prophylactic ICD implantation with coronary artery bypass grafting)
   CAVEAT II (directional coronary atherectomy versus PTCA)
   Circadian Anti-Ischemic Progress in Europe (CAPE)
   GISSI-2 thrombolytic
   Leiden Intervention
   Lipid Research Clinics Coronary Primary Prevention
   MADIT (Multicenter Automatic Defibrillator Implantation)
   MIAMI (intravenous metoprolol in acute myocardial infarction)
   Multicenter Unsustained Tachycardia (MUSTT)
   Multiple Risk Factor Intervention (MRFIT)
   PROMISE
   San Francisco Arteriosclerosis Specialized Center of Research (SCOR) Intervention
   SAVE (Survival and Ventricular Enlargement)
   SWIFT (Should We Intervene Following Thrombolysis)
   TAMI (Thrombolysis and Angioplasty in Myocardial Infarction)
   Urokinase Pulmonary Embolism (UPET)
triamterene/hydrochlorothiazide
triangle
   Burger scalene
   cardiohepatic

triangle *(cont.)*
   carotid
   Einthoven
   femoral
   Garland
   Gerhardt
   internal jugular
   Koch
   Korányi-Grocco
   Scarpa
   supraclavicular
   Todaro
triangular area of dullness
triangulation of Carrel
triatriatum, cor
triatriatum dextrum, cor
triaxial reference system
tributary veins
tributary, venous
Trichinella myocarditis
Trichinella spiralis infection
trichinosis
trichinous embolism
Trichosporon beigelii
Tricor (micronized fenofibrate)
tricuspid aortic valve
tricuspid atresia
tricuspid incompetence
tricuspid murmur
tricuspid orifice regurgitation
tricuspid regurgitation
tricuspid stenosis
tricuspid valve (TV)
tricuspid valve abnormalities
tricuspid valve anuloplasty
tricuspid valve anomaly
tricuspid valve anulus
tricuspid valve closure
tricuspid valve converted to bicuspid
tricuspid valve deformity
tricuspid valve disease
tricuspid valve incompetence

tricuspid valve insufficiency
tricuspid valve obstruction
tricuspid valve regurgitation
tricuspid valve repair, Danielson
   method of
tricuspid valve stenosis
tricuspid valvuloplasty
tricyclic antidepressants
trifascicular block
trifascicular disease
trifascicular heart block
trifid precordial motion
trifurcates
trifurcation
   patent
   popliteal
Trifusion catheter
trigeminal pattern
trigeminus distention of neck veins
trigeminy
triggered activity
triggered by physical exertion
triggering mechanism
trigger, recognizable
triggering ventricular contraction
triglycerides (neutral fat)
   serum
   familial elevated
trigone
   fibrous
   left fibrous
   right fibrous
trigonum caroticum
Triguide guide catheter
triiodothyronine
trilayer appearance
trileaflet
triloculare biatriatum, cor
Trilogy DC+ pacemaker
trilogy, Fallot
Trilogy SR+ single-chamber pacemaker

trimellitic anhydride pneumonitis
trimmed on the bias
Trios M pacemaker
triphasic
triphasic contour of QRS complex
triple A (AAA, abdominal aortic
   aneurysm)
triple-dose gadolinium-enhanced MR
   imaging without MT (magnetization transfer)
triple-drug therapy
triple extrastimuli
triple-lumen catheter
triple-lumen central catheter
triple-lumen central venous catheter
triple-lumen line
triple rhythm
triple ripple
triplet beat
tripod position
tripolar electrode catheter
tripolar tined endocardial lead
tripolar transvenous screw-in electrode
trisomy 11q syndrome
trisomy 13(D) syndrome
trisomy 13-15 syndrome
trisomy 18(E) syndrome
trisomy 21 (Down) syndrome
trisomy 22 syndrome
Triumph-I vascular port
Triumph VR pacemaker
TriVex transilluminated powered
   phlebectomy procedure for
   varicose vein removal
trivial mitral regurgitation
Trocan disposable CO_2 trocar and
   cannula
trocar
   blunt-tip
   Davidson thoracic
   Entree thoracoscopy
   floating tip

trocar *(cont.)*
   Hancock
   Hurwitz thoracic
   L-shaped
   Nelson thoracic
   thoracoscopy
   Trocan disposable CO_2 (and
      cannula)
trocar cannula
trocar wound
TRON 3 VACI cardiac imaging
   system
trophic skin changes
tropical endomyocardial fibrosis
tropical eosinophilia
tropical eosinophilia syndrome
tropical eosinophilic lung
tropomyosin
troponin I
troponin level
troponin T
troponin T test
troubleshooting
trough level of drug
trough of venous pulse
trough
   systolic
   X
   Y
Trousers, Medical Anti-Shock
   (MAST)
Trousseau dilator
Trousseau phenomenon
Trousseau sign of superficial thrombophlebitis
Trousseau syndrome
Tru-Area Determination wound-
   measuring device
Tru-Close wound drainage system
true lumen
true polycythemia
true posterior wall myocardial
   infarction

true truncus arteriosus
true vocal cords
Trufill n-BCA liquid embolic system
truncal artery
truncal congenital vascular defect
truncal valve
truncal venous defects
truncal venous malformations
truncated atrial appendage
truncated exponential simultaneous
   monophasic waveforms
truncation of peak flow
truncus arteriosus
   common
   persistent
   true
truncus arteriosus communis
trunk
   brachiocephalic
   common
   peroneal-tibial
   pulmonary
   saphenous
   single arterial
   supra-aortic
   tibial-peroneal
   twin
   vagus
trunk of atrioventricular bundle
Trusler repair
Trusler rule for pulmonary artery
   banding
Trusler technique to reconstruct aortic
   valve
TruWave pressure transducer
TruZone PFM (peak flow meter)
Trypanosoma cruzi
trypanosomiasis, African
TS (tricuspid stenosis)
T-Span tissue expander
TST (treadmill stress test)
tsutsugamushi disease

TSV (total stroke volume)
T system (sarcolemma)
TTE (transthoracic echocardiography)
TTI (tension-time index)
TTM (transtelephonic electrocardio-
    gram monitoring)
TTN (transient tachypnea of the new-
    born)
T2 relaxation time (in MRI)
T2-weighted image
T12 needle
T12 suture
TU wave
Tubbs mitral valve dilator
tube
    Andrews Pynchon suction
    angled 24F pleural
    angled pleural
    apically directed chest
    atelectasis following removal
        of chest
    Argyle chest
    Argyle Sentinel Seal chest
    bilateral pleural
    Bivona tracheostomy
    Blakemore-Sengstaken tube
    Broncho-Cath endotracheal
    chest
    cuffed endotracheal
    double-lumen endobronchial
    endotracheal
    Endotrol tracheal
    Endo-Tube
    ETT (endotracheal)
    fenestrated
    fenestrated tracheostomy
    Frazier suction
    Haldane-Priestley
    Heimlich
    Hi-Lo Jet tracheal
    Holter
    J-shaped

tube *(cont.)*
    large-caliber
    Lindholm tracheal
    Lo-Pro tracheal
    Miser
    nasogastric
    nasotracheal
    oroendotracheal
    Pleur-evac suction
    pleural
    polyethylene
    Rehfuss
    right-angle chest
    rubber
    Sarns intracardiac suction
    Shiley tracheotomy
    Silastic
    straight chest
    suction
    Thora-Klex chest
    tracheostomy
    Tracheotwist tracheostomy
    water-seal chest
    Yankauer suction
tube drainage
tube endograft
tube graft (see *graft*)
tube guide
tube thoracostomy
tubercle
tubercle bacillus
tubercle of a rib
tubercles, noncaseating
tubercular empyema
tubercular infection
tuberculin reaction
tuberculin Mono-Vacc test
tuberculin test, intermediate
Tuberculin Tine test, Old
tuberculosis (TB)
    acute
    adult

tuberculosis *(cont.)*
  aerogenic
  anthracotic
  atypical
  avian (transmissible to humans)
  basal
  bovine (transmissible to humans)
  caseating
  cavitary
  cestode
  cestoid
  childhood
  disseminated
  endobronchial
  extrapulmonary
  exudative
  fulminant
  hilus
  inhalation
  miliary
  multidrug-resistant (MDR-TB)
  open
  postprimary
  primary
  pulmonary
  reinfection
  tracheobronchial
tuberculosis infection, atypical
tuberculosis of bronchial glands
tuberculosis of serous membranes
tuberculosis reactivation, corticosteroid-
  administration-related
tuberculous bronchiectasis
tuberculous constrictive pericarditis
tuberculous pericarditis
tuberculous pneumothorax
tuberosa, chorditis
tuberosum simplex, xanthoma
tuberous sclerosis syndrome
tubing, extension
tubular breath sounds
tubular breathing

tubular graft, horseshoe
tubular lesion
tubular segment
tubular stenosis
tubular ventricle
Tuffier rib spreader
Tuffier test
tumor
  alveolar cell
  amelioration of
  benign bronchial
  benign peripheral
  carcinoid (of bronchus)
  friable
  granular cell (of the heart)
  Hürthle cell
  juxtaglomerular cell
  macroscopically evident
  mediastinal
  metastatic myocardial
  metasynchronous
  mobile pedunculated left atrial
  Pancoast
  parenchymal
  pulmonary sulcus
  Purkinje cell
  renin-secreting
  vascular
  Wilms
tumor blush
tumor embolism
tumor embolization, cardiac
tumorlike shadow
tumor marker, DNA polymerase-alpha
tumor necrosis factor alpha (TNFa)
tumor of heart
tumor of neural crest origin
tumor plop sound
tumor prolapsed through mitral valve
  orifice
tumor pseudocapsule
tungsten carbide disease

tunica adventitia
tunica intima
tunica media
tunnel
    aortic-left ventricular
    aortico-left ventricular
    aortopulmonary
    baffled
    retroperitoneal
    subaortic stenosis
    subcutaneous
tunnel operation
tunnel repair
tunnel subaortic stenosis
tunnel subvalvular aortic stenosis
tunnel (verb), tunneled
tunneler, hollow
tunneling instrument
tunneling, retroperitoneal
Tuohy-Borst introducer
Tuohy-Borst Y adapter
turbid effusion
turbid fluid
Turbinaire
turbinates, nasal
Turbuhaler
turbulence
turbulent blood flow
turbulent intraluminal flow
turbulent signal
turgor
turgor pressure
Turkish sabre syndrome
Turner syndrome
turning-point morphology (TPM)
turnover
    erythrocyte iron (EIT)
    plasma iron (PIT)
    red blood cell iron (RBC IT)
Turpin syndrome
turtle (modern-day iron lung)
tussive fremitus

tussive syncope
Tuttle thoracic forceps
TV (tricuspid valve)
TVC (total vital capacity)
T vector
T wave, T waves
    biphasic
    broadened
    depressed
    diphasic
    enlarged
    flattened
    flipped
    hyperacute
    inverted
    inverted in V_1 and V_3
    ischemic
    Pardee
    persistently upright
    pseudonormalization of inverted
    tall
    tent-shaped
    upright
T-wave alternans
T-wave amplitude, increased
T-wave changes
T-wave deflection
T-wave flattening
T-wave inversion, terminal
12-lead electrocardiogram
22q11.2 deletion syndrome (22q11DS)
24-hour urine creatinine concentration
24-hour urine potassium concentration
24-hour urine sodium concentration
24-hour urinary secretion of VMA
    (vanillylmandelic acid)
twiddler's syndrome
Twin Cath multilumen peripheral
    catheter
Twin Cath multiple peripheral catheter
TwinFix suture anchor
Twin Jet nebulizer

twinned beats
twin transfusion syndrome
twin-to-twin transfusion
twin trunk
twin-twin transfusion syndrome
twister, wire
TwistLock Cath-Gard
2+ pitting edema
2-D (two-dimensional)
2-D echocardiogram
2-D echocardiography
2-D format
2-D IVUS (two-dimensional intravascular ultrasound)
two-dimensional echocardiography (sector scan)
two-dimensional intravascular ultrasound (2-D IVUS)
two-frame gated imaging
two-layer latex and Marlex closure technique
two-pillow orthopnea
two-stage prothrombin time
two-stage venous cannulation
two-step exercise test
two-stick or three-stick technique
two-turn electrode
two-vessel runoff

Tycron suture (also Ti-Cron)
Tygon catheter
tympanitic percussion note
tympanitic sound
tympany, Skoda
"tynoid" (see *phthinoid*)
type and crossmatch
type A dissections
type A personality
type B dissections
type B personality
type I (supracristal) ventricular septal defect
type II (infracristal) ventricular septal defect
type III (canal type) ventricular septal defect
type IV (muscular) ventricular septal defect
typhoid endocarditis
typhoid pleurisy
typhus, scrub
typical angina
typing, HLA
tyramine response
"tysis" (see *phthisis*)
T–Y tracheobronchial stent

U, u

UAC (umbilical artery catheter)
ubiquitous sound
UCG (ultrasonic cardiography)
Uhl anomaly
Uhl syndrome
ulcer
   atheromatous
   craterlike (with jagged edges)
   decubital
   decubitus
   heel
   hypertensive ischemic
   indolent
   ischemic skin
   penetrating atherosclerotic aortic
   stasis
   stress
   toe
   varicose
   venous stasis
ulcerated atheromatous plaque
ulcerated lesion
ulcerated plaque
ulceration
   arteriolar ischemic
   ischemic

ulceration *(cont.)*
   penetrating
   penetrating aortic
   penetrating atherosclerotic
   toe
ulcerative endocarditis
ulcerative pharyngitis
ulcerative rhinitis
ulcus varicosum
Ullrich-Noonan syndrome
ulnar pulse
U loop
ULP (ultra low profile) catheter
Ultec hydrocolloid dressing
ultracardiography
UltraCision ultrasonic knife
Ultracor prosthetic valve
Ultra 8 balloon catheter
ultrafast imaging
ultrafast train pacing
ultrafiltration, extracorporeal
ultrafine carbon particle
ultrafine particle deposition
Ultraflex intra-aortic balloon catheter
Ultraflex self-expanding stent
UltraKlenz wound cleanser

UltraLite flow-directed microcatheter
ultra-low profile fixed-wire balloon
   dilatation catheter
Ultramark 4 ultrasound
Ultramark 8 transducer
ultrarapid pacing
ultrasonic aortography
ultrasonic cardiogram (UCG)
ultrasonic nebulization system
ultrasonic nebulizer (USN)
ultrasonic scalpel
ultrasonic tomographic image
ultrasonography (also *ultrasound*)
   B-mode
   B-scan
   color duplex
   compression
   continuous wave
   Doppler
   duplex B-mode
   duplex pulsed-Doppler
   endoscopic
   endovascular
   fetal
   gray-scale
   HDI 1000
   Hewlett-Packard
   intracaval endovascular (ICEUS)
   intracoronary
   intravascular (IVUS)
   Irex Exemplar
   Nicolet Elite Doppler
   pulsed
   pulsed Doppler
   real-time
   real-time 4-D ultrasound
   Site-Rite
   Site-Rite II
   Smart-Inflate diagnostic
   Synthetic Aperture Focusing Tech-
      nique (SAFT) in intravascular
      ultrasound imaging

ultrasonography *(cont.)*
   3-D IVUS (three-dimensional
      intravascular ultrasound)
   transcranial color-coded
      sonography (TCCS)
   transcranial Doppler
   transthoracic
   two-dimensional intravascular
      (2-D IVUS)
   Ultramark 4
   VingMed
ultrasound (see *ultrasonography*)
ultrasound-guided compression
ultrasound-guided percutaneous
   thrombin injection
ultrasound-guided pseudoaneurysm
   compression
ultrasound-guided tattooing procedure
ultrasound-guided transthoracic needle
   aspiration
ultrasound nebulizer
   DeVilbiss
   Varic
ultrathin bronchoscope
Ultravas device
Ultravent nebulizer
umbilical artery
umbilical artery catheter (UAC)
umbilical artery catheterized
umbilical tape
umbilical vein, Biograft stabilized
   human
umbilical vein catheterized
umbilical vein graft, modified human
umbilical venous approach
umbrella
   atrial septal
   Bard Clamshell Septal
   Bard PDA
   Mobin-Uddin
umbrella closure of patent ductus
   arteriosus, percutaneous

umbrella filter, Mobin-Uddin
UMI catheter
UMI dilator (*not* HUMI)
UMI needle
unbuttoning of device
uncoiled aortic arch
uncompensated
uncomplicated convalescence
uncomplicated, non-Q-wave
    myocardial infarction
uncomplicated pneumothorax
uncomplicated Q-wave myocardial
    infarction
unconscious
unconsciousness
uncontrolled bronchospasm
uncooperative patient
under fluoroscopic guidance
underdetection
underdrive pacing
underdrive termination
underloading, ventricular
underperfused, underperfusion
undersensing of pacemaker
underventilation
underwater seal and suction
underwater-seal drainage
undulant impulse
undulating or scalloped contour
undyed braided polyglycolic acid
    suture
uneven murmur
uneventful recovery
unfavorable prognosis
unfolded aorta
ungrafted vessels
unicommissural aortic valve
unicommissural valves
unicusp
unicusp with central raphe
unicuspid aortic valve, stenosis of
unidirectional lead configuration

unifascicular block
Uniflex polyurethane adhesive surgical
    dressing
unifocal
unifocalization operations
Unigrip safety adaptor for stent
    delivery system
Unilab Surgibone
unilateral lung volume reduction
    surgery
unilateral aortofemoral graft
unilateral emphysema
unilateral hyperlucent lung
unilateral loss of pulse
unilateral overinflation
unilateral pulmonary emphysema
UNILINK anastomotic device
Unilith pacemaker
unilocular hydatid disease
unimodal
unipolar coil electrode
unipolar lead
unipolar limb lead
unipolar mode
unipolar pacemaker
unipolar pacing
unipolar programmable rate-response
    pacemaker generator
Uniprost (prostacyclin)
unit
    acute coronary care
    BICAP
    coronary care (CCU)
    critical care (CCU)
    progressive care (PCU)
    stepdown
    surgical intensive care
    Wood (of pulmonary vascular
        resistance)
unit of measure, centistoke
Unity-C pacemaker
univariate logistic regression

Univas device
univentricular heart
universal biocompatibility protection
universal IAB catheter
universal pacemaker
universal pacing mode
universal precautions
universale, angiokeratoma corporis
    diffusum
University of Akron artificial heart
University of Wisconsin solution for
    donor heart preservation
unloaded hyperpnea
unmasked by ductus arteriosus closure,
    pulmonary hypoperfusion
unmitigated (unrelieved)
unmodulated radiofrequency current
unmodulated sine wave
Unna boot
Unna-Flex compression dressing and
    wrap
unoxygenated blood
unrelenting pain
unreliable marker
unremitting pain
unresectable pulmonary metastases
unresponsive
unresponsive hypotension
unresponsive programming
unroof
unroofed coronary sinus syndrome
unsaturated fats
unsaturation
    arterial blood oxygen
    oxygen
unstable angina
unstable blood pressure
unstable lesion
untoward event
untreated hypertension
untriggered mode
U-Pass balloon catheter

up-biting biopsy cup forceps
updraft therapy
updraft treatment
upper airway neoplasm
upper airway obstruction, foreign body
upper and lower extremities blood
    pressure discrepancy
upper extremity in situ bypass
upper-limb cardiovascular syndrome
upper lobe vein prominence on chest
    x-ray
upper rate behavior
upper rate interval
upper rate limit
upper respiratory infection (URI)
upper respiratory tract disease
upper respiratory tract infection
    (URTI)
upright T wave
upright tilt-testing electrocardiogram
upright U wave
Upshaw-Schulman syndrome
upsloping ST segment
upsloping ST segment depression
upstairs-downstairs heart
upstream sampling method
upstroke
    brisk carotid
    carotid pulse
    weak carotid
upstroke and falloff
upstroke phase of cardiac action
    potentials
uptake
    ^{11}C (C-11) palmitate
    diffuse myocardial
    increased lung
    increased RV
    localized myocardial
    observed maximal oxygen
    predicted maximal oxygen
upward retraction of left costal margin

urea nitrogen, blood (BUN)
uremic cardiac syndrome
uremic pericarditis
uremic pneumonitis
ureteral stent placed prior to surgery
URI (upper respiratory infection)
urinary creatinine
urinary metanephrine
urine creatinine concentration, 24-hour
urine potassium concentration, 24-hour
urine sodium concentration, 24-hour
urokinase recanalization
urokinase thrombolysis
URTI (upper respiratory tract
  infection)
urticaria
USAFSAM treadmill exercise protocol
USCI angioplasty guiding sheath
USCI angioplasty Y connector
USCI arterial sheath

USCI Bard catheter
USCI cannula
USCI Goetz bipolar electrodes
USCI guidewire
USCI guiding catheter
USCI Mini-Profile balloon dilatation
  catheter
USCI NBIH bipolar electrode
USCI Probe balloon-on-a-wire
  dilatation system
USCI Sauvage EXS side-limb
  prosthesis
USCI sheath
USCI shunt
USN (ultrasonic nebulizer)
Utah TAH (total artificial heart)
UVC (umbilical vein catheter)
uvulopalatopharyngoplasty
U-wave inversion
U wave, prominent

618

V, v

V (lung volume)
V (ventilation)
V (ventricular)
V (volts)
V_A (alveolar ventilation)
VA (ventriculoatrial)
VA block cycle length
vaccine
    bacillus Calmette-Guérin (BCG)
    flu
    FluMist influenza virus
    influenza
    mixed respiratory (MRV)
    pneumonia
    7-valent
V-A conduction
Vaclok syringe
Vacor Rat Killer
VACTERL (vertebral, anal, cardiac
    tracheal, esophageal, renal, limb)
    anomaly
V_2–A_2 curve
Vacutainer
VAD (ventricular assist device)
VAG (Vectra vascular access graft)
vagal carotid sinus syncope
vagal influence

vagally-induced reflex
vagal reaction
vagal reflexes
vagal response
vagal stimulation
vagal syncope syndrome
vagovagal syncope
vagus nerve
vagus pulse
vagus trunk
V–A interval
Vairox high compression vascular
    stockings
Valdes-Cruz method
valley fever
Valsalva maneuver
Valsalva release
Valsalva sinus aneurysm
Valsalva strain
Valsalva test for pneumothorax
valvar aortic stenosis
valvar congenital aortic stenosis
valve (see also *prosthesis*)
    absent pulmonary
    anterior semilunar
    anuloplasty
    aortic (AV)

valve *(cont.)*
- aortocoronary
- aortofemoral
- artificial cardiac
- atrioventricular (AV) left or right
- atrioventricular (mitral and tricuspid)
- ball
- ball-and-cage prosthetic
- ball-and-seat
- ball-cage
- ball-occluder
- ball poppet of prosthetic
- bileaflet heart
- bileaflet tilting-disk prosthetic
- bicommissural aortic
- bicuspid
- bicuspid aortic
- bicuspid atrioventricular
- bicuspid pulmonary
- bileaflet
- billowing mitral
- biological tissue
- bioprosthesis heart
- bovine
- bovine heart
- butterfly heart
- caged ball occluder prosthetic
- caged disk occluder prosthetic
- calcification of mitral
- calcified
- calcified aortic
- cardiac
- C-C (convexo-concave) heart
- cleft mitral
- commissural pulmonary
- competent
- composite aortic
- conduit
- congenital absence of pulmonary
- congenital anomaly of mitral (CAMV)

valve *(cont.)*
- congenital bicuspid aortic
- congenitally bicuspid aortic
- congenitally quadricuspid aortic
- congenital unicuspid
- cryopreserved allograft heart
- disk-type
- doming of
- double velour knitted Dacron
- dysplastic
- early opening of
- eccentric monocuspid tilting-disk prosthetic
- echo-dense
- eustachian
- extirpation of
- femorofemoral crossover
- fibrotic distortion of
- fibrotic mitral
- flail mitral
- flexible cardiac
- floppy
- floppy aortic
- floppy mitral
- glutaraldehyde-tanned porcine heart
- golf T-shaped polyvinyl
- hammock
- hammocking of
- hammock mitral
- healed
- heart
- heterograft
- hockey-stick tricuspid
- hypoplastic
- incompetent
- intact
- integral hemostasis
- intraluminal sutureless
- leaky
- left semilunar
- midsystolic buckling of mitral
- midsystolic closure of aortic

valve *(cont.)*
  mitral (MV)
  monocusp
  narrowed
  native
  native aortic
  neoaortic
  noncoronary seating of the
  notching of pulmonic
  one-way (of catheter)
  outflow tract
  parachute mitral
  pericardial
  porcine heart
  porcine heterograft
  posterior semilunar
  premature closure of
  premature mid-diastolic closure
    of mitral
  prosthetic heart
  pulmonic (PV)
  pulmonary (PV)
  quadricuspid pulmonary
  regurgitation of mitral
  rheumatic mitral
  right atrioventricular
  right semilunar
  seating of
  semilunar (aortic and pulmonary)
  stenosis of mitral
  stenotic
  stent-mounted allograft
  stentless
  stentless porcine aortic valve
  straddling atrioventricular
  synthetic
  systolic anterior motion of mitral
  thebesian
  thickened mitral
  three-way (of catheter)
  tilting-disk valve
  track

valve *(cont.)*
  tricuspid (TV)
  tricuspid aortic
  trileaflet aortic
  truncal
  unicommissural
  unicommissural aortic
  vegetation of
  venous
  xenograft
valve area
valve calcification
valvectomy
valve coaptation site
valvectomy, total
valve cusps
valved conduit
valve dehiscence
valved venous transplant
valve excision
valve function, pulmonary and
  tricuspid
valve incision
valve incompetence
valve leaflets
valve of coronary sinus
valve of foramen ovale
valve of Vieussens
valve outflow strut
valve plane
valve pockets
valve prosthesis (see *valve*)
valve replacement
valve scarring
valve strut
valve thickening and scarring
valve tip
valviform
valvotomy
  anterograde percutaneous aortic
  aortic
  balloon

valvotomy *(cont.)*
  balloon mitral
  closed transventricular aortic
  double-balloon
  mitral
  open
  percutaneous balloon aortic
  percutaneous balloon pulmonary
  percutaneous mitral balloon (PMV)
  pulmonary
  single-balloon
  transcatheter anterograde
  transventricular aortic
  transventricular closed
valvular aortic insufficiency
valvular aortic stenosis
valvular apparatus
valvular atresia
valvular cardiac defect
valvular damage
valvular disease
valvular dysfunction
valvular heart disease
valvular incompetence
valvular opening
valvular orifice
valvular pneumothorax
valvular pulmonic stenosis
valvular pulmonic stenosis murmur
valvular regurgitant lesion
valvular regurgitation
valvular stenosis
valvulitis
  chronic
  rheumatic
valvuloplasty
  aortic
  bailout
  balloon
  balloon aortic
  balloon mitral
  balloon pulmonary (BPV)

valvuloplasty *(cont.)*
  Carpentier tricuspid
  catheter balloon (CBV)
  double-balloon
  Kay tricuspid
  percutaneous aortic (PAV)
  percutaneous aortic balloon
  percutaneous balloon (PBV)
  percutaneous balloon mitral
  transcarotid balloon
  percutaneous balloon aortic
  percutaneous mitral balloon (PMV)
  prosthetic valve
  pulmonary
  pulmonary balloon
  retrograde simultaneous double-
    balloon
  retrograde simultaneous single-
    balloon
  single-balloon
  tricuspid
valvulotome
  expanding
  Gerbode mitral
  Himmelstein
  Leather venous
  Mills pulmonary
  spade-shaped
valvulotome in intraluminal Hall valve
  disruption technique
valvulotomy (valvotomy)
valvutome (see *valvulotome*)
VAN (vein, artery, nerve)
Van Andel catheter
van den Bergh test of concentration of
  bilirubin in blood
vanillylmandelic acid (VMA)
vanishing lung
vanishing lung syndrome (on x-ray)
Vanlev (omapatrilat)
Van Tassel pigtail catheter
VAP (ventilator-associated pneumonia)
  cholesterol test

vaporization of abnormal blood vessels
vaporization of atheromatous plaque
vaporization of plaque material
vapor massage
vapotherapy
Vaquez-Osler syndrome
variability
   beat-to-beat
   peak flow
variable intensity
variable murmur
variable response rate
variable threshold angina
variant
   electrocardiographic
   Kussmaul-Maier
   Loeffler (Löffler)
   orthostatic hypotension
variant angina pectoris
varicella-associated focal angiitis
varices (pl. of varix)
   aneurysmal
   arterial
   arteriovenous
   bilateral saphenous
   esophageal
   pelvic
   saphenous
   scrotal
   sublingual
   vulval
varicography
varicose aneurysm
varicose bronchiectasis
varicose veins
   familial
   primary
varicosity (pl. varicosities)
varicosum, ulcus
Varic ultrasound nebulizer
Vari/Moist wound dressing
variola (smallpox)

Varivas R denatured homologous vein
varix (pl. varices)
varying P-R interval
vasa vasorum (of artery)
Vas-Cath catheter
Vasconnect device
Vascor porcine prosthetic valve
VascuCoil peripheral vascular stent
Vascu-Guard patch
vascular access device, nb200
vascular access graft (see *graft*)
vascular access port (see *port*)
vascular anastomosis
vascular and airway modeling
   on CT scan
vascular atrophy
vascular attachments
vascular bed, pulmonary vascular
vascular brachytherapy
vascular bud
vascular bundle
vascular catastrophe
vascular channels, aberrant
vascular cirrhosis
vascular clamp, atraumatic
vascular compromise
vascular congestion
vascular dementia
vascular disease, peripheral
vascular embolization device
vascular endothelial growth factor
   (VEGF)
vascular engorgement
vascular graft (see *graft*)
vascular graft flushing
vascular hemophilia
vascular heterograft
vascular impedance
vascular insult
vascularis, plexus
vascularity
   decreased
   lung

vascular ligation, selective
vascular lumen
vascular malformation
vascular markings
vascular nephritis
vascular network
vascular obstruction
vascular occlusion clamp
vascular occlusion clip
vascular pedicle
vascular plexus
vascular redistribution
vascular resistance
  coronary
  increased pulmonary
  raised
vascular ring
vascular ring syndrome
vascular sling
vascular smooth muscle cells (VSMC)
vascular spasm
vascular syndrome
vascular systemic resistance
vascular tape
vascular tone
vascular wall damage
vascular xenograft
vasculature
  pulmonary
  splanchnic
VascuLink vascular access graft
vasculitic angiitis
vasculitis (pl. vasculitides)
  allergic
  Churg-Strauss
  hypersensitivity
  leukocytoblastic
  livedo
  necrotizing
  nodular
  polyarteritis-like systemic
  postperfusion pulmonary

vasculitis *(cont.)*
  renal
  segmented hyalinizing
  systemic
  systemic necrotizing
  toxic
vasculopathy
Vasculour prosthesis
Vascutek Gelseal knitted and woven
  vascular graft
Vascutek Gelseal vascular graft
Vascutek Gelsoft
Vascutek knitted vascular graft
Vascutek woven vascular graft
vasoactive medication
vasoactive response
vasoconstriction
  hypoxic pulmonary
  peripheral
  peripheral circulatory
  peripheral cutaneous
  pulmonary arteriolar
  spontaneous transient
  systemic arterial
vasoconstriction
vasoconstrictor response
vasoconstrictors
vasodepressive
vasodepressor carotid sinus syncope
vasodepressor reaction (VDR)
vasodepressor response
vasodepressor syncope
vasodilatation or vasodilation
  breakthrough
  judicious
  peripheral
vasodilate
vasodilation (vasodilatation)
vasodilator, peripheral
vasodilator plus exercise (VEX)
  treadmill test
vasodilatory effect

vasodilatory response
vasomotion, coronary
vasomotor paresthesia
vaso-occlusive angiotherapy (VAT) in
    congenital vascular malformations
vasopressor
vasoreactivity, pulmonary
vasorelaxation of epicardial vessels
vasorum, vasa (of artery)
VasoSeal VHD (vascular hemostatic
    device)
vasospasm
vasospastic angina
Vasotec (enalaprilat maleate)
Vasotrax blood pressure monitor
VasoView balloon dissection system
VasoView Uniport endoscopic
    saphenous vein harvesting system
vasovagal arrest
vasovagal attack
vasovagal bradyarrhythmia
vasovagal episode
vasovagal orthostatism
vasovagal phenomenon
vasovagal syncope, malignant
vasovagal syndrome
Vas recorder
vastus medialis muscle
VAT (vaso-occlusive angiotherapy)
VAT (ventricular activation time)
VAT (video-assisted thoracoscopy)
VATER (vertebral anomalies, anal atre-
    sia, tracheoesophageal fistula, radial
    and renal anomalies) syndrome
VATS (video-assisted thoracic surgery)
Vaughan-Williams antiarrhythmic
    effect
Vaughan-Williams classification of
    antiarrhythmic drugs
Vaxcel peripherally inserted central
    catheter
VC (vital capacity)

VCAB (ventriculocoronary artery
    bypass)
VCAB (ventricle-to-coronary artery
    bypass)
VCAB revascularization procedure
VCB (ventricular capture beat)
VCDF (volume-cycled decelerating-
    flow ventilation)
VCF (ventricular contractility func-
    tion)
VCF (velocardiofacial) syndrome
VCFS (velocardiofacial syndrome)
VCG (vectorcardiogram)
VCO_2 (venous CO_2 production)
VCS clip adapter
VCS clip applier (used in performing
    anastomoses)
VD (valvular disease)
VDD pacing mode
VDI (venous distensibility index)
VDR (vasodepressor reaction)
VEA (ventricular ectopic activity)
VEB (ventricular ectopic beat)
vector
    mean cardiac
    mean QRS
    P
    QRS
    ST
    T
    T-wave
vectorcardiogram, vectorcardiography
    Frank
    frontal plane
    sagittal plane
    spatial
    transverse plane
vector EKG
Vector large-lumen guiding catheter
vector lead
vector loop
VectorX large-lumen guiding catheter

Vectra vascular access graft (VAG)
Veg. (vegetation)
vegetation
  bacterial
  friable
  necrotic fibrinoid
  valvular
vegetation of valve
vegetative endocarditis
vegetative symptoms
VEGF (vascular endothelial growth
  factor)
veil, tissue
Veillonella
vein, veins
  antecubital
  anterior cardiac
  autogenous
  azygos
  blind percutaneous puncture of
    subclavian
  Boyd perforating
  brachiocephalic
  cannulated central
  capacious
  cephalic
  communicating
  congenital stenosis of pulmonary
  cutdown over cephalic
  deep
  dilated
  distended neck
  distention of neck
  Dodd perforating group of
  endoscopic division of incompetent
    perforating
  engorged
  external jugular
  familial varicose
  feeder
  flat neck
  great cardiac

vein *(cont.)*
  great saphenous
  harvest a
  harvested
  hemiazygos
  high ligation of varicose
  IJ (internal jugular)
  iliofemoral
  inferior pulmonary
  inferior thyroid
  infradiaphragmatic
  innominate
  intercostal
  internal jugular
  internal thoracic
  jugular
  leaking
  lesser saphenous
  lobe of azygos
  marginal
  Marshall
  middle cardiac
  necrosed the
  parent
  peroneal
  posterior interventricular
  pulsating
  renal
  reversed greater saphenous
  right internal jugular (IJ)
  saphenous
  scimitar
  small cardiac
  small saphenous
  soleal
  subclavian
  subcutaneous
  superficial
  superficial femoral
  superior intercostal
  superior mesenteric (SMV)
  superior mesenteric-portal (SMPV)

vein *(cont.)*
　superior pulmonary
　thebesian
　Thebesius
　thoracodorsal
　thoracoepigastric
　tortuous
　tributary
　varicose
　vertebral
　visibly distended external jugular
vein graft
　ankle brachial systolic pressure
　　index monitoring of
　blood flow patterns in
　color-flow duplex imaging of
　stenosis of
　thrombosis
　patency of
vein graft failure
vein graft occlusion
Veingard transparent dressing
vein limb
vein nodularity
vein patch angioplasty
vein patch closure
vein patency
veins distended at 45°
veins elevated at 90°
vein sign
vein stripping operation
Velcro rales
Veletri (tezosentan)
velocardiofacial (VCF) syndrome
velocardiofacial syndrome (VCFS)
velocimetry, Doppler
velocity
　blood flow
　closing
　coronary blood flow (CBFV)
　decreased closing
　diastolic regurgitant

velocity　*(cont.)*
　fiber-shortening
　forward
　maximal transaortic jet
　mean aortic flow
　mean posterior wall
　mean pulmonary flow
　meter per second (m/sec)
　peak aortic flow
　peak flow
　peak pulmonary flow
　peak systolic
　peak transmitted
　regurgitant
velocity-encoded magnetic resonance
　imaging
velocity mapping, phase
velocity-time integral of early diastole
velocity-time integral of late diastole
velocity waveforms (VWFs)
velour collar prosthesis
vena cava (pl. venae cavae)
　inferior (IVC)
　superior (SVC)
vena cava clip, Adams-DeWeese
vena cava (or caval) filter
　Bird's Nest
　Gianturco-Roehm Bird's Nest
　Greenfield
　Kimray-Greenfield
　Mobin-Uddin
　Optease permanent
　Timeless Performance
vena caval sieve
vena caval to left atrial communication
vena caval tourniquet
vena cava syndrome
venae cavae (pl. of vena cava)
venae cordis minimae
VenaFlow compression system
VenaFlow vascular graft
Venaport guiding catheter

venarum, sinus
VenaSonix ultrasound catheter
VenaSonix ultrasound therapeutic
    device
Vena Tech percutaneous LGM filter
Venes II medical stockings
Venflon cannula
venipuncture site
venoarterial admixture
venoarterial cannulation
venoarterial shunt
venoarterial shunting
venodilators
Venodyne compression boots
Venodyne compression system
Venofer (iron sucrose)
venofibrosis
venogram, venography
    contrast
    isotope
    lower limb
    radionuclide
    radionuclear
    technetium 99m
Venometer vascular diagnostic and
    monitoring device
veno-occlusive disease (VOD)
venostasis
venosus defect, sinus
venosus, plexus
venotomy, transverse
venotripsy
venous access
venous angioma
venous anomaly
venous avulsion
venous backflow
venous blood, arterialization of
venous blood gas values
venous cannula (see *cannula*)
venous cannulation
venous capillaries

venous catheter (see *catheter*)
venous circulation
venous claudication
venous collaterals
venous congestion
venous coupler
venous cutdown
venous decompensation
venous defects
venous distention
venous Doppler exam
venous dysplasias of infant
venous embolus
venous engorgement, bilateral
venous excursion
venous filling
    early
    late
venous gangrene
venous hum (nun's murmur)
venous hyperemia
venous hypertension
venous insufficiency
venous junction
venous ligation at femoral level
venous malformation (VM)
venous motion, discernible
venous murmur (see *murmur*)
venous obstruction
venous occluder
venous oxygen content
venous phlebitis-gangrene syndrome
venous pooling
venous pressure, elevated
venous pressure increased, inspiratory
venous pulsations 3 cm above the
    sternal angle
venous pulse
    diastolic collapse
    trough of
venous refill time (VRT)
venous reservoir

venous return
    anomalous pulmonary
    total anomalous
venous segment, nonfilling
venous side branch
venous sinus
venous spasm
venous stasis
venous thromboembolism
venous thrombosis (see *thrombosis*)
venous ulcer
venous valve construction
venous valves
venous vascular malformation
venovenous bypass
venovenous cannulation
vent
    aortic
    intracardiac
    left atrial
    left ventricular
    pulmonary arterial
    slotted needle
Ventak AICD (automatic implantable
    cardioverter-defibrillator) pacemaker
Ventak AV III DR cardioverter-
    defibrillator
Ventak ECD (external cardioverter-
    defibrillator)
Ventak ICD (internal cardioverter-
    defibrillator) pacemaker
Ventak Mini II (and III) AICD (auto-
    matic implantable cardioverter-
    defibrillator)
Ventak Prizm implantable defibrillator
Ventak P2 pulse generator
Ventak PRx defibrillation system
Ventak PRx pulse generator
Ventak PRx transvenous ICD
Ventak pulse generator
Ventavis inhaler
VentCheck handheld monitor

vented-electric HeartMate LVAD
Ventex dressing
ventilation
    airway pressure release
    alveolar (V_A)
    assist/control mode
    assisted
    bag-and-mask
    continuous mechanical
    continuous positive pressure
      (CPPV)
    controlled
    excessive
    high minute
    intermittent mandatory (IMV)
    KinetiX ventilation monitor
    low-frequency positive-pressure
    mask
    maximal voluntary (MVV)
    mechanical
    minute
    NIPPV (noninvasive positive
      pressure)
    noninvasive extrathoracic (NEV)
    noninvasive mechanical
    noninvasive positive pressure
      (NIPPV)
    PIP/PEEP
    positive-pressure
    pressure-cycled
    pressure support
    reduced
    reduced alveolar
    synchronized intermittent
      mandatory (SIMV)
    time-cycled
    volume-controlled inverse ratio
    volume-cycled
    volume-cycled decelerating-flow
      (VCDF)
    wasted
    weaned off

ventilation equivalent
ventilation-exchange bougie
ventilation lung scan
ventilation-perfusion (V/Q)
ventilation-perfusion defect
ventilation-perfusion imbalance
ventilation-perfusion, impaired
ventilation-perfusion inequality
ventilation-perfusion lung scan
ventilation-perfusion maldistribution
 and hypoxemia
ventilation-perfusion ratio
ventilation/perfusion scan (V/Q scan)
ventilation pneumonitis
ventilation test
ventilator or respirator
 ACD (active compression-decom-
  pression) resuscitator
 Achieva portable
 assisted-mode
 Avea
 BABYbird respirator
 BABYbird II
 Babyflex
 BagEasy respirator
 Bear Cub infant
 Bennett
 Bennett PR
 Bennett PR-2
 BiPAP
 Bird Mark
 Bird respirator
 Bourns-Bear
 Bourns Bear 1
 Bourns infant
 Cuirass respirator
 Drager Babylog 8000
 Emerson
 Foregger
 Harvard
 high-frequency jet
 high-frequency oscillation

ventilator *(cont.)*
 IMV-Bird
 Infant Star
 iVent
 KinetiX ventilation monitor
 Laerdal resuscitator
 MA-1
 Monaghan; Monaghan 300
 MVV (maximal voluntary
  ventilation)
 noninvasive extrathoracic (NEV)
 Ohio 560
 pneuPAC resuscitator
 Porta-Lung noninvasive extrathoracic ventilator (NEV)
 portable volume ventilator
 pressure-controlled
 Puritan-Bennett
 Sensormedics 3100A
 Siemens Servo
 Siemens Servo 300
 Siemens Servo 900C
 SIMV-PC
 tank-type body
 Vent-Logos pulmonary handheld
 Viasys
 volume
ventilator-associated pneumonia (VAP)
ventilator dependent
ventilatory and perfusion lung scan
ventilatory assistance
ventilatory capacity
ventilatory capacity-demand imbalance
ventilatory defect, restrictive
ventilatory dysfunction
ventilatory effort
ventilatory failure, acute
ventilatory inefficiency
ventilatory muscle training protocol
ventilatory reflex
ventilatory responsiveness
ventilatory support

ventilometric measurements
Ventimask
venting
venting aortic Bengash-type needle
venting of left heart
Ventra catheter for percutaneous
    thromboendarterectomy
ventral aorta
ventral branch
ventral olfactory epithelium
ventricle
    akinetic left
    anterior surface of
    apex of left
    atrialized
    augmented filling of right
    auxiliary
    common
    diaphragmatic surface of
    double-inlet
    double-inlet left
    double outlet left (DOLV)
    double-outlet right (DORV)
    dual
    dysfunctional left
    hypokinetic left
    hypoplastic
    hypoplastic heart
    hypoplastic left
    left (LV)
    Mary Allen Engle
    parchment right
    primitive
    right (RV)
    rudimentary right
    single
    thick-walled
    thrusting
    tubular
ventricle morphology
ventricle-to-coronary artery bypass
    (VCAB)

Ventricor pacemaker
ventricular aberration
ventricular access
ventricular activation time (VAT)
ventricular actuation, direct
    mechanical (DMVA)
ventricular afterload
ventricular aneurysm
ventricular apex
ventricular assist device (VAD)
    abdominal left (ALVAD)
    Abiomed BVS
    ALVAD (intra-abdominal left
        ventricular assist device)
    artificial left (LVAD)
    Berlin Heart
    Bio-Medicus pump
    BiVAD, BVAD (biventricular
        assist device)
    CBAS external or implantable
    DeBakey
    ECG asynchronous
    ECG synchronous
    electrically conditioned and driven
        skeletal muscle
    fully implanted
    HeartHope
    HeartMate 1000 implantable
        pneumatic (IP)
    Hemopump
    Hershey left
    Jarvik 2000
    Jocath
    Jography
    Joguide
    left (LVAD)
    LionHeart left
    mechanical
    MEDOS/HIA
    Medtronic Hemopump
    MicroMed DeBakey
    nonpulsatile

ventricular *(cont.)*
    Novacor
    Penn State
    Pierce-Donachy
    Pierce-Donachy Thoratec
    PUCA (pulsatile catheter) pump
    pulsatile
    right (RVAD)
    Sarns
    TandemHeart
    tethered
    Thermedics
    Thoratec
    Thermocardiosystems
ventricular asynchronous pacemaker
    (VOO)
ventricular burst pacing
ventricular capture beat
ventricular catheter
ventricular cavity
ventricular cavity geometry
ventricular cineangiogram
ventricular compliance
ventricular contraction
ventricular contraction pattern
ventricular couplets
ventricular D-loop
ventricular decompensation
ventricular demand inhibited
    pacemaker
ventricular demand triggered
    pacemaker
ventricular depolarization
ventricular depression
ventricular dilatation
ventricular disproportion
ventricular dysfunction
ventricular dysrhythmias, malignant
ventricular ectopy
ventricular effective refractory period
    (VERP)
ventricular ejection friction

ventricular elastance, maximum
    (EMAX)
ventricular electrical instability
ventricular endoaneurysmorrhaphy
ventricular enlargement
ventricular escape mechanism
ventricular extrastimulation
ventricular fibrillation
    idiopathic
    refractory
ventricular fibrillation pacing
ventricular fibrillation therapy
ventricular filling
ventricular filling sound (third heart
    sound)
ventricular free wall thickness
ventricular function, compromised
ventricular function curve
ventricular function parameters
ventricular fusion beats
ventricular gallop
ventricular gallop rhythm
ventricular gallop sound
ventricular gradient
ventricular hypertrophy
ventricular hypoplasia
ventricular intracerebral hemorrhage
ventricular inversion
ventricular irritability
ventricularization of left atrial
    pressure pulse
ventricularization of pressure
ventricularized morphology
ventricular lead
ventricular left-handedness
ventricular myocardium
ventricular myxoma
ventricular obstruction, intraventricular
    right
ventricular outflow obstruction
ventricular outflow tract obstruction
ventricular overdrive pacing

ventricular paced (V_P) beat
ventricular paced cycle length
ventricular pacing
ventricular paroxysmal tachycardia
ventricular perforation
ventricular pre-excitation
ventricular premature contraction
ventricular premature contraction
   couplets
ventricular premature depolarization
   (VPD)
ventricular pressure, right
ventricular pseudoperfusion beats
ventricular rate
ventricular refractoriness
ventricular refractory period
ventricular remodeling
ventricular repolarization
ventricular response
   atrial fibrillation with high-rate
   fast
   moderate
   rapid
   slow
ventricular resynchronization therapy
ventricular rhythm disturbance
ventricular right-handedness
ventricular segmental contraction
ventricular sensed (V_S) event
ventricular septal (VS)
ventricular septal aneurysm
ventricular septal defect (VSD)
   acquired
   doubly-committed
   flap valve
   infracristal
   juxta-arterial
   juxtatricuspid
   membranous
   perimembranous
   Roger
   subpulmonary

ventricular *(cont.)*
   supracristal
   Swiss cheese
   type I
   type II
   type III
   type IV
ventricular septal rupture
ventricular septal summit
ventricular septum
   intact
   overriding (of aorta)
ventricular single and double
   extrastimulation
ventricular standstill
ventricular status
ventricular stiffness
ventricular synchrony
ventricular systole
ventricular tachyarrhythmia
   malignant
   transient
   reversible
ventricular tachycardia (VT, V tach
   [slang])
   monomorphic
   nonsustained monomorphic
   nonsustained polymorphic
   polymorphic
   recurrent intractable
   refractory
   salvos of
   torsades de pointes
ventricular tachycardia detection
ventricular tachycardia reversal
ventricular tachycardia therapy
ventricular topography
ventricular transposition
ventricular volume load
ventricular wall motion
ventricular wall tension
ventriculoarterial conduit

ventriculoarterial connections,
  discordant
ventriculoarterial discordance
ventriculoatrial (VA) conduction
ventriculoatrial effective refractory
  period
ventriculoatrial time-out
ventriculocoronary arterial fistula
ventriculocoronary artery bypass
  (VCAB) revascularization
ventriculogram
ventriculography
  axial left anterior oblique
  bicycle exercise radionuclide
  biplane
  digital subtraction
  dipyridamole thallium
  exercise radionuclide
  first-pass radionuclide
  gated blood pool
  gated nuclear
  gated radionuclide
  LAO (left anterior oblique)
    projection
  left (LVG)
  radionuclide (RNV)
  RAO (right anterior oblique)
    projection
  retrograde left
  single plane left
  ventriculography
  xenon 133
ventriculoinfundibular fold
ventriculoperitoneal shunt (VP shunt)
ventriculoplasty, Dor remodeling
ventriculoradial dysplasia
ventriculorrhaphy
  linear
  Reed
ventriculotomy
  encircling endocardial
  endocardial

ventriculotomy *(cont.)*
  map-guided partial endocardial
  paracoronary right
  partial encircling endocardial
  transmural
Ventritex Angstrom MD implantable
  cardioverter-defibrillator
Ventritex Cadence ICD
Ventritex Cadence pulse generator
Ventritex defibrillation leads
venturi effect
venturi mask for oxygen administration
venule, venules
  high endothelial
  postcapillary
verapamil HCl (sustained-release
  form)
vera, polycythemia
Verbatim balloon catheter
Verbatim balloon probe
verification of ASD occlusion by echo
  Doppler studies
Veripath peripheral guiding catheter
Verluma (nofetumomab) diagnostic
  imaging agent
vernal edema
vernix membrane
VERP (ventricular effective refractory
  period)
verrucous carditis
verrucous endocarditis
  atypical
  nonbacterial
verrucous hemangioma
verrucous nodules
Versafit stent
Versalab ultrasonic medical device
Versatrax pacemaker
Versatrax pulse generator
Verstraeten bruit
vertebral arterial dissection

vertebral artery
vertebral artery syndrome
vertebral artery system
vertebral-basilar arterial insufficiency
vertebral-basilar artery syndrome
vertebral-basilar ischemia
vertebrobasilar insufficiency
vertebral column
vertebral part of medial surface of
   lung
vertebral pleural reflection
vertebral vein
vertebral venous plexus
vertical axis
vertical heart
vertical long-axis slice
vertiginous syncope
vertigo, laryngeal
very low-density lipoproteins (VLDL)
vesicles, pulmonary
vesiculae pulmonales
vesicular block
vesicular breath sounds
vesicular breathing
vesicular emphysema
vesicular rales
vessel
   angiographically occult
   anomalous
   arcuate
   atherectomized
   brachiocephalic
   caliber of
   circumflex
   codominant
   collateral
   contralateral
   cranial
   cross-pelvic collateral
   culprit
   diminutive
   disease-free

vessel *(cont.)*
   dominant
   eccentric
   great
   infrapopliteal
   intercostal
   interlobular
   lymphatic
   nondominant
   occipital
   patent
   peripelvic collateral
   peripheral
   peroneal
   plump
   posterior lumbar
   runoff
   splanchnic
   tortuous
   transposition of
   wraparound
vessel caliber
vessel closure, abrupt
vessel compression
vessel cutoff of contrast material
vessel loop
vessel loops applied
vessel loops applied
Vesseloops rubber band
vessel rupture
vessel-sizing catheters
vessel test-occluded
vessel topography
VEST ambulatory function monitor
vestibule, laryngeal
vestigial commissure
vestigial left sinoatrial node
VEX (vasodilator plus exercise) treadmill test
VF, V fib (ventricular fibrillation)
VFT (venous filling time)
VG synch period

V-H interval
viability, tissue
viable myocardium
Viagraph computerized exercise EKG
Viasorb wound dressing
Viasys cardiopulmonary exercise
   testing device
Viasys pulmonary function testing
   device
Viasys resuscitation mask
Viasys telemetry
Viasys ventilator
vibrating pulse
vibration
vibratory systolic murmur
vicious cycle
Vickers ring tip forceps
Vicor pacemaker
Vicryl suture
videoangiography, digital
video-assisted thoracic surgery
   (videothoracoscopy)
video-assisted thoracoscopic lung
   metastasectomy
video-assisted thoracoscopic lung
   volume reduction surgery
video-assisted thoracoscopic resection
video-assisted thoracoscopic wedge
   resection
video-assisted thoracoscopy of lung
video-assisted thoracoscopy (VAT)
videodensitometry
videoendoscopic surgical equipment
videolaseroscopy
Vieussens
   circle of
   isthmus of
   limbus of
   loop of
   ring of
   valve of

view (see also *chest x-ray*; *position*)
   anterior
   apical and subcostal four-chambered
   apical four-chamber (echocardio-
      gram)
   apical two-chamber
   biplane orthogonal
   caudal
   cineradiographic
   cranial angled
   four-chamber apical
   hemiaxial (x-ray)
   hepatoclavicular
   ice-pick M-mode echocardiogram
   LAO (left anterior oblique)
   LAO-cranial
   left anterior oblique (LAO)
   long axial oblique
   long-axis parasternal
   parasternal long-axis
   parasternal long-axis echocardio-
      gram
   parasternal short-axis
   RAO (right anterior oblique)
   RAO-caudal
   right anterior oblique (RAO)
   right ventricular inflow
   short-axis
   short-axis parasternal
   sitting-up
   spider x-ray
   steep left anterior oblique
   subcostal four-chamber (echo-
      cardiogram)
   subcostal long-axis (echocardio-
      gram)
   subcostal short-axis (echocardio-
      gram)
   subxiphoid (echocardiography)
   suprasternal notch (echocardiogram)
   weeping willow x-ray

Vigilance CCO/SvO2/CEDV monitor
Vigilon dressing
vigorous manual massage
Vineberg cardiac revascularization
    procedure
Vineberg operation for collateral
    circulation
VingMed ultrasound
violaceous hue
violent sneezing spells
VIPER PTA catheter
viral bronchitis
viral infection
viral myocarditis
viral pericarditis
viral pharyngitis
viral pneumonia
viral tonsillitis
viral toxicity
Virchow perivascular space
Virchow-Robin perivascular space
Virchow thrombosis triad
Virchow triad
viremia
viremic shock
viridans streptococcal infection
viridans streptococci
virology studies
Virtuoso portable three-dimensional
    imaging system
virulent atherosclerosis
virus
    adenovirus
    causative
    coxsackie A
    coxsackie B
    cytomegalovirus
    Epstein-Barr (EB)
    Four Corners
    parainfluenza
    respiratory syncytial (RSV)
    Sin Nombre (SNV)

virus bronchopneumonia
virus-infected cells
Visa II PTCA catheter
VisCath fiberoptic imaging catheter
visceral cholesterol embolization
    syndrome
visceral embolus
visceral heterotaxy
visceralis, pleura
visceral layer
visceral pericardium
visceral pleura, silicotic
visceral pleurisy
visceral rotation incision
visceral situs abnormalities
visceral situs solitus
viscerum inversus, situs
viscid sputum
viscosity
    blood
    increased blood
    plasma
    sputum
viscous resistance
viscous sputum
Visease angiographic catheter
viselike pain
visible anterior motion
visibly distended external jugular veins
Vision 1.5-T Siemens MRI scanner
Vision PTCA catheter
Visitec circular knife
Visitec crescent knife
Vista Brite Tip guiding catheter
Vista pacemaker
Visuflo device to remove unwanted
    blood flow
Visulas Nd:YAG laser
visual disturbance
visualization, inadequate
visualization of the small vessels
visuomotor response

Vitacuff dressing
Vitacuff tissue-interface barrier
Vitagraft arteriovenous shunt
vital capacity (VC)
Vital Cooley microvascular needle-
　holder
Vital-Port vascular access port
Vital Ryder microvascular needle-
　holder
vital signs, stable
vitamin B complex deficiency
vitamin B_{12} (or B12) deficiency anemia
vitamin B_{12} (or B12) injections
vitamin K antagonist therapy
vitamin K deficiency
Vitatrax pacemaker
Vitatron Activity (ACT) sensor
Vitatron catheter electrode
Vitatron Diamond ICD (internal
　cardioverter-defibrillator)
Vitatron Diamond II DDR
Vitatron Diamond II dual sensor
Vitatron Diamond dual chamber
　pacemaker
Vitatron Jade II SSI pacing system
Vitatron QT sensor
Vitatron Ruby II DDD pacing system
Vitatron Selection AFm (atrial fibrilla-
　tion monitor)
Vitatron Topaz II SSIR pacing system
Vitesse E-II eccentric, rapid-exchange
　coronary catheter
Vitex tissue adhesive
vitrector, catheter
VLDL (very-low-density lipoprotein)
VLDL-TG (VLDL-triglyceride)
VLDL-TG/HDL-C ratio
V_1-like ambulatory lead system
V_5-like ambulatory lead system
VLP (ventricular late potential)
VMA (vanillylmandelic acid)
VMax diagnostic device

VM diagnostic device
VNUS Closure catheter
VNUS radiofrequency generator
VNUS Restore catheter
VO_2 (oxygen consumption per unit
　time)
VO_2 (ventilatory oxygen consumption)
VO_2 (whole body oxygen consumption)
VO_2 max (maximum oxygen
　consumption)
vocal fremitus
vocalis muscles
VOD (veno-occlusive disease)
Voda catheter
void, signal
Volkmann contracture of extremity due
　to arterial occlusion
Volkmann retractor
voltage
　battery
　increased (on EKG)
　low (on EKG)
　precordial
　pulse
　R
voltage criteria
voltammetry
volts (V)
volume
　adequate stroke
　alveolar
　atrial emptying
　augmented stroke
　blood
　cavity
　central blood
　chamber
　circulating blood
　circulation
　closing
　decreased stroke
　decreased tidal

volume *(cont.)*
    determination of lung
    diastolic atrial
    diminished lung
    Dodge area-length method for
      ventricular
    end-diastolic
    end-expiratory lung
    endocardial
    end-systolic (ESV)
    end-systolic residual
    epicardial
    expiratory reserve (ERV)
    extracellular fluid
    forward stroke (FSV)
    increased extracellular fluid
    inspiratory reserve (IRV)
    left ventricular
    left ventricular chamber
    left ventricular end-diastolic
    left ventricular inflow (LVIV)
    left ventricular outflow (LVOV)
    left ventricular stroke
    LV (left ventricular) cavity
    mean corpuscular (MCV)
    mean corpuscular red cell
    minute
    pericardial reserve
    plasma
    prism method for ventricular
    pulmonary blood
    pyramid method for ventricular
    radionuclide stroke
    reduced plasma
    reduced stroke
    regurgitant
    regurgitant stroke (RSV)
    residual (RV)
    respiratory
    right ventricular
    right ventricular end-diastolic
    right ventricular end-systolic

volume *(cont.)*
    Simpson rule method for
      ventricular
    stroke (SV)
    systolic atrial
    Teichholz equation for left
      ventricular
    thermodilution stroke
    total stroke (TSV)
    ventricular end-diastolic
    von Recklinghausen test
volume-controlled inverse ratio
    ventilation
volume-controlled ventilator
volume-cycled decelerating-flow
    ventilation (VCDF)
volume-dependent hypertension
volume depletion
    intravascular
    profound
volume infusion
volume loss
volume overload
volume regulation
volume ventilator
voluntary coughing
voluntary hyperventilation, eucapnic
Voluson ultrasound system
Volutrol control apparatus for intra-
    venous infusion
vomitus
von Hippel-Lindau syndrome
Von Rokitansky syndrome
von Willebrand bleeding disorder
von Willebrand blood coagulation
    factor
von Willebrand disease
von Willebrand factor
von Willebrand syndrome
VOO pacemaker
voxel
Voyager aortic device

Vozzle Vacu-Irrigator
VPB (ventricular premature beat)
VPC (ventricular premature complex)
VPC (ventricular premature contraction)
VPD (ventricular premature depolarization)
V peak of jugular venous pulse
VPL thalamic electrode (ventroposterolateral)
VPT (ventricular paroxysmal tachycardia)
V/Q (ventilation-perfusion)
V/Q imbalance
V/Q scan
VRT (venous refill time)
VRT (venous return time)
VS (ventricular septal)
VScore with AutoGate high-quality cardiac imaging
VSD (ventricular septal defect)
VSD and absent pulmonary valve syndrome
VSMC (vascular smooth muscle cells)
VSR (vulcanizing silicone rubber)
VT (ventricular tachycardia)
V tach (slang for ventricular tachycardia)
VTED (venous thromboembolic disease)

V_1 through V_6 (precordial EKG leads)
VT/VF (ventricular tachycardia/ventricular fibrillation)
Vueport balloon-occlusion guiding catheter
vulcanizing silicone rubber
vulnerable myocardium
vulval varices
V_1-V_2 curve
VVI/AAI pacemaker
VVI pacemaker
VVI pacing mode
VVT pacemaker
V wave, augmented
v wave in jugular venous pulse with tricuspid incompetence
v wave of jugular venous pulse
V wave of right atrial pressure
V-wave pressure on left or right atrial catheterization
V-wave blood pressure measurement by cardiac catheterization
V wave on catheterization
V wave on pulmonary capillary wedge tracing
VWFs (velocity waveforms), Doppler
V-Y atrioplasty

W, w

W (whoop)
Waaler-Rose test
Waardenburg syndrome
wafer of endocardium
WAGR (Wilms tumor, aniridia, genito-
    urinary involvement, and retarda-
    tion)
waist in the balloon
Wakabayashi shunt
waking, breathlessness on
waking with chest tightness
Waldhausen and Nahrwold technique
Waldhausen subclavian flap technique
wall
    aortic
    left anterior chest
Wallace Flexihub central venous
    pressure cannula
wall akinesis
wall hypokinesis
wall motion, ventricular
wall thickening
wall thickness
Wallstent (made by Schneider)
Wallstent biliary endoprosthesis
Wallstent endoprosthesis with Unistep
    catheter delivery system

Wallstent spring-loaded stent
wandering atrial pacemaker (WAP)
wandering pacemaker syndrome
wand, programmer
Wang transbronchial needle
waning pain
WAP (wandering atrial pacemaker)
Ward-Romano syndrome
warfarin anticoagulation
warfarin sodium
warm blood cardioplegic induction
    (WBCI)
warm continuous retrograde cardio-
    plegia
warmed heelstick for neonates
warm saline
Warren splenorenal shunt
Warthin sign of increased pulmonary
    sounds in acute pericarditis
Was-Cath catheter for percutaneous
    thromboendarterectomy
washed clot
washed red cell autotransfusion
washings
    bronchial
    cell
washings and brushings

washout
 delayed xenon
 lung
 nitrogen
washout phase
washout time
wasted ventilation
wasting, potassium
watchband incision for endoscopic
  radial artery harvesting
water bottle heart
water-hammer pulse
water retention
watershed region
water, total body
Waterhouse-Friderichsen syndrome
watershed area in lung transplantation
watershed region
Waterston anastomosis
Waterston anastomosis for congenital
  pulmonary stenosis
Waterston-Cooley anastomosis
Waterston groove
Waterston shunt
waterwheel bruit
watery sputum
watt-second
wave (electrocardiogram)
 A
 A larger than V
 alpha
 augmented V
 bifid T
 C
 constant tilt
 CV
 depolarization
 depolarizing
 dicrotic
 F (fibrillary)
 H
 inverted T
 J

wave *(cont.)*
 notched P
 P
 P-on-T
 Osborn (hypothermia)
 palpable A
 PRS
 Q
 Q (in the right precordial leads)
 R
 rapid filling
 recoil wave
 regurgitant CV
 retraction
 S
 slow filling
 standardization
 stationary arterial
 systolic S
 T
 Ta
 tidal
 Traube-Hering
 U
 V
 ventricular
wave (jugular venous pulse)
 A
 c
 cannon
 cannon A
 f
 giant a
 h
 intermittent cannon A
 v
 x
 y
wave form or waveform
 Doppler velocity (VWFs)
 exponential simultaneous
 monophasic
 monophasic shock

wave *(cont.)*
    monophasic truncated exponential
      simultaneous
    simultaneous truncated exponential
    tibial vessel Doppler
    truncated exponential simultaneous
    truncated exponential simultaneous
      monophasic
    velocity (VWFs)
WaveWire high-performance angio-
    plasty guidewire
wax, bone
waxing and waning pain
waxing pain
WCD 2000 system wearable defibrilla-
    tor
WDE (wound dressing emulsion)
weak carotid upstroke
weak signal
weakened arteries
weakness
    profound
    respiratory muscles
    transitory
wean, difficult to
weaned from cardiopulmonary bypass
weaned from IABP
weaned off bronchodilators
weaned off ventilation
weaning from ventilator
Weavenit (and New Weavenit) Dacron
    prosthesis
web
    laryngeal
    lateral
Weber-Osler-Rendu syndrome
Weber protocol (exercise stress testing)
Webster Compli diagnostic catheter
Webster needle holder
Webster orthogonal electrode catheter
Weck clip
wedged

wedge position, pulmonary capillary
wedge pressure, pulmonary venous
wedge resection of lung
wedge resection, video-assisted
    thoracoscopic
wedge-shaped density
wedge-shaped hemorrhagic area
wedge-shaped lobe
Wegener granulomatosis
Wegener syndrome
weight loss therapy
weight on the chest
weight reduction
Weil disease or syndrome
    (Adolf Weil)
Weill sign of pneumonia in infant
    (Edmond Weill)
Weinberg-Himelfarb syndrome
Weingarten syndrome
Weingarten tropical pulmonary
    eosinophilia
Weisenburg syndrome
Weiss-Baker syndrome
Welchol (colesevelam hydrochloride)
welder's lung
welder's siderosis
well, posterior pericardial
well-preserved ejection fraction
Wenckebach AV (atrioventricular)
    block
Wenckebach heart block
Wenckebach incomplete atrio-
    ventricular (AV) heart block
Wenckebach phenomenon
Wenckebach secondary atrioventricular
    heart block
Wenckebach upper rate response
Werlhof autoimmune thrombocyto-
    penia (ATP)
Werlhof disease
Werlhof idiopathic thrombocytopenic
    purpura (ITP)

Werner syndrome
Wesolowski vascular prosthesis
Westermark sign
Western blot test
Westcott scissors
wet cough
wet lung syndrome
wet pleurisy
wet-to-dry dressings
Wexler catheter
wheal (weal), skin
Wheat procedure
Wheatstone bridge
wheat weevil disease
wheeze, wheezes
  asthmatoid
  end-expiratory
  end-inspiratory
  expiratory
  fine
  inspiratory
wheezing
  audible
  breathless when
  diffuse inspiratory and expiratory
  grossly audible
  localized
  paroxysmal
wheezing audible without a stethoscope
wheezing in chest
wheezing respirations
wheezy
whining, expiratory
whiplash technique for repositioning
  a catheter with a trocar under
  fluoroscopy
whispered pectoriloquy
whispering pectoriloquy
whistling rales
whistling respirations
whistling rhonchi
white-appearing blood pool

white blood cell count shift to the left
white clot
white clot syndrome
white-coat hypertension
white cotton umbilical tape
whole lung lavage (WLL)
white lung syndrome
white-noise artifact
white silk suture
white sound
whitish sputum
whole blood infusion
whole blood monoclonal antibody
whole body inflammatory response
Wholey Hi-torque modified J wire
Wholey ("wooley") wire
whoop (W)
  late systolic
  musical
whooping cough
whooping murmur
whorled appearance
whorls
wick (usually gauze)
wide-based blunt-ended right-sided
  atrial appendage
wide-bore needle
widely split second sound
widened heart shadow
widened mediastinum
widened respiratory splitting
widened S_1 or S_2 splitting
widened thoracic outlet
widening, mediastinal
wide pulse
wide splitting of first heart sound
wide splitting of second heart sound
width, pulse
Wiener filter
Wiktor balloon expandable coronary
  stent
Wiktor coronary stent

Wiktor GX coronary stent
Wiktor stent
Wilcoxon rank-sum test (calculation
    for artificial heart)
Willebrand disease (von Willebrand)
Willebrand factor (von Willebrand)
Willebrand syndrome
Williams-Beuren syndrome
Williams-Campbell syndrome
Williams cardiac device
Williams elfin-facies syndrome
Williamson sign or test
Williams sign
Williams syndrome
Willis, circle of
Wilms tumor
Wilson-Mikity syndrome
WinABP ambulatory blood pressure
    monitor
window
    aorticopulmonary
    aortopulmonary
    apical
    esophageal
    gastric
    parasternal
    pericardial
    subcostal
    suprasternal
    systolic-diastolic
window ductus
window into the chest cavity
winged scapula
wing-like protrusion of the scapula
wing sutures
windsock aneurysm
Winiwarter-Buerger disease
Winiwarter-Buerger thromboangiitis
    obliterans
Winiwarter-Manteuffel-Buerger
    syndrome
winter cough

Wintrich sign
Wintrobe hematocrit
Wintrobe sed(imentation) rate
wire
    deflector
    heavy steel
    hydrophilic guide
    Hyperflex guide
    Hyperflex steerable
    magnum guide
    Microven nitinol
    pacing
    parasternal stainless steel
    sensing
    Superstiff
    Wholey Hi-torque modified J
wire insertion tool (quickWIT)
wire-mesh self-expandable stent
wire tightener
wire twister
Wishard catheter
Wiskott-Aldrich syndrome
Wizard cardiac device
Wizard disposable inflation device
Wizdom and Wizdom ST steerable
    guidewire
W. L. Gore vascular graft
WLL (whole lung lavage)
Woakes ethmoiditis
Woakes syndrome
Wolf-Hirschhorn syndrome
Wolff-Parkinson-White (WPW)
    syndrome
Wolff-Parkinson-White syndrome
Wolman disease
Wolvek sternal approximation fixation
    instrument
wood asthma
wood pulp worker's lung disease
Wood units of pulmonary vascular
    resistance
woody mass

Wooler anuloplasty
Wooler-Kay anuloplasty
Wooler-plasty
Wooler-type anuloplasty
woolsorter's inhalation disease
Workhorse percutaneous transluminal
   angioplasty balloon catheter
workload
work, maximal capacity for
worn-out red cells
worsening of asthma, nocturnal
worthlessness
wound
   groin
   missile
   stab
   trocar
wound cleanser
   MicroKlenz
   Puri-Clens
   Saf-Clens chronic
   Sea-Clens
   Shur-Clens
   UltraKlenz
wound contamination

wound dressing emulsion (WDE)
Woun'Dres hydrogel dressing
wound was copiously irrigated
Wound-Span Bridge II dressing
woven Dacron gusset
woven Dacron tube graft
woven Teflon prosthesis
WPW (Wolff-Parkinson-White)
   syndrome
wracking cough
wrap, Angiotech vascular
wraparound graft
wraparound technique
wraparound vessel
wrap-inclusion composite valve graft
   procedure, Bentall
wrapped aneurysmal sac
wrapping of graft
Wright nebulizer
Wright peak flow
Wright stain
wrinkled pleura
Wuchereria bancrofti infection
Wylie carotid artery clamp

X, x

xanthelasma
xanthoma
   eruptive
   palmar
   tendinous
   tuberoeruptive
   tuberous
xanthoma tendinosum
xanthoma tuberosum simplex
xanthomatosis-hypercholesterolemia
x depression of jugular venous pulse
x descent of "a" wave
x descent of jugular venous pulse
XeCT (xenon computed tomography)
X' descent
xenograft (heterograft) (see *graft*)
   discordant cellular xenograft
   discordant organ
   glutaraldehyde-preserved porcine
   porcine
   vascular
xenograft valve
Xenomedica prosthetic valve
xenon chloride (XeCl) excimer
xenon computed tomography (XeCT)
xenon 133 scan (^{133}Xe)

Xenotech prosthetic valve
xenotransplantation
Xeroform ("zero-form") gauze
Xillix LIFE-Lung system
xiphisternal joint
xiphisternal region
xiphoidalgia
xiphoid area
xiphoid cartilage
xiphoid, hypersensitive
xiphoid process syndrome
xiphopubic midline incision
X-linked abnormality
XL-Endograft vascular prosthesis
XMI catheter
Xolair (omalizumab)
XO syndrome (Turner syndrome)
Xpeedior 100 catheter
Xpeedior 60 catheter
Xplorer digital radiography imaging
   system
X-PRESS vascular closure system
x-ray (see also *chest x-ray*; *position*;
   scan; *view*)
   baseline chest
   chest (CXR)

x-ray *(cont.)*
    cineradiographic views
    computerized tomography (CT)
       scan
    contralateral decubitus chest
    megavoltage
    selective coronary arteriography
    soft
    tomograms
X-Sept catheter
X-Sept sheath
X syndrome
XT cardiac device
Xtent catheter
Xtent probe

Xtent stent
Xtent vascular access port
XT radiopaque coronary stent
X-Trode electrode catheter for intra-
    venous insertion into a heart cavity
X trough
XXXY and XXXXX syndrome
x'-wave pressure on right atrial
    catheterization
x waves (negative) on jugular venous
    pulse (JVP) wave tracing
XY plane
Xyrel pacemaker
XYZ lead system

Y, y

Yankauer suction tube
Yasargil artery forceps
Yasargil carotid clamp
yawning
Y configuration, inverted
Y connector, ACS angioplasty
y depression of jugular venous pulse
Y descent
y descent of "a" wave
y descent of jugular venous pulse
Y graft
Yeager formula

yellow plaque, fibrofatty
yellow sputum
Yersinia infection
young female aortic arch arteritis
Young syndrome
Y-shaped graft
Y stenting
Y trough
Y-wave pressure on right atrial
  catheterization
y waves (negative) on jugular pulse
  wave tracing

Z, z

Zaditen (ketotifen)
Zahn
   lines of
   pockets of
Zeek syndrome
Zellweger syndrome
Zemaira (alpha$_1$ proteinase inhibitor, human)
Zener diode
Zenith AAA endovascular graft system
zero diastolic blood pressure
Zestoretic (hydrochlorothiazide, lisinopril)
Zestril (lisinopril)
ZETA coronary stent
Zetia (ezetimibe)
Ziac (hydrochlorothiazide, bisoprolol fumarate)
Ziegler syndrome
Zimmer antiembolism support stockings
Zipper angioplasty catheter
Zipper balloon catheter
Zipper delivery system (for coronary stent)
Zipper stent

zipper scar
Zipzoc stocking compression dressing and wrap
Zitron pacemaker
Z lines
Z-Med catheter
Z mutation
Zoll defibrillator
Zollinger-Ellison syndrome
Zoll NTP noninvasive temporary pacemaker
zone
   arrhythmogenic border
   basal
   clear
   convergence
   ischemic
   lipid
   midlung
   precordial transition
   pyramidal hemorrhagic
   rough
   sonolucent
   transition
Zone diet
zone of fibrosis
zone of hemorrhage

651

zone of ischemia
zone of necrosis
zone of slow conduction (ZSC)
Z point
z point pressure on left (or right) atrial
    catheterization
ZSC (zone of slow conduction)
Zuckerkandl para-aortic bodies at
    bifurcation of aorta

Zucker and Myler cardiac device
Zucker #7 French catheter
Zuma guiding catheter
Zwenger test
Zyderm I or II collagen
zygapophyseal articulation
ZY plane
Zyvox (linezolid)